RHEUMATOLOGY SECRETS

STERLING G. WEST, MD, FACP, FACR

Professor of Medicine
Division of Rheumatology
University of Colorado Health Sciences Center
Denver, Colorado

HANLEY & BELFUS, INC./ Philadelphia
MOSBY/ St. Louis • Baltimore • Boston • Carlsbad • Chicago • London
Madrid • Naples • New York • Philadelphia • Sydney • Tokyo • Toronto

CONTENTS

CONTRIBUTORS

Ramon A. Arroyo, M.D., FACR
Assistant Professor, Department of Medicine, F. Edward Hebert School of Medicine, Bethesda, Maryland; University of Texas Health Sciences Center, San Antonio, Texas

Daniel F. Battafarano, D.O., FACP, FACR
Assistant Chief, Rheumatology Service, Department of Medicine, Brooke Army Medical Center; Clinical Assistant Professor, University of Texas Health Sciences Center, San Antonio, Texas

Nicholas J. Battafarano, M.D., FACAI
Resident, Department of Psychiatry, Tripler Army Medical Center, Honolulu, Hawaii; formerly, Staff Allergist, Fitzsimons Army Medical Center, Aurora, Colorado

Vance J. Bray, M.D., FACR
Arthritis Affiliates, P.C., Colorado Springs, Colorado

Matthew T. Carpenter, M.D., FACR
Assistant Professor, Department of Medicine, F. Edward Hebert School of Medicine, Uniformed Services University of the Health Sciences, Bethesda, Maryland

David Harris Collier, M.D., FACR
Associate Professor, Department of Medicine, University of Colorado Health Sciences Center; Chief of Rheumatology, Denver General Hospital, Denver, Colorado

Gregory J. Dennis, M.D., FACP, FACR
Associate Professor, Department of Medicine, F. Edward Hebert School of Medicine, Uniformed Services University of the Health Sciences, Bethesda, Maryland; Chief of Rheumatology and Clinical Immunology, Walter Reed Hospital, Washington, D.C.

J. Woodruff Emlen, M.D., FACR
Associate Professor, Department of Medicine, University of Colorado Health Sciences Center, Denver, Colorado

Raymond J. Enzenauer, M.D., FACP, FACR
Chief, Rheumatology Service, Department of Medicine, Fitzsimons Army Medical Center, Aurora, Colorado

Alan R. Erickson, M.D., FACR
Assistant Chief, Rheumatology Service, Department of Medicine, Fitzsimons Army Medical Center, Aurora, Colorado

David R. Finger, M.D., FACR
Chief, Rheumatology Service, Department of Medicine, William Beaumont Army Medical Center, El Paso, Texas

Terri H. Finkel, M.D., Ph.D., FACR
Associate Professor, Departments of Pediatrics, Immunology, and Biochemistry, National Jewish Center for Immunology and Respiratory Medicine, University of Colorado Health Sciences Center, Denver Colorado

William R. Gilliland, M.D., FACR
Assistant Professor, Department of Internal Medicine, F. Edward Hebert School of Medicine, Uniformed Services University of the Health Sciences, Bethesda, Maryland

Luis Gonzalez, M.D.
Director, Department of Radiology, Northern Dutchess Hospital, Rhinebeck, New York

Robert A. Hawkins, M.D., FACP, FACR
Associate Clinical Professor, Department of Medicine, Wright State University School of Medicine, Dayton, Ohio

Douglas E. Hemler, M.D., FAAPMR, FAAEM
Clinical Instructor, Physical Medicine and Rehabilitation, University of Colorado Health Sciences Center; Medical Director, Occupational Medicine and Urgent Care, Primera Health Care, Denver, Colorado

J. Roger Hollister, M.D., FACR
Professor, Department of Pediatrics, University of Colorado Health Sciences Center, Denver, Colorado

Edmund H. Hornstein, D.O., FACR
Staff Rheumatologist, Madigan Army Medical Center, Tacoma, Washington

Robert W. Janson, M.D., FACR
Associate Professor, Department of Medicine, Division of Rheumatology, University of Colorado Health Sciences Center, Denver, Colorado

Mark Jarek, M.D., FACR
Staff Rheumatologist, Department of Medicine, William Beaumont Army Medical Center, El Paso, Texas

John Keith Jenkins, M.D., FACR
Assistant Professor, Department of Medicine, Division of Rheumatology/Molecular Immunology, University of Mississippi Medical Center, Jackson, Mississippi

Brian L. Kotzin, M.D., FACR
Professor, Departments of Medicine and Immunology, University of Colorado Health Sciences Center; Professor of Pediatrics and Medicine, National Jewish Center for Immunology and Respiratory Medicine, Denver, Colorado

Elizabeth Kozora, Ph.D.
Assistant Professor, Department of Psychiatry, University of Colorado Health Sciences Center; Department of Medicine, National Jewish Center for Immunology and Respiratory Medicine, Denver, Colorado

James S. Louie, M.D., FACP, FACR
Professor, Department of Medicine, and Chief of Rheumatology, Harbor-UCLA Medical Center, Torrance, California

Mark Malyak, M.D., FACR
Assistant Professor, Department of Medicine, Division of Rheumatology, University of Colorado Health Sciences Center, Denver, Colorado

Michael T. McDermott, M.D., FACP
Clinical Professor, Department of Medicine, University of Colorado Health Sciences Center, Denver, Colorado

Michael A. O'Connell, M.D., FACAI
Assistant Chief and Co-Training Program Director, Allergy-Immunology Service, Fitzsimons Army Medical Center, Aurora, Colorado

James R. O'Dell, M.D. FACP, FACR
Professor of Medicine and Chief of Rheumatology, University of Nebraska Medical Center, Omaha, Nebraska

Steven A. Older, M.D., FACP, FACR
Chief, Rheumatology Service, Department of Medicine, Brooke Army Medical Center; Clinical Associate Professor, Department of Medicine, University of Texas Health Sciences Center, San Antonio, Texas

Kevin M. Rak, M.D.
Chief of Radiology, Divine Savior Hospital, Portage, Wisconsin

John A. Reister, M.D.
Associate Clinical Professor, Department of Orthopedics, Brooke Army Medical Center, San Antonio, Texas

Cynthia Faye Rubio, M.D.
Assistant Director of Medical Education, Internal Medicine Residency Program, Georgia Baptist Medical Center, Atlanta, Georgia

Richard Jay Shea, M.D., FACP
Chief, Medical Consultation Service, Department of Internal Medicine, Fitzsimons Army Medical Center, Aurora, Colorado

James David Singleton, M.D., FACR
Assistant Professor, Department of Medicine, Division of Rheumatology, University of Colorado Health Sciences Center, Denver, Colorado

Robert T. Spencer, M.D., FACR
Assistant Professor, Department of Medicine, Division of Rheumatology, University of Colorado Health Sciences Center, Denver, Colorado

Scott A. Vogelgesang, M.D., FACP, FACR
Assistant Professor, Department of Internal Medicine, Division of Rheumatology, University of Iowa College of Medicine, Iowa City, Iowa

Sterling G. West, M.D., FACP, FACR
Professor, Department of Medicine, Division of Rheumatology, University of Colorado Health Sciences Center, Denver; Clinical Director, Autoimmune Disease Center, National Jewish Center for Immunology and Respiratory Medicine, Denver, Colorado

Danny Claude Williams, M.D., M.S., FRCPC, FACR
Assistant Professor, Department of Medicine, Division of Rheumatology, University of Colorado Health Sciences Center, Denver, Colorado

Dear Reader:

If you would like to contribute question/answer sets for the next edition of *Rheumatology Secrets*, please do so. The questions should be those that medical students and housestaff commonly encounter on rounds, in clinics, and in departmental or "board"-type examinations. Credit will be given if your contributions are used. Please photocopy this page as many times as needed, and submit your question/answer sets to:

Sterling G. West, M.D.
c/o Hanley & Belfus, Inc.
210 South 13th Street
Philadelphia, PA 19107

Question:

Answer:

Reference (optional):

FROM: Name: _____

Address: _____

_____

PREFACE

"Learning without thinking is useless. Thinking without learning is dangerous."

Confucius (551-478 BC)
Analects

Oliver Wendell Holmes correctly points out in his *Medical Essays* that "The bedside is always the true center of medical teaching." Indeed, knowledge gained through the experience of caring for patients is one of the most powerful methods of learning. Our fund of knowledge is further increased when we read about the diseases of the patients we have treated. Yet students and clinicians alike may get lost when trying to sift through all the facts contained in the major textbooks. The information that is most important in helping them care for their patients may be hard to extract. *Rheumatology Secrets* is written to provide medical students, housestaff, fellows, and practicing physicians with "pearls" to help them care for their patients with rheumatic disorders.

Rheumatology Secrets is written in a Socratic question and answer format, which is the hallmark of *The Secrets Series.*® The book's chapters are organized into 16 sections, each with a common theme emphasized by a quotation. Both common and uncommon rheumatic disease problems that we encounter in clinical practice, discuss during teaching rounds, and find on board examinations are covered. Each chapter reviews basic immunology and pathophysiology, important disease manifestations, and practical management issues. The authors have tried to present information, whenever possible, in mnemonics, lists, tables, and pictorial form to help the reader remember the most important points contained in the answers to the questions. We hope that the reader will find *Rheumatology Secrets* both enjoyable and practically useful, with the patient ultimately benefiting the most.

Sterling West, M.D.

ACKNOWLEDGMENTS

As Editor, I want to thank:

All the contributors for their time and effort in writing their chapters,

Mrs. Linda Loehr for her exceptional administrative assistance and great sense of humor throughout the preparation of this book,

Linda Belfus for her help and patience, and for giving me the opportunity to edit *Rheumatology Secrets*,

My patients, teachers, and students for what they have taught me.

I. General Concepts

The rheumatism is a common name for many aches and pains, which have yet no peculiar appellation, though owing to very different causes.
William Heberden (1710–1801)
Commentaries on the History and Cure of Diseases, ch. 79.

1. CLASSIFICATION AND HEALTH IMPACT OF THE RHEUMATIC DISEASES

Sterling West, M.D.

1. What is rheumatology?
A medical science devoted to the study of rheumatic diseases and musculoskeletal disorders.

2. What are the roots of rheumatology?

1st century AD The term *rheuma* first appears in the literature. *Rheuma* refers to "a substance that flows" and probably was derived from *phlegm,* an ancient primary humor, which was believed to originate from the brain and flow to various parts of the body causing ailments.

1642 The word *rheumatism* is introduced into the literature by the French physician, Dr. G. Baillou, who emphasized that arthritis could be a systemic disorder.

1928 The American Committee for the Control of Rheumatism is established in the United States by Dr. R. Pemberton. Renamed American Association for the Study and Control of Rheumatic Disease (1934), then American Rheumatism Association (1937), and finally, American College of Rheumatology (ACR) (1988).

1940s The terms *rheumatology* and *rheumatologist* are first coined by Drs. Hollander and Comroe, respectively.

3. How many rheumatic/musculoskeletal disorders are there?
Over 120.

4. How have these rheumatic/musculoskeletal disorders been classified over the years?
1904 Dr. Goldthwaite, an orthopedic surgeon, makes the first attempt to classify the arthritides. He had five categories: gout, infectious arthritis, hypertrophic arthritis (probably osteoarthritis), atrophic arthritis (probably rheumatoid arthritis) and chronic villous arthritis (probably traumatic arthritis).
1964 American Rheumatism Association (ARA) classification
1983 The ARA classification is revised based on plans to revise the 9th edition of the *International Classification of Disease* (ICD 9). ICD 10 is presently being developed.

5. The 1983 ARA classification is overwhelming. Is there a simpler outline to remember?
Most of the rheumatic diseases can be grouped into 10 major categories:

    I. Systemic connective tissue diseases
   II. Vasculitides
  III. Seronegative spondyloarthropathies
   IV. Arthritis associated with infectious agents
    V. Rheumatic disorders associated with metabolic, endocrine, and hematologic disease
   VI. Bone and cartilage disorders
  VII. Hereditary, congenital, and inborn errors of metabolism associated with rheumatic syndromes
 VIII. Nonarticular and regional musculoskeletal disorders
   IX. Neoplasms and tumorlike lesions
    X. Miscellaneous rheumatic disorders

6. What is the origin and difference between a collagen-vascular disease and a connective tissue disease?

1942   Dr. Klemperer introduces the term *diffuse collagen disease* based on his pathologic studies of systemic lupus erythematosus (SLE) and scleroderma.
1946   Dr. Rich coins the term *collagen-vascular disease* based on his pathologic studies in vasculitis indicating that the primary lesion involved the vascular endothelium.
1952   Dr. Ehrich suggests the term *connective tissue diseases,* which has gradually replaced the term *collagen-vascular diseases.*

In summary, the two terms are used synonymously, although the purist would say that the heritable collagen disorders (Chapter 59) are the only true "diffuse collagen diseases."

7. How common are rheumatic/musculoskeletal disorders in the general population?

Approximately 30% of the population has symptoms of arthritis and/or back pain. Only two-thirds of these patients (i.e., 20% of the population) have symptoms severe enough to cause them to seek medical care. The prevalence of musculoskeletal disorders increases with the age of the patient population.

8. What is the estimated prevalence for the various rheumatic/musculoskeletal disorders in the general population?

Estimated Prevalence of Rheumatic/Musculoskeletal Disorders in the U.S. Population

	PREVALENCE	MILLIONS OF PATIENTS
All musculoskeletal disorders	15–20%	37–50
Arthropathies		
Osteoarthritis	5%	10–15
Rheumatoid arthritis	1%	2–3
Juvenile rheumatoid arthritis	0.06%	0.15
Crystalline arthritis	1%	2–3
Spondyloarthropathies	0.5%	1–1.5
Connective tissue disease		
SLE	0.006%	0.015
Scleroderma	0.002%	0.005
Back/neck pain		
Chronic	5%	10–15
Soft tissue rheumatism	3–5%	5–10
Fibromyalgia	1%	2–3

For comparison, about 20 million people in the general population are being treated for hypertension, and 5 million people have diabetes mellitus.

9. How often are one of the rheumatic/musculoskeletal disorders likely to be seen in an average primary care practice?

About 1 out of every 5–10 office visits to a primary care provider is for a musculoskeletal disorder. Interestingly, 66% of these patients are < 65 years old. The most common problems are osteoarthritis, back pain, gout, fibromyalgia, and tendinitis/bursitis.

10. Discuss the impact of the rheumatic/musculoskeletal diseases on the general population in terms of morbidity and mortality.

Morbidity and Mortality of Rheumatic/Musculoskeletal Diseases

	PERCENT OF POPULATION
Symptoms of arthritis	30%
Symptoms requiring medical therapy	20%
Disability due to arthritis	5–10%
Totally disabled from arthritis	0.5%
Mortality from rheumatic disease	0.02%

Arthritis/back pain is the second leading cause of acute disability (behind respiratory illness) and is the number one cause of chronic disability in the general population. Ten percent of all surgical procedures are for disabilities related to arthritis.

11. What is the economic impact of the rheumatic/musculoskeletal diseases?
The cost of musculoskeletal disorders in healthcare expenditure and lost wages is $149 billion a year, or about 2.5% of the total U.S. gross national product. Over 30% of working-age persons (aged 18–64) with arthritis are either unable to work or cannot work in their usual occupation due to their disease.

BIBLIOGRAPHY

1. Benedek TG: A century of american rheumatology. Ann Intern Med 106:304–312, 1987.
2. Bradley EM: The provision of rheumatologic services. In Klippel JH, Dieppe PA (eds): Rheumatology, London, Mosby, 1994, pp 1-9.1–1-9.10.
3. Decker JL, Glossary Subcommittee of the ARA Committee on Rheumatologic Practice: American Rheumatism Association nomenclature and classification of arthritis and rheumatism. Arthritis Rheum 26:1029–1032, 1983.
4. Pincus T, Mitchell J, Burkhauser R: Substantial work disability and earnings losses in individuals less than 65 with osteoarthritis: Comparisons with rheumatoid arthritis. J Clin Epidemiol 42:449–457, 1989.
5. Reynolds MD: Origins of the concept of collagen—vascular diseases. Semin Arthritis Rheum 15:127–131, 1985.
6. Yelin E, Callahan LF: The economic cost and social and psychological impact of musculoskeletal conditions. Arthritis Rheum 38:1351–1362, 1995.

2. RHEUMATOLOGY'S TEN GOLDEN RULES

Sterling West, M.D.

Rheumatology can be confusing to many physicians during their housestaff training (and beyond!). Although nothing in medicine is 100%, I have found the following "golden rules" valuable when evaluating a patient with a rheumatic/musculoskeletal problem. I have limited the rules to 10, but certainly many others could be added:

1. A good **history** and **physical examination,** coupled with knowledge of musculoskeletal anatomy, is most important when evaluating a patient with a rheumatic disorder. You have to examine the patient!

2. Don't order a **laboratory test** unless you know why you're ordering it and what you will do if it comes back abnormal.

3. All acute inflammatory monoarticular arthritides need a **joint aspiration** to rule out septic arthritis and crystalline arthropathy.

4. Any patient with a chronic inflammatory monoarticular arthritis of > 8 weeks' duration, whose evaluation has failed to define an etiology for the arthritis, needs a **synovial biopsy.**

5. **Gout** usually does not occur in premenopausal women or affect joints close to the spine.

6. Most **shoulder pain** is periarticular (i.e., a bursitis or tendinitis) and most **low-back pain** is nonsurgical.

7. Patients with **osteoarthritis** affecting joints not normally affected by primary osteoarthritis (i.e., metacarpophalangeals, wrists, elbows, shoulder, ankles) need to be evaluated for secondary causes of osteoarthritis (i.e., metabolic diseases, others).

8. Primary **fibromyalgia** does not occur for the first time in patients after the age of 55 years, nor is it likely to be the correct diagnosis in patients with musculoskeletal pain who also have abnormal laboratory values.

9. All patients with a positive **rheumatoid factor** do not have rheumatoid arthritis, and all patients with a positive **antinuclear antibody** do not have systemic lupus erythematosus.

10. In a patient with a known systemic rheumatic disease who presents with fever or multisystem complaints, rule out **infection** and possibly other nonrheumatic etiologies before attributing the symptoms and signs to the underlying rheumatic disease. Clearly, infection causes death of rheumatic disease patients more often than underlying rheumatic disease does.

Remember, nothing is 100%!

3. ANATOMY AND PHYSIOLOGY OF THE MUSCULOSKELETAL SYSTEM

Sterling West, M.D.

1. Name two major functions of the musculoskeletal system.
Structural support and purposeful motion. The activities of the human body depend on the effective interaction between joints and the neuromuscular units that move them.

2. Name the five components of the musculoskeletal system.
(1) Muscles, (2) Tendons, (3) Ligaments, (4) Cartilage, (5) Bone. All of these structures contribute to the formation of a functional and mobile joint.

3. The different connective tissues differ in their composition of macromolecules. List the macromolecular "building blocks" of connective tissue.
Collagen, elastin and adhesins, and proteoglycans.

COLLAGEN

4. How many types of collagen are there? In which tissues is each type most commonly found?
The collagens are the most abundant body proteins and account for 20–30% of the total body mass. There are at least 14 different types of collagen. The unique properties and organization of each collagen type enable that specific collagen to contribute to the function of the tissue of which it is the principal structural component.

Collagen Types and Their Principal Tissue Distributions

COLLAGEN TYPE	COLLAGEN CLASS	TISSUE DISTRIBUTION
I	Interstitial	Bone, tendon, joint capsule and synovium, skin
II	Interstitial	Hyaline cartilage, vitreous of eye
III	Interstitial	Blood vessels, intestine
IV	Basement membrane	Lamina densa of basement membrane
V	Interstitial	Same as type I collagen
VI	Nonfibrillar	Aortic intima, skin, kidney, muscle
VII	Nonfibrillar	Amnion, dermoepidermal anchoring fibrils
VIII	Short-chain	Endothelial cells, Descemet's membrane
IX	FACIT	Same as type II collagen, cornea
X	Short-chain	Growth plate cartilage
XI	Interstitial	Hyaline cartilage
XII	FACIT	Same as type I collagen
XIII	Nonfibrillar	Endothelial cells
XIV	FACIT	Skin, tendon

FACIT = Fibril-associated collagens with interrupted triple helices.

5. Discuss the structural features common to all collagen molecules.
The definitive structural feature of all collagen molecules is the **triple helix.** This unique conformation is due to three polypeptide chains (α-chains) twisted around each other into a right-handed major helix. Extending from the amino and carboxyl terminal ends of both helical domains of the α-chains are nonhelical components called telopeptides. In the major interstitial collagens, the helical domains are continuous, whereas in the other collagen classes (nonfibrillar, short-chain, FACIT), the helical domains may be interrupted by 1 to 12 nonhelical segments.

The primary structure of the helical domain of the α-chain is characterized by the repeating triplet X–Y–Gly. X and Y can be any amino acid but are most frequently proline and hydroxypro-

5

line, respectively. Overall, approximately 25% of the residues in the triple helical domains consist of proline and hydroxyproline. Hydroxylysine is also commonly found. In the most abundant interstitial collagens (i.e., type I, II), the triple helical region contains about 1000 amino acid residues, $(X-Y-Gly)_{333}$.

Diagram of interstitial (fibrillar) collagen molecule demonstrating triple helix configuration with terminal telopeptides.

6. Identify the major collagen classes and the types of collagen included in each class.
- Interstitial (fibrillar) collagens—types I, II, III, V, XI. The most abundant collagen class, these collagens form the extracellular fabric of the major connective tissues. They have the same tensile strength as steel wire.
- Fibril-associated collagens with interrupted triple helices (FACIT)—types IX, XII, XIV. These collagens are associated with the interstitial (fibrillar) collagens and occur in the same tissues.
- Collagens with specialized structures or functions:
  Basement membrane collagen—type IV
  Nonfibrillar collagens—types VI, VII, XIII
  Short-chain collagens—types VIII, X

7. How are the interstitial collagens synthesized?
1. There are at least 20 distinct genes encoding the various collagen chains. The collagen genes studied thus far contain coding sequences (exons) interrupted by large, noncoding sequences (introns). The DNA is transcribed to form a precursor mRNA, which is processed to functional mRNA by excising and splicing which removes mRNA coded by introns. The processed mRNAs leave the nucleus and are transported to the polyribosomal apparatus in the rough endoplasmic reticulum for translation into polypeptide chains.
2. The polypeptide chains are hydroxylated by prolyl hydroxylase and lysine hydroxylase. These enzymes require O_2, Fe^{2+}, α-ketoglutarate, and ascorbic acid as cofactors. Hydroxyproline is critical to the stable formation of the triple helix. A decrease in hydroxyproline content as seen in scurvy (ascorbic acid deficiency) results in unstable molecules that lose their structures and are broken down by proteases.
3. Glycosylation of hydroxylysine residues, which is important for secretion of procollagen monomers (molecules).
4. Formation of interchain disulfide links, followed by procollagen triple-helix formation.
5. Secretion of procollagen into the extracellular space.
6. Proteolysis by procollagen peptidase of amino and carboxyl terminal telopeptides, resulting in conversion of procollagen to collagen.
7. Assembly of collagen monomers (molecules) into fibrils (microfibrils) by quarter-stagger shift, followed by cross-linking of fibrils.
8. End-to-end and lateral aggregation of fibrils to form collagen fiber.
Each collagen molecule is 300 nm in length and 1.5 nm in width and has five charged regions 68 nm apart. The charged regions align in a straight line when the fibrils are formed, even though the individual molecules themselves are staggered a quarter of their lengths in relation to each

other. One can easily see that there are multiple steps where defects in collagen biosynthesis could result in abnormalities leading to disease (see also Chapter 59).

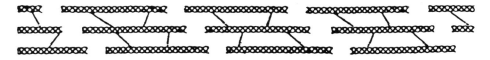

Self-assembly of collagen molecules into fibrils with cross-linking.

8. Which enzymes are important in collagen degradation? How are they regulated?

The most important collagenolytic enzymes responsible for cleavage of type I collagen belong to the **matrix metalloproteinase group.** This enzyme (MMP1) is secreted in latent form and, when activated, cleaves the collagen molecule at a single specific site 75% from the amino terminal end (between residues 775–776 of $\alpha 1(I)$ chain). Gelatinases and stromelysin degrade the unfolded fragments.

Both α_2-macroglobulin and tissue inhibitor of metalloproteases (TIMP) are capable of inhibiting collagenase activity. It is likely that other collagen types have type-specific collagenases capable of degrading them. Serum procollagen peptides, urinary hydroxyproline, and urinary pyridinoline/deoxypyridinoline cross-links are used as measures of collagen turnover.

ELASTIN AND ADHESINS

9. What is elastin and where is it located?

Elastin fibers are connective tissues that can stretch when hydrated and return to their original length after being stretched. They comprise a significant portion of the dry weight of ligaments (up to 70–80%), lungs, larger blood vessels such as aorta (30–60%), and skin (2–5%). Elastin is a polymer of tropoelastin monomers which contain 850 amino acids, predominantly valine, proline, glycine, and alanine. When tropoelastin molecules associate to form a fiber, lysine residues cross-link by forming desmosine and isodesmosine which are unique to elastin. Elastases, which are serine proteases, are capable of degrading elastase. Elastases are located in tissues, macrophages, leukocytes, and platelets. Such elastases may contribute to blood vessel wall damage and aneurysm formation in the vasculitides. Urinary desmosine levels are used as a measure of elastin degradation.

10. List the important adhesins that can be present in intracellular matrices and basement membranes.

Fibronectin — connective tissue
Laminin — basement membrane
Chondronectin — cartilage
Osteonectin — bone
These proteins have specific adhesive and other important properties.

11. What is fibrillin?

Fibrillin is a large glycoprotein coded for by a gene located on chromosome 15. It functions as part of the microfibrillar proteins which are associated with an elastin core. Fibrillin can also be found as isolated bundles of microfibrils in skin, blood vessels, and several other tissues. Abnormalities in fibrillin are thought to cause Marfan's syndrome (see also Chapter 59).

PROTEOGLYCANS

12. How do a proteoglycan and a glycosaminoglycan differ?

Proteoglycans are glycoproteins that contain one or more sulfated glycosaminoglycan (GAG) chains. They are classified according to their core protein, which is coded for by distinct genes.

GAGs are usually classified into five types: chondroitin sulfate, dermatan sulfate, heparan sulfate, heparin, and keratan sulfate. GAGs make up part of proteoglycans.

13. How are proteoglycans distributed?
Proteoglycans are synthesized by all connective tissue cells. They can remain associated with these cells on their cell surface (syndecan, betaglycan), intracellularly (serglycin), or in the basement membrane (perlecan). These cell-associated proteoglycans commonly contain heparin/heparan sulfate or chondroitin sulfate as their major GAGs. Alternatively, proteoglycans can be secreted into the extracellular matrix (aggrecan, visican, decorin, biglycan, fibromodulin). These matrix proteoglycans usually contain chondroitin sulfate, dermatan sulfate, or keratan sulfate as their major GAGs.

14. How are proteoglycans metabolized in the body?
Proteoglycans are degraded by proteinases which release the GAGs. The GAGs are taken up by cells by endocytosis, where they are degraded in lysosomes by a series of glycosidases and sulfatases. Defects in these degradative enzymes can lead to diseases called **mucopolysaccharidoses.**

MUSCULOSKELETAL SYSTEM

15. Discuss the classification of joints.
Synarthrosis: Suture lines of the skull where adjoining cranial plates are separated by thin fibrous tissue.

Amphiarthroses: Adjacent bones are bound by flexible fibrocartilage that permits limited motion to occur. Examples include the pubic symphysis, part of the sacroiliac joint, and intervertebral discs.

Diarthroses (synovial joints): These are the most common and most mobile joints. All have a synovial lining. They are subclassified into ball and socket (hip), hinge (interphalangeal), saddle (first carpometacarpal), and plane (patellofemoral) joints.

16. What major tissues comprise a diarthroidal (synovial) joint?
A diarthroidal joint consists of **hyaline cartilage** covering the surfaces of two or more opposing **bones.** These articular tissues are surrounded by a **capsule** which is lined by **synovium.** Some joints contain **menisci,** which are made of fibrocartilage. Note that the joint cavity is a potential space. The pressure within normal joints is negative (-5.7 cm H_2O) compared to ambient atmospheric pressure.

17. Describe the microanatomy of normal synovium.
Normal synovium contains synovial lining cells which are 1–3 cells deep. Synovium lines all intracapsular structures except the contact areas of articular cartilage. The synovial lining cells reside in a matrix rich in type I collagen and proteoglycans.

There are two main types of synovial lining cells, but these can only be differentiated by electron microscopy. **Type A** cells are macrophage-like and have primarily a phagocytic function. **Type B** cells are fibroblast-like and produce hyaluronate, which accounts for the increased viscosity of synovial fluid.

Other cells found in the synovium include antigen-presenting cells called dendritic cells and mast cells. The synovium does not have a limiting basement membrane. Synovial tissue also contains fat and lymphatic vessels, fenestrated microvessels, and nerve fibers derived from the capsule and periarticular tissues.

18. Why is synovial fluid viscous?
Hyaluronic acid, synthesized by synovial lining cells (type B), is secreted into the synovial fluid, making the fluid viscous. Synovia means "like egg white," which describes the normal viscosity of synovial fluid.

19. What are the physical characteristics of normal synovial fluid from the knee joint?
Color—Colorless and transparent
Amount—Thin film covering surfaces of synovium and cartilage within joint space
Cell count—$< 200/mm^3$ with $< 25\%$ neutrophils
Protein—1.3–1.7 g/dl (20% of normal plasma protein)
Glucose—within 20 mg/dl of the serum glucose level after 6 hours of fasting
Temperature—32°C (peripheral joints are cooler than core body temperature)
String sign (measure of viscosity)—1–2 inches
pH—7.4

20. What is the function, structure, and composition of articular cartilage?
Articular cartilage is **avascular** and **aneural.** It serves as a load-bearing connective tissue that can absorb impact and withstand shearing forces. Its ability to do this relates to the unique composition and structure of its extracellular matrix.

Normal cartilage is composed of a sparse population of specialized cells called **chondrocytes** that are responsible for the synthesis and replenishment of extracellular matrix. This matrix consists mainly of collagen and proteoglycans. Most of the collagen is type II (>90%), which makes up 50–60% of the *dry* weight of cartilage. Collagen forms a fiber network that provides shape and form to the cartilage tissue.

Proteoglycans comprise the second largest portion of articular cartilage. The proteoglycans are large supramolecular aggregates (aggrecan) with molecular weight (MW) of 2–3 million. The proteoglycan aggregate consists of a central hyaluronic acid filament to which multiple proteoglycan monomers (containing mostly keratan sulfate and chondroitin sulfate) are noncovalently attached and stabilized by a link protein.

The entire structure looks like a large "bottle brush" and has a MW of 200 million. These proteoglycans are stuffed into the collagen framework. The negative charge of the proteoglycans causes them to spread out until the elastic forces are balanced by the tensile forces of the collagen. Note that other collagens (types V, VI, IX, X, XI), two proteins (chondronectin, anchorin), and lipid are also in cartilage.

Water is the most abundant component of articular cartilage and accounts for 80% of the tissue *wet* weight. Water is held in cartilage by its interaction with matrix proteoglycan aggregates.

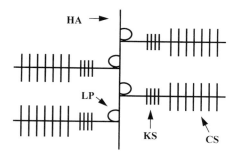

Diagram of proteoglycan aggregate in articular cartilage. Hyaluronate (HA) is the backbone of the aggregate. Proteoglycan monomers (aggrecan) arise at intervals from either side of the hyaluronate core. LP = link protein, KS = keratan sulfate, CS = chondroitin sulfate.

21. What are the four zones of cartilage?
The different molecular components of cartilage are highly organized into a structure which varies with the depth of cartilage. From top to bottom these four zones include:
1. **Superficial (tangential) zone** (10%)—smallest zone. Collagen fibers are thin and are oriented horizontally to subchondral bone. Low GAG content. This zone is called the **lamina splendens.**

2. **Middle (transitional) zone** (50%)—largest zone. Collagen fibers are thicker and start to be arranged into radial bundles. High proteoglycan and water content.

3. **Deep (radial) zone** (20%)—largest collagen fibers arranged radially (perpendicular) to subchondral bone. Many chondrocytes.

4. **Calcified zone**—separates cartilage from subchondral bone. Collagen fibers penetrate into this zone and anchor the cartilage to the bone.

22. Since cartilage doesn't have a blood supply, how do chondrocytes obtain nutrition?
Adult cartilage is avascular, and chondrocytes obtain nutrients through diffusion. The nutrients are derived from the synovial fluid. Diffusion is facilitated during joint loading. With joint loading some of the water in the cartilage is squeezed out into the synovial space. When the joint is unloaded, the hydrophilic properties of the cartilage proteoglycans cause the water to be sucked back into the cartilage. As the water returns to the cartilage, diffusion of nutrients from the synovial fluid is facilitated.

23. If cartilage is not innervated, then why do patients with osteoarthritis have pain?
Patients experience pain due to irritation of the subchondral bone, which is exposed as the cartilage degenerates. Additionally, accumulation of synovial fluid can cause pain through distention of the innervated joint capsule and synovium. Mild synovial inflammation also causes pain.

24. Describe the lubrication of diarthroidal joints.
Diarthroidal (synovial) joints serve as mechanical bearings with coefficients of friction lower than the friction an ice skate generates as it glides over ice. Its three major sources of lubrication are:
- Hydrodynamic lubrication: Loading of the articular cartilage causes compression which forces water out of the cartilage. This fluid forms an aqueous layer that separates and protects the opposing cartilage surfaces.
- Boundary layer lubrication: A small glycoprotein called **lubricin,** which is produced by synovial lining cells, binds to articular cartilage where it retains a protective layer of water molecules.
- Hyaluronic acid: Produced by synovial lining cells, this molecule lubricates the contact surface between synovium and cartilage. It does not contribute to cartilage on cartilage lubrication.

25. Discuss the normal matrix turnover of articular cartilage.
In normal articular cartilage, chondrocytes rarely divide. Chondrocytes synthesize and replace the extracellular matrix components of the major components. Proteoglycans have a faster turnover rate ($t_{1/2}$ of weeks) compared to collagen ($t_{1/2}$ of months). The degradation of these macromolecules is accomplished by proteolytic enzymes. Metalloproteases, such as collagenases and stromelysin, are the most important. Cytokines such as interleukin-1 and tumor necrosis factor-α can upregulate the degradative process, while transforming growth factor-β and insulin-like growth factor-1 have an anabolic effect on chondrocyte metabolism. Assays using monoclonal antibodies to measure type II collagen and proteoglycans (keratan sulfate) in bodily fluids have been used to detect cartilage breakdown.

26. What is the difference between a ligament and a tendon?
A **ligament** is a specialized form of connective tissue attaching one bone to another. It frequently reinforces the joint capsule and provides stability to the joint. A **tendon** attaches a muscle to a bone. Both are comprised mostly of type I collagen.

27. Discuss the types and composition of bone.
Bone is a mineralized connective tissue. It is comprised of two subtypes: **cortical** (or compact) bone and **cancellous** (or trabecular) bone. Cortical bone comprises 80% of the skeleton and is increased in long bone shafts. Cancellous bone is in contact with bone marrow cells and is en-

riched in the vertebral bodies, pelvis, and proximal ends of femora, all of which are subject to osteoporosis and fractures.

Bone comprises mainly type I collagen and contains three cell types: **osteoclasts** which resorb mineralized bone, **osteoblasts** which synthesize the proteins of the bone matrix, and **osteocytes** which are probably osteoblasts that have secreted bone matrix and become buried within it.
Osteocytes communicate with each other through a canalicular system. The skeleton contains
99% of the total body calcium, 80–85% of the phosphorus, and 66% of the magnesium.

28. How many muscles are in the human body?
Approximately 640. Muscles constitute up to 40% of the adult body mass.

29. Discuss the morphology of muscle.
Skeletal muscle consists of cells called **fibers.** Fibers are grouped into **fascicles.**

Muscle fibers are part of **motor units** that consist of a lower motor neuron originating from
a spinal cord anterior horn cell and all the muscle fibers it innervates. All muscle fibers within a
motor unit are of the same type. Different fibers within a single fascicle are innervated by different motor neurons.

Muscle fibers are divided into three types based on their metabolism and response to stimuli:
Types 1, 2a, and 2b. Fiber type can be altered by reinnervation with a different motor neuron type,
physical training (controversial), or disease processes. However, heredity is the most important determinant of fiber type distribution. On average, muscle contains 40% type 1 and 60% type 2 fibers.

Each muscle fiber is surrounded by a plasma membrane called a **sarcolemma.** Fibers contain **myofilaments** called actin, troponin, tropomyosin, and myosin, which are contractile proteins. The myofilaments are bathed in sarcoplasm and organized into **fibrils,** which are enveloped
by the sarcoplasmic reticulum. Communication between the sarcolemma and sarcoplasmic reticulum occurs through a channel network called the **T-tubule system.**

30. Describe the characteristics of the three types of muscle fibers.
- **Type 1** (slow twitch, oxidative fibers) (red fiber): Respond to electrical stimuli slowly. Fa-
  tigue-resistant with repeated stimulation. Many mitochondria and higher lipid content. Endurance training (long-distance running) enhances metabolism of these fibers.
- **Type 2a** (fast twitch, oxidative-glycolytic fibers): Properties intermediate between type 1
  and type 2b.
- **Type 2b** (fast twitch, glycolytic fibers) (white fiber): Respond rapidly and with greater
  force of contraction but fatigue rapidly. These fibers contain more glycogen and have
  higher myophosphorylase and myoadenylate deaminase activity. Strength training (weightlifting, sprinters, jumpers) leads to hypertrophy of these fibers.

31. How does muscle contraction and relaxation occur?
Muscle contraction occurs by shortening of myofilaments within muscle fibers. Stimulation
causes an **action potential** to be transmitted along the sarcolemma, then through the T-tubule system to the sarcoplasmic reticulum. This causes release of calcium into the sarcoplasm. As the calcium concentration increases, **actin** is released from a state of inhibition, allowing actin-myosin
cross-linkage and shortening of the myofilaments. The muscle fiber shortens until calcium is actively pumped back into the sarcoplasmic reticulum, which breaks the cross-links causing the
fiber to relax. ATP, electrolytes (Na, K, Ca, Mg) and three ATPase proteins contribute to normal
fiber contraction and relaxation. (See also Chapter 76.)

BIBLIOGRAPHY

1. The musculoskeletal system. In Schumacher HR Jr (ed): Primer on the Rheumatic Diseases, 10th ed. Atlanta, Arthritis Foundation, 1993, pp 5–15.
2. Structural molecules of connective tissues. In Schumacher HR Jr (ed): Primer on the Rheumatic Diseases,
   10th ed. Atlanta, Arthritis Foundation, 1993, pp 16–26.

II. Scientific Basis of the Rheumatic Diseases

The origin of all science is in the desire to know causes.
William Hazlitt, 1829

Science has been seriously retarded by the study of what is not worth knowing,
and of what is not knowable.
Johann Wolfgang von Goethe, 1825

4. OVERVIEW OF THE IMMUNE RESPONSE

Michael O'Connell, M.D.

1. What are the two broad categories of immunity involved in host defense?

Categories of Immunity

	NATURAL (INNATE) IMMUNITY	ACQUIRED (SPECIFIC) IMMUNITY
Physical barriers	Skin, mucous membranes	Mucosal immune systems
Circulating factors	Complement	Antibody
Cells	Macrophages, neutrophils	Lymphocytes
Cell-derived mediators	Monokines	Lymphokines

2. Acquired immune responses can be active or passive. Describe and differentiate the two.

Active immunity is so named because the host plays an active role in responding to the foreign antigen. The best example of active immunity is **immunization,** whereby a vaccine containing a foreign antigen is administered to a nonimmune host, resulting in active production of specific antibody and lymphocyte-based memory.

Passive immunity refers to transfer of soluble factors (either antibodies or cells) from an immune individual to a nonimmune host. This process confers immunity passively, without the recipient needing prior exposure to the antigen. A good example of passive immunity is parenteral administration of immune serum globulin to travelers as preexposure **prophylaxis** against unusual infections.

3. What are the two main types of lymphocytes? How are they differentiated?

- **T lymphocytes,** or T cells, are **T**hymus-derived and express the T-cell receptor on their surface. They can be separated from other lymphocytes by use of monoclonal antibodies which recognize CD3, a component of the T-cell receptor. The majority of circulating lymphocytes in the bloodstream are T cells.
- **B lymphocytes,** or B cells, are **B**one marrow-derived antibody-secreting cells which express surface immunoglobulin on their surfaces.

4. Specific immune responses can be differentiated into two major categories based on whether B or T cells are primarily involved. What are these two categories?

1. **Humoral immunity** refers to immune responses involving antibody that is produced by mature B cells and plasma cells (terminally differentiated B cells).

2. **Cellular immunity** is mediated by T cells which secrete cytokines and signal effector cells to direct an overall cell-mediated immune response.

5. How does antibody participate in immune and inflammatory responses?
There are three main ways in which antibody is immunologically active:
    1. Antibody can coat and neutralize invading organisms, not allowing the organism access to the host.
    2. Two classes of antibody (IgM and IgG) activate ("fix") complement, resulting in cell chemotaxis, increased vascular permeability, and target cell lysis.
    3. Antibody coats foreign particles (opsonization), increasing the efficiency of phagocytosis by cells which contain surface immunoglobulin receptors (neutrophils and macrophages).

6. Humoral (antibody-mediated) immunity is most important in host defense against which type of infectious organisms?
Bacteria, especially those with a polysaccharide capsule. Patients with severe antibody deficiency (hypogammaglobulinemia) suffer from sinopulmonary infections, especially with encapsulated organisms (e.g., *Pneumococcus, Haemophilus influenzae*).

7. Name the four major classes of antibodies. What specific role does each play in humoral immunity?
The mnemonic is **GAME**:
G—Ig**G**—Highest concentration in serum and excellent penetration into tissues. Crosses the placenta. Fixes complement.
A—Ig**A**—Most important antibody for host defense at mucosal surfaces (sites of antigen entry). Produced locally and often present in a modified form in secretions such as tears and saliva (secretory IgA). Secretory IgA is more resistant to enzymatic degradation.
M—Ig**M**—The first class of antibody made in the primary response to antigen. Vigorously fixes complement and is very important in host defense against blood-borne antigens.
E—Ig**E**—Binds to the surface of mast cells and basophils, and when cross-linked, results in release of granular contents (primarily histamine). Important in allergic diseases and host defense against parasites.
    Pearl: Antibody (immunoglobulin) is also called gamma globulin because it is contained primarily in the gamma fraction when serum proteins are electrophoresed on a gel.

8. What are the different types of T-cells? How are they differentiated?
- Classically, T cells can be functionally classified into helper/inducer, suppressor, and cytotoxic subsets.
- Most helper/inducer T cells express the CD4 cell-surface marker.
- The majority of cytotoxic T cells express the CD8 cell-surface marker.
- Suppressor T cells also classically express the CD8 cell-surface marker, but their existence as a separate distinct T-cell subtype is controversial.

9. Cellular immunity (T-cell mediated) is most important in host defense against which infectious organisms?
Virus, parasites, fungi, and mycobacteria. AIDS patients have a severe dysfunction of T-cell-mediated immunity and suffer from recurrent infections with these agents.

10. What are NK cells, and how are they identified?
NK cells are **natural killer** cells, so named because they are potent cytotoxic cells whose targets are not MHC-restricted (i.e., they are not antigen-specific). They have the appearance on light microscopy of large lymphocytes with numerous cytoplasmic granules and are sometimes called large granular lymphocytes. They classically express the CD16 and CD56 cell-surface markers and do *not* express CD4 or CD8.

11. Using the classification developed by Gel and Coombs, immune responses can be segregated into four main types. Name them.
Type I—IgE-mediated immediate hypersensitivity (e.g., allergic rhinitis or hayfever)
Type II—Antibody-mediated tissue injury, (e.g., autoimmune hemolytic anemia)

Type III—Immune complex (antigen–antibody) formation (e.g., serum sickness, Arthus skin reaction)

Type IV—Delayed-type hypersensitivity (e.g., immune response to mycobacterial antigens, positive PPD skin test)

12. What are MHC molecules and on which cells are they found?
MHC stands for **major histocompatibility complex,** a group of genes located on human chromosome 6. The products of MHC gene loci can be classified into two categories—Class I and Class II MHC molecules:
- Class I MHC molecules are expressed on the surface of all nucleated cells.
- Class II MHC molecules are found mostly on specialized cells called antigen-presenting cells.

13. How do T cells recognize antigen to initiate a specific immune response?
a. Unlike macrophages, neutrophils, and B cells, T cells cannot recognize free soluble antigen.
b. T cells can only "see" antigen via their surface T-cell receptor, which will only bind to antigen bound to ("presented by") an MHC molecule on the surface of a cell.
c. T cells "see" only pieces of large antigens since the antigen-binding groove in a MHC molecule can only accommodate a small peptide. Large protein antigens are digested ("processed") prior to insertion in the groove.

14. Which cells are specialized antigen-presenting cells? Where are they found?

Antigen Presenting Cells

CELL TYPE	LOCATION
Macrophages	
Histiocyte	Connective tissue
Monocyte	Blood
Alveolar macrophage	Lung
Kupffer cell	Liver
Microglia	CNS
Osteoclast	Bone
Dendritic cells	Skin, lymph nodes
Langerhans cells	Skin
B lymphocytes	Lymph nodes

15. Which type of T cells do antigen-presenting cells (APCs) present antigen to?
- APCs are cells that express surface MHC Class II molecules.
- MHC Class II molecules preferentially bind to T-cell receptors associated with the CD4 surface molecule.
- Thus, APCs present antigen to the $CD4^+$ T cells, the helper/inducer subset.

16. Which type of T cell recognizes antigen presented by Class I MHC molecules?
Class I MHC molecules preferentially bind to T-cell receptors associated with the CD8 surface molecule. Thus, antigen presented in the groove of MHC Class I molecules would interact with $CD8^+$ T cells, the cytotoxic/suppressor subset. Class I MHC molecules are present on the surface of all nucleated cells, thus allowing cells to present their internal antigens to cytotoxic T cells. This mechanism is critically important in host defense against intracellular pathogens such as viruses.

17. How do T cells become activated?
T-cell activation requires two signals:
- Engagement of the T-cell receptor by the antigen/MHC complex
- A second signal, usually transduced by direct cognate interaction ("touching") between costimulatory cell-surface molecules on the APC and T cell

T-cell activation resulting from the two signals leads to production of cytoplasmic and nuclear factors, resulting in gene activation and new DNA synthesis.

18. If the T-cell receptor is engaged by an antigen/MHC complex, but the second signal is not given, what happens?
Typically, the T cell is tolerized (made unresponsive) to that antigen or the cell dies by undergoing apoptosis.

19. What is the role of neutrophils in the immune response?
Neutrophils are critically important in phagocytosing and digesting foreign particles at sites of inflammation and antigen entry. Neutrophils kill and dissolve microbes by release of enzymes and bactericidal products from their intracytoplasmic granules and by generation of toxic oxygen radicals and hypohalous acids. Clinical deficiency of leukocytes manifests as recurrent skin and soft-tissue infections with pyogenic organisms and sepsis (as seen in cancer patients receiving toxic chemotherapy).

20. What is the role of eosinophils in the immune response?
Eosinophils are active in immunity against parasites, especially helminths. Eosinophils are specialized leukocytes whose granules contain numerous toxic products, including major basic protein, eosinophil peroxidase, and eosinophil cationic protein. These products are especially toxic to helminths.

21. What is the role of complement in the immune response?
Complement components have immunologic activity both individually and in an activation cascade leading to a polymer formed by C5, C6, C7, C8, and C9 (the membrane attack complex, or MAC) which results in lysis of target cell membranes (see figure). Early classic complement components (especially C3 products) act as opsonins and assist in the phagocytosis of bacterial particles by neutrophils and macrophages. Certain complement split products (C3a and C5a) are chemotactic for phagocytic neutrophils and also act as "anaphylatoxins," which directly stimulate mast cells and basophils to release histamine resulting in increased vascular permeability. Deficiency of early complement components is associated with increased pyogenic infections (C3

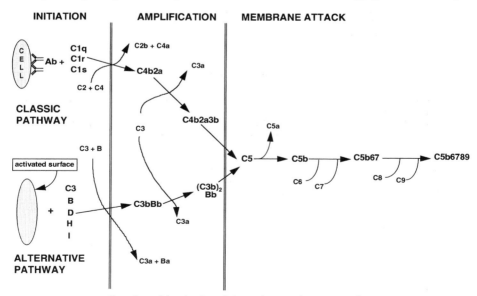

Overview of the classic and alternative complement cascades.

deficiency) and an increased incidence of autoimmune diseases (C1, 4, and 2 deficiency), possibly due to impaired clearance of immune complexes. The MAC appears especially important in host defense against *Neisseria* infection. Deficiency of any one of the terminal complement components can result in recurrent infections with *Neisseria*.

22. Describe the cellular interactions and cytokines involved in the immune response.

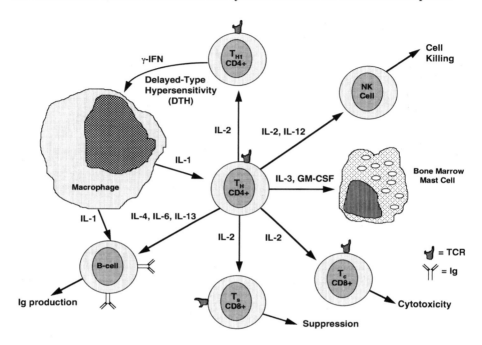

Overview of the framework of cellular immunity, illustrating the central role of the CD4+ T-helper cell. (IL, interleukin; TCR, T-cell receptor; Ig, immunoglobulin; NK, natural killer; IFN, interferon; GM-CSF, granulocyte–macrophage colony-stimulating factor.)

BIBLIOGRAPHY

1. Abbas AK, Lichtman AH, Pober JS: Cellular and Molecular Immunology, 2nd ed. Philadelphia, W.B. Saunders, 1994.
2. Goodman JW: The immune response. In Stites DP, Terr AI, Parslow TG (eds): Basic and Clinical Immunology, 8th ed. Norwalk, CT, Appleton & Lange, 1994, pp 40–49.
3. Johnston RB: The complement system in host defense and inflammation: The cutting edges of a double-edged sword. Pediatr Infect Dis J 12:933–941, 1993.
4. Keller R: The macrophage response to infectious agents: Mechanisms of macrophage activation and tumor cell killing. Res Immunol 144:271–273, 1993.
5. Roitt I, Brostoff J, Male D: Immunology, 3rd ed. St. Louis, Mosby, 1993.

5. OVERVIEW OF THE INFLAMMATORY RESPONSE

Michael O'Connell, M.D.

1. Name the four cardinal signs of inflammation.
Pain, swelling, warmth, and erythema (redness).

2. What are the underlying mechanisms responsible for the signs of inflammation?
Local arteriolar dilation produces the redness and warmth. Permeability increases in the postcapillary venules, allowing vascular fluid to leak into the surrounding tissue to produce swelling (edema). Pain is a result of the action of numerous inflammatory mediators and inflammatory cell-derived products on local nerves.

3. Inflammatory responses can be either detrimental or beneficial to the host. Give examples of each.

Detrimental
- Allergic diseases in which IgE-mediated (Type 1) inflammatory reactions resulting from exposure to an allergen cause significant symptoms (e.g., rhinitis, anaphylaxis) despite the fact that the inciting agent is often of no threat to the host (e.g., pollen).
- Autoimmune diseases in which immunologically mediated inflammation is misdirected against host tissues, resulting in injury and destruction.

Beneficial
- In infection by foreign microorganisms, increased vascular permeability enhances the ability of immune defensive cells (e.g., neutrophils, lymphocytes) to egress the bloodstream and enter tissues invaded by foreign pathogens.
- In infection, increased local blood flow enhances delivery of oxygen to stressed tissues.

4. What three types of inflammatory cells are involved in the majority of inflammatory reactions?
Neutrophils, macrophages, and lymphocytes. Neutrophils predominate in acute inflammatory reactions whereas lymphocytes are the key cell in chronic inflammatory processes. Other inflammatory cells are critically important in special types of inflammatory responses. Mast cells and basophils are the principal cells involved in IgE-mediated hypersensitivity (allergic) reactions. Eosinophils play a principal role in the host response to parasitic infection.

5. What advantageous properties of neutrophils allow them to play a critical role in acute inflammatory responses to a foreign pathogen?
Neutrophils are attracted by several types of chemotactic stimuli to sites of tissue injury, regardless of its cause. This property permits a rapid cellular response to many different types of injury, including infection, trauma, foreign body penetration, and burns. Additionally, since large numbers of neutrophils are constantly circulating in the blood, large numbers of cells can be mobilized quickly in response to an injury. These properties make neutrophils the cellular "first line of defense."

6. How do neutrophils attack foreign substances that enter the body?
Neutrophils are active phagocytic cells that can engulf foreign particles efficiently. Their cell membranes contain receptors for antibody and complement fragments, dramatically increasing the efficiency of phagocytosis of opsonized particles. Once the foreign particle is engulfed, neutrophils release granular contents, including degradative enzymes and microbicidal products. This results in killing/degradation of the foreign particle and local remodeling of the tissues—the first step in wound healing.

7. Macrophages are also potent phagocytic cells. How is their role unique in the inflammatory response from that of the neutrophil?
Macrophages possess three key properties that distinguish them from neutrophils:
1. They express MHC Class II on their cell surface and function as antigen-presenting cells.
2. They produce/secrete a number of important proinflammatory and costimulatory cytokines, including tumor necrosis factor (TNF), interleukin 1 (IL-1), IL-6, and IL-8, which drive the so-called acute phase response.
3. Macrophages respond to certain cytokines (notable gamma-interferon derived from T cells) which cause their activation, dramatically increasing their phagocytic capacity and causing aggregation into granulomas and multinucleated giant cells.

8. How do lymphocytes participate in chronic inflammatory responses?
T lymphocytes are the master controllers of the specific immune response. After antigen stimulation via antigen-presenting cells, T cells secrete cytokines which (1) direct and activate effector cells (e.g., macrophages) in a specific fashion, and/or (2) direct B cells to produce antigen-specific antibody. These processes are long-lived due to the nature of the cells involved and the fact that certain T and B cells differentiate into memory cells with extremely long lifespans.

9. What are the major classes of inflammatory mediators?

Vasoactive mediators
Histamine
Arachidonic acid products
  Prostaglandins
  Leukotrienes
Platelet-activating factor (PAF)
Kinins
Enzymes
Tryptase
Chymase

Chemotactic factors
Complement products (C3a, C5a)
Leukotriene B_4
Platelet-activating factor
Cytokines (IL-8)
Proinflammatory cytokines
Interleukins 1, 6, and 8
Tumor necrosis factor
Gamma-interferon

10. How does histamine promote inflammation?
Histamine is a preformed mediator rapidly released from mast cell and basophil granules after activation. Histamine interacts with specific cellular receptors (called H1, H2, and H3), resulting in increased vascular permeability, smooth muscle contraction, and increased glandular mucous secretion. This results clinically in sneezing, wheezing, itching, and edema. Antihistamine drugs block the receptors and limit or prevent symptom development.

11. How are prostaglandins and leukotrienes formed?
Unlike histamine (which is a preformed and stored mediator), prostaglandins and leukotrienes require active synthesis. The initial source molecule is arachidonic acid, which is liberated from cell membrane phospholipids. Once formed, arachidonic acid can be metabolized by either of two enzyme pathways (see figure on next page):
1. Cyclo-oxygenase pathway—results in prostaglandins
2. Lipoxygenase pathway—results in leukotrienes

12. How do prostaglandins and leukotrienes promote inflammation?
Prostaglandins (especially prostaglandin D_2) induce local vasodilation and increased vascular permeability. Leukotrienes (LT) fall into two classes: LTC_4, LTD_4, and LTE_4 induce smooth muscle contraction, bronchoconstriction, and mucous secretion. They were once collectively called slow reacting substance of anaphylaxis (SRS-A). LTB_4 has none of the above properties but is a potent chemotactic factor for leukocytes.

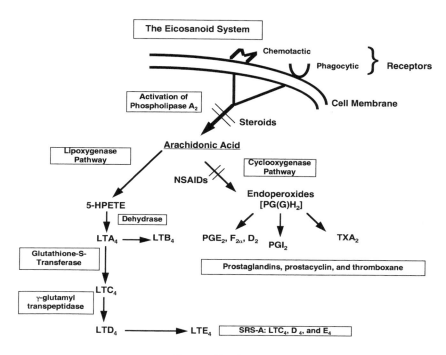

Eicosanoid pathways.

13. By what mechanism are the anti-inflammatory effects of aspirin and NSAIDs mediated?

- Both aspirin and NSAIDs block the activity of cyclo-oxygenase, resulting in decreased synthesis of prostaglandins.
- Drugs that block leukotriene synthesis are currently in experimental trials.

14. What is the acute phase response? What blood proteins are involved?

The acute phase response is a complex cascade of primarily liver-synthesized proteins which rise in response to a variety of infectious or immunologic stimuli. This response results in multiple metabolic and cellular alterations which contribute to host defense and a return to homeostasis.

Major acute phase proteins include alpha-1-antitrypsin, C3, ceruloplasmin, C-reactive protein, fibrinogen, haptoglobin, and serum amyloid A.

15. What mechanisms are involved in the initiation of an acute phase response?

Macrophages and monocytes appear to be the principal cells involved (though T cells may also play a role). When activated by antigen or other stimuli, macrophages secrete IL-1, 6, and TNF. IL-6 is a potent hepatocyte-stimulating factor resulting in increased synthesis of acute phase proteins. IL-1 generally enhances the effects of IL-6 on hepatocytes.

BIBLIOGRAPHY

1. Ballou S, Kushner I: C-reactive protein and the acute phase response. Adv Intern Med 37:313–336, 1992.
2. Dinarello CA, Wolff SM: The role of interleukin-1 in disease. N Engl J Med 328:106–113, 1993.
3. Holtzman MJ: Arachidonic acid metabolism. Am Rev Respir Dis 143:188–203, 1991.
4. Johnson RB: The complement system in host defense and inflammation: The cutting edges of a double-edged sword. Pediatr Infect Dis J 12:933–941, 1993.

5. Keller R: The macrophage response to infectious agents: Mechanisms of macrophage activation and tumor cell killing. Res Immunol 144:271–273, 1993.
6. Sox H, Liang M: The erythrocyte sedimentation rate—Guidelines for rational use. Ann Intern Med 104:515–523, 1986.
7. Terr AI: Inflammation. In Stites DP, Terr Al, Parslow TG (eds): Basic and Clinical Immunology, 8th ed. Norwalk, CT, Appleton & Lange, 1994, pp 137–150.

6. IMMUNOGENETICS OF THE RHEUMATIC DISEASES

Nicholas J. Battafarano, M.D.

1. What three types of molecules enable the immune system to bind specific antigen?
Immunoglobulins, T-cell receptors (TCRs), and major histocompatibility complex class I and II molecules (MHC I and II).

Each of these molecular classes displays its own unique associations with the rheumatic diseases. However, the associations between certain autoimmune diseases and the expression of specific MHC molecules provide insights into disease susceptibility and pathogenesis.

2. What is the MHC and what does it do?
The major histocompatibility complex (MHC) is located on the short arm of chromosome 6 in a region stretching approximately 4 million base pairs. There are three regions that encode for three different classes of proteins—MHC Classes I, II, and III (see figure).

The largest stretch, approximately 2 million base pairs, encodes the MHC Class I molecules, while a shorter stretch, approximately 1 million base pairs, encodes Class II molecules. The role of these two classes of molecules is to enable presentation of antigen to T cells. The remainder of the MHC complex stretches between the Class I and II regions and encodes various proteins that are not capable of presenting antigen. However, many of these MHC Class III proteins are in-

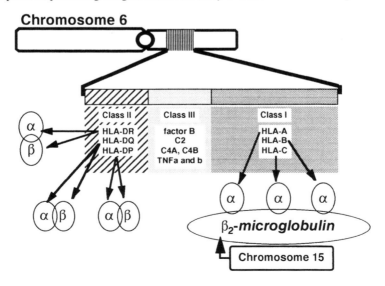

The major histocompatibility complex.

volved in the regulation of the immune response, and some have rheumatic disease associations. These include C2, C4, and factor B of the complement system, the tumor necrosis factors (TNF) α and β, and some of the heat-shock proteins. Both MHC Class I and II molecules are dimers. While the MHC encodes both the α- and β- chains of the Class II molecules, it encodes only the MHC Class I α-chain. β_2-Microglobulin, the β-chain shared by all MHC Class I molecules, is encoded by a relatively invariant allele on chromosome 15.

3. Is there a difference between MHC and HLA?

For many practical purposes, MHC and HLA (human leukocyte antigen) are used as interchangeable terms. However, technically, they are different. MHC specifically refers to the major histocompatibility complex of genes located on chromosome 6. MHC encodes HLA. HLA specifically describes the molecular products of the MHC genes—i.e., HLA molecules are the cell-surface proteins that are encoded by the different MHC genetic loci. Because these proteins, like most cell-surface proteins, can be specifically recognized by T-cell receptors and immunoglobulins, they are antigens. Since these proteins were first described on white blood cells, they were referred to as human leukocyte antigens (HLA). However, we now know that their distribution is considerably broader than just leukocytes. From a technical standpoint then, MHC and HLA are not identical, but rather, MHC leads to HLA.

4. Why is the MHC complex so unusual when compared with the rest of our genome?

The **diversity** enabled by the MHC is unparalleled in the remainder of the genome. There are a variety of factors responsible for this diversity. First, the MHC contains many genetic loci that can encode for the same class of molecule. In addition, the MHC is distinguished by its polymorphism, linkage disequilibrium, and codominant pattern of inheritance.

5. What does polymorphism mean?

An **allele** is one of the alternative forms of a gene that can be inherited at a specific locus. The prevalence of allelic alternatives for most of the MHC Class I and II gene loci exceeds the frequency that would occur secondary to mutation alone. Furthermore, unlike the single residue allelic differences that characterize other proteins, such as immunoglobulins, MHC allelic polymorphism is characterized by differences at multiple residues. So, instead of a protein gene product that differs by one to three amino acids at just one site, MHC molecules may differ by >10% of their amino acids. These differences occur in several areas of MHC molecules, but most of the variation occurs in three specific areas, hypervariable regions 1, 2, and 3. These areas just happen to be responsible for the specific binding of the peptide fragments to be presented. This genetic polymorphism is no accident. Rather, it is probably the result of positive selection to help us survive against the multiple antigens to which humans are exposed.

Examples of polymorphism include the HLA-A α-chain locus, for which approximately 50 different alleles have been identified; HLA-B locus, 100 alleles; HLA-C locus, 35 alleles; and HLA-DRβ chain locus, 100 alleles. Each individual, however, only inherits 2 alleles for each locus—one from mom, one from dad.

6. What is the significance of linkage disequilibrium?

The combination of alleles on a single chromosome is called a **haplotype.** Two combinations of chromosome 6 alleles, i.e., two haplotypes, are inherited by an individual—one maternal, one paternal. Analysis of MHC haplotypes shows linkage disequilibrium; i.e., certain combinations of alleles in the MHC are inherited with striking frequency, more frequently than their chance inheritance based on the individual allele frequencies in the population.

As an example, many diseases are associated with HLA-DR3. There are a number of alleles in linkage disequilibrium with HLA- DR3. For example, Caucasian HLA-DR3 haplotypes contain the same HLA-DQA1 and HLA-DQB2 alleles. If we identify an HLA-DR3 association with a disease, then the gene most responsible for the association may be any of a number of genes that are commonly in linkage disequilibrium with HLA-DR3.

7. What is the significance of codominant inheritance?

For each locus along the MHC, an individual receives a paternal and maternal allele. Rather than one alternative or the other being expressed, both alleles are expressed. This again increases the number of possible combinations of MHC molecules. The effects of each of the molecules expressed are dominant. Therefore, a person heterozygous for a particular disease-associated HLA molecule has increased vulnerability to that disease.

8. What do the letters appearing with HLA mean—e.g. HLA-A, HLA-B, etc.?
When you have HLA followed by a hyphen and one letter, such as HLA-A, it describes the specific gene location (region) within the MHC that codes for a particular HLA molecule. For example, HLA-A, HLA-B, and HLA-C describe the most important individual MHC I gene loci.

9. Why does HLA-D get the extra letters—R, P, Q?
The letter D describes the entire MHC Class II region, not just a single gene locus. Therefore, to describe an actual gene locus, you need more letters. For example, HLA-DP, -DQ, and -DR get you closer to the gene loci that code for the most important Class II molecules.

To make matters worse, each MHC Class II molecule consists of two separate polypeptide chains, designated α and β. So, when you see HLA-DRA or HLA-DRB, it is describing the locus for the HLA-DR α- or β-chain, respectively.

10. How do I know which letters (regions)—A, B, C, D, etc.—belong to which MHC class?

Major MHC Class I and II Molecules

MHC CLASS I	MHC CLASS II
HLA-A	HLA-DR
HLA-B	HLA-DP
HLA-C	HLA-DQ

HLA-A, -B, and -C are the most important MHC Class I molecules. All HLA-D molecules are MHC Class II molecules, and HLA-DP, -DQ, and -DR are the most important ones. There are other letters—E, F, G, H, M, N, O—but these are all Class I and of less importance. Just know:
- If it's HLA anything **without a D** in it, it's MHC Class I.
- If it's HLA-**D** anything, it's MHC Class II.

11. How does the antigen bind?
Each antigen-binding site has on a similar configuration. It consists of a groove, the walls of which are α-helical structures. A series of anti-parallel strands of the molecule form the floor of the groove, a β-pleated sheet. In TCR and MHC II, this configuration is formed by the interaction between the amino termini of both the α and the β-chains. For immunoglobulins, the antigen-binding site is formed by the interaction of the amino termini of the heavy and light chains. MHC I differs in that the antigen-binding site is formed by the interaction between the two amino terminal domains of the same chain, the α-chain.

The antigen binds at points on both the α-helical walls and the β-pleated floor. When the TCR

Antigen binding site.

embraces the MHC-peptide complex, it recognizes the unique conformation and charge of the antigen peptide and α-helices. Unlike the antigen, the TCR cannot "see" the unique determinants of the β-pleated floor.

The three areas of greatest genetic diversity (hypervariable regions) are expressed in segments of each of the α-helices and the β-pleated sheet. This genetic variation very specifically affects, or "selects," which antigens can bind to specific molecules. In addition, it specifically "selects" which TCRs can interact with specific combinations of MHC-antigen complex, often referred to as the trimolecular interaction.

These same areas correlate with the predisposition to certain diseases. In rheumatoid arthritis, for example, a specific sequence of amino acids in the hypervariable region is strongly associated with disease susceptibility — between amino acids from position 67–74 of the HLA-DR β-chain.

12. How are the four molecules that specifically recognize antigen constructed?

Immunoglobulins, T-cell receptors (TCR), and MHC Class I and Class II molecules all are expressed as transmembrane, cell-surface molecules (see figure). Each has two or more associated chains, which means each is expressed as a "dimer." Each of the chains is based on a similar repeating structure that is derived from a common primordial gene known as the "immunoglobulin supergene." For each molecule, the furthest extracellular extension is the **amino terminus;** the intracellular end is the **carboxy terminus** (COOH). The site of antigen binding is located near the amino terminus of each molecule. In each of these molecules, the genes encode for extraordinary diversity at the **antigen-binding site.** More specifically, most of the diversity occurs in three **hypervariable regions** (HVRs 1, 2, and 3) near the amino terminus, with the greatest diversity occurring in HVR3. In contrast to these regions of marked diversity, the remainder of the structure is remarkably conserved to facilitate antigen binding and, in the case of the MHC and TCR molecules, MHC-TCR recognition.

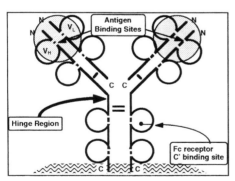

Surface Immunoglobulin

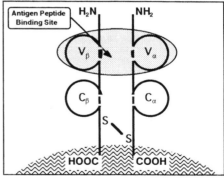

T Cell Receptor

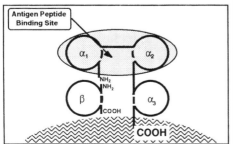

MHC Class I

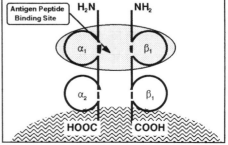

MHC Class II

13. If the MHC Class I and II molecules share so much in common, why are they classified separately?
While both are dimeric cell-surface molecules, the MHC Class II molecules show more diversity than MHC Class I molecules. Both the α and β chains of the MHC Class II are encoded by the Class II region of the MHC. However, while the α chains of the MHC Class I molecules are encoded by MHC Class I alleles, they all share a common β chain, β_2-microglobulin.

14. How do the MHC Class I and II molecules differ in function?
They differ in their cellular distribution, the antigenic peptide fragments they present, and the type of T cell that recognizes and responds to the complex they present.

Function of MHC Class I and II Molecules

	MHC CLASS I	MHC CLASS II
Cellular distribution	All nucleated cells and platelets	Certain immune system cells, particularly if they serve as "professional" antigen-presenting cells: B Cells Monocytes/macrophages Dendritic cells Thymic epithelial cells Some activated T cells Some cells in which MHC Class II expression can be induced, particularly during chronic inflammatory processes: Endothelial cell Synovial cells
Antigen size	8–13 amino acids in length	13–25 amino acids in length
Antigen type	Antigenic peptide fragment endogenous to the cytoplasm or nucleus of the cell that is expressing the MHC molecule (e.g., endogenous or "self"-peptides; peptides of obligate intracellular pathogens such as viruses and chlamydia; tumor antigens)	Antigenic peptide fragment present in lysosomal compartments as a result of phagocytosis or receptor-mediated endocytosis (e.g., exogenous or foreign infectious material [bacteria])
T-cell recognition	$CD8^+$ T cell	$CD4^+$ T cell
Resultant T-cell response	Cell-mediated killing or suppression of the MHC Class I-presenting cell	T cell-coordinated phagocytic and/or antibody response to eradicate the antigen that was presented

15. Is the total number of your potential and actual MHC Class II molecules greater than the total number of MHC Class I molecules?
Yes. The possibilities of HLA-A and HLA-B MHC molecules approximate 50 and 100, respectively; the number of HLA-C possibilities is almost 40. However, even in an individual heterozygous at each MHC Class I α-chain allele, the total number of MHC Class I molecules expressed will be 6—3 from mom, 3 from dad (see figure).
For MHC II, only the HLA-DR α-chain alleles are limited in variation. However, the polymorphism at the HLA-DP and -DQ α-chain loci and the HLA-DP, -DQ, and -DR β-chain loci is extraordinary. As a result, the number of possible combinations is staggering. Individuals with the greatest diversity will express 2 HLA-DR, 4 HLA-DP, and 4 HLA-DQ molecules. That is, with different alleles at each MHC Class II locus, except the HLA-DR α locus which is relatively invariant, a total of 10 types of MHC Class II molecules can be expressed.

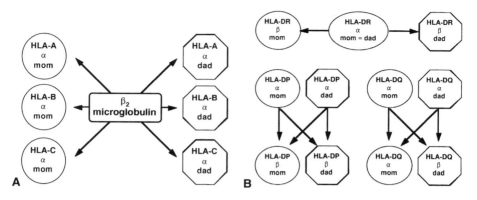

A, Inherited MHC I molecule possibilities in a given individual. B, Inherited MHC II possibilities in a given individual.

16. What are some of the commonly recognized associations of MHC molecules with diseases?

HLA–Antigen Associations

HLA-A3	Idiopathic hemochromatosis	HLA-DR3	Systemic lupus erythematosus
HLA-A26	Pemphigus vulgaris (Jews)		Sjögren's syndrome
HLA-B5	Beçhet's disease		Gluten-sensitive enteropathy
	Ulcerative colitis		Chronic active hepatitis
	Polycystic kidney disease		Dermatitis herpetiformis
HLA-B8	Graves' disease		Graves' disease
	Myasthenia gravis		Insulin-dependent diabetes mellitus
HLA-B14	Idiopatic hemochromatosis		Idiopathic membranous glomeru-
HLA-B27	Seronegative spondyloarthropathies		lonephritis
HLA-B38	Psoriatic arthritis		Gold/penicillamine nephropathy
HLA-DR1	Rheumatoid arthritis	HLA-DR4	Rheumatoid arthritis
HLA-DR2	Narcolepsy		Pemphigus vulgaris (Jews)
	Multiple sclerosis		Insulin-dependent diabetes mellitus
	Goodpasture's syndrome		IgA nephropathy
		HLA-DR5	Pauciarticular juvenile rheumatoid
			arthritis
			Pernicious anemia
			Hashimoto's thyroiditis
		HLA-DR7	Congenital adrenal hyperplasia
		HLA-DQ3.2	Insulin-dependent diabetes mellitus

17. If T cells coordinate chronic inflammatory responses, what role do MHC molecules play in predisposing to the development of rheumatic diseases?
- MHC molecules are pivotal in the process by which the immune system decides whether infant T cells are allowed to survive and develop or whether they must die.
- MHC molecules control what T cells can see. Remember, T cells are "blind" and cannot recognize antigens alone. The agents that T cells can specifically recognize, and therefore respond to, are MHC–peptide complexes.

18. How do the MHC molecules control what the T cells see?
They do this in two ways:
- The sequence of amino acids in an MHC molecule determines which antigenic peptide fragments can bind to that molecule. Only those "selected" antigenic peptides that can

bind to one of an individual's MHC molecules have the potential to be specifically recognized.

- Not all T cells can see all the MHC molecules. The peptides presented in the context of MHC Class I molecules can only be seen by T cells that have CD8 molecules associated with their TCR, while the peptides presented in the context of MHC Class II molecules can only be seen by T cells that have CD4 molecules associated with their TCR.

19. So a person inheriting HLA-DR4 will develop rheumatoid arthritis, just like with other hereditary diseases. Right?

No. Unlike many diseases in which autosomal dominant or recessive genes actually transmit or cause the diseases with which they are associated (e.g., an absent or mutant gene might result in deficient production of a vital enzyme), most HLA-associated diseases cannot be explained in that way. Certainly, none of the rheumatic disease associations fits such an explanation. Some HLA molecules neither cause nor confer susceptibility to the disease with which they are associated, but instead they are associated just because they are commonly inherited in association with another gene that actually confers susceptibility to the disease—the phenomenon of **linkage disequilibrium.** In several instances, however, particular HLA molecules do appear to confer susceptibility to the diseases with which they are associated.

20. If a gene for an HLA molecule is not actually causing a disease, then maybe there is simply another gene—one that we don't know about yet—that directly causes the disease? How can we tell?

Identical twin studies provide us with the clearest response to this question. If an inherited gene directly caused the disease under study, then identical twins would always suffer from the disease. It is clear that identical twins who express HLA-DR4, which is genetically associated with rheumatoid arthritis, both have a significantly higher risk of developing rheumatoid arthritis. However, many HLA-DR4-positive individuals never develop rheumatoid arthritis, even though their identical sibling suffers from the disease.

Additional studies compel us to believe that many of the HLA molecules are more than inherited "bystanders." In looking at penetrance of disease in heterozygotes versus homozygotes, we know that HLA molecules are "dominant" in their effects, because even heterozygotes display enhanced disease rates. However, individuals who are homozygous for a particular gene are clearly more vulnerable to the development of a particular disease than heterozygotes. Such studies of MHC **codominant expression** reinforce the belief that HLA associations are important in the pathophysiology of autoimmune diseases.

"Designer" rats may provide the most compelling information supporting a true immunopathogenetic relationship between HLA and disease. These rats—transgenic B27 Lewis rats—are genetically designed to express HLA-B27 on their cells. As a consequence, they spontaneously develop gut, skin, nail, joint, urethral, and spine problems similar to the seronegative spondyloarthropathies associated with HLA-B27 in humans.

21. Why should we believe that a gene associated with a rheumatic disease does not cause the disease but does confer susceptibility?

Although we know that some HLA molecules are associated with particular diseases, clearly not everyone who expresses that HLA molecule necessarily develops the disease. Thus, certain genes may confer susceptibility to certain diseases, even though they do not independently cause them. We also know that nongenetic factors, such as infections, have been clearly associated with the development of some HLA-associated diseases. Thus, there appear to be other factors, involving the host and its environment, that may "select" the development of a disease in a person who is genetically susceptible.

22. By what mechanism do they confer susceptibility?

That is the $64 million question regarding these genes. While that question remains unanswered, the cost of treatment of these diseases dwarfs that $64 million figure.

23. How do you determine the strength of these associations? How susceptible to diseases are people with HLA associations?

The risk of patients developing an HLA-associated disease is conventionally expressed as their **relative risk.** For example, relative risk describes the odds that an HLA-DR4-positive person will get rheumatoid arthritis compared to a person who is not HLA-DR4 positive:

$$\text{Relative risk} = \frac{(\%\text{antigen-positive patients}) \ (\%\text{antigen-negative controls})}{(\%\text{antigen-negative patients}) \ (\%\text{antigen-positive controls})}$$

The relative risk estimates vary somewhat based on the ethnicity of the population studied. For example, the relative risk of rheumatoid arthritis in HLA-DR4-positive whites of Northern European extraction is much greater than that in HLA-DR4-positive Jewish people.

24. How do you determine a person's HLA type?

HLA-DR3 or HLA-DR4 specificities are referred to as "serologic" specificities. These are determined by using transplantation or pregnancy sera in which the antibodies against MHC molecules have previously been identified. There are sera, for example, that contain antibodies only against HLA-DR2, HLA-DR3, or HLA-DR4, etc. Combinations of these sera are then used to "type" or characterize an individual's MHC molecules. While this method has been extremely valuable over the years, especially in transplantation biology, more genetically specific methods are now available to characterize the MHC identity of individuals and so investigate immunogenetic associations with diseases.

25. What is cross-reactivity in serologic typing?

Antibodies obtained from human sera that are directed against HLA molecules can bind to molecules that are very similar, but not identical. When serologic specificities were developed, the antibodies against the MHC molecules were not defined as being specific for that small area of the molecule that predisposes to autoimmune disease. If most but not all HLA-DR4 molecules are identical at the particular site that enhances the susceptibility to rheumatoid arthritis (RA), then most but not all HLA-DR4-positive individuals would have enhanced susceptibility to RA. In contrast, two individuals, one HLA-DR4-positive and the other HLA-DR1-positive, might both have enhanced susceptibility to RA if they share the site that enhances susceptibility to RA, even though their serologic specificities differ.

26. Is it really this confusing? Can there really be people who are HLA-DR4-positive who are not predisposed to rheumatoid arthritis? Can there be people who are HLA-DR4-negative, but HLA-DR1-, DR6-, or DR10-positive who are predisposed?

Yes. This cross-reactivity, and therefore compromised specificity of serotyping, clarified the need for more genetically pure typing. Techniques have been developed that can define the nucleotide sequences of the MHC genetic loci—designated, for example, by DRB*0402. They can be more specific for that special area of the HLA molecule that predisposes to the disease—the **shared epitope.** These methods provide improved estimates of relative risk.

The issue of cross-reactivity has created significant confusion in the study of RA. In different ethnic groups, HLA-DR1, -DR4, -DR6, and -DR10 molecules have been associated with RA. HLA-DR4 molecules share marked homology in the first and second hypervariable regions (HVRs), which align them according to serologic typing (note the striking homology in the HVRs 1 and 2 which characterize the upper four sequences in the figure on the next page). Some HLA-DR4, -DR1, -DR6, and -DR10 alleles, while very different in HVRs 1 and 2, share crucial amino acid homology in the HVR3 (see the homology in the HVR3 regions of the lower six sequences in the figure). This "shared epitope" in HVR3 appears to predispose to RA. In contrast, the HLA-DRB*0402 sequence (top sequence in the figure) does not predispose to RA. In the DRB*0402 allele, there are the amino acids isoleucine (I), aspartic acid (D), and glutamic acid (E) at positions 67, 70, and 71, respectively. The predisposition to RA seems to require a leucine (L) at position 67, glutamine (Q) or arginine (R) at position 70; arginine (R) or lysine (K) at position 71; and alanine (A) at position 74.

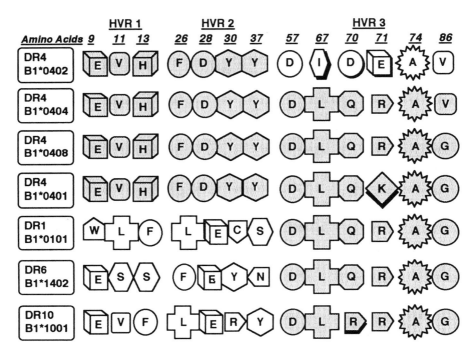

Amino acid sequence in the three hypervariable regions (HVR) of several different allelic forms of the HLA-DRβ chain.

BIBLIOGRAPHY

1. Abbas AK, Lichtman AH, Pober JS: The major histocompatibility complex. In Abbas AK, Lichtman AH, Pober JS (eds): Cellular and Molecular Immunology, 2nd ed. Philadelphia, W.B. Saunders 1994, pp 96–115.
2. Carson DA: Genetic factors in the etiology and pathogenesis of autoimmunity. FASEB J 6:2800–2805;1992.
3. Goodman JW: Antigen presentation and the major histocompatibility complex. In Stites DP, Terr AI, Parslow TG (eds): Basic and Clinical Immunology, 8th ed. Norwalk, CT, Appleton & Lange, 1994, pp 58–65.
4. Nepom BS, Nepom GT: Immunogenetics of the rheumatic diseases. In Kelley WK, Harris ED, Ruddy S, Sledge CB (eds): Textbook of Rheumatology, 4th ed. Philadelphia, W.B. Saunders, 1993, pp 89–107.
5. Nepom BS: The role of the major histocompatibility complex in autoimmunity. Clin Immunol Immunopathol 67:S50–S55, 1993.
6. Robinson DM, Nepom GT: The major histocompatibility complex and disease susceptibility. Immunol Allergy Clin North Am 13:255–272, 1993.
7. Salazar M, Yunis EJ: MHC: Gene structure and function. In Frank MM, Austen KF, Claman HN, Unanue ER (eds): Samter's Immunologic Diseases, 5th ed. New York, Little, Brown and Company, 1994, pp 101–106.
8. Weyand CM, Goronzy JJ: Functional domains on HLA-DR molecules: Implications for the linkage of HLA-DR genes to different autoimmune diseases. Clin Immunol Immunopathol 70:91–98, 1994.
9. Winchester RJ: Immunogenetics. In Schumacher HR (ed): Primer on the Rheumatic Diseases, 10th ed. Atlanta, Arthritis Foundation, 1993, pp 35–40.
10. Winchester RJ: The molecular basis of susceptibility to rheumatoid arthritis. Adv Immunol 65:389–466, 1994.

7. TOLERANCE AND AUTOIMMUNITY

Nicholas J. Battafarano, M.D.

1. What is tolerance?

The healthy immune system must be able to recognize and eradicate certain antigens that would otherwise cause damage or death to the organism. An equally vital requirement is the ability to recognize, but not eradicate, the antigens it needs. **Tolerance** is the term used to describe the phenomenon of **antigen-specific unresponsiveness.** That is, the immune system encounters certain antigens that it specifically does not eradicate.

2. Is tolerance innate or acquired?

Tolerance is characterized by specificity and memory. That is, the immune system "learns" to be tolerant of some specific antigens, just as it learns to be "intolerant" of many foreign antigens. When discussing autoimmune disorders, we often narrow our perspective to the tolerance of **autoantigens,** such as an individual's own nucleoproteins or cell-surface molecules. However, the phenomenon of tolerance is not limited to autoantigens. In fact, tolerance to **exogenous antigens,** such as dietary proteins, is just as crucial for the survival of an individual as "self-tolerance." Valuable insights into the development and loss of tolerance in autoimmune disorders, as well as creative therapeutic approaches, emerge from our understanding of tolerance to exogenous proteins.

3. What is autoimmunity?

The term *autoimmunity* is commonly employed to describe conditions in which an individual becomes the victim of his or her own immune response. As it relates to tolerance, autoimmunity can be defined as the **absence of healthy self-tolerance.** Just like immunity to foreign antigens, autoimmune disorders are antigen-driven processes that are characterized by specificity and memory. In contrast, however, an autoimmune process involves the immune system's recognition of an antigen—foreign or self—followed by an assault on its own self-antigens (i.e., autoantigens). Typically, these processes develop in an individual who previously displayed tolerance to the same antigens that are now targeted by the immune response. Therefore, most autoimmune processes are better described not simply as an absence of tolerance but as a **loss of tolerance.**

4. If autoimmune processes involve a loss or absence of tolerance which leads to a chronic antigen-driven immune response against autoantigens, shouldn't the key to their control involve preventing the loss of tolerance or re-establishing tolerance?

Many investigators believe this. However, effective implementation of this hypothesis presumes an understanding of the development and maintenance of tolerance. We have many observations confirming that tolerance is, indeed, developed, maintained, and can be pathologically lost. Unfortunately, our understanding of these processes is limited. In other words, we have several pieces of the puzzle, but we do not know quite how they fit together. Therefore, current therapies for these disorders are directed at pieces of the process that have been observed.

5. What are the major factors that influence the development of specific immune responses?

- Characteristics of the antigen involved in the specific immunologic response
- Characteristics of the accessory cells that initially interact with the antigen
- Nature of the responding lymphocytes and the cytokines that they produce

6. How can the characteristics of the antigen favor the development of tolerance rather than autoimmunity?

The antigen can "select" certain types of immune responses based on its **chemical composi-**

tion, the initial **amount** to which an individual is exposed, the initial **route** by which the antigen is introduced to the immune system, and the **milieu** within which the antigen encounters the immune system. Two important aspects of that milieu include the level of development of the immune system at initial antigen presentation and the presence or absence of surrounding inflammation when the antigen is presented.

TOLERANCE	IMMUNE RESPONSE
Polysaccharide	Protein
IV or oral route	SC or ID route
Large dose	Small dose
Immunologic immaturity	Surrounding inflammation

For example, we are more likely to develop an immune response against a protein than to a polysaccharide. Small subcutaneous (SC) or intradermal (ID) doses are more likely to evoke an immune response than large intravenous (IV) or oral doses of the same antigen. If an inflammatory response is generated in the same locale as an antigen is introduced (e.g., by employing an adjuvant) an antigen-specific response is more likely to develop. If, on the other hand, no inflammation is present or the exposed immune cells are immature at the time of antigen presentation, tolerance is favored.

7. Discuss the role of the MHC molecules in the development of autoimmune disease.

First, the vast majority of antigens targeted in autoimmune diseases are proteins. Antigen-specific memory responses to proteins—be they humoral, phagocytic, or cytotoxic—are coordinated by T cells. However, T cells can only recognize protein antigens presented to them in the context of MHC molecules. MHC molecules serve several important roles at this level:

1. They translate the immunologically nonspecific responses of cells into specific immunologic responses.

2. MHC molecules are used to communicate antigen-specific experiences. For example, antigen-specific B cells, which recognize an antigen via their surface immunoglobulin receptor, translate that specific experience to T cells via their MHC molecules.

This places MHC molecules at the crux of the development or absence of an immune response. If something goes awry at the level of the MHC, development and maintenance of tolerance would be expected to be affected. Thus, it makes sense that the MHC molecules provide the strongest genetic link with the development of autoimmune diseases.

8. How do variations in an antigen's amino acid sequence influence the development of autoimmune disease?

It is not simply that antigens are proteins, but also the sequence of their amino acids that is important. When MHC Class I and II molecules present peptide to T cells, only a small peptide fits in the antigen-binding cleft—8–13 amino acids for MHC Class I and 13–25 amino acids for MHC Class II. It is clear that individual amino acid positions in the MHC molecules can be crucial for the binding of certain complementary peptide amino acid sequences.

9. How can the primary structure of an antigen lead to a loss of tolerance?

First, the peptide sequence of a foreign antigen may resemble a self-antigen. If that happens, untoward sequelae may develop. Rheumatic heart disease is the classic example of such a situation. Myocardial autoantigens—myosin and sarcolemmal membrane proteins—resemble the streptococcal M protein structure. Part of the pathogenesis, supported by autoantibodies, may be secondary to innocent myocardial tissue becoming the target of immune response products evoked by M protein. Subsequently, the myocardial autoantigens could continue to drive the process.

In another example, there are peptides derived from some pathogens that have stretches of amino acids whose sequence is identical to the sequences in the antigen-binding cleft of certain MHC molecules themselves, For example, a string of five amino acids in a peptide (plasmid) of *Shigella flexneri* that is identical to a sequence within HLA-B27 has been identified from bacteria infecting patients with dysentery and Reiter's syndrome. Similar homology has been shown or predicted to exist for a number of other pathogen-derived products.

These are two examples of cross-reactivity in which the products of the immune response to a foreign antigen might inappropriately engage an individual's own antigens. This pathologic confusion is commonly referred to as **molecular mimicry.** The T- and B-cell clones that were initially "turned on" by the foreign antigen might continue to be stimulated by the cross-reactive autoantigens. It is conceivable that autoantigen-driven immune responses might persist long after the foreign antigen which initiated the process has been eliminated.

10. Discuss therapeutic experiments using the amount and route of antigen exposure to induce immunologic responses.

Large doses of either protein or polysaccharide have been shown to select T- or B-cell tolerance, respectively. In the appropriate cellular interactions, low-dose peptide presentation may evoke T-cell tolerance.

Recently, investigators have attempted therapeutic trials that employ oral doses of an antigen in an effort to induce tolerance to endogenous antigens. For example, in experimental allergic encephalomyelitis, an animal model similar to multiple sclerosis, myelin basic protein (MBP) is the target autoantigen. Therapy with oral MBP in these animals has reduced the severity of their disease. As a consequence, human therapeutic trials with oral doses of MBP, perhaps the autoantigen in multiple sclerosis, have been initiated. A similar approach with oral collagen administration in patients with rheumatoid arthritis has been attempted to take advantage of the same tolerogenic phenomenon.

11. What are superantigens? Do these lead to autoimmunity?

Superantigens are foreign antigens, particularly of bacterial or retroviral origin, that are capable of binding to the T-cell receptor (TCR) and MHC Class II molecule outside the antigen-binding groove and, in turn, bind the two together (see figure). These antigens are not as restricted in their effects as typical antigens. They do not need to be processed and subsequently presented in the antigen-binding cleft of MHC molecules in order to stimulate T-cell activation. The superantigen is specific for a segment in the variable (v) region of the TCR β-chain, the Vβ region. Up to 10% of T cells may share a common Vβ region for which the superantigen is specific. This results in the activation of extremely large numbers of different antigen-specific clones of T cells.

Although they are implicated in the pathology of staphylococcal-associated toxic shock syndrome, T-cell superantigens do not appear to mediate the classic rheumatic diseases. Bacterial lipopolysaccharide (LPS) functions as a polyclonal activator of B cells, including autoreactive B cells. LPS may play some role in the pathogenesis of the autoimmune diseases, at least at certain points in the course of the disease. This role has not been established.

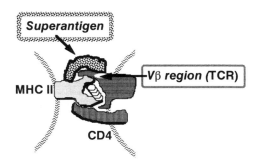

Superantigen specificity for the TCR Vβ region external to the conventional MHC–peptide antigen-binding cleft.

12. How does the milieu affect the development of immunologic responses?

It has long been recognized that the effectiveness of immunization can be enhanced by the use of adjuvants. However, autoantigens to which an individual previously has been tolerant are sometimes "innocently" presented to lymphocytes in an area where inflammation is already established. This can be the result of enhanced and aberrant presentation of autoantigens because of cytokine stimulation of antigen-presenting cells. Such an event can lead to a loss of tolerance. This might then be followed by an autoantigen-driven specific immune response that persists long after the trigger of the initial inflammatory process has been eliminated.

13. What is determinant spreading?

This term is used to describe the phenomenon introduced in Question 12. A juicy marital argument serves as a good analogy to the process in which an acute inflammatory response can proceed to the development of a more severe and chronic inflammatory response. When cool heads prevail, a discussion can stay focused on and effectively resolve a very specific conflict. However, sometimes a discussion turns into an irrational, long-standing battle. Suddenly, every point that is presented in this milieu becomes threatening. Issues that have come up thousands of times, but to which the individuals had previously been tolerant, are now responded to with a vengeance. Frequently, the event that triggered the dispute is long forgotten, while each of the little issues has taken on a life of its own. The previously acquired tolerance to these many "innocuous" factors can be extremely difficult to recover.

Determinant spreading describes the loss of tolerance—and thus an active, ongoing, autoantigen-driven specific immune response—to a number of antigens that are presented in the milieu of acute and chronic inflammation. There is evidence of maturing autoreactive T- and B-cell-mediated responses to a variety of autoantigens during the course of chronic autoimmune disease.

14. What is meant by the term "hidden antigens"?

Hidden antigens are potential antigens for which an individual may never have developed specific recognition. Therefore, these particular antigens, typically intracellular contents, have the potential to evoke either an aggressive or tolerant response from the immune system.

Continuing the previous analogy, timing may be everything! The events associated with first impressions can be crucial. If in the midst of an argument regarding finances, a remote extramarital affair is disclosed for the first time, a long-standing violent assault may ensue. This can happen, even though that particular issue presents no direct threat to the current relationship. Particularly if there is continued cellular breakdown secondary to the ongoing inflammatory response, previously hidden antigens may persistently resurface and be responded to as foreign.

15. How can accessory cells favor the development of tolerance rather than autoimmunity?

Antigen-presenting cells (APCs) are often referred to as "accessory cells"—i.e., these cells are looked upon as being supportive to the lymphocytes. Of course, the T lymphocytes are really doing the worthwhile work, but from the perspective of the APC, the notion of lymphocytes, particularly the T cell, as the favorite cell is undoubtedly comical. Is the T cell really in control? APCs respond, "We let them think so." APCs only disclose exactly what they want to disclose and when they want to disclose it. They present information only in a context that they determine so that they can limit what is seen and by whom. Not only that, but in almost all cases they must authorize the lymphocytic response—a phenomenon known as **costimulation.** (This T-cell–APC relationship bears a striking resemblance to the illusions that attending physicians maintain regarding their relationship with their housestaff.)

APCs play a major role in the selection of the T-cell repertoire and the lifelong maintenance of tolerance. They influence this via their methods and choice of processing and presenting antigens, the MHC context within which they present it, the intensity within which they present it, and the costimulatory signals they provide. If APCs do not function properly or are misunderstood, autoimmunity may indeed be enhanced.

16. Summarize the potential roles of MHC molecules in autoimmune processes.

There are many postulated mechanisms. No one mechanism alone explains autoimmunity.

Potential Roles of MHC Molecules in Autoimmune Disorders

ROLE IN AUTOIMMUNITY	EXPLANATION
T-cell selection bias	The T-cell population that is selected via the inherited disease-associated MHC molecules may include more autoreactive T cells or disease-specific autoreactive T cells.
Pathogenic receptor function	Certain disease-associated MHC molecules may function as a receptor for certain pathogens that cause autoimmune disease.
Unique peptide presentation	Disease-associated MHC molecules may be uniquely capable of presenting certain peptides that evoke the autoimmune response. This is supported by the shared epitope hypothesis.
Molecular mimicry	A foreign antigen or another MHC + foreign peptide may resemble the disease-associated MHC molecule, with or without bound peptide. This may be followed by: • An appropriate immunologic response followed by pathologic autoreactivity, or • The immune system, tolerized to its own MHC molecule with or without bound peptide, cannot mount an appropriate response to the cross-reactive foreign antigen. That foreign antigen may go on to cause the chronic disease.
Inappropriate peptide presentation	Presentation of self-antigens when the APC is also expressing costimulating molecules or when the cytokine milieu will stimulate a response. Presentation of improperly processed peptides. Increased presentation of peptides that do not require a response may result from APC activation by cytokine stimulation.

17. What is clonal deletion?

Clones of T lymphocytes are not useful if they cannot recognize "self-MHC" or if they recognize but then try to eradicate it. In other words, the recognition by the T-cell receptor (TCR) for the MHC-peptide complex cannot be "too hot" or "too cold"; it has to be "just right." If it is not just right, the T cells are often instructed to kill themselves. **Clonal deletion** refers to the intrathymic process during which immature T cells whose TCRs cannot get it "just right" are told to kill themselves. These cells and their potential progeny are then deleted from the T-cell repertoire.

18. How are T cells selected to survive or die in the thymus?

Current observations are consistent with the existence of at least two processes:

1. The cells must be **positively selected.** That is, the TCR must recognize "self-MHC + peptide" enough to be able to respond when necessary. Those whose TCRs do recognize the MHC + peptide survive; if not, they die.

2. T cells must be **negatively selected.** That is, they must not have such a strong affinity for the MHC that they respond by eradicating self-MHC + peptide. Those whose interaction is "too hot" have to be either deleted or inactivated.

19. How can cells be activated to kill themselves? If they don't kill themselves on command, does that result in autoimmune disease?

Recent investigations strongly support the notion that autoreactive T cells may not be eliminated because they cannot be effectively commanded to commit suicide. One mechanism by which this programmed cell death, termed **apoptosis,** can be initiated is by cross-linking of a cell-surface molecule called Fas/APO1 (CD95). A defect in Fas-mediated apoptosis appears to be the genetic defect in a murine model of systemic lupus erythematosus, the MRL-*lpr/lpr* mouse. A recent report suggests that aberrant Fas-mediated apoptosis may also be involved in human SLE.

20. What is clonal anergy?

We know that thymic T-cell selection and education are not foolproof. There are a lot of potentially autoreactive T cells out in the circulation and secondary lymphoid tissues. **Clonal anergy** refers to the processes, implemented either centrally in the thymus or in the peripheral tissues, whereby autoreactive T cells are functionally inactivated but not destroyed. That is, processes by which autoreactive T cells are inactivated or "learn" that they are permitted to recognize but not respond.

21. How does clonal anergy happen?

Of course, we don't exactly know. However, a recurrent theme in immunology is repetitive signaling. Most cell activation responses, especially antigen-specific responses, require more than one signal. Evidence suggests that some anergy processes include an interaction of the MHC–peptide complex with an autoreactive TCR during which costimulatory signals are *not* provided to the autoreactive T cell.

22. Does the term "suppressor T cell" describe some form of T-cell tolerance?

The concept of the suppressor T cell is a controversial one. There is a continued vigilance for the T-suppressor cell because investigators have demonstrated transfer of antigen-specific immunologic suppression via passive transfer of T cells. The controversy surrounds the belief that there is a unique type of T cell that mediates *only* suppressor functions.

The phenomenon of antigen-specific suppression of immunologic responses is *in*consistent with the technical definition of tolerance because it would require a specific T-cell-activation response to mediate the suppression. Technically, immunologic tolerance describes the lack of cell activation, despite antigen-specific recognition. From a nontechnical standpoint, antigen-specific T-cell-suppressive effects, perhaps via release of TGF-β, may well modify autoreactivity. It has been difficult to establish this effect as the role of a unique T cell.

23. Is there such a thing as B-cell tolerance?

Yes, B cell tolerance definitely exists. Mechanisms of B-cell tolerance are actively being investigated. Current evidence suggests that immature B cells that are specific for self-antigen are more than likely developmentally blocked rather than killed. High doses of polysaccharides, in contrast to peptides for T cells, can foster B-cell tolerance. Encounter with antigen in the absence of specific T-cell help, particularly during early development, is probably responsible for some B-cell tolerance. It has recently been proposed that *loss* of B-cell tolerance may be able to occur without direct T-cell help. While T-cell anergy appears to be long-lasting, maintenance of B-cell anergy appears to require more frequent exposure to antigen.

24. Where do autoantibodies fit into the picture?

As previously mentioned, the presence of autoreactive lymphocytes, B cells as well as T cells, is well recognized. It is also common for the production of autoantibodies (rheumatoid factors and antinuclear antibodies) to increase transiently in the face of immune activation. This up-regulation appears to be a relatively normal phenomenon. With increasing age, autoantibody production increases, perhaps reflecting some loss in the maintenance of tolerance. This increase does parallel the increased prevalence of autoimmune diseases with advancing age but does *not* implicate autoantibodies in the pathogenesis of all autoimmune diseases.

25. Describe some diseases in which autoantibodies appear to play a major pathogenic role.

- Autoantibodies appear to deliver the major cytopathic lesion in some hemolytic anemias and autoimmune thrombocytopenias.
- In insulin-resistant diabetes mellitus, myasthenia gravis, and pernicious anemia, autoantibodies directed against cellular receptors directly lead to pathologic cellular responses.
- In Goodpasture's syndrome and bullous pemphigoid, antibodies directed against basement membrane components result in the major pathologic lesions of those diseases.
- In systemic lupus erythematosus and post-streptococcal glomerulonephritis, immune complexes involving autoantibodies appear to be responsible for glomerular damage.
- In other diseases, the association of certain autoantibodies with specific diseases or particular manifestations of diseases may or may not directly lead to the pathology.

BIBLIOGRAPHY

1. Abbas AK, Lichtman AH, Pober JS: Immune-mediated tissue injury and disease. In Abbas AK, Lichtman AH, Pober JS (eds): Cellular and Molecular Immunology, 2nd ed. Philadelphia, W.B. Saunders, 1994, pp 393–408.
2. Abbas AK, Lichtman AH, Pober JS: Self tolerance and autoimmunity. In Abbas AK, Lichtman AH, Pober JS (eds): Cellular and Molecular Immunology, 2nd ed. Philadelphia, W.B. Saunders, 1994, pp 376–392.
3. Fowlkes BJ, Ramsdell F: T-cell tolerance. Curr Opin Immunol 5:873–879, 1993.
4. Holman HR: Thought barriers to understanding rheumatic diseases. Arthritis Rheum 37:1565–1572, 1994.
5. Kotb M: Infection and autoimmunity: A story of the host, the pathogen, and the copathogen. Clin Immunol Immunopathol 74:10–22, 1995.
6. Lasalle JM, Hafler DA: T cell anergy. FASEB J 8:601–608, 1994.
7. Mountz JD, Wu J, Cheng J, Zhou T: Autoimmune disease. A problem of defective apoptosis. Arthritis Rheum 37:1415–1420, 1994.
8. Nemazee D: Promotion and prevention of autoimmunity by B lymphocytes. Curr Opin Immunol 5:866–872, 1993.
9. Ridgway WM, Weiner HL, Fathman CG: Regulation of autoimmune response. Curr Opin Immunol 6:946–955, 1994.
10. Schwartz BD. Structure, function, genetics of the HLA complex in rheumatic disease. In McCarty DJ, Koopman WJ (eds): Arthritis and Allied Conditions: A Textbook Of Rheumatology, 12th ed. Philadelphia, Lea & Febiger, 1993, pp 509–523.
11. Sercarz EE, Datta SK: Mechanisms of autoimmunization: Perspective from the mid 90's. Curr Opin Immunol 6:875–881, 1994.
12. Shur PH. Arthritis and autoimmunity. Arthritis Rheum 37:1818–1825, 1994.
13. Steinberg AD. Mechanisms of disordered immune regulation. In Stites DP, Terr AI, Parslow TG (eds): Basic and Clinical Immunology, 8th ed. Norwalk, CT, Appleton & Lange, 1994, pp 380–386.

III. Evaluation of the Patient with Rheumatic Symptoms

> *Specialism is a natural and necessary result of the growth of accurate knowledge, inseparably connected with the multiplication and perfection of instruments of precision. It has its drawbacks, absurdities even. . . . . A few years ago a recent graduate and ex-hospital intern asked me, apparently seriously, to give him the name of a specialist in rheumatism. We can afford to laugh at these things. . . . .*
> Frederick Shattuck, 1897
> Professor of Medicine
> Harvard Medical School

---

8. HISTORY AND PHYSICAL EXAMINATION

Danny C. Williams, M.D.

---

1. What symptoms or signs should your history include when interviewing a patient for connective tissue disease?

Fever

Weight loss

Fatigue

Headache

Alopecia

Rash

Photosensitivity

Nodules

Raynaud's phenomenon

Arthralgias/arthritis

Myalgias/myositis

Anemia

Leukopenia

Autoimmune antibodies

Xerophthalmia

Xerostomia

Ocular inflammation

Visual disturbance

Mucositis

Serositis

Carditis

Nephritis

Colitis

Urethritis

Cognitive disturbance

Seizures

Neuropathy

Fetal loss

Thrombosis

2. Define photosensitivity.

In rheumatology, *photosensitivity* refers to the development of **rash following sun exposure** in patients (30–60%) with cutaneous or systemic lupus erythematosus. *Photophobia* is the term reserved for **ocular sensitivity** to light.

3. What historical or physical features are essential for the diagnosis of Raynaud's phenomenon?

Raynaud's phenomenon is a vascular disorder characterized by transient, stress-induced (e.g., cold temperature) ischemia of the digits, nose-tip, and/or ears. As a result of vasospastic alterations in blood flow, a triphasic color response is observed. The initial color is **white** (ischemic pallor), then **blue** (congestive cyanosis), and finally **red** (reactive hyperemia). The diagnosis of Raynaud's phenomenon *best* correlates with the initial "dead-white" pallor of ischemia.

4. What historical symptoms enable you to categorize a rheumatic disorder as inflammatory or mechanical (degenerative)?

FEATURE	INFLAMMATORY	MECHANICAL
Morning stiffness	>1 hr	<30 min
Fatigue	Profound	Minimal
Activity	Improves symptoms	Worsens symptoms
Rest	Worsens symptoms	Improves symptoms
Systemic involvement	Yes	No
Corticosteroid response	Yes	No

5. List the five cardinal signs of inflammation.
Swelling (*tumor*)
Warmth (*calor*)
Erythema (*rubor*)
Tenderness (*dolor*)
Loss of function (*functio laesa*)

6. Which signs of inflammation are suggestive of acute synovitis in a joint?
In the absence of corticosteroids, most joints affected by an inflammatory arthritis exhibit warmth and limitation of range. The best indicator of synovitis, however, is the presence of **joint-line tenderness** elicited by direct palpation. Swelling, even effusions, may occur in the noninflammatory arthritides (e.g., osteoarthritis). Furthermore, most inflamed joints are not typically erythematous, with exception of acute septic and crystalline arthritis. If you encounter red, hot joints, particularly in a monarticular distribution, your first thought should be "where's the needle?" in order to perform a joint aspiration.

7. How do "active" and "passive" range of motion (ROM) differ? Why compare the two maneuvers?
Active ROM—performed by the patient.
Passive ROM—performed by the examiner with the patient at rest.
These maneuvers are useful in differentiating articular versus periarticular rheumatism. Discrepancy (e.g., decreased active, normal passive ROM) between "active" and "passive" ROM suggests a soft tissue origin, whereas agreement (decreased active *and* passive ROM) implicates the true joint. Supraspinatus tendinitis is an exception to this rule.

8. In a patient with an inflammatory arthritis, what history is useful in assessing disease activity?
Subjective status, duration of morning stiffness, and **degree of fatigue.** These subjective parameters, along with the joint count, are useful in assessing disease progression and treatment efficacy.

9. How much pressure should you apply when palpating a joint for synovitis? How do you "stress" a joint for demonstration of synovitis?
A good "rule of thumb" is to palpate with enough pressure to blanche your thumbnail (4 kg/cm^2). This standardizes the joint exam and ensures that adequate pressure is being applied to detect sy-novitis. Obviously, with overtly inflamed joints, this degree of pressure may be excessive. The tender points characteristic of fibromyalgia may be similarly palpated.
Applying stress to joints is a technique reserved for those occasions when synovitis is suspected but not evident by direct palpation. "Stressing" a joint is easily accomplished by gently forcing the joint toward its limitation of range. Any discomfort generated by this maneuver is suggestive of synovitis.

10. Which joints are included in a joint count?

Peripheral joints

Hand	Foot
Distal interphalangeal (DIP)	Interphalangeal
Proximal interphalangeal (PIP)	Metatarsophalangeal (MTP)
Metacarpophalangeal (MCP)	Talocalcaneal (subtalar)
Thumb carpometacarpal (CMC)	
Wrist	Ankle
Elbow	Knee

Axial joints

Shoulder	Spine
Glenohumeral	Cervical
Acromioclavicular	Thoracic
Sternoclavicular	Lumbar
Hip	Temporomandibular
Sacroiliac	

11. Describe the STWL system for recording the degree of arthritic involvement of a joint.

The STWL system records the degree of **swelling, tenderness, warmth,** and **limitation of motion** in a joint based on a quantitative estimate of severity. A score of 0 (normal), 1 (trace), 2 (mild), 3 (moderate), or 4 (severe) can be assigned to the S, T, and W categories. Limitation of motion is scored as 0 (normal), 1 (25% loss of motion), 2 (50% loss), 3 (75% loss), or 4 (ankylosis). For example, Rt. 2nd MCP S2T2W1L2 means the right second MCP joint has mild synovitis, mild tenderness, trace warmth, and a 50% loss of normal range of motion.

12. What is crepitus? What does it signify?

Crepitus is an audible or palpable "grating" emanating from a joint in motion. The **fine** crepitus of inflamed synovium is of uniform intensity and perceptible only with a stethoscope. In contrast, **coarse** crepitus is easily detected, of variable intensity, and transmitted from damaged cartilage and/or bone. Crepitus may be elicited by compressing a joint throughout its range of motion.

13. How do a tender point and trigger point differ?

FEATURE	TENDER POINT	TRIGGER POINT
Disorder	Fibromyalgia	Myofascial pain syndrome
Distribution	Widespread	Regional
Abnormal tissue	No	Yes
Tenderness	Focal	Focal
Referred pain	No	Yes

14. What rheumatic disorders, other than rheumatoid arthritis, may exhibit subcutaneous nodules?

Systemic lupus erythematosus	Lupus profundus
Rheumatic fever	Sarcoid
Tophaceous gout	Vasculitis
Juvenile chronic arthritis	Panniculitis
Scleroderma (calcinosis)	Type II hyperlipoproteinemia
Erythema nodosum	Multicentric reticulohistocytosis

15. Describe the examination for a patient with suspected median nerve entrapment of the wrist (carpal tunnel syndrome).

Thenar atrophy is a reliable sign of carpal tunnel syndrome (CTS) but only occurs as a consequence of chronic disease. Acute CTS symptoms are typically sensory (the median nerve supplies sensory innervation to the palmar surface of the thumb, index finger, middle finger, and radial half of the ring finger). Its symptoms may be reproduced by the provocation tests of Tinel and Phalen. **Tinel's test** is best performed with the wrist in extension. The full width of the transverse carpal ligament is then percussed using a broad-headed, reflex hammer. In contrast, **Phalen's test** is performed by gently positioning the wrist at full flexion for 60 seconds. Nerve conduction velocity studies are useful in confirming the clinical diagnosis of CTS.

16. In the examination of an arthritic hand, what features enable you to differentiate rheumatoid arthritis from osteoarthritis?

Clinical Features of Rheumatoid Arthritis Versus Osteoarthritis

FEATURE	RHEUMATOID ARTHRITIS	OSTEOARTHRITIS*
Symmetry	Yes	Occasional
Synovitis	Yes	Sometimes[†]
Nodules	Yes	No
Bony hypertrophy	No	Yes
Joint involvement		
DIP	No	Heberden's nodes
PIP	Yes	Bouchard's nodes
MCP	Yes	No[‡]
CMC	No	Thumb
Wrist	Yes	No[§]
Deformity	Swan neck	Lateral flexion
	Boutonniere	
	Subluxation	
Digital infarcts	Seldom	No

*Osteoarthritis may occur secondary to any inflammatory arthritis.
†Synovitis can occur in inflammatory erosive osteoarthritis.
‡Osteoarthritis of the index and middle finger MCP joints is a feature of hemochromatosis.
§Osteoarthritis of the wrist may occur secondary to trauma or crystalline arthritis.

17. What is Finkelstein's test?
Finkelstein's test is a useful adjunct to direct palpation in the clinical diagnosis of deQuervain's tenosynovitis. The test is initially performed by asking the patient to make a fist enclosing the thumb. While stabilizing the patient's forearm, the examiner gently bends the fist toward the ulnar styloid. If extreme discomfort occurs at the "anatomic snuffbox," then deQuervain's tenosynovitis of the **abductor pollicis longus** and **extensor pollicis brevis** tendons is present.

18. How do you diagnose "tennis elbow" (lateral epicondylitis)?
In addition to direct palpation, tennis elbow may be diagnosed by stressing the wrist extensor muscles at their origin, the lateral epicondyle. This provocation maneuver requires the patient to form a fist and maintain the wrist in extension. The examiner then flexes the wrist against resistance, while supporting the patient's forearm. Pain arising from the lateral epicondyle confirms the diagnosis.

19. When examining a swollen, inflamed elbow, how can you physically differentiate olecranon bursitis from true arthritis?
Differentiation may be difficult due to swelling, pain, and limitation of range (extension and flexion). Rotation of the forearm, with the elbow flexed at 90°, is the one maneuver that can differentiate the two disorders. True arthritis of the elbow will inhibit pronation and supination of the radiohumeral joint, whereas in olecranon bursitis, the joint moves freely.

20. In the evaluation of shoulder pain, what single maneuver can differentiate glenohumeral joint involvement from that of the periarticular tissues?
Significant glenohumeral joint pathology can be excluded if normal **passive external rotation** of the shoulder is demonstrated.

21. What does the "painful arc" sign mean?
A "painful arc" encountered while assessing shoulder abduction is usually indicative of supraspinatus tendinitis and/or subacromial bursitis. Painful interruption of abduction typically devel-

ops at about 70° in active range of motion (normal shoulder range of abduction is 0–180°). Occasionally, the shoulder may be passively abducted beyond 120° with abrupt relief of symptoms. Subacromial impingement of an inflamed bursa and/or supraspinatus tendon during abduction produces this "painful arc" of 50°. A second "painful arc" may also be demonstrated in patients with acromioclavicular joint disease, starting at 140° of abduction.

22. Name the four shoulder muscles comprising the rotator cuff. How do you physically assess their integrity?
The rotator cuff is comprised of the **SITS** muscles. Function of these muscles is tested by resistance maneuvers. Resistance is best performed with the patient's arm against the side and the elbow flexed to 90°.

MUSCLE	RESISTANCE MANEUVER
Supraspinatus	Abduction
Infraspinatus	External rotation
Teres Minor	External rotation
Subscapularis	Internal rotation

23. How do you perform Adson's test to evaluate vascular compromise in thoracic outlet syndrome?
While the examiner palpates the radial pulse, the patient's arm is abducted, extended and externally rotated. The patient is then asked to look *toward* the side being tested and inhale deeply. Diminution or loss of the radial pulse with development of a supraclavicular bruit is suggestive of significant subclavian artery compression.

24. When a patient has true hip joint pathology, where does he or she perceive the pain?
Despite misconceptions of the lay public, the origin of true hip pain is the **groin,** not the waist, lateral flank, or buttock. Hip pain may occasionally radiate from the groin to the thigh, greater trochanter, buttock, and knee. Assessment of hip mobility may help differentiate hip pathology from other causes of groin pain (e.g., adductor tendinitis).

25. What simple screening maneuver can exclude true hip pathology as a source of hip pain?
The **log roll** maneuver is performed with the leg in extension. While grasping the thigh and shin, the examiner rotates the entire limb back and forth, using the hip joint as a pivot. Groin pain or inhibition of internal or external rotation is suggestive of true hip joint pathology.

26. What does a positive Trendelenburg's test indicate?
A positive Trendelenburg's test reveals weakness of the **gluteus medius** muscle, implicating hip joint pathology. The test is performed by observing the patient from behind as he or she stands on one leg. Normally, gluteus medius contraction of the ipsilateral, weight-bearing limb will elevate the contralateral pelvis. In contrast, a weakened gluteus medius muscle cannot support the contralateral pelvis, and thus it will remain level or drop. Neurogenic causes (i.e., L5 nerve root compression) of gluteus medius weakness should also be excluded.

27. Describe the physical findings of a patient with meralgia paresthetica.
Meralgia paresthetica (lateral femoral cutaneous nerve syndrome) results from entrapment of the lateral femoral cutaneous nerve as it passes under the inguinal ligament medial to the anterior pelvic brim. Typical symptoms include burning dysesthesias and pain over the anterolateral thigh. In some patients, these symptoms may be elicited by performing **Tinel's test** at the site of entrapment.

28. How do you diagnose trochanteric bursitis?
The diagnosis of trochanteric bursitis is best made by direct palpation of the soft tissues overlying the greater trochanter of the femur. In addition to focal tenderness, the examiner may find that the bursal area is "boggy," particularly in slender individuals. Trochanteric bursa pain may also be elicited by hip flexion and external rotation.

29. When examining a swollen knee, how can you tell if it is inflamed?

In absence of erythema, **warmth** may be the best indicator of inflammation in a swollen knee. Knee temperature is generally cooler than the pretibial skin in normal individuals. Thus, if comparative palpation reveals the anterior knee skin to be warmer, then inflammation is likely.

30. When examining a swollen knee, how can you tell if there is an effusion?

Two methods are available for the detection of fluid within the knee joint. The patellar **bulge** test is most useful when evaluating minimal effusions. In contrast, a successful patellar **tap** test is dependent on moderate to large effusions.

To perform the **bulge** test, the palm is used to "milk" a potential effusion from the *medial* knee to the suprapatellar compartment. A reverse, similar maneuver is then performed on the *lateral* side, starting from the suprapatellar surface. If rapid filling of the *medial* patellar fossa occurs, then the bulge test is positive.

The **tap** test is initially performed by anterior compression of the suprapatellar compartment. This maneuver forces a potential effusion into the retropatellar space, thus "floating" the patella. Fingertip ballottement of the patella, with a resultant "knock" against the femoral condyles, constitutes a positive tap test.

31. What is the patellofemoral compression test?

This test is used to evaluate damage (e.g., osteoarthritis) to the retropatellar surface. With the knee in extension, the examiner compresses the patella against the femoral condyles. The patient is then asked to extend their knee forcefully, thus contracting the quadriceps muscle. With quadriceps contraction, the patella will be displaced proximally against the femur. If this maneuver produces **pain**, the test is positive.

32. How do you differentiate prepatellar bursitis from arthritis when evaluating an inflamed knee?

Unlike in the elbow, rotational movement of the knee is quite limited and useless for differentiating the two disorders. A typical feature of acute, inflammatory arthritis of the knee is loss of extension. This feature is not characteristic of prepatellar bursitis. Thus, if an inflamed knee demonstrates full extension without "stress" pain, then the disease is likely extra-articular.

33. When evaluating an unstable knee, how do you perform Lachman's test?

Lachman's test is a type of drawer test used to evaluate the integrity of the anterior cruciate ligament. It is best performed by holding the knee in 15–20° of flexion. While stabilizing the thigh with one hand, the examiner uses the other hand to pull the tibia forward. A mild "give," or forward subluxation, is suggestive of anterior cruciate laxity or tear. Congenital laxity (hypermobility) must be excluded by comparison of both knees.

34. Why examine a patient for leg-length inequality?

Leg-length discrepancy is associated with several "mechanical" disorders, such as chronic back pain, trochanteric bursitis, and degenerative hip disease. **True** leg-length discrepancy reflects measurable differences (congenital or acquired) of both limbs using the anterior, superior iliac spines and lateral malleoli as landmarks. **Apparent** or functional leg-length discrepancy is primarily a measure of "pelvic tilt" typically induced by scoliosis or hip contractures. This apparent inequality is determined by measuring the distance from the umbilicus to each lateral malleoli. True leg-length measurement is usually *equal* in disorders of apparent leg-length discrepancy. Correction of significant inequality (>1 cm) with a simple shoe lift can be therapeutic.

BIBLIOGRAPHY

1. Doherty M, Doherty J: Clinical Examination in Rheumatology. London, Wolfe Publishing Ltd., 1992.
2. Doherty M, Hazelman BL, Hutton CW, et al: Rheumatology Examination and Injection Techniques. London, W.B. Saunders, 1992.
3. Hoppenfeld S: Physical Examination of the Spine and Extremities. Norwalk, CT, Appelton-Century-Crofts, 1976.

4. Kelly WN, Harris ED, Ruddy S, Sledge CB (eds): Textbook of Rheumatology, 4th ed. Philadelphia, W.B. Saunders, 1993.
5. Klippel JH, Dieppe PA (eds): Rheumatology. London, Mosby, 1994.
6. Polley HF, Hunder GG: Rheumatologic Interviewing and Physical Examination of the Joints, 2nd. ed. Philadelphia, W.B. Saunders, 1978.

9. LABORATORY EVALUATION

Woodruff Emlen, M.D.

1. Which laboratory tests are used most commonly in the clinical assessment of ongoing inflammation?

Most clinicians follow the erythrocyte sedimentation rate (ESR) and/or C-reactive protein levels. These tests are nonspecific but may be useful for monitoring disease activity in rheumatoid arthritis, giant cell arteritis, polymyalgia rheumatica, and some other vasculitides.

2. What is the erythrocyte sedimentation rate? How is it measured, and what influences its result?

The ESR is a measurement of the distance in millimeters that red blood cells (RBCs) fall within a specified tube (Westergren or Wintrobe) over 1 hour. The ESR is an indirect measurement of alterations in acute-phase reactants and quantitative immunoglobulins. Acute-phase reactants are a heterogeneous group of proteins (fibrinogen, protease inhibitors, others) that are synthesized in the liver in response to inflammation. The inflammatory cytokine, interleukin-6, is the most potent mediator stimulating production of acute-phase proteins by the liver. Any condition that causes a rise in the concentration of these acute-phase proteins or hypergammaglobulinemia (polyclonal or monoclonal) will cause an elevation of the ESR by increasing the dielectric constant of the plasma. This results in dissipation of inter-RBC repulsive forces, leading to closer aggregation of RBCs and causing them to fall faster. Increasing age, female sex, and pregnancy are noninflammatory conditions that can elevate the sedimentation rate.

Normal Values for Erythrocyte Sedimentation Rates

	AGE <50 YRS	AGE >50 YRS
Westergren method (mm/hr)		
Male	<15	<20
Female	<25	<30
Wintrobe method (mm/hr)		
Male	<10	<20
Female	<15	<25

Pearl: A rough rule of thumb is that the age-adjusted upper limit of normal for ESR is:

Male = age/2   Female = (age + 10)/2

3. How do the Westergren and Wintrobe methods differ?

The Westergren method uses a 200-mm tube, has a dilution step that corrects for the effect of anemia, and is the preferred method. The Wintrobe method uses a 100-mm tube and has no dilutional step. Due to its longer tube, only the Westergren method can detect an ESR > 50–60 mm/hr.

4. What causes an extremely high or extremely low ESR?

Markedly elevated ESR (> 100 mm/hr)

    Infection, bacterial (35%)

    Connective tissue disease: giant cell arteritis, polymyalgia rheumatica, SLE, other vasculitides (25%)

Malignancy: lymphomas, myeloma, others (15%)
Other causes (22%)
Unknown (3%)
Markedly low ESR (0 mm/hr)
Afibrinogenemia/dysfibrinogenemia
Agammaglobulinemia
Extreme polycythemia (hematocrit > 65%)
Increased plasma viscosity

5. Describe your approach to the evaluation of an elevated ESR.

1. Complete history and physical examination and routine screening laboratories (complete blood count, chemistries, liver enzymes, urinalysis).
2. If there is no clear association after step 1, consider the following:
   - Repeat ESR to ensure it is still elevated and there was no laboratory error.
   - Review medical record to compare with any previously obtained ESR.
   - Measure fibrinogen, serum protein electrophoresis (SPEP), and CRP for evidence of an acute-phase response.
   - Check SPEP and quantitative immunoglobulins to rule out myeloma or polyclonal gammopathy.
3. If still no obvious explanation, recheck ESR in 1–3 months. Up to 80% of patients will normalize. Follow patient for development of other symptoms or signs of disease if ESR remains elevated.

6. What is the C-reactive protein?

CRP is a pentameric protein comprised of five identical, non-covalently bound subunits, arranged in cyclic symmetry in a single plane. Its function is to bind to cell wall components, C1q complement component, and receptors on neutrophils and monocytes to help initiate and facilitate the inflammatory response. CRP is produced as an acute-phase reactant by the liver in response to interleukin-6 and other cytokines. Elevation occurs within 4 hours of tissue injury with peaks within 24–72 hours. CRP is measured by ELISA, radioimmunodiffusion, or nephelometry. A normal value is typically < 0.08 mg/dl. Levels > 8–10 mg/dl should suggest bacterial infection or systemic vasculitis.

7. When should you order a CRP instead of an ESR?

Both tests measure components of the acute-phase response and are useful in measuring generalized inflammation. The ESR is affected by multiple variables and, as such, is somewhat imprecise. Nevertheless, it is inexpensive and easy to perform. The CRP test measures a specific acute-phase reactant, and thus it is more specific. It rises more quickly and falls more quickly (decreases by 50% in 24 hours) than the ESR, which tends to remain elevated for a longer time (decreases by 50% in 1 week) after inflammation subsides. The major drawback of the CRP is its increased cost relative to the ESR.

8. When is it appropriate to order an antinuclear antibody (ANA) test?

An ANA should be ordered when the clinical assessment of the patient suggests the presence of an autoimmune disease. An ANA should generally not be used as a screening test or as part of a "fishing expedition" to work-up a confusing case.

9. How are antinuclear antibodies measured?

The major method currently in use is fluorescence microscopy. Permeabilized cells are fixed to a microscope slide and incubated with the patient's serum, allowing ANAs to bind to the cell nucleus. After washing, a fluoresceinated second antibody is added, which binds to the patient's antibodies (which are bound to the nucleus). Cells are visualized through a fluorescence microscope to detect nuclear fluorescence. The amount of ANAs in a patient's serum is determined by diluting the patient's serum prior to adding the serum to the fixed cells—the greater the dilution (titer) at which nuclear fluorescence is detected, the greater the amount of ANAs present in the patient's serum.

Most laboratories use HEp-2 cells (a proliferating cell line derived from a human epithelial tumor cell line) for the substrate to detect ANAs instead of frozen sections of rodent organ cells (mouse liver/kidney). This is because rapidly growing and dividing cells contain a larger array and higher concentration of nuclear antigens (such as SS-A and centromere antigens). Recently, enzyme-linked immunoassay methods (ELISA) have become available to detect ANAs. These assays vary among manufacturers and may not detect certain ANAs that are detected by the immunofluorescent method. However, because of the ease of performing these ELISA methods, they may gradually replace fluorescent ANA methods.

10. What is an LE cell?

The LE cell (lupus erythematosus cell) *was* the major method of measuring ANAs in the 1950s and 1960s. In this test, a bare nucleus stripped of cytoplasm is incubated with the patient's serum, allowing ANAs to bind to the nucleus. Normal polymorphonuclear leukocytes (PMNs) are then added, and if sufficient antibodies have been bound to the nucleus, the nucleus is opsonized and the PMNs engulf the nuclear material. A PMN containing phagocytosed nuclear material is known as an LE cell. This test is relatively insensitive in detecting ANAs and may be difficult to interpret. It therefore has been replaced by the fluorescent ANA.

11. At what point is an ANA test considered positive?

A positive ANA is arbitrarily defined as that level of antinuclear antibodies which exceeds the level seen in 95% of the normal population. Each laboratory must determine the level that it considers positive, and this level may vary significantly among labs. In most laboratories, this level is a titer of 1:40 to 1:80. In laboratories where HEp-2 cells are used as substrate to detect an ANA, clinically significant titers are usually $\geq$ 1:160.

12. What is the clinical significance of a positive ANA?

It depends on the clinical context. A positive ANA in isolation does not make a specific diagnosis, and a negative ANA does not absolutely exclude autoimmune diseases. The ANA should be used primarily as a confirmatory test when the physician strongly suspects systemic lupus erythematosus (SLE) or other autoimmune disease.

13. Can a positive ANA occur in a normal individual?

Yes. A positive ANA is defined as the level (titer) of ANA that exceeds the level found in 95% of normal individuals. Thus, up to 5% of normals can be ANA-positive. In these individuals, titers are usually $\leq$ 1:320, and the nuclear staining pattern is most often speckled or homogenous. The incidence of these ANAs is higher among women and older individuals.

14. Can a patient with SLE ever be ANA-negative?

Yes. A very few patients (1–2%) with active, untreated SLE will have a negative ANA. These patients usually have antibodies to the nuclear antigen SS-A and are ANA-negative because the substrate used in the fluorescent ANA test did not contain sufficient SS-A antigen to allow detection of those antibodies. In addition, a larger number of SLE patients (10–15%) will become ANA-negative with treatment or as their disease becomes inactive. SLE patients with end-stage renal disease on dialysis frequently become ANA-negative (40–50%).

15. What medical conditions are associated with a positive ANA?

CONDITION	% ANA-POSITIVE
SLE	95–99
Healthy relatives of SLE patients	15–25
Rheumatoid arthritis	50–75
Mixed connective tissue disease (MCTD)	95–100
Progressive systemic sclerosis	95
Polymyositis	80
Sjögren's syndrome	75–90
Cirrhosis (all causes)	15
Autoimmune liver disease (autoimmune hepatitis, primary biliary cirrhosis)	60–90
Normals	3–5
Normal elderly (> 70 yrs)	20–40
Neoplasia	15–25

16. Can the ANA titer be used to follow disease activity in patients with SLE or other autoimmune diseases?

No. There is no evidence that variations in ANA titer (level) as measured by the screening ANA correlate with disease activity.

17. What is the significance of ANA patterns?

ANA patterns refer to the patterns of nuclear fluorescence observed under the fluorescence microscope. Certain patterns of fluorescence are associated with certain diseases, although these associations are not specific:

Homogenous (diffuse)	SLE, drug-induced LE, other diseases
Rim (peripheral)	SLE, chronic active hepatitis
Speckled	SLE, MCTD, Sjögren's, scleroderma, other diseases
Nucleolar	Scleroderma
Centromere	Limited scleroderma (CREST)

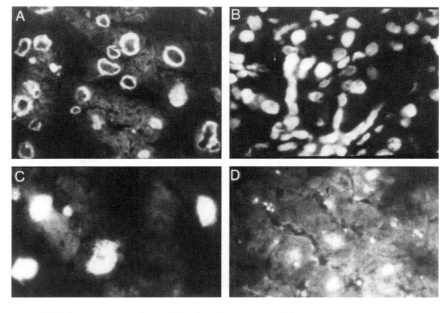

Patterns of ANA fluorescence: *A,* rim (peripheral); *B,* homogenous (diffuse); *C,* speckled; *D,* nucleolar. (From the Clinical Slide Collection on the Rheumatic Diseases. Atlanta, American College of Rheumatology, 1991; with permission.)

Different patterns reflect the differences in ANA content in different sera. Readings of ANA patterns has largely been replaced by identification of specific antinuclear antibodies through the ANA profile (*see* Questions 20 and 21).

18. Is the ANA a good screening test for SLE?

No. Simple mathematics indicate that if 5% of the *normal* American population is ANA-positive, then 12.5 million normal individuals have a positive ANA. In contrast, even if 100% of SLE patients are ANA-positive, because the prevalence of SLE is only approximately 3/1000, there are only 750,000 individuals with SLE who are ANA-positive. Thus, if the entire population were screened for ANA, more normal individuals would be detected who are ANA-positive than SLE individuals. The clinical value of an ANA test can be tremendously enhanced by ordering an ANA when there is a reasonable pre-test probability (i.e., clinical suspicion) of an autoimmune disease.

19. Can drugs induce a positive ANA?

Common	**Unusual**
Procainamide	Up to 60 different drugs have been
Hydralazine	implicated as unusual causes
Phenothiazines	of a positive ANA
Diphenylhydantoin	
Isoniazid	
Quinidine	

The clinical syndrome of drug-induced lupus occurs in only a small percentage of patients with drug-induced ANAs (see Chapter 21). ANA may remain positive months to years after discontinuing the drug. The ANA is usually directed against the epitope formed by the (H2A-H2B)–DNA complex, although hydralazine causes an ANA primarily against the H3–H4 histone dimer.

20. What is meant by an "ANA profile"?

An ANA profile consists of a battery of tests that measure ANAs specific for certain nuclear antigens. The standard profile includes tests to measure antibodies to double-stranded DNA, ribonuclear protein (RNP), Smith antigen (Sm), SS-A (Ro), SS-B (La), and centromere. Other disease-specific antinuclear antibodies [SCL-70 (topoisomerase I), PM-SCL (PM-1), histones] and ancytoplasmic antibodies (Jo-1, ribosomal P, mitochondrial) have to be ordered individually.

21. Which diseases are associated with the different antibodies measured in the ANA profile?

	dsDNA	RNP	SM	SS-A	SS-B	CENTROMERE
SLE	60%	30%	30%	30%	15%	Rare
Rheumatoid arthritis	–	–	–	Rare	Rare	–
Mixed connective tissue disease	–	>95% (high titer)	–	Rare	Rare	Rare
Progressive systemic sclerosis	–	(low titer)	–	Rare	Rare	10–15%
Limited scleroderma (CREST)	–	–	–	–	–	60–90%
Sjögren's syndrome	–	Rare	–	70%	60%	–

– = negative. Numbers indicate the percentage of patients with the indicated disease who will test positive for the antibody.

22. When is it appropriate to order an ANA profile?

An ANA profile should be ordered when the screening ANA is positive and when additional information is desired regarding the type of autoimmune disease. Occasionally, antibodies to SS-A are detected on the ANA profile even in the face of a negative immunofluorescent ANA. Therefore, if the physician has a strong suspicion of SLE or another SS-A-associated disease, antibodies to SS-A should be ordered even despite a negative ANA.

23. What syndromes are associated with antibodies to SS-A?
SLE
Primary Sjögren's syndrome
Subacute cutaneous lupus (SCLE) (a variant of lupus characterized by prominent photo-sensitivity and rash)
Neonatal lupus
Congenital heart block
Secondary Sjögren's syndrome (rarely)

24. In some diseases, antibodies against cytoplasmic antigens can be more helpful diagnostically than antibodies against nuclear antigens. Which diseases?

Autoimmune Diseases Associated with Anticytoplasmic Antibodies

DISEASE	CYTOPLASMIC ANTIGEN	FREQUENCY
Polymyositis	tRNA synthetase (anti-Jo-1, others)	20–30%
SLE	Ribosomal P	5–10%
Wegener's granulomatosis	Serine protease-3 (seen only in neutrophils)	90%
Microscopic polyarteritis and some other vasculitides	Myeloperoxidase, others (see only in neutrophils)	70%
Primary biliary cirrhosis	Mitochondria	80%

Patients with polymyositis, Wegener's granulomatosis, microscopic polyarteritis, or primary biliary cirrhosis accompanied by an anticytoplasmic antibody frequently lack antibodies to nuclear antigens and hence are ANA-negative. Consequently, the specific anticytoplasmic antibody should be ordered when these diseases are suspected.

25. Which of the ANAs measured in the ANA profile are useful to follow disease activity?
Antibodies to DNA usually parallel disease activity in SLE. High titers of antibody to DNA are associated with lupus nephritis, and increases in DNA antibody levels are frequently predictive of a flare of lupus activity. Other antibodies included in the ANA profile are markers of disease subsets but do not fluctuate with disease activity.

26. Which antibodies are useful in a patient who is suspected of having progressive systemic sclerosis (scleroderma)?
Anticentromere antibodies are seen in 60–90% of patients with the limited form of scleroderma (CREST syndrome), and antibodies to SCL-70 (anti-topoisomerase I) are seen in 20–33% of patients with diffuse systemic sclerosis.

27. What is the significance of antibodies to ribonuclear protein (RNP)?
Antibodies to RNP produce a speckled pattern on immunofluorescent ANA and are seen in a number of autoimmune diseases, including SLE, progressive systemic sclerosis, mixed connective tissue disease (MCTD). The presence of very high levels of anti-RNP (level should be determined by each lab) is highly suggestive of MCTD, a syndrome of overlapping disease manifestations with features of progressive systemic sclerosis, SLE and polymyositis.

28. What are rheumatoid factors, and how are they measured?
Rheumatoid factor (RF) is the general term used to describe an autoantibody directed against antigenic determinants on the Fc (crystallizable) fragment of immunoglobulin G. RF may be of any isotype: IgM, IgG, IgA, or IgE. IgM RF is the only one routinely measured by clinical laboratories. A titer of ≥ 1:160 is usually considered significant if done by the latex agglutination technique. Recently, many laboratories have begun using nephelometry and ELISA techniques to measure IgM RF.

29. Describe how the ANA pattern and antigen specificity are used in the diagnosis of the connective tissue diseases.

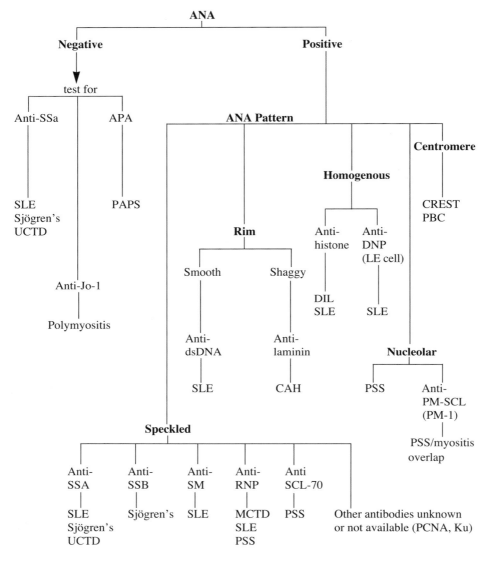

APA = antiphospholipid antibodies (lupus anticoagulant, anticardiolipin antibodies); CAH = chronic active hepatitis; DIL = drug-induced lupus; MCTD = mixed connective tissue disease; PAPS = primary antiphospholipid antibody syndrome; PSS = progressive systemic sclerosis (scleroderma); SCL-70 = topoisomerase I; UCTD = undifferentiated connective tissue disease.

30. How would you evaluate an unexplained positive ANA in a patient with nonspecific arthralgias?

- History and physical examination: Look for signs of a connective tissue disease and particularly occult Sjögren's syndrome.
- Obtain an ANA profile: ANA titers ≥ 1:160 or the presence of disease-specific autoantibodies usually indicate the ANA is significant.
- Obtain additional studies looking for evidence of immune hyperactivity:
  CBC: Look for anemia of chronic disease, neutropenia, and thrombocytopenia.

Liver enzymes: If elevated, consider chronic active hepatitis.
C3, C4: Look for hypocomplementemia.
SPEP: Look for polyclonal gammopathy.
RF, ESR, ribonuclear protein: Look for false-positives.
Electrolytes, creatinine, urinalysis for completeness.

If any of the above are abnormal, the ANA may be indicative of an evolving autoimmune disease, and the patient will need to be followed closely.

31. In a patient with a known clinical diagnosis of rheumatoid arthritis (based on history and physical examination), what is the value of measuring rheumatoid factor?
It should be emphasized that a positive RF does not make the diagnosis of rheumatoid arthritis. However, once rheumatoid arthritis has been diagnosed, patients who are RF-positive tend to have more severe disease. Joint inflammation is more severe and more frequently leads to joint destruction in these patients than in patients who are RF-negative. Patients with high-titer RF are at increased risk to develop extra-articular manifestations of rheumatoid arthritis, including nodules, pulmonary disease, cutaneous ulcers, vasculitis, and Felty's syndrome.

32. Do changes in rheumatoid factor level reflect changes in rheumatoid arthritis disease activity?
No. Disease activity of rheumatoid arthritis is best determined by clinical assessment.

33. What are the causes of a positive rheumatoid factor?
The common denominator for the production of RF is **chronic immune stimulation.** The most common diseases associated with RF production are: **CHRONIC,** as the mnemonic indicates:

CH Chronic disease, especially hepatic and pulmonary diseases
 R Rheumatoid arthritis, 80–85% of patients
 O Other rheumatic diseases, such as SLE (15–35%), scleroderma (20–30%), MCTD (50–60%), Sjögren's (75–95%), polymyositis (5–10%), sarcoid (15%)
 N Neoplasms, especially after radiation or chemotherapy
 I Infections, e.g., AIDS, mononucleosis, parasitic infections, chronic viral infections, chronic bacterial infections (tuberculosis, subacute bacterial endocarditis, others)
 C Cryoglobulinemia, 40–100% of patients

34. Rheumatoid factors are present in some normal people, especially the elderly. What are the false-positive rates?
In normal individuals who are RF-positive, males and females are affected equally, and in only 20% of cases is the RF titer $\geq$ 1:160.

Frequency of Positive RF in Normal Individuals of Different Ages

AGE	FREQUENCY OF RF
20–60 yrs	2–4%
60–70 yrs	5%
>70 yrs	10–25%

35. What are anti-neutrophilic cytoplasmic antibodies (ANCA)?
Antibodies directed against specific antigens present in the cytoplasm of neutrophils. There are two different types of ANCAs.

ANCA reactive with myeloperoxidase (MPO), elastase, or lactoferrin give a perinuclear pattern of staining on immunofluorescence of ethanol-fixed neutrophils and are termed perinuclear or **P-ANCA.** Antibodies to serine proteinase-3 give diffuse cytoplasmic staining on immunofluorescence and are called cytoplasmic or **C-ANCA.**

36. Which diseases are associated with ANCAs?
ANCA are most strongly associated with necrotizing vasculitis. Disease associations differ for C-ANCA and P-ANCA:

C-ANCA	P-ANCA
Wegener's granulomatosis	Microscopic polyarteritis
Microscopic polyarteritis	Pauci-immune glomerulonephritis
Churg-Strauss vasculitis (rare)	Churg-Strauss vasculitis
	Ulcerative colitis (MPO negative)
	Autoimmune liver disease
	HIV infection
	Certain other infectious or neoplastic diseases (rare)

37. Do ANCA titers fluctuate with disease activity?
In Wegener's granulomatosis, the titer of C-ANCA does correlate with disease activity (in 60% of cases) and has been used to predict flares of disease. However, it remains controversial as to whether changes in C-ANCA titers should be used as the sole basis for changes in therapy. There is little evidence that P-ANCA titers fluctuate with disease activity.

38. What are the causes of decreased circulating complement components?
Serum complement may be decreased as a result of:

1. Decreased production, due to either a hereditary deficiency or liver disease (complement components are synthesized in the liver)

2. Increased consumption (proteolysis), due to complement activation. A major cause of complement consumption is increased levels of circulating immune complexes.

39. What clinical conditions are associated with hereditary complement deficiencies?

COMPLEMENT COMPONENTS	DISEASE
Early (C1, C2, C4)	SLE-like disease
	Glomerulonephritis
Mid (C3, C4)	Recurrent pyogenic infections
	SLE-like disease
Terminal (C5–C9)	Recurrent infections (especially gonococci and meningococci)
Regulatory (C1 INH)	Angioedema (hereditary or acquired)

40. Can a patient with increased complement consumption due to circulating immune complexes have a normal complement level?
Yes. The serum level of complement components represents a balance between consumption and production. Complement components are acute-phase reactants, and therefore production by the liver increases when an individual is acutely ill. Therefore, despite increased consumption of complement components, increased production may keep pace with consumption, resulting in a normal level of complement. Clinically, this means that while a decreasing level of complement is confirming evidence for complement consumption, normal complement levels cannot exclude complement consumption.

41. What autoimmune and acquired diseases are associated with hypocomplementemia?
Rheumatic diseases
SLE
Systemic vasculitis (especially polyarteritis nodosum, urticaria)
Cryoglobulinemia
Rheumatoid arthritis with extra-articular manifestations

Infectious diseases
Subacute bacterial endocarditis
Bacterial sepsis (pneumococcal, gram-negative)
Viremias (especially hepatitis B)
Parasitemias
Glomerulonephritis
Post-streptococcal
Membranoproliferative

42. Why should you order three complement components (C3, C4, and CH50) rather than just one?
By measuring three complement components, you can assess the activity of both the classical and alternative pathways as well as screen for complement deficiencies. In complement consumption by the classical pathway (immune complexes), all three components are decreased. If complement is activated by the alternative pathway (as seen with glomerulonephritis due to C3 nephritic factor), C3 and CH50 are decreased, but C4 (in the classical pathway) remains normal. Finally, CH50, which requires all components of the complement pathway to be present, is a good screen for complement deficiency. A CH50 level of 0 or "unmeasurable" is suggestive of a hereditary complement deficiency.

BIBLIOGRAPHY

1. Fernandez-Madrid F, Mattioli M: Antinuclear antibodies (ANA): Immunologic and clinical significance. Semin Arthritis Rheum 6:83, 1976.
2. Fritzler MJ: Antinuclear antibodies in the investigation of rheumatic disease. Bull Rheum Dis 35:127–136, 1987.
3. Fritzler MJ, Rubin RL: Drug-induced lupus. In Wallace DJ, Hahn BH (eds): Dubois' Lupus Erythematosus. Philadelphia, Lea & Febiger, 1993, pp 442–454.
4. Goeken JA: Antineutrophil cytoplasmic antibody—A useful serological marker for vasculitis. J Clin Immunol 11:161–174, 1991.
5. Homburger HA: Cascade testing for autoantibodies in connective tissue diseases. Mayo Clin Proc 70:183–184, 1995.
6. Molden DP, Nakamuras RM, Tan EM: Standardization of the immunofluorescence test for autoantibody to nuclear antigens (ANA): Use of reference sera of defined antibody specificity. Am J Clin Pathol 82:57–66, 1984.
7. Reichlin M, Harley J: Antinuclear antibodies: An overview. In Wallace DJ, Hahn BH (eds): Dubois' Lupus Erythematosus. Philadelphia, Lea & Febiger, 1993, pp 188–194.
8. Roberts DE: Antineutrophil cytoplasmic autoantibodies. Lab Immunol 12:85–97, 1992.
9. Schur PH: Complement and systemic lupus erythematosus. In Wallace DJ, Hahn BH (eds): Dubois' Lupus Erythematosus. Philadelphia, Lea & Febiger, 1993, pp 120–127.
10. Shmerling RH, Delbanco TL: The rheumatoid factor: An analysis of clinical utility. Am J Med 91:528–534, 1991.
11. Sox HC, Liang MH: The erythrocyte sedimentation rate: Guidelines for rational use. Ann Intern Med 104:515–523, 1986.
12. Tan EM: Antinuclear antibodies: Diagnostic markers for autoimmune diseases and probes for cell biology. Adv Immunol 44:93, 1989.

10. ARTHROCENTESIS AND SYNOVIAL FLUID ANALYSIS

Robert T. Spencer, M.D.

1. When should arthrocentesis be performed?
Without doubt, the single most important reason to perform arthrocentesis is to check for **joint infection.** Timely identification and treatment of a patient with septic arthritis are of paramount importance to clinical outcome. In addition, arthrocentesis is generally indicated to gain diagnostic information through synovial fluid (SF) analysis in the patient with a mono- or polyarticular arthropathy of unclear etiology characterized by joint pain and swelling.

2. When is arthrocentesis contraindicated?
When the clinical indication for obtaining SF is strong, such as in the patient with suspected septic arthritis, there is no absolute contraindication to joint aspiration. Relative contraindications include **bleeding diatheses,** such as hemophilia, anticoagulation therapy, or thrombocytopenia; however, these conditions frequently can be treated or reversed prior to arthrocentesis. **Cellulitis** overlying a swollen joint can make the approach to the joint space difficult, but this rarely precludes the ability to perform the procedure. Allergy to lidocaine or topical antiseptics is easily remedied by using alternatives.

3. What techniques should be used when performing arthrocentesis?
The procedure should be performed using **aseptic technique.** A topical antiseptic, such as povidone-iodine, should be applied to the area. Nonsterile gloves should always be worn as part of universal precautions. Sterile gloves should be used if palpation of the area is foreseen subsequent to antiseptic prep and prior to placement of the needle. A 25-gauge needle should be used to administer a local anesthetic (e.g., 1% lidocaine). The aspiration itself should be performed using an 18-gauge, 1.5-inch needle, when possible, and a 10–30-ml syringe. Aspiration techniques for individual joints are described in other references.

4. What are the potential complications of arthrocentesis?
- Infection (risk <1 in 10,000)
- Bleeding/hemarthrosis
- Vasovagal syncope
- Pain
- Cartilage injury

5. What studies should be performed for synovial fluid analysis?
Because the single most important determination of SF analysis is for the presence of infection, **Gram stain** and **culture** should be performed on samples from joints with even relatively low suspicion for infection. Determining **total leukocyte count** and **differential** helps in differentiating between noninflammatory and inflammatory joint conditions. Lastly, **polarized microscopy** should be done to evaluate for the presence of pathologic crystals. Chemistry determinations, such as glucose, total protein, and lactate dehydrogenase, are unlikely to yield helpful information beyond that obtained by the previous studies, and therefore they should not be routinely ordered.

6. How should the SF sample be handled?
Once fluid has been obtained, samples should be allocated into sterile vacuum tubes and sent for analysis. Fluid for culture and Gram stain may be sterilely transferred to a red-top tube. Fluid for crystal analysis may be place in a red- or green-top tube, depending on the lab's preference. Fluid for cell count and differential should be placed in a purple-top tube.

7. What if no SF is obtained (a "dry tap")?

Even if no fluid is aspirated into the syringe, frequently one or two drops of fluid and/or blood can be found within the needle and its hub. This amount is sufficient for culture, in which case the syringe with capped needle should be submitted to the microbiology lab. If one extra drop can be spared, it can be placed on a microscope slide with a coverslip for polarized microscopy. When microscopy is completed, the coverslip can be removed and the specimen may then serve as a smear for Gram stain. The specimen remaining on the coverslip may be an adequate smear on which to perform a Wright's stain, allowing determination of leukocyte differential. Thus, two drops of fluid can yield the same important diagnostic information as that obtained from a larger specimen, with the exception of a leukocyte count. The lesson to be learned from this is that when a "dry tap" is encountered, the needle and syringe should *not* be reflexively discarded!

8. Within what time frame should SF analysis occur?

SF should be analyzed as soon as possible after the fluid is drawn. If it is delayed more than 6 hours, results may be spuriously altered. Problems that can arise include:

- Decrease in leukocyte count (due to cell disruption)
- Decrease in number of crystals (primarily calcium pyrophosphate dihydrate)
- Appearance of artifactual crystals

9. Describe the classification based on SF analysis.

Synovial Fluid Classification

FLUID TYPE	APPEARANCE	TOTAL WBC COUNT/MM³	% PMNS
Normal	Clear, pale yellow	0–200	<10%
Group 1 (noninflammatory)	Clear to slightly turbid	200–2000	<20%
Group 2 (inflammatory)	Slightly turbid	2000–50,000	20–70%
Group 3 (pyarthrosis)	Turbid to very turbid	>50,000	>70%

WBC, white blood cell (leukocyte); PMN, polymorphonuclear cell.

10. Name some causes of noninflammatory (group 1) joint effusions.

Osteoarthritis, joint trauma, mechanical derangement, pigmented villonodular synovitis, and avascular necrosis.

11. Group 2 (inflammatory) synovial fluid is typical for which rheumatic disorders?

Rheumatoid arthritis
Gout
Pseudogout
Psoriatic arthritis
Ankylosing spondylitis
Reiter's syndrome
Juvenile rheumatoid arthritis
Rheumatic fever
Systemic lupus erythematosus
Polymyalgia rheumatica
Giant cell arteritis
Wegener's granulomatosis
Hypersensitivity vasculitis

Polyarteritis nodosum
Familial Mediterranean fever
Sarcoidosis
Infectious arthritis
   Viral (hepatitis B, rubella, HIV,
     parvovirus, others)
   Bacterial (gonococci)
   Fungal
   Mycobacterial
   Spirochetal (Lyme disease, syphilis)
Subacute bacterial endocarditis
Palindromic rheumatism

12. Other than joint sepsis, which conditions are associated with a group 3 fluid (pyarthrosis)?

When a group 3 fluid is discovered, septic arthritis *must* be assumed until proved otherwise by SF culture. A few disorders may cause noninfectious pyarthrosis, sometimes referred to as joint **pseudosepsis.**

Gout
Reiter's syndrome
Rheumatoid arthritis

13. List some causes of a hemarthrosis.

- Trauma
- Bleeding diatheses
- Tumors
- Pigmented villonodular synovitis
- Hemangiomas

- Scurvy
- Iatrogenic (post-procedure)
- Arteriovenous fistula
- Intense inflammatory disease
- Charcot's joint

14. Compare the polarized light microscopic findings of synovial fluid from a joint with gout and one with pseudogout.

	GOUT	PSEUDOGOUT
Crystal	Urate	Calcium pyrophosphate dihydrate (CPPD)
Shape	Needle	Rhomboid or rectangular
Birefringence	Negative	Positive
Color of crystals parallel to axis of red-plate compensator	Yellow	Blue

Pearl: For the crystal color, use the mnemonic **ABC** (**A**lignment, **B**lue, **C**alcium). If the crystal aligned with the red-plate compensator is blue, then it is calcium pyrophosphate dihydrate. Urate crystals are the opposite, being yellow when parallel to the compensator.

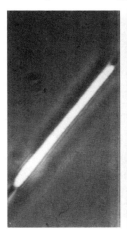 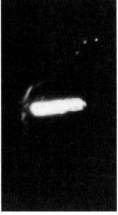

Left, Urate crystal of gout, showing needle shape. *Right,* CPPD crystal of pseudogout, showing rhomboid shape.

15. How may synovial fluid WBC count be estimated by "wet drop" examination?
At the time polarized microscopy is performed, the synovial fluid WBC count can be easily estimated. The finding of 2 or fewer WBCs per high power field (40×high dry objective) confidently suggests a noninflammatory fluid (<2000 WBCs per mm³). If greater than 2 WBCs per high power field are seen, there is a significant chance the synovial fluid is inflammatory and formal determination of the WBC count should be ordered.

BIBLIOGRAPHY

1. Clayburne G, Daniel DG, Schumacher HR: Estimated synovial fluid leukocyte numbers on wet drop preparations as a potential substitute for actual leukocyte counts. J Rheumatol 19:60, 1992.
2. Cohen MG, Emmerson BT: Crystal arthropathies: Gout. In Klippel JH, Dieppe PA (eds). Rheumatology. London, Mosby, 1994.
3. Doherty M: Crystal arthropathies: Calcium pyrophosphate dihydrate. In Klippel JH, Dieppe PA (eds): Rheumatology. London, Mosby, 1994.
4. Doherty M, Hazelman BL, Hutton CW, Maddison PJ, Perry JD (eds): Rheumatology Examination and Injection Techniques. Philadelphia, W.B. Saunders, 1992.

5. Hasselbacher P: Arthrocentesis, synovial fluid analysis, and synovial biopsy. In Schumacher HR, Klippel JH, Koopman WJ (eds): Primer on the Rheumatic Diseases, 10th ed. Atlanta, Arthritis Foundation, 1993.
6. Kerolus G, Clayburne G, Schumacher HR: Is it mandatory to examine synovial fluids promptly after arthrocentesis? Arthritis Rheum 32:271, 1989.
7. Schumacher HR: Synovial fluid analysis and synovial biopsy. In Kelley WN, Harris ED, Ruddy S, Sledge CB (eds): Textbook of Rheumatology, 10th ed. Philadelphia, W.B. Saunders, 1993.
8. Shmerling RH, et al: Synovial fluid tests: What should be ordered? JAMA 264:1009, 1990.

11. RADIOGRAPHIC AND IMAGING MODALITIES

Kevin M. Rak, M.D.

1. Describe the radiographic modalities available in the assessment of arthritis.

Plain film radiographs are the cornerstone of radiologic diagnosis in the arthritides. They typically define the character and distribution of bone erosions, abnormalities of the cartilaginous space, malalignment, soft-tissue swelling, or calcifications. Conventional radiography is the least expensive modality available and readily depicts the extent of disease as well as progression of disease.

Computed tomography (CT) permits cross-sectional images to be displayed with excellent contrast resolution. CT is helpful in diagnosis of arthritides in complex joints (e.g., sacroiliac, subtalar, and sternoclavicular joints), in evaluation of bone tumors (e.g., osteoid osteoma), and in assessment of trauma, particularly in the spine and pelvis, as it defines and characterizes fractures better than plain radiographs.

Arthrography has been replaced somewhat by MRI in the assessment of intra-articular disorders. In the knee, arthrograms are rarely performed, except in cases of prior meniscectomy. Arthrography is still performed in other joints, such as the shoulder, wrist, ankle, and hip, particularly if MRI results are inconclusive. Aspiration arthrography is certainly indicated in a patient with a painful hip or knee prosthesis, to differentiate infection from aseptic loosening.

Magnetic resonance imaging (MRI) has no radiation, is noninvasive, and permits imaging in any plane or axis. It has outstanding sensitivity but, unfortunately, commonly lacks specificity. The excellent contrast resolution provided by MRI has made it the study of choice in evaluating internal disorders of the knee, rotator cuff tears, avascular necrosis, herniated nucleus pulposus, and spinal stenosis. In osteomyelitis, MRI is complementary to nuclear medicine scans, but its superior spatial resolution permits depiction of the full extent of marrow infection or edema. MRI also may be effective with contrast enhancement in determining the degree of synovial proliferation accompanying arthritides.

Ultrasound in the musculoskeletal system has a somewhat limited role. It is useful for evaluating superficial soft tissue structures. It is largely operator-dependent but, in experienced hands, can be effective in identifying and characterizing joint effusions and abnormalities of tendons, ligaments, and muscle.

2. Does nuclear medicine have a role in musculoskeletal imaging?

Bone scanning is routinely performed with ^{99m}Tc-labeled diphosphonates, which are adsorbed onto the surface of bone proportional to the local osteoblastic activity and skeletal vascularity. Bone scans are therefore sensitive in detecting bone abnormalities but somewhat nonspecific, as tumor, trauma, infection, or other pathology can all cause increased tracer uptake. Bone scanning is the screening examination of choice for evaluating bony metastatic disease, as it images the entire skeleton. Bone scanning will commonly detect metastatic disease or osteomyelitis while plain radiographs are still normal, since up to 50% of bone must be decalcified for plain film detection of tumor or infection versus 1% for bone scanning. Bone scanning can also detect stress fractures earlier than plain radiographs and may detect avascular necrosis or bone infarcts not seen by MRI.

In arthritis, there is increased concentration of radionuclide in the bone adjacent to affected joints. This increased tracer uptake may be due to synovitis with increased vascularity, or the periarticular uptake may be due to direct bone involvement. Although the various forms of arthritis cannot be distinguished except by distribution of uptake, the bone scan is helpful in diagnosis and in documenting extent of disease. Other common indications for bone scanning are in the evaluation of Paget's disease or metabolic bone disease.

3. What are the relative costs of the radiographic procedures used in musculoskeletal imaging of a specific joint (e.g., the shoulder)?

Plain radiograph	$100	Bone scan	470
Ultrasound	190	CT scan	590
Arthrography	320	MRI scan	800

4. Is there a pattern approach to interpreting a radiograph for arthritis?
In assessing a skeletal radiograph, a pattern approach using **ABCDES** can be very helpful:

A —Alignment. Rheumatoid arthritis (RA) and systemic lupus erythematosus (SLE) are characterized by deformities such as ulnar deviation at metacarpophalangeal joints.
— Ankylosis. Seronegative spondyloarthropathies frequently cause ankylosis.
B —Bone mineralization. Periarticular osteoporosis is typical of RA or infection, and is rare in crystal diseases, seronegative spondyloarthropathies, and degenerative joint disease.
— Bone formation. Reactive bone formation (Periostitis) is the hallmark of seronegative spondyloarthropathies. Osetophytosis is seen in degenerative joint disease and calcium pyrophosphate disease and can be present in any end-stage arthritis.
C —Calcifications. Soft tissue calcifications may be seen in gouty tophi, SLE, or scleroderma. Cartilage calcification is typical of calcium pyrophosphate disease.
— Cartilage space. Symmetric and uniform cartilage or joint-space narrowing is typical of inflammatory disease. Focal or nonuniform joint-space loss in the area of maximal stress in weight-bearing joints is the hallmark of osteoarthritis.
D —Distribution of joints. For example, RA usually has symmetric distribution of affected joints, whereas seronegative spondyloarthropathies are asymmetric. Also, target sites of involvement may permit differentiation of arthritides.
— Deformities. Swan neck or boutonniere deformities of the hands are typical of RA.
E —Erosions. In addition to their presence or absence, the character of erosions may be diagnostic, such as overhanging edges and sclerotic margins in gout.
S —Soft tissue and nails. Look for distribution of soft tissue swelling, nail hypertrophy in psoriasis, and sclerodactyly in scleroderma.
— Speed of development of changes. Septic arthritis will rapidly destroy the affected joint.

Pearl: When obtaining radiographs on patients with arthritis, always order weight-bearing radiographs to evaluate joint-space narrowing in lower extremity joints (i.e., hip, knee, ankles).

5. Describe the radiographic features of an inflammatory arthritis.
1. Soft tissue swelling
2. Periarticular osteoporosis
3. Uniform loss of cartilage (i.e., diffuse joint-space narrowing)
4. Bony erosion in "bare" areas

Synovial inflammation causes soft tissue swelling. The inflammation also results in hyperemia which, coupled with the inflammatory mediators released (such as prostaglandin E_2), causes periarticular (juxta-articular) osteoporosis. With chronicity, inflammatory arthritis may lead to more diffuse osteoporosis due to disuse (and other factors) of the joints due to pain. As the inflammation leads to synovial hypertrophy and pannus formation, the pannus erodes into the bone. These erosions occur first in the marginal "bare areas" where synovium abuts bone that does not possess protective cartilage (see figure). The pannus ultimately extends over the cartilaginous surface and/or erodes through the bone to the undersurface of the cartilage. Cartilage destruction results either by enzymatic action of the inflamed synovium and/or by interference with normal cartilage nutrition. Due to its generalized nature, this cartilage destruction is radiographically seen as uniform or symmetric, diffuse joint-space narrowing observed best in weight-bearing joints.

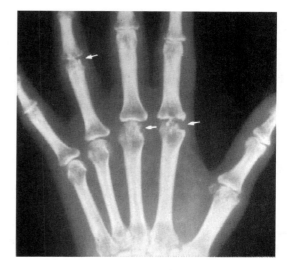

Radiograph of hand showing periarticular osteoporosis and bony erosions (*arrows*) compatible with an inflammatory arthritis. Patient had rheumatoid arthritis.

6. What is the "bare area"? Why do the earliest erosions begin here?

In synovial articulations, hyaline articular cartilage covers the ends of both bones. The articular capsule envelopes the joint cavity and is composed of an outer fibrous capsule and a thin inner synovial membrane. The synovial membrane typically does not extend over cartilaginous surfaces but lines the nonarticular portion of the synovial joint and also covers the intracapsular bone surfaces which are not covered by cartilage. These unprotected bony areas occur at the peripheral aspect of the joint and are referred to as "bare areas" (see figure).

In these areas, the bone does not have a protective cartilage covering. Consequently, the in-

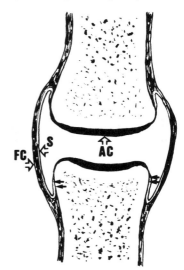

Diagram of typical synovial joint. Small black *arrows* point to "bare areas" where bone is exposed to synovium without protective cartilage covering. AC, articular cartilage; S, synovium; FC, fibrous capsule.

flamed synovial pannus, which occurs in inflammatory arthritides such as rheumatoid arthritis, comes in direct contact with bone, resulting in marginal erosions. These "bare areas" are where you should look for the earliest evidence of erosions. With progression of disease, the pannus proliferates to cover the cartilage surfaces, resulting in cartilage destruction (joint-space narrowing) and more diffuse bony erosions.

7. List the rheumatic disease categories which typically cause radiographic features of an inflammatory arthritis.
- Rheumatoid arthritis (adult and juvenile)
- Connective tissue diseases (SLE)
- Seronegative spondyloarthropathies
- Septic arthritis

8. Describe the radiographic features of noninflammatory, degenerative arthritis.
1. Sclerosis/osteophytes
2. Nonuniform loss of cartilage (focal joint-space narrowing in area of maximal stress in weight-bearing joints)
3. Cysts/geodes

The causes of degenerative arthritis are multifactorial. However, the primary problem and end result is cartilage degeneration. As the cartilage degenerates, the joint space narrows. However, in contrast to uniform, diffuse narrowing seen with inflammatory arthritides, the noninflammatory, degenerative arthritides tend to have nonuniform, focal joint-space narrowing, being most pronounced in the area of the joint where stresses are more concentrated (e.g., superolateral aspect of hip, medial compartment of the knee) (see figure).

Following cartilage loss, subchondral bone becomes sclerotic or eburnated, due to trabecular compression and reactive bone deposition. With denudation of cartilage, synovial fluid can be forced into underlying bone, forming subchondral cysts or geodes with sclerotic margins. As an attempted reparative process, the remaining cartilage undergoes endochondral ossification to develop osteophytes. Such osteophytes commonly occur first at margins or nonstressed aspects of the joint (e.g., medial and lateral aspects of the distal femur and proximal tibia of the knee). Teleologically, osteophytes are felt to be the way the body attempts to restrict motion of a degenerating joint and a way to further spread forces across a joint.

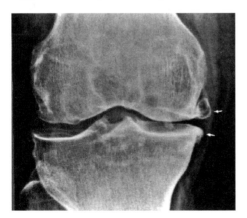

Knee radiograph demonstrating osteophytes (*arrows*) and medial joint-space narrowing consistent with degenerative arthritis.

9. List the rheumatic disease categories that typically cause radiographic features of a noninflammatory arthritis.
- Degenerative joint disease (e.g., primary ortheoarthritis and secondary causes of ortheoarthritis, such as traumatic arthritis, congenital bone diseases, others)
- Metabolic or endocrine disease (e.g., diseases associated with calcium pyrophosphate deposition, ochronosis, acromegaly)
- Miscellaneous (e.g., hemophilia, avascular necrosis)

10. What are the typical sites of joint involvement in primary (idiopathic) osteoarthritis compared to secondary causes of noninflammatory, degenerative arthritis?

Primary (idiopathic) osteoarthritis can cause noninflammatory, degenerative arthritic changes in the following joints:

Hands
  Distal interphalangeal joints (DIPs)
  Proximal interphalangeal joints (PIPs)
  First carpometacarpal joint (CMC) of thumb
Acromioclavicular joint of shoulder
Cervical, thoracic, and lumbosacral spine
Hips
Knees
Feet
  First metatarsophalangeal joints (MTP)

Secondary causes of degenerative arthritis can result in noninflammatory, degenerative changes in any joint (not just those for primary disease). Consequently, if a patient has degenerative changes in any of the following joints, you must consider secondary causes of orteoarthritis:

* Hands
   MCPs (see figure)
* Wrist (see figure)
* Elbow
* Glenohumeral joint of shoulder
* Ankle
* Feet, other than first MTP

If the degenerative changes involve only one joint, consider traumatic arthritis. If multiple joints are involved, consider a metabolic or endocrine disorder which has caused the cartilage to degenerate in several joints. Note that the end stage of an underlying inflammatory arthritis which has destroyed the cartilage can result in degenerative changes superimposed on the inflammatory radiographic features.

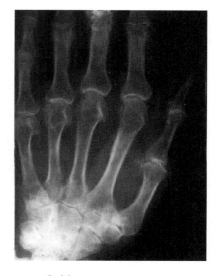

Hand radiograph with degenerative arthritis of MCPs and wrist. Patient had hemochromatosis.

11. Describe the radiographic features of chronic gouty arthritis.
* Erosions with sclerotic margins and an overhanging edge (see figure next page). These are caused by tophaceous deposits in the synovium slowly expanding into bone. The bone reacts and forms a sclerotic margin around the erosion.

- Relative preservation of joint space until late in disease
- Relative lack of periarticular osteoporosis for the degree of erosion seen
- Nodules in soft tissue (i.e., tophi). Unlike rheumatoid nodules, tophi can become calcified.

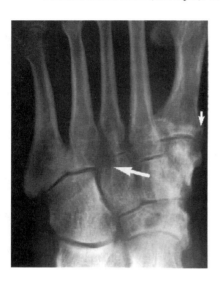

Radiograph of foot showing gouty erosions (*arrows*). One erosion demonstrates the characteristic overhanging edge (*small arrow*).

12. What other diseases can give radiographic features similar to those of chronic gouty arthritis?
Mycobacterium tuberculosis and some fungal infections
Pigmented villonodular synovitis
Amyloidosis
Multicentric reticulohistiocytosis
Synovial osteochondromatosis

13. Compare the radiographic features of inflammatory and noninflammatory spinal arthritis.
Inflammatory spinal arthritis is typically related to either infection or a seronegative spondyloarthropathy. Hematogenous spread of infection usually results in **osteomyelitis** originating near the endplate regions with subsequent spread to the intervertebral disc. The typical radiographic appearance of osteomyelitis is disc-space narrowing with poorly defined cortical endplates and destruction of the adjacent vertebrae (see figure). Although this appearance is very suggestive of infection, other inflammatory arthropathies, such as RA, seronegative spondyloarthropathies, and calcium pyrophosphate deposition disease can *rarely* give a similar appearance.

Ankylosing spondylitis (AS) is associated with squared anterior vertebral bodies with sclerotic anterior corners, syndesmophytes (ossification of the annulus fibrosus), discovertebral erosions, and vertebral and apophyseal fusion (see figure). Psoriasis or Reiter's syndrome may cause spinal changes similar to AS; however, more typical is the presence of paravertebral ossifications or large, nonmarginal syndesmophytes near the thoracolumbar junction. Radiographic sacroiliitis will also be present in spondyloarthropathy patients who have inflammatory spinal disease (see Chapters 38–41).

Noninflammatory lumbar arthritis is characterized by disc-space narrowing and vacuum phenomenon, osteophytosis, and bony sclerosis in the absence of sacroiliitis (see figure). Degenerative diseases of the vertebral column can affect cartilaginous joints (discovertebral junction),

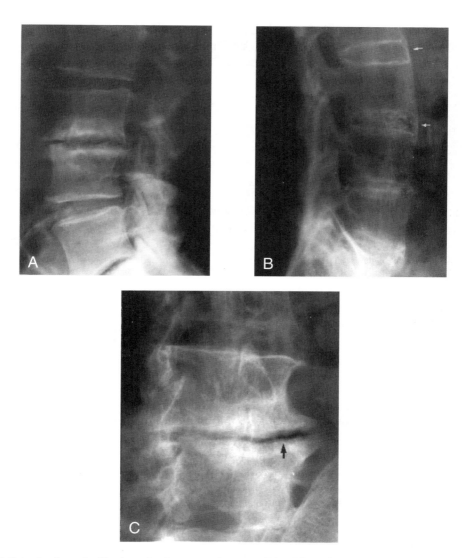

A, Lateral radiograph of lumbar spine demonstrated osteomyelitis at L3–4 with erosive/destructive changes of the adjoining cortical endplates. *B,* Lateral radiograph of lumbar spine demonstrating ankylosing spondylitis with anterior squaring of vertebrae and syndesmophytes (*arrows*). *C,* Oblique radiograph of lumbar spine showing degenerative disc disease, vacuum sign (*arrow*), and osteophytes.

synovial joints such as apophyses, or ligaments (enthesopathy). Typically, dehydration of the disc results in cartilage fissuring, with subsequent diminution in height and vacuum phenomenon (gas within the disc) and ultimately, bony sclerosis (intervertebral osteochondrosis). Osteophytosis (spondylosis deformans) is generally felt to be initiated by annulus fibrosus disruption. Ligamentous degeneration also occurs; ligamentum flavum hypertrophy may contribute to spinal stenosis, while ossification of the anterior longitudinal ligament is characteristic of diffuse idiopathic skeletal hyperostosis (DISH) (see Chapter 55).

Radiographic Features of Inflammatory versus Noninflammatory Spinal Arthritis

	INFLAMMATORY		NONINFLAMMATORY
	INFECTION	SPONDYLOARTHROPATHY	
Sacroiliac joints	Normal	Erosions	Normal
Vertebral bodies	Irregular, eroded endplates	Squaring ± erosions	Sclerosis
Disc space	Narrowed	May be destroyed or convex	Narrowed, vacuum
	One site	Multiple sites	
Syndesmophytes	–	+	–
Osteophytes	–	–	+
Osteoporosis	+	+	–
Soft tissue mass	+	–	–

14. What is the difference between an osteophyte and a syndesmophyte?

FEATURE	*OSTEOPHYTE*	*SYNDESMOPHYTE*
Disorder	Osteoarthritis	Spondyloarthropathy*
Vertebral involvement	Lower cervical	Lower thoracic
	Lumbar	Upper lumbar
		Cervical
Vertebral orientation	Horizontal	Vertical
Pathogenesis	Endochondral ossification	Outer annulus fibrosus
	"Bony spurs"	calcification
		"Vertebral bridging"
Complications	Radiculopathy	Ankylosis
	Vertebrobasilar ischemia	"Bamboo spine"
		Fracture

*Includes Ankylosing spondylitis, psoriatic arthritis, Reiter's syndrome, inflammatory bowel disease arthritis.

15. What rheumatic disease categories typically have unique radiographic features and are difficult to categorize using the inflammatory, noninflammatory, or gout-like patterns of radiographic changes?

     Collagen vascular disease (e.g., scleroderma, SLE)

     Endocrine arthropathies (e.g., hyperparathyroidism, acromegaly, hyperthyroidism)

     Miscellaneous (sickle cell disease, hemophilia, Paget's disease, avascular necrosis, Charcot joints, sarcoidosis, hypertrophic osteoarthropathy)

     Tumors (e.g., synovial osteochondromatosis)

16. List the most common diseases associated with the following radiographic changes seen in the hands.

     Extensive arthritis of multiple DIP joints

         Primary osteoarthritis

         Psoriatic arthritis

         Multicentric reticulohistiocytosis (MRH)

     First CMC joint arthritis

         Primary osteoarthritis

     Second and third MCP joint arthritis

         Hemochromatosis and acromegaly if degenerative arthritis with hook-like osteophytes

         Rheumatoid arthritis or psoriatic arthritis if erosive changes

     Arthritis mutilans of the hands (or feet)

         Psoriatic arthritis

         Rheumatoid arthritis

         Chronic gouty arthritis

         Other less common diseaes (MRH)

17. Outline the approach to the radiographic diagnosis of a patient with peripheral arthritis.

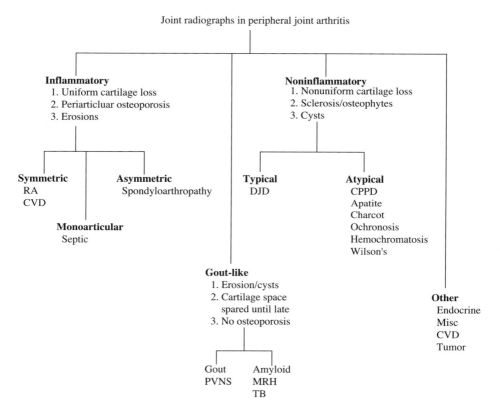

Joint radiographs in peripheral joint arthritis

Inflammatory
1. Uniform cartilage loss
2. Periarticluar osteoporosis
3. Erosions

Noninflammatory
1. Nonuniform cartilage loss
2. Sclerosis/osteophytes
3. Cysts

Symmetric
RA
CVD

Asymmetric
Spondyloarthropathy

Typical
DJD

Atypical
CPPD
Apatite
Charcot
Ochronosis
Hemochromatosis
Wilson's

Monoarticular
Septic

Gout-like
1. Erosion/cysts
2. Cartilage space spared until late
3. No osteoporosis

Other
Endocrine
Misc
CVD
Tumor

Gout   Amyloid
PVNS   MRH
          TB

CVD, collagen vascular disease; DJD, degenerative joint disease; CPPD, calcium pyrophosphate deposition disease; PVNS, pigmented villonodular synovitis; MRH, multicentric reticulohistiocytosis; TB, tuberculosis.

18. List the most common diseases associated with the following radiographic changes seen in the upper extremity and shoulder.
   Radioulnar joint arthritis
      Rheumatoid arthritis
      Juvenile rheumatoid arthritis
      Calcium pyrophosphate deposition disease (CPPD)
   Swan neck and/or ulnar deviation deformities
      Rheumatoid arthritis if erosive changes and nonreversible deformities
      SLE if nonerosive and reversible deformities
   Elbow nodules in soft tissue
      Rheumatoid arthritis
      Tophaceous gout (particularly if contains calcium deposits)
      Scleroderma-associated calcium deposits
   "Pencilling" of clavicle distal end
      Rheumatoid arthritis
      Hyperparathyroidism

19. Outline an approach to the radiographic diagnosis of a patient with arthritis of the back.

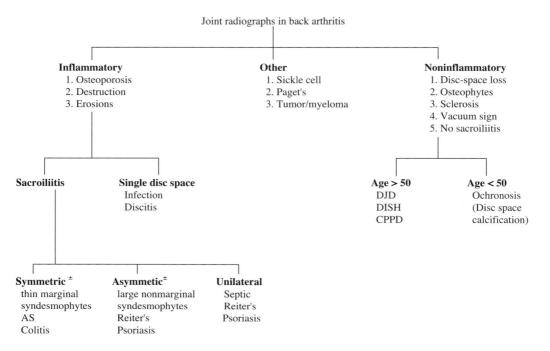

AS, ankylosing spondylitis; DISH, diffuse idiopathic skeletal hyperostosis.

20. List the most common diseases associated with the following radiographic changes seen in the feet.

Destructive arthritis of great-toe interphalangeal joint
Reiter's syndrome
Psoriatic arthritis
Gout and rheumatoid arthritis, less commonly

Destructive arthritis at great-toe MTP joint
Rheumatoid arthritis
Chronic gouty arthritis
Reiter's and psoriatic arthritis, less commonly
Primary osteoarthritis if noninflammatory degenerative changes

MTP joint erosive arthritis
Reiter's or psoriatic if asymmetric distribution
Rheumatoid arthritis if symmetric distribution

Calcaneal spurs
Traction spurs (noninflammatory)
Seronegative spondyloarthropathies (inflammatory spurs)

21. In the spine?
Vacuum disc sign
Degenerative disc disease (essentially this sign excludes infection at this disc level)

Disc space calcification at multiple levels
Ochronosis if patient young (<30 yrs)
CPPD and others
Sacroiliitis
Ankylosing spondylitis (usually symmetric sacroiliitis)
Enteropathic arthritis (usually symmetric sacroiliitis)
Reiter's syndrome (frequently asymmetric sacroiliitis)
Psoriatic arthritis (frequently asymmetric sacroiliitis)
Infection (unilateral sacroiliitis)
Syndesmophytes
Ankylosing spondylitis and enteropathic arthritis (thin, marginal bilateral syndesmophytes)
Reiter's syndrome and psoriatic arthritis (large, nonmarginal, asymmetric syndesmophytes)
[Don't get fooled by DISH with its calcification of the anterior longitudinal ligament (sacroiliac joints will be normal).]

22. **And other places (or everywhere)?**
Chondrocalcinosis
Idiopathic CPPD
Hyperparathyroidism
Hemochromatosis
Others, but they are rare diseases
Erosions (hallmark of inflammatory synovial-based arthritis)
Rheumatoid arthritis or juvenile rheumatoid arthritis
Seronegative spondyloarthropathies
Chronic gouty arthritis
Septic (infectious) arthritis
Others (SLE rarely, mixed connective tissue disease, multicentric reticulohistiocytosis, pigmented villonodular synovitis)
Isolated patellofemoral degenerative arthritis
CPPD

23. **Give the characteristic radiographic features of the different arthritides.**
Rheumatoid arthritis—**Symmetric, erosive** arthritis, uniform joint-space narrowing. Most common sites are small joints of hands and feet (MCPs, PIPs, wrists, MTPs) and cervical spine. Soft tissue nodules that do not calcify. Swan-neck deformities and ulnar deviation.
Juvenile chronic arthritis—Osteoporosis, but joint-space narrowing and erosions typically absent until late. Periosteal reaction and **bony fusion** (carpus, facets in cervical spine) may distinguish it from RA. Whenever it looks as if someone has fused the wrist with a blow-torch, think juvenile rheumatoid arthritis.
Ankylosing spondylitis—bilateral, symmetric sacroiliitis with ankylosis. **Bilateral, thin, marginal** syndesmophytes in the spine may cause spinal fusion (bamboo spine). Peripheral arthropathy affects axial joints (shoulders, hips).
Reiter's syndrome—Can be bilateral or **unilateral, asymmetric sacroiliitis.** Peripherally, there is a predilection for **lower extremities** (especially the interphalangeal joint of great toe), with erosions and fluffy periostitis. Enthesopathy with erosions and calcifications at tendon insertions into calcaneus. Frequently, asymmetric joint involvement. Large, asymmetric, nonmarginal (jug-handle) syndesmophytes.
Psoriatic arthritis—Axial arthropathy similar to Reiter's. Peripherally, it has an **upper extremity predilection; DIP or PIP fusion. "Pencil-in-cup" deformity.** Enthesopathy and periostitis. **Erosions of several joints of a single digit** (MCP, PIP, and DIP of one finger). Frequently, asymmetric joint involvement. Acro-osteolysis. Jug-handle syndesmophytes.

Gout—**Erosions with overhanging edge and sclerotic margins.** Preserved joint space. Soft tissue tophi which can contain calcium.

Calcium pyrophosphate dihydrate deposition (CPPD)—Osteoarthritic changes at sites **atypical for degenerative joint disease (DJD)** (MCPs, elbow, radiocarpal, ankle, shoulder). **Chondrocalcinosis.** Uniform joint-space narrowing despite being a cause of degenerative arthritis. **Isolated patellofemoral DJD.**

Degenerative joint disease (primary osteoarthritis)—Nonuniform joint-space narrowing, sclerosis, **osteophytosis,** cysts. Most common sites include the DIPs, PIPs, first CMC, knees, hips, and spine.

Neuropathic joint (Charcot)—Destruction, disorganization, density (i.e., sclerosis), debris, dislocation (**the 5 Ds**).

Systemic lupus erythematosus (SLE)—**Reversible swan neck and ulnar deviation deformity and subluxation,** but absence of erosions.

Scleroderma—Tapered, atrophic soft tissues (**sclerodactyly**) with soft tissue calcifications. Acro-osteolysis of terminal phalanges.

Hemochromatosis—Chondrocalcinosis. **Degenerative changes at MCPs** (especially second and third) with "hook-like" spurs. Cystic changes of radiocarpal joint of wrist.

Ochronosis—**Vertebral disc calcification,** chondrocalcinosis, osteoarthritis in multiple joints (especially spine) at young age.

Acromegaly—**widened joint and disc spaces.** Large spurs at bases of distal phalanges (**spade phalanges**).

Hyperparathyroidism—**subperiosteal resorption** at radial side of middle phalanges. Soft tissue calcifications, chondrocalcinosis, **"salt and pepper" skull,** ligament and tendon ruptures.

Avascular necrosis—**crescent sign, stepoff sign.** Hips and shoulders are most commonly affected.

24. What is the difference between T1- and T2-weighted images on MRI?

T1- or T2-weighting typically refers to the spin echo MR sequence. TR is the repetition time, or time between 90° radiofrequency pulses, whereas TE is the echo time, or time between the 90° pulse and the time the signal is received. **T1-weighted images** are short TR (300–1000 ms) and short TE (10–30 ms) and provide excellent anatomic detail. In contrast, **T2-weighted images** are long TR (1800–2500 ms) and long TE (40–90 ms), sensitive for detecting edema. The TR and TE numbers are printed in the corner of the MRI film so that you can tell if the image is T1- or T2-weighted.

Two other sequences commonly used are gradient echo and STIR (short tau inversion recovery). **Gradient echo** sequences can be either T1- or T2-weighted and permit very rapid acquisition with thin-section, high-quality images. **STIR** is effectively a fat-suppression technique, very sensitive in detection of fluid or edema. These images greatly aid in detection of marrow and soft tissue disease, and we routinely rely on these sequences for detecting pathology such as muscle tears, osteomyelitis, bone marrow edema, or tumor involvement.

25. Describe the appearances of the various tissues on T1- and T2-weighted MR images.

STRUCTURE	T1 INTENSITY	T2 INTENSITY
Fat, fatty marrow	High	Lower
Hyaline cartilage	Intermediate	Intermediate
Muscle	Intermediate	Intermediate
Fluid, edema	Low	High
Neoplasm	Low	High
Cortical bone	Very low	Very low
Tendon, ligaments	Very low	Very low

High appears white on MRI; low appears black on MRI.

26. In which clinical situations is CT scan superior to MRI and vice versa?
Plain radiographs should be obtained before a CT scan or MRI when evaluating muscu-
loskeletal disorders. If the plain radiographs do not delineate the abnormality, then CT scan and
MRI may add further information.

CT scan is superior to MRI in:

Acute trauma (fracture and dislocations)	Sacroiliac joint erosions
Tarsal coalition	Intra-articular osteocartilaginous loose bodies
Sternoclavicular joint arthritis	

MRI scan is superior to CT scan in:

Cervical spine disease or instability	Osteomyelitis
Spinal stenosis	Soft tissue tumors
Internal derangement of knee	Pigmented villonodular synovitis (PVNS)
Rotator cuff tears and tendinitis	Inflammatory sacroiliitis
Avascular necrosis	Synovitis and tenosynovitis (rarely needed)

MRI is complementary to CT scan and bone scintigraphy when evaluating bone tumors.

27. What imaging features are typically seen in infections of bones or joint spaces?
In acute osteomyelitis, the earliest radiographic abnormality is **soft tissue swelling** with obliteration of normal tissue planes. Hyperemia results in osteoporosis, and bone destruction or periostitis may not be visualized for 7–14 days. Thus, nuclear medicine scanning or MRI are much more
sensitive for detection of early osteomyelitis. MRI is particularly helpful in defining the full extent of osteomyelitis, particularly when amputation is a therapeutic option (see figure). Subacute
osteomyelitis is frequently referred to as a Brodie's abscess, usually in the metaphysis of tubular
bones. A well-marginated **lucent defect** (commonly elongated) is seen surrounded by a thick
band of sclerosis. With chronic osteomyelitis, radiodense spicules of necrotic bone, referred to as
sequestra, may be seen within the lucent defect.

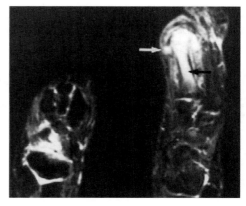

STIR MR image depicts the high-signal edema
(*black arrow*) corresponding to osteomyelitis involving the entirety of the first metatarsal. Focus
of high signal in the adjacent soft tissues represents an abscess (*white arrow*).

BIBLIOGRAPHY

1. Battafarano DF, West SG, et al: Comparison of bone scan, computed tomography and magnetic resonance imaging in the diagnosis of sacroiliitis. Semin Arthritis Rheum 23:161–176, 1993.
2. Bloem JL, Sartoris DJ (eds): MRI and CT of the Musculoskeletal System. Baltimore, Williams &
   Wilkins, 1992.
3. Early PJ, Sodee DB: Principles and Practice of Nuclear Medicine. St. Louis, Mosby, 1994.
4. Rafii M (ed): The Shoulder. Magn Reson Imag Clin North Am 1(1): 1993.
5. Resnick D: Bone and Joint Imaging. Philadelphia, W.B. Saunders, 1989.
6. Schumacher HR (ed): Primer on Rheumatic Disorders, 10th ed. Atlanta, Arthritis Foundation, 1993.
7. Stark DD, Bradley WG: Magnetic Resonance Imaging. Chicago, Mosby–Yearbook, 1992.
8. Weissman BN (ed): Imaging of rheumatic diseases. Rheum Dis Clin North Am 17(3):1991.
9. Weissman BN (ed): Syllabus: A Categorical Course in Musculoskeletal Radiology. Chicago, Radiolog-
   ical Society of North America, 1993.

12. SYNOVIAL BIOPSIES

Sterling West, M.D.

1. What are the indications to do a synovial biopsy?

The main indication for synovial biopsy is a chronic (> 6–8 weeks), nontraumatic, inflammatory (synovial fluid WBC count > 2000 cells/mm^3) arthritis limited to one or two joints in which the diagnosis has not been made by history, physical examination, laboratory studies, or synovial fluid analysis with culture (including for fungi and mycobacteria).

2. What diseases can be diagnosed with a synovial biopsy?

- Chronic infections
  Fungal arthritis
  Mycobacterial arthritis
  Spirochetal arthritis (Lyme disease, syphilis)
  Whipple's disease
- Chronic sarcoidosis
- Infiltrative/deposition diseases*
  Amyloidosis
  Ochronosis
  Hemochromatosis
  Crystal-induced arthritis

- Tumors
  Pigmented villonodular synovitis
  Synovial osteochondromatosis
  Synovial cell sarcoma
  Leukemia/lymphoma
  Metastatic disease to the joint
- Others
  Multicentric reticulohistiocytosis
  Plant thorn and other foreign-body
    synovitis

*Synovial biopsy is usually not necessary in these diseases.

3. Does a synovial biopsy help in the diagnosis of a systemic connective tissue disease such as rheumatoid arthritis?

No. Although biopsy of the synovium in a patient with rheumatoid arthritis may be compatible with the diagnosis, it is not pathognomonic. Clearly, spondyloarthropathy can produce synovial biopsies that look very much like those obtained from rheumatoid arthritis patients.

4. How can synovial tissue be obtained?

METHOD	SIZE OF HOLE
Closed-needle biopsy	14-gauge needle
(Parker-Pearson or other needle)	(1.6 mm)
Needle arthroscopy	1.8 mm
Arthroscopy	4–5 mm
Open surgical biopsy	Several inches

5. List the advantages and disadvantages of the different methods of synovial biopsy.

Comparison of Synovial Biopsy Techniques

	ADVANTAGES	DISADVANTAGES
Needle biopsy	Least expensive Least traumatic One skin incision	Small biopsy specimens
Needle arthroscopic biopsy	Minimally invasive Direct visualization	Two skin incisions Moderately expensive
Arthroscopic biopsy	Direct visualization Large biopsy specimen	Expensive Invasive

Open surgical biopsy	Direct visualization
	Large biopsy specimen
	Best if suspected tumor
	  or foreign body
	Can be done on any joint
		Expensive
		Most invasive
		Longest postop
		  recovery time

6. Which joints can be biopsied with a closed-biopsy needle?
Usually large joints, most commonly the knee.

7. How many specimens must be obtained by a closed-biopsy needle to minimize sampling error?
Five to eight specimens from the joint being biopsied.

8. Who invented arthroscopy?

1918	Japanese physician, Dr. Takagi, performs first knee arthroscopy with a cystoscope.
1930s	German rheumatologist, Dr. Vaupel, proposes use of arthroscopy to follow the course of arthritis.
1957	Dr. M. Watanabe performs first partial meniscectomy through arthroscope.
1969	Dr. N. Matsui performs first arthroscopic synovectomy.

BIBLIOGRAPHY

1. Arnold W: Arthroscopy in the diagnosis and therapy of arthritis. Hosp Pract 27:43–53, 1992.
2. Gibson T, Fagg N, Highton J, et al: The diagnostic value of synovial biopsy in patients with arthritis of unknown cause. Br J Rheumatol 24:232–241, 1985.
3. Schumacher HR: Needle biopsy of the synovial membrane: Experience with the Parker-Pearson technique. N Engl J Med 286:416–419, 1972.
4. Schumacher HR: Synovial fluid analysis and synovial biopsy. In Kelley WK, Harris ED, Ruddy S, Sledge CB (eds): Textbook of Rheumatology, 4th ed. Philadelphia, W.B. Saunders Co., 1993; pp 570–576.

13. ELECTROMYOGRAPHY AND NERVE CONDUCTION STUDIES

Douglas E. Hemler, M.D.

1. What is an EMG?
EMG, or **electromyography,** is a specific type of analysis performed on the neural control mechanism of muscle (the motor unit), in which the resting and voluntary muscle activity are recorded electrically. It is also a global term applied to the entire spectrum of tests performed in electrodiagnostic medicine.

2. What is the motor unit?
The anatomic unit of function for the motor portion of the peripheral nervous system. It includes the **motor neuron** found within the anterior horn of the spinal cord, its **axon,** the **neuromuscular junction,** and the **muscle fibers** supplied by the peripheral nerve. The electrodiagnostic physician can utilize a combination of EMG, nerve conduction studies (NCS), repetitive stimulation, and other electrophysiologic tests to assess individual components of the motor unit.

3. What is an innervation ratio?
For each efferent motor axon, there is a variable number of terminal axons and muscle fibers. Depending on the specific requirement of control, the ratio may be quite low or extremely high. The innervation ratio of the extraocular muscles is typically 1:3, due to the fine control required for binocular vision. Conversely, the innervation ratio of the gastrocnemius can be as high as 1:2000, since most movements involving the plantar flexors of the ankle are relatively large motions requiring more force than accuracy.

4. Name some other types of electrodiagnostic tests.

- **Nerve conduction studies** (NCS), sometimes called nerve conduction velocities (NCVs), are used to assess the amplitude and velocity of signals carried within the peripheral nerve.
- **Repetitive stimulation studies** are utilized for the evaluation of the neuromuscular junction (i.e., myasthenia gravis).
- **Somatosensory evoked potentials** are used to evaluate conduction within the spinal cord and brain.
- Other less frequently used tests include single-fiber EMG, motor-evoked potentials, and nerve root stimulation.

5. What are the clinical indications for ordering an EMG? An NCS?

An EMG is ordered to determine the localization and severity of neuropathic disorders and/or to document myopathic disorders. NCSs are ordered to localize anatomic abnormalities of the peripheral motor and sensory nervous systems and to assess the severity of axonal or demyelinating pathology.

6. Describe the components of a normal EMG.

Resting muscle: Normal **insertional activity** is the brief discharge of single muscle fibers during insertion of the EMG needle. This does not indicate an abnormality unless it is increased in amount. There should be no **spontaneous activity** due to involuntary firing of single motor neurons (fibrillations, positive sharp waves) when the muscle is at rest.

Mild muscle contraction: The patient slightly contracts the muscle to generate isolated **motor unit action potentials** (MUAP). A normal MUAP waveform has a duration of 5–15 msec, 2–4 phases (usually 3), and an amplitude of 0.5–3 mV (depending on the muscle stimulated).

Maximal muscle contraction: The patient fully contracts the muscle. Normally, a sufficient number of motor units are recruited so that MUAPs overlap each other, resulting in obliteration of the resting baseline. This is called a normal or "full" **interference** or **recruitment pattern.**

7. What is an incremental response?

Both the sensory and motor components of the nervous system function in an all-or-none fashion. For example, when the anterior horn cell of a single motor unit is activated, the entire motor unit depolarizes. Gradients or values of sensory or motor response are assessed or controlled by the CNS by the progressive addition of incremental responses. For example, when one motor unit is firing, a muscle may have little or no assessable change in tone. As additional motor units discharge, muscle tone increases to the point of visible contraction with progressively more force. Recruitment is an important assessment tool for the electromyographer which takes both visible and auditory training and skills.

8. How do fasciculations, fibrillations, and positive sharp waves differ on EMG?

A **fasciculation** is an involuntary firing of a single motor neuron and all its innervated muscle fibers. This is seen as spontaneous activity at rest on EMG and is clinically visible in the patient as a brief irregular undulation of muscle. This is the hallmark of amyotrophic lateral sclerosis (Lou Gehrig's disease).

A **fibrillation** is an involuntary contraction of single motor units. It does not cause muscle movement but can be seen under the skin as with a fasciculation. Fibrillations indicate denervation and occur due to spontaneous firing of muscle fibers which have developed an increased number of acetylcholine receptors on their surfaces following denervation (Cannon's law). Any extraneous acetylcholine in the area causes the muscle fiber to contract, generating electrical activity that is seen as a spontaneous fibrillation on the resting muscle EMG.

Positive sharp waves are also seen with denervation and appear as downward waveforms on the resting muscle EMG in contrast to the upward waveforms seen with fibrillations.

9. How do normal EMG findings compare with the findings seen in a denervated muscle?

EMG	NORMAL	DENERVATED MUSCLE	REINNERVATED MUSCLE
Rest			
Insertional activity	Normal	Increased	Normal to increased
Spontaneous activity	None	Fibrillations, positive sharp wave	None
Mild contraction			
MUAP	Normal	Normal, limited recruitment	Large, polyphasic, limited recruitment
Maximal contraction			
Interference pattern	Full	Reduced	Reduced

Note that fibrillations and positive sharp waves are not seen in resting muscles until 7–14 days after the onset of axonal degeneration. Full reinnervation of the denervated musclel, resulting in large, polyphasic motor unit action potentials (MUAPs), may take 3–4 months.

10. Compare normal EMG findings with the findings seen in myopathic processes.

EMG	NORMAL	MYOPATHY	INFLAMMATORY MYOSITIS
Rest			
Insertional activity	Normal	Normal	Increased
Spontaneous activity	None	None	Fibrillations, positive sharp waves
Mild contraction			
MUAP	Normal	Small units, early recruitment	Small units, early recruitment
Maximal contraction			
Interference pattern	Full	Full, low amplitude	Full, low amplitude

Up to 30% of patients with a noninflammatory myopathy may have a normal EMG. Inflammatory myositis (i.e., polymyositis) causes both neuropathic and myopathic EMG abnormalities. The fibrillations and positive sharp waves seen on EMG are due to inflammation affecting the nerve endings in the muscle, causing features of denervation. The inflammation will also injure muscle fibers, causing a low-amplitude MUAP which is a feature of myopathic processes.

11. Is the amplitude of a normal sensory nerve action potential (SNAP) higher or lower than a normal MUAP?
The SNAP varies depending on the size and accessibility of distal nerves. It ranges from 10 to 100 μV, which is about 1/20th the size of a normal MUAP.

12. Is the normal nerve conduction velocity (NCV) the same throughout the length of the nerve?
NCVs vary among nerves and along their lengths. Normally, proximal nerve conduction is faster than distal nerve conduction. This is due to the increased temperature as the nerve travels toward the trunk which more closely approximates core temperature. Additionally, nerve fibers are larger in the proximal segments of the nerve. This difference in NCV is most readily noted in the difference between normal values for the upper and lower extremities: upper extremity, 45–75 m/sec, vs lower extremity, 38–55 m/sec.

13. Why is temperature recorded during the course of an electrodiagnostic examination?
NCVs change by 2.0–2.4 m/sec *per* °C reduction in both sensory and motor nerves. These changes can be significant, particularly in cooler climates. An astute question for a non-electromyographer to ask when results are borderline is, "What was the patient's temperature during the examination, or was the limb warmed before the NCV measurements were obtained?" Failure to warm the limb can result in false-positive studies, leading to a misdiagnosis of carpal tunnel syndrome or generalized sensory motor neuropathy.

14. What are the H-reflex and F-wave? How are they clinically useful?

The **H-reflex** is the electrical counterpart of the ankle jerk and gives information on the S1 afferent–efferent reflex arc. The H-reflex may be abnormal in neuropathies, S1 radiculopathies, or sciatic mononeuropathies.

The **F-wave** is a delayed motor potential following the normal MUAP and represents the antidromic response seen when a motor nerve is powerfully stimulated. An F-wave can be obtained on any peripheral motor nerve and gives information about the proximal part of the nerve, since stimulation travels proximally and returns down the nerve to contract the muscle.

15. How are sensory and motor portions of the peripheral nervous system tested?

Sensory and motor nerve conduction studies are the primary means to test the peripheral nerves. The amplitude of the waveform, its point of onset, and its peak are compared with standardized normal values and with those from the opposite extremity. The waves created are summations of incremental depolarization of individual axonal fibers. Late responses (F-waves and H-reflexes) provide assessment of the more proximal, anatomically difficult-to-reach portions of the peripheral nervous system. These tests are also utilized to assess nerve conduction over a long segment of nerve fiber. F-waves, in particular, are an important screening test in the diagnosis of Guillain-Barré syndrome. Other less common techniques for assessing the peripheral nerves include somatosensory evoked potentials, dermatomal somatosensory evoked potentials, and selected nerve root stimulation.

16. What disorders are characteristic of the peripheral nerve?

Functionally, the peripheral nerve starts in the vicinity of the neural foramen, where sensory and motor fibers join. At its most proximal level, peripheral nerve injury in the form of **radiculopathy** is caused by compression of the nerve root by a herniated disc or bony fragment. **Plexus involvement** by disease or injury may occur in the upper (brachial plexus) or lower extremity (lumbar or lumbosacral plexopathy).

Peripheral nerve conditions can be acquired or congenital. Congenital anomalies include the hereditary senory and motor neuropathies (e.g., Charcot-Marie-Tooth types I and II). Acquired conditions can include neuropathic disorders, such as diabetes, or those caused by toxins or metabolic insufficiencies.

Focal neural entrapment can be caused by carpal tunnel syndrome, ulnar neuropathy, or tarsal tunnel syndrome, to name just a few. It is very important for the electrodiagnostic physician to have taken a good history prior to commencing the examination.

17. Describe the three main types of nerve injury.

Nerves sustain a gradient of injury, which was originally defined by Seddon:

1. **Neurapraxia** is the functional loss of conduction without anatomic change of the axon. Demyelination may occur, however; with remyelination, NCV returns to normal.

2. In **axonotmesis,** the axonal continuity is lost. With its loss, wallerian degeneration occurs in the distal segment. Recovery, which is frequently not complete, occurs as a result of axonal regrowth at a rate of 1–3 mm/day.

3. **Neurotmesis** results from separation of the entire nerve, including its supporting connective tissue. Regeneration frequently does not occur. Nerves with this degree of trauma frequently need surgical attention for any recovery to occur.

18. Do the three types of nerve injuries ever occur together?

Neurapraxia and axonotmesis commonly occur as a result of the same injury. When compression is relieved from the involved segment of nerve, two periods of healing typically occur. One is relatively immediate, from hours to weeks, as the neurapraxia resolves. A second period of healing, from weeks to months, may occur as a result of axonal regrowth.

19. How can a demyelinating peripheral neuropathy and an axonal peripheral neuropathy be differentiated by EMG and NCS?

Demyelinating neuropathies show moderate to severe slowing of motor conduction, with temporal dispersion of the MUAP, normal distal amplitudes, reduced proximal amplitudes, and delayed distal latencies. **Axonal neuropathies** show a milder slowing in NCV, with generally low MUAP amplitudes at all sites of stimulation. The EMG shows denervation abnormalities early in axonal neuropathies and only later in demyelinating neuropathies, when axons begin to degenerate.

20. Which systemic diseases cause predominantly a demyelinating peripheral neuropathy? An axonal peripheral neuropathy?

Peripheral polyneuropathies due to systemic disease can be classified (1) as acute, subacute, or chronic in onset; (2) as affecting predominantly sensory or motor nerves; and (3) as causing an axonal or demyelinating injury. Note that over time, most axonal neuropathies will develop myelin degeneration subsequently.

Characteristic Polyneuropathies in Systemic Disease*

DISEASE	AXONAL		DEMYELINATING	
	ACUTE	SUBACUTE/CHRONIC	ACUTE	SUBACUTE/CHRONIC
Diabetes mellitus	–	S,SM	–	S,SM
Uremia	–	SM	–	–
Porphyria	M	–	–	–
Vitamin deficiency	–	SM	–	–
		S (B12 def.)		
Amyloidosis	–	SM	–	–
Carcinoma	–	S (breast),	–	–
		SM (lung)	–	–
Lymphoma	–	SM	–	SM
Myeloma	–	SM	–	SM
Cryoglobulinemia and vasculitis	SM	SM	–	–
Diphtheria toxin	–	–	SM	–

S = sensory, SM = sensorimotor, M = motor. In addition to these diseases, several drugs and environmental toxins can produce a polyneuropathy.

21. How is EMG/NCS used in diagnosing carpal tunnel syndrome? Ulnar nerve entrapment at the elbow?

Carpal tunnel syndrome (CTS) is the most common entrapment neuropathy, affecting 1% of the population. NCVs are abnormal in 90–95% of patients. Sensory nerve action potential latencies of the median nerve (palmar latency) are delayed twice as often as motor latencies, although with increasing severity, motor latencies will be affected. Needle EMG is of limited value and, when abnormal, shows denervation of the thenar muscles, which is a late finding indicating advanced CTS.

In **ulnar nerve entrapment** at the elbow, motor and sensory NCVs are abnormal in 60–80% of cases. An EMG is useful in demonstrating the degree of denervation in the muscles of the hand and forearm, which are innervated by the ulnar nerve.

22. What is a double crush syndrome?

A double crush syndrome may be present when carpal tunnel syndrome occurs in association with degenerative cervical spine disease. The initial peripheral nerve entrapment occurs at the cervical root level, causing a disruption in axoplasmic flow in both afferent and efferent directions. A second point of entrapment occurs more proximally, usually at the carpal tunnel, resulting in a second physiologic insult along the course of the axon. While electromyographers speak of the syndrome, it is very difficult to quantify and document as an actual clinical entity.

23. Which other entities can be differentiated by EMG/NCS from the common peripheral nerve syndromes?

PERIPHERAL NERVE SYNDROME	DIFFERENTIAL DIAGNOSIS
CTS	Pronator teres syndrome
	Other areas of median nerve entrapment
Ulnar entrapment at the elbow	C8 radiculopathy
	Brachial plexus lesion
Radial nerve palsy	C7 radiculopathy
Suprascapular nerve lesion	C5–6 radiculopathy
Peroneal nerve palsy	L4–5 radiculopathy
Femoral nerve lesion	L3 radiculopathy

24. How is EMG used in the diagnosis and prognosis of myasthenia gravis, myotonic dystrophy, and Bell's palsy?

Myasthenia gravis. Slow repetitive nerve stimulation of a motor nerve at 2–3 Hz will show a 10% or greater decremental motor response in 65–85% of patients. Single-fiber EMG, which measures the delay in transmission between terminal nerve fibers and their muscle fibers, is abnormal in 90–95% of patients.

Myotonic dystrophy. EMG shows MUAPs that vary in amplitude and frequency and are heard on the loud speaker as "dive bombers."

Bell's palsy. Facial NCS, done 5 days after the onset of palsy can indicate the prognosis for recovery. If NCV latencies and amplitudes are normal at this time, the prognosis for recovery is excellent.

BIBLIOGRAPHY

1. Ball RD: Electrodiagnostic evaluation of the peripheral nervous system. In DeLisa JA (ed): Rehabilitation Medicine: Principles and Practice, 2nd ed. Philadelphia, J.B. Lippincott, 1993, pp 269–307.
2. MacCaen IC (ed): Electromyography: A Guide for the Referring Physician. Phys Med Rehabil Clin North Am 1:1–160, 1990.
3. Dumitru D: Electrodiagnostic Medicine. Philadelphia, Hanley & Belfus, 1995.
4. Goodgold J, Eberstein A (eds): Electrodiagnosis of Neuromuscular Diseases, 3rd ed. Baltimore, Williams & Wilkins, 1983.
5. Johnson EW (ed): Practical Electromyography. Baltimore, Williams & Wilkins, 1980.
6. Kimura J (ed): Electrodiagnosis in Diseases of Nerve and Muscle: Principles and Practice, 2nd ed. Philadelphia, F.A. Davis, 1989.
7. Robinson LR (ed): New Developments in Electrodiagnostic Medicine. Phys Med Rehabil Clin North Am 5(3):1994.
8. Weichers DO, Johnson EW: Electrodiagnosis. In Kottke FJ, Lehmann JF (eds): Krusen's Handbook of Physical Medicine and Rehabilitation, 4th ed. Philadelphia, W.B. Saunders, 1990, pp 72–107.

14. APPROACH TO THE PATIENT WITH MONOARTICULAR SYMPTOMS

Robert A. Hawkins, M.D.

1. What conditions can be mistaken for a monoarticular process?

Several common inflammatory processes occur in the soft tissues *around,* but not in, the joints. These conditions can be painful and may mimic arthritis. Examples include rotator cuff tendinitis of the shoulder, olecranon bursitis of the elbow, and prepatellar bursitis of the knee. It is important to distinguish these disorders from true joint disease because their management is often quite different from that of monoarticular arthritis. Careful history and physical examination usually allows correct identification of the affected region. (*See also* Chapter 66.)

2. List the diseases that commonly present with monoarthritis.

Diseases Causing Monoarticular Symptoms

Septic	Traumatic
Bacterial	Fracture
Mycobacterial	Internal derangement
Lyme disease	Hemarthrosis
Crystal deposition diseases	Other
Gout	Osteoarthritis
Calcium pyrophosphate deposition (CPPD)	Juvenile rheumatoid arthritis
disease (pseudogout)	Coagulopathy
Hydroxyapatite deposition disease	Avascular necrosis of bone
Calcium oxalate deposition disease	Foreign-body synovitis
	Pigmented villonodular synovitis
	Synovioma

3. What polyarticular diseases occasionally present with a monoarticular onset?

Rheumatoid arthritis	Reiter's syndrome
Juvenile rheumatoid arthritis	Psoriatic arthritis
Viral arthritis	Enteropathic arthritis
Sarcoid arthritis	Whipple's disease

4. What is the most critical diagnosis to consider in the patient with monoarticular symptoms?

Joint infection, one of the few rheumatologic emergencies! The septic joint must be diagnosed quickly and managed aggressively. Bacterial infections, especially those due to gram-positive organisms, can destroy the joint cartilage within a few days. Prompt and proper treatment of the septic joint will usually leave it without permanent structural damage. Additionally, as the septic joint is usually the result of hematogenous spread of infection from another body site, early recognition of the joint process allows more timely diagnosis and treatment of the primary infection. When evaluating a patient with acute monoarticular arthritis, a good rule of thumb is to assume that the joint is infected until proven otherwise.

5. What nine questions should you ask when obtaining a history from a patient with monoarticular arthritis?

1. Did the pain come on suddenly, in seconds or minutes? (Consider fracture and internal derangement.)
2. Did the pain come on over several hours or 1–2 days? (Consider infection, crystal deposition diseases, inflammatory arthritis syndromes, and palindromic rheumatism.)
3. Did the pain come on insidiously over days to weeks? (Consider indolent infections, such as mycobacteria and fungi, osteoarthritis, tumor, and infiltrative diseases.)
4. Has the joint been overused or damaged, either recently or in the past? (Consider traumatic causes.)
5. Is there a history of intravenous drug abuse? Has the patient had a recent infection of any kind? (Consider infection.)
6. Has the patient ever experienced previous acute attacks of joint pain and swelling that resolved spontaneously in any joint? (Consider crystal deposition diseases and other inflammatory joint syndromes.)
7. Has the patient recently been treated with a prolonged course of corticosteroids for any reason? (Consider infection or osteonecrosis of bone.)

8. Has the patient had symptoms, such as a skin rash, low-back pain, diarrhea, urethral discharge, conjunctivitis, or mouth sores? (Consider Reiter's syndrome, psoriatic arthritis, or enteropathic arthritis.)
9. Is there a history of a bleeding diathesis? Is the patient being treated with anticoagulants? (Consider hemarthrosis.)

6. Is the age of the patient useful in the differential diagnosis?
Yes! With the exception of infection (which occurs in all age groups), some joint diseases presenting as monoarthritis are more likely to occur at certain ages.
- In children, consider congenital dysplasia of the hip, slipped capital femoral epiphysis, or a monoarticular presentation of juvenile rheumatoid arthritis. Children are unlikely to have crystalline arthritis.
- In young adults, consider seronegative spondyloarthropathy, rheumatoid arthritis, or internal derangement of the joint. They are less likely to have crystalline arthritis.
- Older adults are more likely to have crystalline arthritis, osteoarthritis, osteonecrosis, or internal derangement of the joint.

7. Is fever a useful sign?
Yes, but it can be misleading. Fever is often present in infectious arthritis, but it may be absent. Fever, however, can also be a feature of acute attacks of gout and CPPD disease, rheumatoid arthritis, juvenile rheumatoid arthritis, sarcoidosis, and Reiter's syndrome. Many clinicians have been fooled by a gout attack masquerading as cellulitis or a septic joint.

8. How does the presentation of gonococcal arthritis differ from that of nongonococcal bacterial arthritis?
Gonococcal arthritis is often **polyarticular** and **migratory** in its earliest phase. It then progresses, in many instances, to a **monoarticular** joint phase. Two other characteristic features of disseminated gonococcal infection are tenosynovitis and skin involvement. **Tenosynovial inflammation** usually involves the dorsum of the hands and feet, wrists, and Achilles tendons. The **skin lesions** are unique to this septic arthritis and include tender vesicopustular lesions on an erythematous base and hemorrhagic papules.

9. What are the most likely diagnoses in hospitalized patients who develop acute monoarticular arthritis following admission for another medical or surgical disease?
Acute gout, pseudogout, and infection are by far the most common causes of acute attacks of such monoarthritis. These patients are often middle-aged or elderly, the primary age range for the crystalline arthropathies. In addition, they often have hospitalization-related risk factors known to provoke gout or pseudogout attacks: trauma, surgery, hemorrhage, infection, or medical stress such as renal failure, myocardial infarction, and stroke. One must be especially careful to exclude infection in these hospitalized patients.

10. What is the single most useful diagnostic study in the initial evaluation of monoarthritis?
Synovial fluid analysis.

11. List the most common indications for arthrocentesis and synovial fluid analysis.
   1. **Suspicion of infection.** As little as 2 ml of fluid are sufficient for Gram stain, culture, and white blood cell (WBC) count and differential. A positive Gram stain will allow for rapid initiation of appropriate therapy. A positive culture will provide a definitive diagnosis. As previously stressed, failure to initiate timely and appropriate therapy can be disastrous for a septic joint.
   2. **Suspicion of crystal-induced arthritis.** The sensitivity of polarizing microscopy in identifying birefringent crystals approaches 90% in acute gout and 70% in acute pseudogout. The benefits of joint aspiration in crystal-induced arthritis include exclusion of concomitant infection and the therapeutic effects of aspiration. Precise diagnosis of crystal deposition diseases also allows the most appropriate institution of both acute and chronic therapy in gout. It also prevents the use of inappropriate therapy (allopurinol, probenecid) in pseudogout.

3. Suspicion of hemarthrosis. Bloody joint fluid is characteristic of traumatic arthritis, clotting disorder, and pigmented villonodular synovitis.

4. Differentiating inflammatory from noninflammatory arthritis. The degree of elevation of synovial fluid WBC count can be useful in narrowing the list of possible causes of monarthritis in a given patient. (*See also* Chapter 10.)

12. If gonococcal arthritis is suspected, what special procedures should be performed?

Neisseria gonorrhoeae and *N. meningitidis* are unusually fragile organisms outside the human host. Fewer than 25% of gonorrhea-infected joint aspirates grow in culture. This rate can be improved by plating the joint fluid at the bedside or by informing the laboratory that they should immediately inoculate the specimen on chocolate agar. Cervical, urethral, anal, and pharyngeal cultures for gonococci should also be obtained, as directed by the history of sexual contact.

13. Does a crystal-proven diagnosis of gout or pseudogout rule out infection?

No. Either gout or pseudogout can coexist with a septic joint.

14. What other diagnostic studies are most useful in the initial evaluation of monoarthritis?

Almost always indicated

1. *Radiograph of the joint and contralateral joint:* Although frequently normal, the radiograph may disclose important information. It may diagnose unsuspected fracture, osteonecrosis, osteoarthritis or juxtaarticular bone tumor. The presence of chondrocalcinosis, a radiologic feature of CPPD disease, increases suspicion for a pseudogout attack. Tumor, chronic fungal or mycobacterial infection, and other indolent destructive processes may be revealed. The contralateral joint radiograph serves as a basis for comparison.
2. *Complete blood count:* Leukocytosis supports the possibility of infection.

Indicated in selected patients

1. *Cultures of blood, urine,* or other possible primary sites of infection: Mandatory when a septic joint is being considered.
2. *Serum prothrombin and partial thromboplastin time:* Useful if the patient is receiving anticoagulation or if a coagulation disorder is suspected.
3. *Erythrocyte sedimentation rate:* Although results are often nonspecific, significant elevation may suggest an inflammatory process.

Rarely indicated

1. *Serologic tests for antinuclear antibodies and rheumatoid factor:* However, the antinuclear antibody determination is frequently positive in the pauciarticular form of juvenile rheumatoid arthritis.
2. *Serum uric acid levels:* Notoriously unreliable in making or excluding the diagnosis of gout. These levels may be spuriously elevated in acute inflammatory conditions not related to gout and may be acutely diminished in a true gout attack. Also, by their uricosuric action, analgesics such as aspirin, which may have been taken by patients during the acute attack of arthritis, may lower serum uric acid levels into the normal range.

15. If infection cannot be adequately ruled out by initial diagnostic studies, what should you do?

The patient should be hospitalized and treated presumptively for a septic joint until culture results become available. This is usually indicated in the patient with synovial fluid findings suggesting a highly inflammatory process (synovial fluid WBC count > 50,000/mm^3) but with a negative synovial fluid Gram stain and no obvious primary source of infection. To lessen confusion regarding response to therapy, anti-inflammatory drugs should be withheld during this period.

16. A diagnosis is always established by the end of the first week of onset of acute monoarticular arthritis. Right?

No. Many patients defy initial attempts at diagnosis despite appropriate evaluation. A few achieve spontaneous remission, leaving the physician frustrated about the diagnosis, but relieved. Many patients, however, continue to have symptoms.

17. The initial evaluation is unrevealing and the arthritis persists. What should be done?
If the initial evaluation was carefully accomplished, a period of watchful waiting is often useful at this time. As noted previously, some processes will resolve spontaneously. Others become poly-articular, and the differential diagnosis will change to reflect the new joint involvement. New find-ings, such as the skin rash of psoriasis, occasionally emerge to aid in diagnosis. In a small number of patients, the monoarthritis persists.

18. What is the definition of chronic monoarticular arthritis? Why is it useful to consider this as a category separate from acute monoarticular arthritis?
Chronic monoarticular arthritis can be arbitrarily defined as **symptoms persisting within a sin-gle joint for > 6 weeks.** The differential diagnosis shifts away from some important and common causes of acute arthritis, such as pyogenic infection and acute crystal deposition diseases. In pa-tients with an inflammatory synovial fluid, the likelihood of chronic inflammatory syndromes, such as mycobacterial or fungal septic arthritis, or a seronegative spondyloarthropathy increases. In patients with a noninflammatory process, a structural abnormality or internal derangement is a possibility.

19. Name the most likely causes of chronic monoarticular arthritis.

INFLAMMATORY	NONINFLAMMATORY
Mycobacterial infection	Osteoarthritis
Fungal infection	Internal derangement of the knee
Lyme arthritis	Avascular necrosis of bone
Monoarticular presentation of rheumatoid arthritis	Pigmented villonodular synovitis
Seronegative spondylarthropathies	Synovial chondromatosis
Sarcoid arthritis	Synovioma
Foreign-body synovitis	

20. What seven questions should you ask when obtaining a history from a patient with chronic monoarticular arthritis?
1. Did the pain come on insidiously over days to weeks? (Consider indolent infections, such as mycobacteria and fungi, osteoarthritis, tumor, and infiltrative diseases.)
2. Is there a history of tuberculosis or a positive tuberculin skin test? (Consider mycobacte-rial disease.)
3. Is the patient a farmer, gardener, or floral worker or have a similar exposure to soil or de-caying vegetation? (Consider sporotrichosis.)
4. If the knee is involved, has the joint been damaged in the past? Does it ever "lock" in flex-ion? (Consider internal derangement and osteoarthritis.)
5. Has the patient ever experienced previous acute attacks of joint pain and swelling that re-solved spontaneously in any joint? (Consider inflammatory joint syndromes.)
6. Has the patient recently been treated with a prolonged course of corticosteroids for any reason? (Consider osteonecrosis of bone.)
7. Has the patient had symptoms such as a skin rash, low-back pain, diarrhea, urethritis, con-junctivitis, or uveitis? (Consider the spondyloarthropathies.)

21. What physical findings are useful in the differential diagnosis of a chronic monoarticu-lar arthritis?
1. Extra-articular features of the spondyloarthropathies, such as skin rashes (psoriasis, ker-atoderma blennorrhagicum), oral ulcers, conjunctivitis, uveitis
2. Erythema nodosa, a feature of sarcoidosis and inflammatory bowel syndrome
3. A positive McMurray maneuver in the knee examination, suggesting internal derangement

22. In evaluating chronic monoarthritis, what initial studies should be obtained?
Almost always indicated
1. *Radiograph of the joint* and, if not initially obtained, radiograph of the contralateral joint: Although radiographs are frequently normal in acute arthritis, they are often revealing in

chronic arthritis. Chronic infections by mycobacteria and fungi often cause radiographically detectable abnormalities. Osteoarthritis, avascular necrosis of bone, and other causes of noninflammatory chronic arthritis also have characteristic radiographic appearances.

2. *Synovial fluid analysis,* if at all possible: This analysis is extremely useful in dividing possible causes of the joint process into the two broad diagnostic categories, inflammatory and noninflammatory arthritis. The presence of a bloody synovial effusion points to pigmented villonodular synovitis, synovial chondromatosis, or synovioma. Cultures of synovial fluid may demonstrate mycobacterial or fungal infection.

Indicated in selected patients

1. *Erythrocyte sedimentation rate:* Although results are often nonspecific, significant elevation may suggest an inflammatory process.
2. *Radiograph of sacroiliac joints:* This may demonstrate asymptomatic sacroiliitis in young males presenting with a chronic monoarticular arthritis as an initial manifestation of a spondyloarthropathy.
3. *Chest radiograph:* To detect evidence of a prior mycobacterial disease or to assess for pulmonary sarcoidosis.
4. *Skin test reaction to tuberculin:* A negative test is useful in excluding mycobacterial infection.
5. *Serologic tests for Lyme disease* (Borrelia burgdorferi), *rheumatoid factor, and antinuclear antibody.*

23. Are other diagnostic studies useful in the evaluation of chronic monoarthritis?

1. **Arthroscopy:** Arthroscopy allows direct visualization of many important articular structures and provides the opportunity for synovial biopsy in all large and some medium-sized joints. It is particularly useful for diagnosing internal derangement of the knee.
2. **Synovial biopsy:** Microscopic evaluation with culture of synovial tissue is useful in the diagnosis of:

Tumors	Sarcoid arthritis
Pigmented villonodular synovitis	Foreign-body synovitis
Synovial chondromatosis	Fungal and mycobacterial infection
Synovioma	

3. **Magnetic resonance imaging of the joint**

Avascular necrosis	Internal derangement of the knee
Osteomyelitis	Destruction of periarticular bone

4. **Bone scan**

Avascular necrosis	Osteomyelitis

24. How often is a specific diagnosis made in patients with chronic monoarthritis?

Appropriate evaluation yields a diagnosis in approximately two-thirds of patients. Fortunately, the most serious and treatable diseases yield to diagnosis if a carefully reasoned clinical approach is taken.

BIBLIOGRAPHY

1. Baker DG, Schumacher HR: Acute monoarthritis. N Engl J Med 329:1013–1020, 1992.
2. Bomalaski JS: Acute rheumatologic disorders in the elderly. Emerg Med Clin North Am 8:341–359, 1990.
3. Carias K, Panush RS: Acute arthritis. Bull Rheum Dis 43(7):1–4, 1994.
4. Fries JF, Mitchell DM: Joint pain or arthritis. JAMA 235:199–202, 1976.
5. Goldenberg DL, Reed JI: Bacterial arthritis. N Engl J Med 312:764–771, 1985.
6. Ho G, DeNuccio M: Gout and pseudogout in hospitalized patients. Arch Intern Med 153:2787–2790, 1993.
7. Katz WA: Diagnosis of monoarticular and polyarticular rheumatic disorders. In Katz WA (ed): Diagnosis and Management of Rheumatic Diseases. Philadelphia, J.B. Lippincott Co., 1977, pp 751–761.
8. Liang MH, Sturrock RD: Evaluation of musculoskeletal symptoms. In Klippel JH, Dieppe PA (eds): Rheumatology. London, Mosby-Year Book Europe Ltd., 1994, pp 2-1.1–2-1.18.

9. Mankin HJ: Nontraumatic necrosis of bone (osteonecrosis). N Engl J Med 326:1473–1479, 1992.
10. McCarty DJ: Gout without hyperuricemia. JAMA 271:302–303, 1994.
11. Nissenbaum MA, Adamis MK: Magnetic resonance imaging in rheumatology: An overview. Rheum Dis Clin North Am 20:343–360, 1994.
12. O'Rourle KS, Ike RW: Diagnostic arthroscopy in the arthritis patient. Rheum Dis Clin North Am 20:321–342, 1994.
13. Panush RS, Kisch A: Gonococcal arthritis. In Hurst W (ed): Medicine, 3rd ed. Boston, Butterworths, 1992, pp 215–217.
14. Shmerling RH: Synovial fluid analysis: A critical reappraisal. Rheum Dis Clin North Am 20:503–512, 1994.

15. APPROACH TO THE PATIENT WITH POLYARTICULAR SYMPTOMS

Robert A. Hawkins, M.D.

1. What are the most important tools that the clinician can use on a patient with polyarticular symptoms?

A careful history and physical examination. Laboratory testing and radiographic or other imaging studies provide definitive answers in only a few instances. Tests are often most useful in confirming the suspected diagnosis or in providing prognostic information. When confronted with a patient with polyarticular symptoms, an inexperienced clinician often will slight the most important, the history and physical examination, opting instead for "shotgun" laboratory testing. While tests such as rheumatoid factor, uric acid, ASO titers, and antinuclear antibodies may be indicated in many instances, the history and physical examination will reveal 75% of the information required for diagnosis.

2. How are the many diseases causing polyarticular symptoms classified?

No single classification scheme can be used to differentiate the wide variety of diseases presenting with polyarticular symptoms. A few diseases have a single descriptive finding that is essentially diagnostic, such as a positive synovial fluid culture in gonococcal polyarthritis, a high serum titer of anti-double-stranded DNA in systemic lupus erythematosus (SLE), or the rash of psoriasis in psoriatic arthritis. Most polyarticular diseases, however, are diagnosed by their characteristic clinical findings, such as the triad of urethritis, conjunctivitis, and oligoarticular arthritis in Reiter's syndrome, or the symmetrical synovitis and morning stiffness involving the small joints of the hands in rheumatoid arthritis.

In most instances, the clinician uses several variables in combination to reduce the number of diagnostic possibilities. These variables include:

   Acuteness of onset of the process
   Degree of inflammation of the joints
   Temporal pattern of joint involvement
   Distribution of joint involvement
   Age and sex of the patient

Additionally, many systemic diseases with polyarticular involvement have characteristic extra-articular features that contribute substantially to the diagnosis. As previously stressed, these variables are often identified by the medical history and physical examination. The clinician can apply selected tests to the few remaining likely diseases to confirm the diagnosis.

3. Which diseases commonly present with acute polyarticular symptoms?

Infection	Other inflammatory
Gonococcal	Rheumatoid arthritis
Meningococcal	Polyarticular and systemic juvenile
Lyme	rheumatoid arthritis
Acute rheumatic fever	Systemic lupus erythematosus
Bacterial endocarditis	Reiter's syndrome
Viral (esp. rubella, hepatitis B,	Psoriatic arthritis
parvovirus, Epstein-Barr, HIV)	Polyarticular gout
	Sarcoid arthritis
	Serum sickness

4. Which diseases commonly present with chronic (persisting > 6 weeks) polyarticular symptoms?

Inflammatory

Rheumatoid arthritis	Enteropathic arthritis
Polyarticular juvenile rheumatoid arthritis	Polyarticular gout
Systemic lupus erythematosus	Calcium pyrophosphate deposition
Progressive systemic sclerosis	(CPPD) disease
Polymyositis	Sarcoid arthritis
Reiter's syndrome	Vasculitis
Psoriatic arthritis	Polymyalgia rheumatica

Noninflammatory

Osteoarthritis	Fibromyalgia
Calcium pyrophosphate deposition	Benign hypermobility syndrome
(CPPD) disease	
Polyarticular gout	Hemochromatosis
Paget's disease	

5. How do polyarthritis, polyarthralgias, and diffuse aches and pains differ?

Polyarthritis is definite inflammation (swelling, tenderness, warmth) of ≥ 5 joints demonstrated by physical examination. (A patient with 2–4 involved joints is said to have pauci- or oligoarticular arthritis.) The acute polyarticular diseases (see Question 3) and chronic inflammatory diseases (see Question 4) commonly present with polyarthritis. Most of the chronic noninflammatory diseases do not manifest significant joint inflammation. The exceptions are CPPD disease and polyarticular gout, which can present with either polyarthritis or polyarthralgia.

Polyarthralgia is defined as pain in ≥ 5 joints without demonstrable inflammation by physical examination. SLE, systemic sclerosis, vasculitis, polymyalgia rheumatica, and the chronic noninflammatory arthritides commonly present with polyarthralgias.

Diffuse aches and pains are poorly localized symptoms originating in joints, bones, muscles, or other soft tissues. The joint examination does not reveal inflammation. Polymyalgia rheumatica, fibromyalgia, SLE, polymyositis, and hypothyroidism commonly present with these symptoms.

6. Describe the three characteristic temporal patterns of joint involvement in polyarthritis.

1. **Migratory pattern:** Symptoms are present in certain joints for a few days and then remit, only to reappear in other joints. Rheumatic fever, gonococcal arthritis, and the early phase of Lyme disease are famous examples.

2. **Additive pattern:** Symptoms begin in some joints and persist, with subsequent involvement of other joints. This pattern is nonspecific, being common in rheumatoid arthritis, SLE, and many other polyarticular syndromes.

3. **Intermittent pattern:** This pattern is typified by repetitive attacks of acute polyarthritis

with complete remission between attacks. A prolonged observation may be necessary to establish this phenomenon. Rheumatoid arthritis, polyarticular gout, sarcoid arthritis, Reiter's syndrome, and psoriatic arthritis may present in this manner.

7. How is the distribution of joint involvement helpful in the differential diagnosis of polyarthritis?

Different diseases characteristically affect different joints. Knowledge of the typical joints involved in each disease is a cornerstone of diagnosis in polyarthritis. In practice, knowledge of which joints are *spared* in each form of arthritis is also quite useful.

Distribution of Joint Involvement in Polyarthritis

DISEASE	JOINTS COMMONLY INVOLVED	JOINTS COMMONLY SPARED
Gonococcal arthritis	Knee, wrist, ankle, hand IP	Axial
Lyme arthritis	Knee, shoulder, wrist, elbow	Axial
Rheumatoid arthritis	Wrist, MCP, PIP, elbow, glenohumeral, cervical spine, hip, knee, ankle, tarsal, MTP	DIP, thoracolumbar spine
Osteoarthritis	First CMC, CIP, PIP, cervical spine, thoracolumbar spine, hip, knee, first MTP, toe IP	MCP, wrist, elbow, glenohumeral, ankle, tarsal
Reiter's syndrome	Knee, ankle, tarsal, MTP, toe IP, elbow, axial	
Psoriatic arthritis	Knee, ankle, MTP, toe IP, wrist, MCP, hand IP, axial	
Enteropathic arthritis	Knee, ankle, elbow, shoulder, MCP, PIP, wrist, axial	
Polyarticular gout	First MTP, instep, heel, ankle, knee	Axial
CPPD disease	Knee, wrist, shoulder, ankle, MCP, hand IP, hip, elbow	Axial
Sarcoid arthritis	Ankle, knee	Axial
Hemochromatosis	MCP, wrist, knee, hip, feet, shoulder	

Joints: IP, interphalangeal; MCP, metacarpophalangeal; PIP, proximal interphalangeal; CMC, carpometacarpal; DIP, distal interphalangeal; MTP, metatarsophalangeal.

8. Name the two most common causes of chronic polyarthritis.

1. **Osteoarthritis:** The prevalence of osteoarthritis rises steeply with age. Between 10–20% of people 40-years-old have evidence of osteoarthritis, and 75% of women over age 65 have osteoarthritis. This very high prevalence makes osteoarthritis the single most likely diagnosis in older patients complaining of polyarticular pain who have noninflammatory signs and symptoms.

2. **Rheumatoid arthritis:** The prevalence in U.S. whites is approximately 1%, making it the most common chronic inflammatory joint disease.

9. What are the most likely diagnoses in women aged 25–50 who present with chronic polyarticular symptoms?

Osteoarthritis, rheumatoid arthritis, systemic lupus erythematosus, fibromyalgia, and benign hypermobility syndrome.

10. What are the most likely diagnoses in men aged 25–50 who present with chronic oligoarticular or polyarticular symptoms?

Gonococcal arthritis, Reiter's syndrome, ankylosing spondylitis, osteoarthritis, and hemochromatosis.

11. And in patients over age 50 presenting with chronic polyarticular symptoms?

Osteoarthritis, rheumatoid arthritis, CPPD disease, polymyalgia rheumatica, and paraneoplastic polyarthritis.

12. What is morning stiffness? How is it useful in sorting out the causes of polyarticular symptoms?

Morning stiffness refers to the amount of time it takes for patients with polyarthritis to "limber up" after arising in the morning. This rough measure is useful in differentiating inflammatory from noninflammatory arthritis. In inflammatory arthritis, morning stiffness lasts > 1 hour. In untreated rheumatoid arthritis, it averages 3.5 hours and tends to parallel the degree of joint inflammation. In contrast, noninflammatory processes, such as osteoarthritis, may produce transient morning stiffness that lasts < 15 minutes.

13. List the differential diagnosis of fever and polyarthritis.

Infectious arthritis: septic arthritis, bacterial endocarditis, Lyme disease, acid-fast bacterial or fungal arthritis, viral arthritis

Reactive arthritis: enteric infections, Reiter's syndrome, rheumatic fever, inflammatory bowel disease

Systemic rheumatic diseases: rheumatoid arthritis, SLE, Still's disease, systemic vasculitis

Crystal-induced arthritis: gout, pseudogout

Miscellaneous disease: malignancy, familial Mediterranean fever, sarcoidosis, dermatomyositis, Behçet's disease, Henoch-Schönlein purpura, Kawasaki's, erythema nodosum, erythema multiforme, pyoderma gangrenosum, pustular psoriasis

14. Define tenosynovitis. How is its presence useful in the differential diagnosis of polyarticular symptoms?

Tenosynovitis is inflammation of the synovial-lined sheaths surrounding tendons in the wrists, hands, ankles, and feet. Physical examination usually reveals tenderness and swelling along the track of the involved tendon *between* the joints. It is a characteristic feature of rheumatoid arthritis, gout, Reiter's syndrome, gonococcal arthritis, and tuberculous and fungal arthritis. It is distinctly uncommon in other causes of polyarticular disease.

15. List skin lesions that can be useful in the diagnosis of acute or chronic polyarthritis.

Erythema chronicum migrans (Lyme arthritis)
Erythema nodosum (sarcoid arthritis, enteric arthritis)
Psoriatic plaques (psoriatic arthritis)
Keratoderma blennorrhagicum (Reiter's syndrome)
Erythema marginatum (acute rheumatic fever)
Palpable purpura (vasculitis)
Livedo reticularis (vasculitis)
Vesicopustular lesions or hemorrhagic papules (gonococcal arthritis)
Butterfly rash, discoid lupus, or photosensitive rash (SLE)
Thickening of the skin (systemic sclerosis)
Heliotrope rash on eyelids, upper chest, and extensor aspects of joints (dermatomyositis)
Gottron's papules overlying the extensor aspects of the MCP and IP joints of the hands (dermatomyositis)
Gray/brown skin hyperpigmentation (hemochromatosis)

16. Which rheumatic diseases should be considered in a patient with Raynaud's phenomenon and polyarticular symptoms?

Progressive systemic sclerosis (prevalence of 90%)
Systemic lupus erythematosus (prevalence of 20%)
Polymyositis/dermatomyositis (prevalence of 20–40%)
Vasculitis (variable prevalence, depending on the particular syndrome)

17. What other systemic features are seen in diseases causing polyarthritis?

Extra-articular Organ Involvement in Polyarticular Rheumatic Diseases

DISEASE	LUNG	PLEURA	PERI-CARDIUM	HEART MUSCLE	HEART VALVE	KIDNEY	GI TRACT	LIVER
Acute rheumatic fever		•	•	•	•			
Viral arthritis								•
Bacterial endocarditis					•	•		
Rheumatoid arthritis	•	•	•	•	•			
Polyarticular JRA								
SLE	•	•	•	•	•	•		
Systemic sclerosis	•	•	•	•		•	•	•
Polymyositis/ dermatomyositis	•	•	•	•				
Reiter's syndrome					•		•	
Psoriatic arthritis								
Enteropathic arthritis							•	•
Polyarticular gout						•		
Sarcoid arthritis	•							•
Serum sickness						•		
Vasculitis								
Polymyalgia rheumatica								•
Hemochromatosis				•				•

JRA, juvenile rheumatoid arthritis.

18. Which tests are most useful in evaluating a patient with chronic polyarticular symptoms?

Complete blood count
Erythrocyte sedimentation rate
Antinuclear antibodies (ANA)
Rheumatoid factor
Liver enzymes
Serum creatinine
Serum uric acid

Urinalysis
Others to consider
   Thyroid stimulating hormone
   Iron studies
   Synovial fluid analysis
   Radiographs

19. What is the significance of a positive ANA in a patient with chronic polyarticular symptoms?

A patient with polyarthralgia or polyarthritis who has a significantly elevated ANA titer often will have one of the following diseases: SLE (including drug-induced lupus), rheumatoid arthritis, Sjögren's syndrome, polymyositis, systemic sclerosis, or mixed connective tissue disease.

The history and physical examination should be directed toward the clinical findings in these diseases. A careful medication history may reveal that the patient has received procainamide or hydralazine, two common causes of drug-induced lupus (see Chapter 12 for other drugs known to induce positive ANA). Finally, it must be stressed that a positive ANA is a feature of several other chronic diseases and can also be found in normal healthy individuals, although usually in low titer. (See also Chapter 9.)

20. Why should a rheumatoid factor *not* be ordered in the evaluation of patients with acute polyarticular symptoms?

Rheumatoid factor (RF) has a low sensitivity and specificity for rheumatoid arthritis in patients with acute polyarticular symptoms. Serum RF is frequently positive in acute infectious syndromes caused by hepatitis B, Epstein-Barr, influenza and other viruses but disappears as the viral syndrome resolves. Although RF will eventually become positive in 75–85% of patients with rheumatoid arthritis, it is positive in early rheumatoid arthritis in 25–70% of patients.

21. Which chronic polyarticular diseases are most likely to be associated with low serum complement levels?

SLE and several of the vasculitis syndromes. Low serum complement levels (C3, C4, and total hemolytic complement) usually suggest the presence of immune complex disease. In SLE and in many diseases causing vasculitis, immune complexes often activate the complement cascade, resulting in consumption of individual complement components. In many instances, the liver is unable to produce these components as rapidly as they are consumed, resulting in a fall in serum levels.

22. When should arthrocentesis for synovial fluid analysis be considered in the evaluation of polyarthritis?

When the diagnosis has not been established *and* joint fluid can be obtained. Both of these requirements need to be met. For example, a patient with obvious osteoarthritis established by history and physical examination does *not* require a diagnostic aspiration of an uncomplicated knee effusion.

If it can be obtained, synovial fluid analysis can be useful in the diagnosis of bacterial joint infection and crystal-induced arthritis. Even if a specific diagnosis is not forthcoming, synovial fluid analysis reduces the list of diagnostic possibilities by categorizing the process as either inflammatory or noninflammatory.

23. Should radiographs of affected joints always be obtained?

Not always. As a general rule, patients with acute polyarticular arthritis will not benefit from joint radiographs. Radiographs are most valuable in evaluating chronic arthritis that has been relatively long-standing and that has resulted in characteristic changes in joints. Osteoarthritis, chronic rheumatoid arthritis, psoriatic arthritis, gout, CPPD disease, systemic sclerosis, and sarcoidosis all have specific appearances on radiographs that are very useful in diagnosis. Remember, though, that osteoarthritis is so common that it may coexist with other arthritis syndromes, and radiographic changes may be a mixture of both types of arthritis in a given patient.

24. Why should the rheumatologist think in "geologic" time?

Because many chronic polyarticular diseases require months or years to diagnose, tremendous and profound patience is often required. This prolonged period often seems like "geologic" time to many patients who may expect an accurate diagnosis in one or two visits. The characteristics of many chronic polyarticular diseases require this extraordinary degree of patience, in that:

- Many present insidiously with few objective findings for prolonged times.
- Many initially masquerade as other diseases before finally settling into their usual pattern. Rheumatoid arthritis, for example, can present as a monoarticular arthritis before assuming its more typical polyarticular course.
- Characteristic laboratory abnormalities may require months or years to develop. Patients with rheumatoid arthritis may have symptoms for a prolonged period before the development of RF in serum.
- The joint symptoms of many conditions precede the extra-articular features of the disease in some patients by months or years. The skin plaques of psoriasis and the bowel symptoms of inflammatory bowel disease may be the last and final diagnostic features of these arthritis syndromes.
- Joint radiographs may not show characteristic changes of the arthritis for months or years.

BIBLIOGRAPHY

1. Hughes RA, Keat AC: Reiter's syndrome and reactive arthritis: A current view. Semin Arthritis Rheum 24:190–210, 1994.
2. Bomalaski JS: Acute rheumatologic disorders in the elderly. Emerg Med Clin North Am 8:341–359, 1990.
3. Carias K, Panush RS: Acute arthritis. Bull Rheum Dis 43(7):1–4, 1994.
4. Goldenberg DL, Reed JI: Bacterial arthritis. N Engl J Med 312:764–771, 1985.
5. Katz WA: Diagnosis of monoarticular and polyarticular rheumatic disorders. In Katz WA (ed): Diagnosis and Management of Rheumatic Diseases. Philadelphia, J.B. Lippincott, 1977, pp 751–759.
6. Liang MH, Sturrock RD: Evaluation of musculosketetal symptoms. In Klippel JH, Dieppe PA (eds): Rheumatology. London, Mosby-Year Book Europe, 1994, pp 2,1.1–2,1.18.
7. Panush RS, Kisch A: Gonococcal arthritis. In Hurst W (ed): Medicine, 3rd ed. Boston, Butterworths, 1992, pp 215–217.
8. American College of Rheumatology Ad Hoc Committee on Clinical Guidelines: Guidelines for the initial evaluation of the adult patient with acute musculoskeletal symptoms. Arthritis Rheum 39:1–8, 1996.
9. Pinals RS: Polyarthritis and fever. N Engl J Med 330:769–774, 1994.

16. APPROACH TO THE PATIENT WITH NEUROMUSCULAR SYMPTOMS

Robert A. Hawkins, M.D.

1. Discuss the relationship between rheumatic diseases and neuromuscular disease.
Many primary rheumatic diseases, such as systemic lupus erythematosus, rheumatoid arthritis, and systemic vasculitis, are frequently complicated by neurologic or myopathic disease. Chronic synovitis, joint contractures, and deformities seen in rheumatoid arthritis lead to muscle atrophy and weakness. Other rheumatic diseases such as polymyositis are dominated by immune-mediated inflammation of muscle, and the differential diagnosis of myopathy is quite broad. Neuromuscular manifestations of rheumatic diseases may present as early and dominant findings, or as late complications of well-established diseases. They may also be complications of therapy for rheumatic diseases, as with the use of corticosteroids or D-penicillamine.

2. What are the cardinal symptoms of neuromuscular lesions?
Weakness and/or **pain** are the most common symptoms reported by patients. Weakness should be separated from complaints of fatigue and malaise. Fatigue differs from weakness in that fatigue is a loss of strength with activity which recovers with rest. Malaise is a subjective feeling of weakness without objective findings.

3. Many patients complain of weakness. What is the best way to determine the cause of weakness in a given patient?
The first step is to exclude **systemic causes** of fatigue or weakness, such as cardiopulmonary disease, anemia, hypothyroidism, malignancy, or depression. Many of these patients complain of malaise rather than weakness, and their examination usually fails to reveal true weakness if they give their best effort. The carefully directed history and physical examination, combined with focused laboratory testing, are usually effective in eliminating these causes of weakness.

Common Systemic Causes of Weakness or Fatigue

Cardiopulmonary disease	Hypothyroidism	Malignancy
Anemia	Hyperthyroidism	Depression
Chronic infection	Poor physical conditioning	Chronic inflammatory disease

4. Once systemic causes of weakness have been excluded, what is the next step?
The **neuromuscular causes** of weakness should be considered. A very useful method of categorizing neuromuscular diseases is by their customary level of anatomic involvement, beginning with the spinal cord and proceeding distally through nerve roots, peripheral nerves, neuromuscular junctions, and muscle.

Diseases Affecting Neuromuscular Structures, by Level of Anatomic Involvement

SPINAL CORD	NERVE ROOT	PERIPHERAL NERVE	NEUROMUSCULAR JUNCTION	MUSCLE
Amyotrophic lateral sclerosis	Herniated nucleus pulposus	Vasculitis	Myasthenia gravis	Polymyositis
Transverse myelitis	Cervical spondylosis	Guillain-Barré syndrome	Eaton-Lambert syndrome	Hypothyroidism
Vasculitis	Lumbar spondylosis	Collagen vascular diseases		Hyperthyroidism
Collagen vascular diseases		Nerve compression		Muscular dystrophy
		Amyloidosis		Corticosteroid use
				Vasculitis
				Collagen vascular diseases

5. Many patients complain of pain. What historical features are most useful in the differential diagnosis of pain?

Neurologic lesions may or may not cause pain, depending on the level of involvement and the cause of the abnormality. Pure spinal cord lesions generally do not produce pain, although occasionally painful flexor muscle spasms will occur. Nerve root compression commonly produces pain in the affected nerve distribution. Peripheral nerve disease is often manifest by numbness, tingling, and paresthesias (pins and needles sensation). Some diseases such as Guillain-Barré syndrome, on the other hand, affect primarily the motor aspect of the peripheral nerve. Their predominant manifestation is weakness rather than pain. Diseases of the neuromuscular junction are not painful.

Myopathies may or may not be painful. In sorting them out, the following concepts are useful:
- Inflammatory myopathies are usually dominated by weakness, not pain. The exception to this rule is when the inflammatory myopathy has a fulminant onset, when pain may be as dominant a feature as weakness.
- Muscle pain on exertion is suggestive of claudication (vascular insufficiency) or rarer diseases of muscle metabolism.
- Myopathies do not produce numbness or paresthesias.

6. How does the distribution of weakness or pain aid in differentiating neurologic from muscular lesions?

Myopathies tend to cause *proximal* and *symmetrical* (bilateral) weakness or pain involving the shoulder girdle and hip girdle. Patients with proximal upper extremity weakness will note difficulty in combing hair or brushing their teeth. Patients with lower extremity weakness will complain of difficulty in rising from a chair or climbing stairs. If present, pain may be reported as aching or cramping.

Peripheral neuropathies, as a rule, cause *distal* (hands and feet) weakness and/or pain that is often *asymmetrical*. Typically, patients report their upper extremity weakness as clumsiness of the hands or a tendency to drop things. Lower extremity distal weakness is often manifest by foot dragging or tripping over rugs or rough surfaces. Asymmetrical peripheral weakness points toward a regional neurologic condition, such as median nerve compression in carpal tunnel syndrome.

Nerve root compression causes asymmetric weakness and pain that may be either proximal or distal, depending on the level of the involved nerve root.

Spinal cord lesions usually are associated with a distinct sensory level described as a tightness bilaterally around the trunk or abdomen. Distal spastic weakness, often with loss of bowel and bladder sphincter function, is also a feature of spinal cord disease.

7. How does the temporal pattern of weakness or pain aid in diagnosis?

1. **Abrupt onset** of weakness is characteristic of Guillain-Barré syndrome, poliomyelitis, and hypokalemic periodic paralysis.

2. **Intermittent** weakness may occur with myasthenia gravis, the rare causes of metabolic myopathy, and hypokalemic periodic paralysis.

3. **Gradual onset** of weakness or pain is typical of most muscle diseases, including inflammatory myopathies, the muscular dystrophies, and endocrine myopathies, as well as most neuropathies. It may also occur with myasthenia gravis.

8. What is meant by fatigability? How is it useful in diagnosing neuromuscular disease?

Fatigability is defined as progressive weakness of muscle with repetitive use, followed by recovery of strength after a brief period of rest. It is a classic finding in myasthenia gravis. Eaton-Lambert syndrome is often referred to as reverse myasthenia gravis due the paradoxical increase in muscle strength observed with repetitive muscle contraction.

9. How does the family history aid in diagnosis?

Many of the muscular dystrophy syndromes have strong patterns of inheritance.

Duchenne muscular dystrophy	X-linked
Limb-girdle muscular dystrophy	Autosomal recessive or dominant
Facioscapulohumeral muscular dystrophy	Autosomal dominant
Myotonic dystrophy	Autosomal dominant
Peroneal muscular atrophy (Charcot-Marie-Tooth disease)	Autosomal dominant

10. Name three hormones whose deficiency or excess is associated with myopathy.
   Thyroxine (hypothyroidism or hyperthyroidism)
   Cortisol (Addison's disease or Cushing's disease)
   Parathyroid hormone (hypoparathyroidism or hyperparathyroidism)

11. Which drugs are most commonly responsible for neuromuscular symptoms?

Corticosteroids	Alcohol	D-Penicillamine	Clofibrate, lovastatin,
Emetine	Chloroquine	Colchicine	other cholesterol-
Zidovudine	Hydroxychloroquine	Cocaine	lowering agents

12. What toxins should be sought in the evaluation of neuromuscular symptoms?
   - **Organophosphates:** These esters are used in pesticides, petroleum additives, and modifiers of plastic. Their toxicity affects peripheral nerves. With progression of the neuropathy, pyramidal tract signs and spasticity may develop.
   - **Lead:** Lead toxicity can result in encephalopathy and psychiatric problems (children), abdominal pain, and peripheral neuropathy appearing in the hands before the feet (adults).
   - **Thallium:** This toxin is used in rodenticides and industrial processes. Patients present with a sensory and autonomic neuropathy. Alopecia usually develops at the onset of symptoms.
   - **Arsenic, mercury** (electrical and chemical industry), and industrial solvents containing aliphatic compounds can also cause neuromuscular symptoms.

13. What are the key elements of the physical examination in the evaluation of neuromuscular symptoms?

System	Examine for:
General	Cardiopulmonary disease, infection, thyroid disease, malignancy
Joints	Synovitis, deformities, contractures
Muscles	Muscle bulk, tenderness, weakness, fasciculations
Neurologic	Sensory abnormalities, deep tendon reflexes, weakness

14. What is Gower's sign?
A patient attempts to rise from a seated position by climbing up their legs with their hands. It is seen in patients with proximal lower extremity muscular weakness due to myopathy.

15. How is muscle weakness graded by the physical examiner?
   The most commonly accepted scale is the Medical Research Council Grading System. Because there is a wide range of muscle strength between grades 5 and 4, it is common to assign intermediate values such as 5− or 4+ to many muscle groups in the examination.

Grade	Degree of Strength
5	Normal strength
4	Muscle contraction possible against gravity plus some examiner resistance
3	Muscle contraction possible against gravity only
2	Muscle contraction possible only with gravity removed
1	Flicker of muscle contraction observed but without movement of extremity
0	No contraction

16. How are deep tendon reflexes graded by the physical examiner?

Grade	Strength of Contraction
+4	Clonus
+3	Exaggerated
+2	Normal
+1	Present but depressed
0	Absent

17. Can alterations in deep tendon reflexes aid in differentiation of neuromuscular diseases?
The following generalizations are useful:
- Spinal cord lesions (above L2) and upper motor neuron disease usually produce exaggerated deep tendon reflexes and pathologic plantar reflexes.
- Nerve root and peripheral nerve lesions usually produce depressed or absent reflexes.
- Primary muscle diseases do not usually *present* with altered deep tendon reflexes. Late in the disease process, however, substantial muscle atrophy may cause reduction or loss of the reflex.
- Hyperthyroidism produces exaggerated tendon reflexes.
- Hypothyroidism produces depressed deep tendon reflexes with slow relaxation phase.
- Many people over age 60 experience a natural loss of their ankle reflexes.

18. Which screening laboratory tests can evaluate for systemic causes of neuromuscular symptoms?

Complete blood count	Erythrocyte sedimentation rate	Thyroid function tests
Serum electrolytes, calcium, magnesium, phosphorus	Serum liver enzyme tests	Chest radiograph
Serum muscle enzymes	Serum renal function tests	Electrocardiogram

19. Which serum enzymes are elevated in muscle disease?

Serum Enzyme	Clinical Utility
Creatine kinase (CK)	Most sensitive and specific for muscle disease
Aldolase	Elevated in muscle, liver, and erythrocyte diseases
Lactic dehydrogenase	Elevated in muscle, liver, erythrocyte, and other diseases
Aspartate aminotransferase (AST)	Most specific for inflammatory muscle disease

20. What are other causes of elevation of serum creatine kinase besides myopathy?
Intramuscular injections
Muscle crush injuries
Recent strenuous exercise
Myocardial infarction
Race of individual (healthy blacks have significantly higher CK levels than the "normal" values derived from the entire population).

21. Are additional specific tests useful in the evaluation of neuromuscular symptoms?

SPECIFIC TEST	SUSPECTED DISEASE PROCESSES
Serum antinuclear antibodies	Inflammatory myopathy, vasculitis
Serum rheumatoid factor	Inflammatory myopathy, vasculitis
Serum complement assay	Inflammatory myopathy, vasculitis
Serum cryoglobulins	Vasculitis
Hepatitis B surface antigen and hepatitis C antibody	Vasculitis
Anti-neutrophil cytoplasmic antibodies	Vasculitis
Acetylcholine receptor antibodies	Myasthenia gravis
Serum parathyroid hormone	Parathyroid disease
Electromyography and nerve conduction tests	Disease of nerve roots, peripheral nerves, or myopathies
Muscle biopsy	Inflammatory or metabolic myopathies, vasculitis
Nerve biopsy	Vasculitis
Magnetic resonance scan	Spinal cord, nerve root, and myopathic processes

22. What is mononeuritis multiplex?

Mononeuritis multiplex is a pattern of motor and sensory involvement of multiple individual peripheral nerves that is a classic neurologic presentation of systemic vasculitis. First, one peripheral nerve becomes involved (usually with burning dysesthesias), followed by other individual nerves, often with motor dysfunction as well. The patchy nature of nerve involvement reflects the patchy vasculitis of the vasa nervorum which is the underlying cause of the neuropathy.

23. Is mononeuritis multiplex seen only in patients with vasculitis?

No. The differential diagnosis of mononeuritis multiplex also includes:

Vasculitis	Sarcoidosis
Diabetes mellitus	Wartenburg's relapsing sensory neuritis
Lead neuropathy	

24. Is mononeuritis multiplex the only pattern of neuropathy seen in vasculitis?

No. Two patterns of peripheral neuropathy are usually seen. Although mononeuritis multiplex is the most famous pattern, a **stocking-glove** pattern of neurologic involvement is seen more frequently. A stocking-glove pattern involves both feet, the calves, and hands. Most patients with vasculitic neuropathy will have an overlap of mononeuritis multiplex and a stocking-glove neuropathy.

25. What are the most common causes of proximal shoulder girdle and hip girdle aches, pains and/or weakness? How are they differentiated?

Six diseases are responsible for >90% of diffuse, proximal aches or weakness. The first step is to decide which is the dominant clinical finding, pain or weakness. To determine if true weakness is present, the examiner should ask the patient to ignore any pain that may occur during muscle strength testing so that a true measure of muscle strength can be determined. Although patients with fibromyalgia syndrome and polymyalgia rheumatica may complain of weakness in addition to pain, they are not truly weak on physical examination.

DISEASE	PAIN	WEAKNESS	ESR	SERUM CK	SERUM T4
Fibromyalgia	Yes	No	Normal	Normal	Normal
Polymyalgia rheumatica	Yes	No	Marked elevation	Normal	Normal
Polymyositis	Usually none	Yes	Usually normal	Elevated	Normal
Corticosteroid myopathy	No	Yes	Normal	Normal	Normal
Hyperthyroidism	No	Yes	Normal	Normal	Elevated
Hypothyroidism	Yes	No	Normal	Elevated	Depressed

ESR—erythrocyte sedimentation rate; T4—thyroxine.

26. What is the diagnostic significance of "strokes in young folks"? What rheumatic syndromes should be considered in the differential diagnosis of cerebrovascular disease?

Most cerebrovascular disease occurs in patients over age 50 due to long-standing hypertension, atherosclerosis, and cardiac emboli. When ischemic cerebrovascular disease occurs in patients under age 50, the possibility of several rheumatic syndromes should be especially considered:

Systemic lupus erythematosus	Isolated angiitis of the CNS
Antiphospholipid antibody syndrome	Polyarteritis nodosa
Takayasu's arteritis	Wegener's granulomatosis

BIBLIOGRAPHY

1. Bohlmeyer AHB, et al: Evaluation of laboratory tests as a guide to diagnosis and therapy of myositis. Rheum Dis Clin North Am 19:845–856, 1994.
2. Bresnihan B: Arthritis and muscle weakness or neuropathy. In Klippel JH, Dieppe PA (eds): Rheumatology. London, Mosby-Year Book Europe Ltd, 1994, pp 2,7.1–2,7.8.

3. Brick JE, Brick JF: Neurologic manifestations of rheumatic disease. Neurol Clin 7:629–639, 1989.
4. Kissel JT, Mendell JR: Vasculitic neuropathy. Neurol Clin 10:761–781, 1992.
5. Miller ML: Weakness. In Kelly WM, Harris ED, Ruddy S, Sledge CB (eds): Textbook of Rheumatology, 4th ed. Philadelphia, W.B. Saunders, 1993, pp 389–397.
6. Nissenbaum MA, Adamis MK: Magnetic resonance imaging in rheumatology: An overview. Rheum Dis Clin North Am 20:343–360, 1994.
7. Plotz PH: Not myositis: A series of chance encounters. JAMA 268:2074–2077, 1992.
8. Tervaert JWC, Kallenberg C: Neurologic manifestations of systemic vasculitides. Rheum Dis Clin North Am 19:913–940, 1994.
9. Wolf PL: Abnormalities in serum enzymes in skeletal muscle diseases. Am J Clin Pathol 95:293–296, 1991.
10. Wortmann RL: Inflammatory disease of muscle. In Kelly WM, Harris ED, Ruddy S, Sledge CB (eds): Textbook of Rheumatology, 4th ed. Philadelphia, W.B. Saunders, 1993, pp 1159–1182.
11. Wortmann RL: Muscle disease symptoms: Evaluation and significance. Bull Rheum Dis 43(6):1–4, 1994.

17. HEALTH STATUS MEASUREMENTS

Sterling West, M.D.

1. What are the most important concerns of a patient with a newly diagnosed chronic rheumatic disease?
- Why did this happen to me?
- How well can my pain and other symptoms be controlled?
- Will I become disabled and lose the ability to be independent?

2. What should be the primary goal of health care for a patient with a chronic rheumatic disease?
The goal of health care for patients with any chronic disease is to maintain, or restore, the individual's ability to function successfully in personal, family, and community life.

3. How do physicians traditionally assess rheumatic disease activity and/or response to therapy?
History: How well is the patient doing compared to the last evaluation, including the amount of pain.
Physical examination: Number of tender and swollen joints; joint range of motion; document deformities; neuromuscular and other organ-specific examination.
Laboratory (sedimentation rate, other) and **radiographic** tests.
From this evaluation, the physician documents impairments (i.e., loss of range of motion, demonstrable deformities, others) and disease activity. This evaluation, however, does not necessarily tell the physician anything about the patient's functional disabilities.

4. How do you determine the overall functional status of a patient with a chronic rheumatic disease (or any chronic disease for that matter)?
In addition to a history, physical examination, and laboratory evaluation, other assessments that should be done include:
Physical function assessment
Psychological/cognitive function assessment
Social function assessment

5. What "open-ended" questions can you ask a rheumatic disease patient to get an idea of his or her functioning?
1. Are you able to do the things you want to?
2. What's the most difficult thing for you to do?
3. What do you need to do that you can't do or have difficulty doing?

4. What do you want to do that you can't do or have difficulty doing?
5. During a typical day, what limitations do you have to overcome?
6. How do you function in your family?
7. Do you have trouble sleeping and/or bathing?

6. What is involved in the assessment of physical function?
The assessment of physical function consists of evaluating the following areas:
- Ability to perform activities of daily living (ADLs)
- Recreational (avocational) or leisure-time activities
- Occupational (vocational) activities, including job, housework, and schoolwork
- Sexual activities
- Sleep

7. What aspects are assessed when evaluating a patient's ability to perform activities of daily living?
ADLs include the ability to do personal (self) care, which assesses upper-extremity function, as well as the ability to be mobile and ambulate, which assesses lower-extremity function.
Personal care assessment
    Bed/bedroom—bed activities and dressing
    Bathroom—toileting, bathing, grooming
    Kitchen—eating, cooking
    Other household activities—reaching, gripping
Mobility and ambulation assessment
    Walking
    Climbing stairs
    Transfers/rising from a seated or supine position

8. List the areas involved in the assessment of psychological function.
Cognitive function, affective function (depression, anxiety, mood), coping skills, compliance with treatment plan

9. Which areas are evaluated in the assessment of social function?
- Social support systems (with family, friends, and community)
- Interpersonal relationships (with family, friends, and community)
- Social integration (with family, friends, and community)
- Ability to fulfill social roles
- Family functioning
- Socioeconomic/financial

10. What methods can be used in clinical practice to assess a rheumatic disease patient's overall functioning?
Several multidimensional health status questionnaires have been developed that can measure simultaneously multiple areas of functional status and disease activity at one point in time. Many of these questionnaires can be filled out by the patient or administered by trained personnel and take only a few minutes to complete. These questionnaires can be used to identify functional disabilities that are a problem for the patient and need to be further evaluated and treated. They also can be administered over time to detect changes in clinical and functional status and to help assess how well a patient is responding to a specific therapy.

11. Name some multidimensional health status questionnaires commonly used to evaluate patients with chronic rheumatic diseases.
    General health status questionnaires
        Sickness Impact Profile (SIP)
        Medical Outcomes Study 36-Item Short-Form Health Survey (SF-36)

Rheumatic disease-specific questionnaires
Rheumatoid arthritis and/or osteoarthritis
Arthritis Impact Measurement Scales (AIMS 1 and 2)
Stanford Health Assessment Questionnaire (HAQ)
Modified HAQ (MHAQ)
McMaster-Toronto Arthritis Questionnaire (MACTAR)
Spondyloarthropathy
HAQ-Spond
Childhood rheumatic disorders
Juvenile HAQ
Systemic lupus erythematosus (SLE)
British Isles Lupus Assessment Group (BILAG) Index
SLE Disease Activity Index (SLEDAI)
SLE Activity Measure (SLAM)
Pain
Visual analogue pain scale (VAPS)
McGill Pain Questionnaire
Roland Disability in Low-Back Pain Questionnaire
The AIMS and HAQ have also been adapted for use in many rheumatic diseases other than rheumatoid arthritis. Some of these multidimensional health status questionnaires are available in foreign languages. Note that these questionnaires can identify functional limitations but cannot determine the *etiology* of that disability.

12. What are some problems with the use of multidimensional health status questionnaires in clinical practice?
- Intrapatient variability in filling out self-reported forms.
- Inter-rater variability in filling out forms administered to the same patient.
- Ability of questionnaires to detect change over time and agreement on what degree of change in score is significant clinically
- Length of time to administer

13. Describe the American College of Rheumatology criteria for classification of global functional status.
Class I: Able to perform usual ADLs (self-care, vocational, and avocational).
Class II: Able to perform usual self-care and vocational activities but limited in avocational activities.
Class III: Able to perform usual self-care activities but limited in vocational and avocational activities.
Class IV: Limited in ability to perform usual self-care, vocational, and avocational activities.
In this classification, a patient is assigned to a specific functional class by a physician depending on an evaluation.

BIBLIOGRAPHY

1. American College of Rheumatology Glossary Committee: Dictionary of the Rheumatic Diseases: Vol III. Health Status Measurement. Atlanta, American College of Rheumatology, 1988.
2. Calkins DR, Rubenstein LV, Cleary PD, et al: Failure of physicians to recognize functional disability in ambulatory patients. Ann Intern Med 114:451–454, 1991.
3. Hochberg MC, et al. The American College of Rheumatology 1991 revised criteria for classification of global functional status in rheumatoid arthritis. Arthritis Rheum 35:498–502, 1992.
4. Meenan RF: Health status assessment. In Schumacher HR Jr. (ed): Primer on the Rheumatic Diseases, 10th ed. Atlanta, Arthritis Foundation, 1993, pp 81–82.
5. Meenan RF, Mason JH, Anderson JJ, et al. AIMS 2: The content and properties of a revised and expanded Arthritis Impact Measurement Scales health status questionnaire. Arthritis Rheum 35:1–10, 1992.
6. Ramey DR, Raynauld JP, Fries JF: The Health Assessment Questionnaire 1991: Status and review. Arthritis Care Res 5:119–129, 1992.
7. Ware JE, Sherbourne CD: The Medical Outcomes Study 36-Item Short-Form Health Survey (SF-36): Conceptual framework and item selection. Med Care 30:473–483, 1992.
8. Wolfe F: Health status questionnaires. Rheum Dis Clin North Am 21:445–464, 1995.

18. PREOPERATIVE ASSESSMENT OF PATIENTS WITH RHEUMATIC DISEASE

Richard J. Shea, M.D.

1. Why is it important for rheumatic disease patients to be evaluated preoperatively?

In general, rheumatic disease patients who go to surgery do not have postoperative complications related to the procedure performed or the anesthetic used, but to exacerbations of antecedent medical conditions. Patients with rheumatic diseases can have unique problems because of advanced disease, complications of medical therapy, and limitations in functional status. The preoperative evaluation can identify those factors that may contribute to surgical risk so that appropriate action can be taken to avoid complications.

2. List the essential items to review in the preoperative evaluation of a patient with a rheumatic disease.

A comprehensive evaluation should include the "ABCDE'S":

    A—adjust medications
    B—bacterial prophylaxis
    C—cervical spine disease
    D—deep vein thrombosis prophylaxis
    E—evaluate extent and activity of disease
    S—stress-dose steroid coverage

3. How are patients "cleared" for surgery?

The term "clearance" was formerly used at a time when the goal of the preoperative assessment was to crudely divide patients into those able to tolerate surgery ("cleared") and those unable to tolerate surgery. The term is archaic since today patients are rarely excluded from being considered for an operative procedure on the basis of their underlying medical conditions, but they may be at increased risk for a complication. A more appropriate goal of the preoperative assessment is risk stratification.

4. What laboratory tests are routinely required for patients with rheumatic diseases scheduled for elective surgery?

As a minimum, a complete blood count, blood urea nitrogen, creatinine, and urinalysis with culture should be obtained on all patients. Other tests in *asymptomatic* patients include:

TEST	ORDER IN A PATIENT WITH:
Liver function tests	NSAID, gold, methotrexate use
Prothrombin time/partial thromboplastin time	Liver disease or bleeding disorder
	Antiphospholipid antibody syndrome
Electrocardiogram	Age > 40
	Coronary disease
Bleeding time	Controversial; possibly in recent NSAID users
Chest x-ray	Long-standing arthritis
	Pulmonary or cardiovascular disease
	Thoracic surgery
	Age > 60
Pulmonary function tests/arterial blood gases	Same as chest x-ray
Cervical spine x-ray	Rheumatoid arthritis, juvenile rheumatoid arthritis

5. Are patients with rheumatic diseases at increased risk for perioperative complications compared to other patients?

Patients with rheumatic diseases may have a higher incidence of postoperative wound infections and impaired wound healing than nonrheumatic patients, usually due to the medications used to treat their diseases.

6. Should rheumatoid patients with active synovitis be taken to elective surgery?

No. Postoperatively, patients with active synovitis will have significant pain from their arthritis, which can impair functional status, impede progress with rehabilitation, and prolong hospitalization. Patients with active synovial disease and its consequent disability should have the inflammation controlled as much as possible prior to elective surgical procedures.

7. Why is it important to evaluate patients with rheumatoid arthritis (RA) for cervical spine disease prior to surgery?

Instability of the cervical spine may be found in up to 25% of patients with RA awaiting elective surgical procedures. Proliferative synovitis along the articular surfaces of the cervical vertebrae can lead to erosion of surrounding bone and destruction or laxity of the supporting ligaments. In particular, **atlanto-axial subluxation** can occur due to weakening of the transverse ligament which holds the odontoid process of C2 against the anterior arch of C1. Manipulation of the neck during intubation and transport of the patient, especially extreme flexion or extension, can cause compression of the spinal cord by the odontoid process.

8. What factors increase the risk for cervical spine disease in patients with rheumatoid arthritis?

C—corticosteroid use
S—seropositive RA
P—peripheral joint destruction
I—involvement of cervical nerves (paresthesias, neck pain, weakness)
N—nodules (rheumatoid)
E—established disease (present > 10 ys)

Most anesthesiologists advocate preoperative radiographs for all RA patients, because significant disease may be present but asymptomatic.

9. How is atlanto-axial instability diagnosed?

Instability of C1–C2 is diagnosed when the odontoid process is found to be displaced > 3 mm from its normal position against the anterior arch of the atlas in the lateral flexion and extension radiographs.

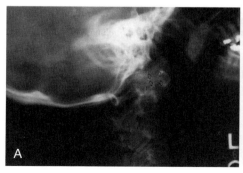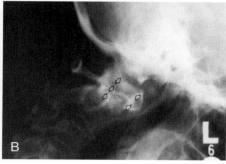

Atlanto-axial instability. Arrows show wide separation of the odontoid process of C2 from the anterior arch of C1 in extension (*panel A*) and flexion (*panel B*) in a patient with severe RA.

10. How are patients with cervical spine disease managed?
Symptomatic patients should have surgical stabilization performed before the planned procedure. Patients with asymptomatic or mild disease may be considered for intubation with fiberoptic assistance to minimize the extremes of motion associated with routine intubation. A soft cervical collar worn throughout the perioperative period will serve as a visual reminder that these patients should be handled with care, but it does not offer support to an unstable spine.

11. What is cricoarytenoid disease? How can it impact on anesthetic complications?
The cricoarytenoid (CA) joint is a true diarthrodial articulation and is subject to the same destructive changes that occur in other small joints in patients with RA. Proliferative synovium can spread across the articular surface of the CA joint during episodes of disease activity and impair the mobility of the vocal cords, giving symptoms of tracheal pain, dysphonia, stridor, dyspnea, and dysarthria. Other patients can have minor symptoms related to synovitis but over time develop fibrous replacement of the normal cartilage and ankylosis across the joint space. In the latter group, the diagnosis of CA disease may be clinically silent until attempts at endotracheal intubation by standard techniques result in trauma to the adducted vocal cords, with subsequent edema, inflammation, and airway obstruction.

12. Who is at risk for developing cricoarytenoid disease?
The degree of involvement correlates with the extent and activity of the peripheral joint disease. The prevalence of laryngeal abnormality noted by laryngoscopy is as high as 25%, though clinically significant disease is rare.

13. How is cricoarytenoid disease managed?
Preoperative fiberoptic laryngoscopy is recommended for all patients with symptoms of CA disease. Mild cases may be treated preoperatively with systemic steroids (prednisone, 20 mg orally three times daily) or injection of the CA joint with triamcinolone acetonide. Intubation under fiberscopic guidance is also recommended at the time of surgery. Patients with severe disease should be considered for elective tracheostomy if the vocal cords are found to be chronically adducted.

14. Should aspirin be discontinued preoperatively in rheumatic disease patients?
Patients treated with aspirin and salicylate-containing medications may be at risk for increased surgical bleeding, because these drugs impair platelet aggregation for the life of the platelet (7–10 days). However, the clinical significance of the excess blood loss and the ability of a preoperative bleeding time (BT) to predict it have been questioned. Regardless, it is the practice of most surgeons to recommend discontinuation of salicylate-containing medications 7–10 days prior to a planned surgical procedure. Short-acting NSAIDs (ibuprofen, 800 mg three times daily, held the day prior to surgery) or prednisone (5–10 mg daily) may be used to control disease activity during the perioperative period. Aspirin may be restarted 3–4 days postoperatively.

15. What about other nonsteroidal anti-inflammatory drugs (NSAIDs)?
NSAIDs affect platelet aggregation in the same way as aspirin, but their effects are reversible with discontinuation of the medicine. These drugs have also been associated with more frequent episodes of gastrointestinal bleeding when given perioperatively. All NSAIDs should be held preoperatively for a time equal to four to five half-lives of the drug to allow return of normal platelet function, and they may be restarted 2–3 days postoperatively (*See also* Chapter 84).

16. How does the normal adrenal gland respond to surgery?
In a baseline state, the adrenal gland secretes the equivalent of 30 mg of hydrocortisone (7.5 mg of prednisone) per day, but with stress, it may produce the equivalent of 200–400 mg of hydrocortisone (50–100 mg of prednisone) per 24-hour period. Cortisol levels typically peak within 24 hours of the time of surgical incision and return to normal after 72 hours if no other factors contribute to perioperative stress.

17. What causes perioperative adrenal insufficiency?
The administration of exogenous corticosteroids can interfere with the normal dynamics of the hypothalamic-pituitary-adrenal axis and blunt endogenous cortisol excretion. With stress, the

adrenal output may become inadequate to support physiologic demands, leading to hemodynamic instability, fever, nausea, and other signs of adrenal insufficiency. A routine part of the preoperative evaluation should be to consider whether the patient is at risk for adrenal insufficiency.

18. Who is at risk for adrenal insufficiency?
   1. Patients treated with daily administration of supraphysiologic doses of prednisone (> 10 mg) for > 1 week during the 12 months preceding surgery.
   2. Patients who overuse steroid inhalers to treat inflammatory lung disease.
   3. Rarely, patients who receive intra-articular steroid injections.

19. How can patients at risk for adrenal insufficiency be tested preoperatively?
The Cortrosyn (cosyntropin) stimulation test is a simple and reliable method to evaluate the adrenal gland's ability to respond to stress. After a baseline cortisol level is obtained, 25 units of Cortrosyn (an ACTH analogue) is injected intravenously, and a cortisol level is collected after 60 minutes. Patients with a normal hypothalamic-pituitary-adrenal axis should demonstrate a stimulated value of > 20 μg.

20. How are stress-dose steroids given?
Guidelines for steroid dosing in patients at risk for adrenal insufficiency are given below. Because the risks of coverage are minimal, and the complications avoided can be life-threatening, it is best to err on the side of safety when considering steroid administration.
   Major surgery
   100 mg hydrocortisone IV on call to the OR, *then*
   100 mg hydrocortisone IV q 6–8 hrs × 3 doses, *then*
   50 mg hydrocortisone IV q 6–8 hrs × 3 doses, *then*
   25 mg hydrocortisone IV q 6–8 hrs × 3 doses, *then* Stop.
   Minor surgery
   100 mg hydrocortisone IV on call to the OR, *then*
   100 mg hydrocortisone IV q 6–8 hrs for 24 hrs, *then* Stop.
   Elaborate tapering schedules are not required unless postoperative complications prolong stress after surgery. Patients on oral steroids preoperatively may resume their normal dose after this protocol is complete. The oral prednisone equivalent can be given once the patient can take oral medications (1 mg prednisone = 4 mg hydrocortisone).

21. Name the two most common organisms to infect a prosthetic joint at the time of surgery.
Staphylococcus aureus
Staphylococcus epidermidis

22. What is standard antibiotic prophylaxis for prosthetic joint surgery?
   • Cefazolin, 1 gm IV within 60 min of incision, then every 4–8 hrs during the procedure
   • Vancomycin, 1 gm IV every 12 hrs, in penicillin-allergic patients
Prophylactic antibiotics should not be continued for > 48 hours postoperatively.

23. Should patients who have prosthetic joints have antibiotic prophylaxis prescribed before undergoing dental procedures?
There is not yet a consensus among orthopedic surgeons, dentists, and primary care providers as to the utility of antibiotic prophylaxis during dental procedures in patients with prosthetic joints.
   For
   1. The risk of prosthetic joint infections is similar to that for prosthetic heart valves, in which prophylactic antibiotics have significantly reduced morbidity following dental procedures.
   2. Animal models confirm the occurrence of hematogenous seeding of prosthetic joints.
   3. Numerous case reports of prosthetic joint infections following dental procedures have been documented.
   4. Consequences of infection are severe, including removal of the prosthesis, prolonged sepsis, and death.
   5. Routine antibiotic administration would be cost-effective, even allowing for the cost of adverse drug reactions.

Against

1. Prosthetic joints are not similar to prosthetic heart valves in terms of their likelihood of being infected following dental manipulation, and there is no evidence to support routine prophylaxis.

2. The inoculum used during animal studies was large (half the animals died of septicemia or shock) and was not representative of the transient bacteremia induced by dental procedures.

3. A review by Thyne and Ferguson of the published cases of prosthetic joint infections thought secondary to dental procedures concluded that only one or two episodes fulfilled the criteria to establish causality, while the others were considerably less convincing.

4. Episodes of adverse reactions to antibiotics, including fatal anaphylaxis, would impose a risk of administration that would far outweigh the benefits of reduced numbers of infections.

5. Routine antibiotic administration to an unselected population would not be cost-effective.

I agree with the latter argument against the routine use of prophylaxis. However, it has been recognized that several clinical factors, including a history of RA, corticosteroid use, diabetes, and operations for prosthesis replacement, may increase the risk of prosthetic joint infection. Antibiotics prescribed for these select patients would probably provide benefit without excess risk. In the absence of good data, erythromycin, cephalexin, or cephradine, 1000 mg orally 1 hour before and 500 mg 4 hours after the procedure, appear to be rational choices.

24. What are the options for deep vein thrombosis prophylaxis in patients undergoing joint replacement procedures?

- Coumadin, 10 mg the day before surgery, then 5 mg the evening of surgery, then dose by sliding scale to a target prothrombin time of 16–18 sec (INR 2–3) until time of discharge
- Heparin, 3500 units subcutaneously prior to surgery, then 3500 units every 8 hrs after surgery, then adjust by sliding scale every other day to maintain the adjusted partial thromboplastin time at the upper limit of normal until discharge.
- Pneumatic compression devices, worn on the lower extremities at all times, until the patient is ambulatory or discharged.

Low-molecular weight heparins are still under investigation.

25. Should cytotoxic/remittive agents be stopped prior to elective surgery?

Data and Recommendations on Remittive Agents in the Perioperative Period

DRUG	TOXICITY	INCREASED INFECTION	WOUND HEALING	RECOMMEND
Hydroxychloroquine	Retina	No data: unlikely	No data: unlikely	Continue when patient is eating
Oral gold	Gastrointestinal, hematologic, renal, rare hepatic	No data	No data	Continue when patient is eating
Intramuscular gold	Hematologic, renal, pulmonary, skin, hepatic	No data	No data	Continue
Penicillamine	Hematologic, renal, pulmonary, rare myasthenia gravis	No data	Data conflict	? Hold 1–2 wks; no data
Methotrexate	Hepatic, hematologic, pulmonary	Maybe*	Maybe*	Continue; if very concerned, then hold 1 wk preoperatively and restart 1 wk postoperatively

From Sorokin R: Management of the Patient with Rheumatic Diseases Going to Surgery. Philadelphia, W.B. Saunders, 1993, p 456; with permission.

Most drugs are safe to continue perioperatively. Several studies suggest that methotrexate should be discontinued 1–4 weeks before a planned procedure. This is a reasonable strategy if the patient's disease can be controlled during this time with the addition of NSAIDs or low-dose prednisone. I recommend discontinuation of methotrexate the week of surgery and the week after surgery.

26. A patient with RA is found to have a swollen, warm, and tender knee on postoperative day 4 after a cholecystectomy. Should the patient have an arthrocentesis performed?
Yes. An acutely inflamed joint postoperatively should always be aspirated to exclude a septic joint. Do not assume that the symptoms are due to a flare of RA, especially if the involved joint seems "out of synch" with the rest of the patient's disease activity.

27. A patient with chronic tophaceous gout has the acute onset of left knee pain and swelling postoperatively. Aspiration reveals negatively birefringent needle-shaped crystals. Can you be certain of the diagnosis of acute gouty arthritis?
Not yet. Patients with chronic gout can have uric acid crystals seen on synovial fluid aspirated from an asymptomatic joint, and so in this case their presence is not diagnostic. Sepsis and gout can also occur simultaneously, so Gram stain and culture of the fluid are mandatory.

28. What predisposes patients to postoperative gout attacks?
Dehydration
Increased uric acid production due to adenosine triphosphate breakdown (energy utilization) during surgery.
Medicines (diuretics, heparin, cyclosporine)
Minor trauma to the joint during surgery and transport
Infections
Hyperalimentation
Surgical stress

29. What are the options for treating patients with acute gouty arthritis postoperatively when they are NPO?
- Indomethacin, 50 mg three times daily per nasogastric tube or suppositories per rectum.
- Colchicine, 2 mg in 20 ml of normal saline, infused over 20 min. May repeat with 1 mg every 6 hrs for two additional doses. (No oral colchicine for 7 days after intravenous use.) Reduce the colchicine dose if renal or liver disease is present.
- ACTH, 20 units intravenous slowly, or 40 units intramuscularly.
- Triamcinolone acetonide, 40 mg intramuscularly.
- Triamcinolone preparation injected into the joint if you are sure it is not infected.

BIBLIOGRAPHY

1. Antimicrobial prophylaxis in surgery. Med Lett Drugs Ther 34:5–8, 1992.
2. Connelly CS, Panush RS: Should nonsteroidal anti-inflammatory drugs be stopped before elective surgery? Arch Intern Med 151:1963–1966, 1991.
3. Dockery KM, Sismanis A, Abedi E: Rheumatoid arthritis of the larynx: The importance of early diagnosis and corticosteroid therapy. South Med J 84:95–96, 1991.
4. Goldman DR: Surgery in patients with endocrine dysfunction. Med Clin North Am 71:499–509, 1987.
5. Merli GJ, Weitz HH (eds): Medical Management of the Surgical Patient. Philadelphia, W.B. Saunders, 1992.
6. Schneller S: Medical considerations for perioperative care for rheumatoid surgery. Hand Clin 5:115–126, 1989.
7. Segreti J: The role of prophylactic antibiotics in the prevention of prosthetic device infections. Infect Dis Clin North Am 3:357–370, 1989.
8. Sorokin R: Management of the patient with rheumatic diseases going to surgery. Med Clin North Am 77:453–464, 1993.
9. Thyne GM, Ferguson JW: Antibiotic prophylaxis during dental treatment in patients with prosthetic joints. J Bone Joint Surg Br 73B:191–194, 1991.
10. White RH: Preoperative evaluation of patients with rheumatoid arthritis. Semin Arthritis Rheum 14:287–299, 1985.

IV. Systemic Connective Tissue Diseases

The wolf, I'm afraid, is inside tearing up the place.
Letter to Sister Mariella Gable from Flannery O'Connor, a
sufferer of systemic lupus erythematosus, July 5, 1964

[P.S.] Prayers requested. I am sick of being sick.
Letter to Louise Abbot from Flannery O'Connor, May 28,
1964

19. RHEUMATOID ARTHRITIS

James O'Dell, M.D.

1. What is rheumatoid arthritis?

Rheumatoid arthritis (RA) is a chronic, systemic, inflammatory disorder of unknown etiology that is characterized by its pattern of diarthrodial joint involvement. Its primary site of pathology is the synovium of the joints. The synovial tissues become inflamed and proliferate, forming **pannus** which invades bone, cartilage, and ligament and leads to damage and deformities. Rheumatoid factor positivity and extra-articular manifestations commonly accompany the joint disease, but arthritis represents the major manifestation.

2. List the criteria for the classification of RA.

The 1987 Revised Criteria for the Classification of Rheumatoid Arthritis

1. Morning stiffness in and around joints lasting at least 1 hour before maximal improvement*
2. Soft-tissue swelling (arthritis) of 3 or more joint areas observed by a physician*
3. Swelling (arthritis) of the proximal interphalangeal (PIP), metacarpophalangeal (MCP), or wrist joints*
4. Symmetric arthritis*
5. Subcutaneous nodules
6. Positive test for rheumatoid factor (RF)
7. Radiographic erosions or periarticular osteopenia in hand or wrist joints

*Present for at least 6 weeks.
From Arnett FC, Edworthy SM, Bloch DA, et al: The American Rheumatism Association 1987 revised criteria for the classification of rheumatoid arthritis. Arthritis Rheum 31:315–324, 1988, with permission.

To be classified as having RA, a patient must meet 4 or more criteria. The criteria demonstrate a 92% sensitivity and 89% specificity for RA when compared to control subjects with non-RA rheumatic disease. These new criteria also have been used to diagnose of RA (controversial).

It is important to point out that the first five criteria are all obtained by history or physical examination. Thus, the diagnosis of RA is an extremely clinical one. Most patients with RA have a **symmetric polyarthritis** involving the small joints of the hands (MCPs, PIPs), wrists, and frequently the feet metatarsophalangeals, (MTPs). Up to 85% of patients are RF-positive (titer ≥1:160), and most develop periarticular erosions of the small joints within the first 2 years of disease.

3. What other diseases should be excluded before making the diagnosis of RA?
Common diseases

Seronegative spondylarthropathies	Calcium pyrophosphate deposition disease
Connective tissue diseases (SLE, sclero- derma, polymyositis, vasculitis, MCTD, polymyalgia rheumatica	Osteoarthritis Viral infection (paravovirus, rubella, hepatitis B, etc.)
Polyarticular gout`	Fibromyalgia

Uncommon diseases

Hypothyroidism	Relapsing polychondritis
Subacute bacterial endocarditis	Rheumatic fever
Hemochromatosis	Sarcoidosis
Hypertrophic pulmonary osteoarthropathy	Lyme disease
Hyperlipoproteinemias (types II, IV)	Amyloid arthropathy
Hemoglobinopathies	

Rare diseases

Familial Mediterranean fever	Whipple's disease
Multicentric reticulohistiocytosis	Angioimmunoblastic lymphadenopathy

A clinician should consider a diagnosis other than RA particularly in patients who have an asymmetric arthritis, predominantly large-joint arthritis, back disease, renal disease, RF-negative status, leukopenia, hypocomplementemia, or no erosions on radiographs after many months of disease.

4. Discuss the epidemiologic characteristics of RA.
- Race—worldwide, all races
- Sex distribution—females >males 3:1
- Age—peak age 35–45 years old
- Occurs in about 1% of adults in the United States. The prevalence increases with age.

5. Is RA a genetic disease?
RA is definitely associated with HLA-DR4 and, to a lesser extent, HLA-DR1 positivity. Over 90% of patients have one of these HLA antigens, especially those patients with severe disease (extra-articular features, those requiring joint replacement surgery, etc.). Patients who are homozygous or complex heterozygous for these so-called at-risk alleles have the most severe disease.

However, HLA-DR4 positivity also occurs in 20–30% of the general population, and therefore genetics does not completely explain the pathogenesis of RA. Other factors must be present for the disease to develop. These other factors or triggers are not well understood but are the subject of active research and debate.

6. How does RA usually have its onset?
It usually has a subacute (20%) or insidious (70%) onset with arthritic symptoms of pain, swelling, and stiffness, with the number of joints involved increasing over weeks to months. About 10% of patients have an acutely severe onset, and a few start with episodic symptoms that progress to persistent disease.

7. Which joints are commonly affected in RA?

Most Common Joints Involved During the Course of RA

MCP	90–95%	Ankle/subtalar	50–80%
Wrist	80–90%	Cervical spine (esp. C1–2)	40–50%
PIP	65–90%	Hip	40–50%
Knee	60–80%	Elbow	40–50%
MTP	50–90%	Temporomandibular	20–30%
Shoulder	50–60%		

The joints most commonly involved *first* are the MCPs, PIPs, wrists, and MTPs. Larger joints generally become symptomatic after small joints. Patients may start out with only a few joints involved (oligoarticular onset) but progress to involvement of multiple joints (polyarticular) in **symmetric distribution** within a few weeks to months.

Involvement of the thoracolumbar, sacroiliac, or hand distal interphalangeal (DIP) joints is very rare in RA and should suggest another diagnosis, such as a seronegative spondyloarthropathy (sacroiliac joints), psoriatic arthritis (DIP joints), or osteoarthritis (lumbar spine, DIP joints).

8. What is meant by symmetrical involvement of joints?

The most obvious meaning is that both sides of the body are involved similarly. Additionally, in RA, the whole joint surface is involved, as compared with osteoarthritis which usually involves only the weight-bearing areas of the joint.

9. What is pannus?

The synovium is the primary site for the inflammatory process in RA. The inflammatory infiltrate consists of mononuclear cells, primarily T lymphocytes, as well as activated macrophages and plasma cells (some making RF). The synovial cells proliferate, and the inflamed synovium becomes boggy and edematous and develops villous projections. This proliferative synovium is called **pannus**, and it is capable of invading bone and cartilage, causing destruction of the joint.

It is important to note that few if any polymorphonuclear leukocytes (PMNs) are found in the synovium, whereas the predominant cell in the inflammatory synovial fluid of RA patients is the PMN. Degradative enzymes from these synovial fluid PMNs also contribute to destruction of the joint cartilage.

10. What are the common deformities of the hand in RA?

Fusiform swelling—Synovitis of PIP joints, causing them to appear spindle-shaped.

Boutonniere deformity—Flexion of the PIP and hyperextension of the DIP joint, caused by weakening of the central slip of the extrinsic extensor tendon and a palmar displacement of the lateral bands. This deformity resembles a knuckle being pushed through a buttonhole.

Swan-neck deformity—Results from contraction of the flexors of the MCPs, resulting in flexion contracture of the MCP joint, hyperextension of PIP, and flexion of the DIP joint.

Ulnar deviation of fingers with subluxation of MCP joints.

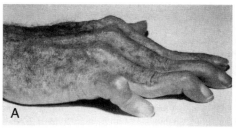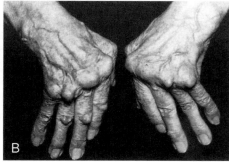

A, Swan neck (2nd to 4th fingers) and boutonniere (5th finger) deformities. *B*, Ulnar deviation of fingers (note rheumatoid nodules). (From the Revised Clinical Slide Collection on the Rheumatic Diseases. Atlanta, American College of Rheumatology, 1991; with permission.)

11. What are the most common the deformities seen in the foot in RA?

Inflammation of the MTP joints leads to subluxation of the metatarsal heads and ultimately to the most common deformity in the foot of RA patients: the **claw toe**, or **hammer toe** deformity. When this problem occurs, the patient has problems fitting his or her toes into the shoe because the tops of the toes rub on the shoe box, which results in callous or ulcer formation. Additionally, because the soft tissue pad that normally sits underneath the metatarsal heads is displaced, the heads of the metatarsal bones are no longer cushioned and become very painful to walk on, frequently resulting in calluses on the inferior surface of the foot (patients complain that it feels as though they are walking on pebbles or stones). Arthritic involvement of the tarsal joint and subtalar joint can result in flattening of the arch of the foot and hindfoot valgus deformity.

12. **Describe the radiographic features of RA.**
   The mnemonic **ABCDE'S** is a convenient way to remember these:
   A—Abnormal *alignment*; no *ankylosis*
   B—*Bones*—periarticular (juxta-articular) osteoporosis; no periostitis or osteophytes
   C—*Cartilage*—uniform (symmetric) joint-space loss in weight-bearing joints; no cartilage or soft tissue calcification
   D—*Deformities* (swan neck, ulnar deviation, boutonniere) with symmetrical distribution
   E—Marginal *erosions*
   S—*Soft-tissue swelling;* nodules without calcification
   The radiographic changes in RA take months to develop. Juxta-articular osteopenia is seen early in the course of the disease, followed later by more diffuse osteopenia. Joint erosions typically occur at the margins of small joints. Later, joint-space narrowing and deformities develop.

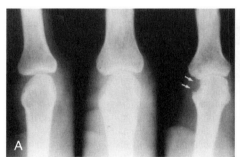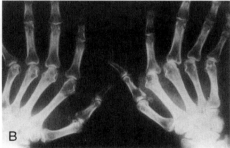

A, Progressive marginal erosions (*arrows*) of an MCP joint. *B*, MCP joints demonstrate erosions, joint-space narrowing, and ulnar deviation. From the Revised Clinical Slide Collection on the Rheumatic Diseases. Atlanta, American College of Rheumatology, 1991; with permission.

13. **Compare the radiographic features of RA with those of osteoarthritis (OA).**

	RA	OA
Sclerosis	±	++++
Osteophytes	±	++++
Osteopenia	+++	0
Symmetry	+++	+
Erosions	+++	0
Cysts	++	++
Narrowing	+++	+++

14. **What are the typical features of the synovial fluid in RA?**
The synovial fluid is inflammatory, with WBC counts typically between 5,000–50,000/mm^3. Generally the differential shows a predominance (> 50%) of PMNs. The protein level is elevated, and the glucose level may be low compared to serum values (40–60% of serum glucose). There are no crystals in the fluid, and cultures are negative. Unfortunately, there are no specific findings in the synovial fluid that allow a definitive diagnosis of RA.

15. How is the cervical spine involved in RA?
The cervical spine is involved in 30–50% of the RA patients. All levels can be involved, but C1–2 is the most commonly involved level. Because arthritic involvement of the cervical spine can lead to instability with potential impingement of the spinal cord, it is important for the clinician to obtain radiographs of the cervical spine prior to surgical procedures that may require intubation. The patterns of cervical spine involvement include:

C1–2 involvement (20–40% of patients)
- Anterior atlantoaxial subluxation resulting in >3 mm between the arch of C1 and the odontoid of C2. This is caused by synovial proliferation around the articulation of the odontoid process with the anterior arch of C1. This leads to stretching and rupture of the transverse ligament and alar ligaments, which keep the odontoid in contact with the arch of C1.
- Vertical atlantoaxial subluxation occurs due to collapse of the lateral articulations between C1 and C2. This causes settling of the arch downward with upward migration of the odontoid. The odontoid can impinge on the brainstem. Although this occurs in less than 5% of RA patients, it has the worst prognosis neurologically.
- Lateral atlantoaxial (rotary) subluxation occurs with collapse of one of the lateral articular masses between C1 and C2, leading to rotation of C1 on C2 and a head tilt.
- Posterior atlantoaxial subluxation

Subaxial involvement (10–20% of patients)
- Subaxial subluxation occurring at one or more levels leading to a stepladder appearance. This is due to arthritic involvement of the facet joints. The C2–3 and C3–4 levels are most commonly involved.
- Vertebral endplate erosions and disc-space narrowing. This rheumatoid discitis is due to pannus eroding into the disc from the joints of Luschka.

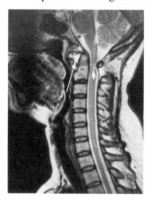

MRI of the cervical spine demonstrating pannus formation of the C1–2 articulation (*long arrow*) and impingement of the odontoid on the spinal cord (*arrow*).

16. What are the typical findings of the complete blood count in RA patients?
Most patients with active RA have an anemia of chronic disease. The severity of the anemia correlates with the activity of the disease, so that if therapy for the RA is successful, the anemia often improves. Platelet counts are often elevated in RA patients and again correlate with the activity of the disease. WBC counts are generally normal but may be low in patients with Felty's syndrome.

17. Which laboratory tests correlate with activity of disease?
Clearly, the degree of **anemia** and the degree of **thrombocytosis** may correlate with the activity of the disease. However, the best correlation is found with the **erythrocyte sedimentation rate** (ESR) and **C-reactive protein**. When choosing a laboratory test to follow in patients with RA, you would probably select one of these indicators, keeping in mind that both are very nonspecific.

18. What is rheumatoid factor? How commonly is it found in RA patients?
RF is a series of antibodies that recognize the Fc portion of an IgG molecule as their antigen. RFs can be of any isotype (IgM, IgG, IgA, IgE), but their distinguishing feature is the recogni-

tion of IgG as their antigen. Most of the RFs that are measured clinically are, in fact, IgM RFs. Teleologically, RFs probably developed in humans as a mechanism to help remove immune complexes from the circulation. Therefore, many conditions associated with chronic inflammation are also associated with RF positivity. In RA patients, approximately 70% are RF-positive at disease onset, and an additional 10–15% (overall 85%) become RF-positive over the first 2 years after onset.

19. What is the significance of RF in RA patients?
RF positivity is associated with more severe disease, with extra-articular manifestations including subcutaneous nodules, and with increased mortality.

20. Are antinuclear antibodies (ANAs) found in patients with RA?
About 25% of RA patients have ANA, but these ANAs are not directed against any of the antigens typically tested for in the ANA profile (SS-A, SS-B, Sm, RNP, DNA). These patients with ANAs tend to have more severe disease and a poorer prognosis than RA patients who are ANA-negative.

21. Are complement levels abnormal in RA?
C3, C4, and CH50 levels are usually normal or elevated. Hypocomplementemia is rare and seen only in patients with severe vasculitis associated with RA.

22. List some of the extra-articular manifestations of RA.

General	**Cardiac**
Fever	Pericarditis
Lymphadenopathy	Myocarditis
Weight loss	Coronary vasculitis
Fatigue	Nodules on valves
Dermatologic	**Neuromuscular**
Palmar erythema	Entrapment neuropathy
Subcutaneous nodules	Peripheral neuropathy
Vasculitis	Mononeuritis multiplex
Ocular	**Hematologic**
Episcleritis	Felty's syndrome
Scleritis	Large granular lymphocyte syndrome
Choroid and retinal nodules	Lymphomas
Pulmonary	**Others**
Pleuritis	Sjögren's syndrome
Nodules	Amyloidosis
Interstitial lung disease	
Bronchiolitis obliterans	
Arteritis	

23. Which patients with RA are most likely to get extra-articular manifestations?
Patients who are RF-positive or HLA-DR4-positive are more likely to have extra-articular manifestations. It is important for clinicians to rule out other causes (infection, malignancy, medications, etc.) for an extra-articular manifestation before ascribing it to RA, especially if the patient is RF-negative.

24. How commonly do fever and lymphadenopathy occur in RA patients?
They are uncommon and generally seen only in those patients with severely active disease. Infection and lymphoreticular malignancy should always be considered in an RA patient with these symptoms.

25. What are rheumatoid nodules? Where are they found?
Rheumatoid nodules are subcutaneous nodules that have the characteristic histology of a central area of fibrinoid necrosis surrounded by a zone of palisades of elongated histiocytes and a pe-

ripheral layer of cellular connective tissue. They occur in about 20–35% of RA patients, who typically are RF-positive and have severe disease. They tend to occur on the extensor surface of the forearms, in the olecranon bursa, over joints, and over pressure points. They frequently develop and enlarge when the patient's RA is active and may resolve when disease activity is controlled. Methotrexate therapy has caused increased nodulosis in some RA patients, even when the disease is well-controlled.

26. Which diseases should be considered in a patient with subcutaneous nodules and arthritis?

Rheumatoid arthritis	Xanthoma
Gouty tophi	SLE (rare)
Amyloidosis	Rheumatic fever (rare)
Sarcoidosis	

27. Which cutaneous disorder can cause lesions that pathologically are similar to rheumatoid nodules?

Granuloma annulare lesions have been called "benign" rheumatoid nodules. Patients with granuloma annulare do not have arthritis and are RF-negative.

28. What are the ocular manifestations of RA?

Both episcleritis and scleritis can occur as extra-articular manifestations of RA. If scleral inflammation persists, scleral thinning and scleromalacia perforans can occur. Sicca symptoms of dry eyes frequently accompany coexistent Sjögren's syndrome.

29. Discuss the pulmonary manifestations of RA.

Pleural disease: Pleurisy and pleural effusions can occasionally be the first manifestations of RA. Pleural effusions are characterized as cellular exudates with high protein and lactate dehydrogenase levels, a low glucose level, and frequently a low pH (suggesting an infection).

Nodules: Rheumatoid nodules in the lung may be solitary or multiple and can cavitate or resolve spontaneously. Caplan's syndrome involves multiple rheumatoid nodules occurring in the lungs of RA patients who are coal miners.

Interstitial fibrosis: Fibrosing alveolitis occurs commonly in RA patients but is symptomatic and progressive in <10%. Patients can have progressive dyspnea, Velcro rales, and fibrosis primarily in the lower lobes on chest radiography.

Bronchiolitis obliterans: Patients have dyspnea, hyperinflated chest x-ray, and small airways obstruction on pulmonary function tests. This condition can be rapidly fatal. Penicillamine therapy has occasionally been associated with causing this disease.

30. Why is the glucose level low in RA pleural effusions?

There is a defect in the transport of glucose across the pleura into the fluid.

31. What are the clinical consequences of the cardiac manifestations of RA?

Pericarditis	Pain (1% of RA patients)
	Tamponade (rare)
	Constriction (uncommon)
Nodules	Conduction abnormalities
	Valvular problems
Coronary arteritis	Myocardial infarction
Myocarditis	Congestive heart failure

Pericarditis is the most common cardiac manifestation of RA. It usually manifests as asymptomatic pericardial effusions which may be found by echocardiography in up to 50% of patients. These effusions are rarely large enough to cause tamponade but may result in constrictive pericarditis late in the course of the disease. RA may also cause nodules to form in and around the heart, leading to conduction defects and occasionally valvular insufficiency.

32. Which types of vasculitis occur in RA patients?

Vasculitis most commonly occurs in RA patients with long-standing disease, significant joint involvement, high-titer RF, and nodules. The types of vasculitis are:

- **Leukocytoclastic vasculitis**—Usually presents as palpable purpura and results from inflammation of postcapillary venules.
- **Small arteriolar vasculitis**—Presents as small infarcts of digital pulp and frequently is associated with a mild distal sensory neuropathy caused by vasculitis of vasa nervorum.
- **Medium-vessel vasculitis**—Can resemble polyarteritis nodosa with visceral arteritis, mononeuritis multiplex, and livedo reticularis.
- **Pyoderma gangrenosum**

33. What three findings make up the classic triad of Felty's syndrome?

Rheumatoid arthritis in combination with **splenomegaly** and **leukopenia.** Felty's syndrome is usually seen in RA patients who have RF and subcutaneous nodules as well as other extra-articular manifestations. Almost all patients are HLA-DR4 positive. The leukopenia in Felty's is generally a neutropenia ($<2000/mm^3$). The major complications of Felty's syndrome include bacterial infections and chronic nonhealing leg ulcers. Severe bacterial infections correlate with WBC counts of $<100/mm^3$. Additionally, thrombocytopenia may occur.

Most patients with Felty's syndrome do not require treatment other than that indicated for their joint disease. However, if severe, recurrent bacterial infections or chronic nonhealing leg ulcers develop, splenectomy may be indicated. Unfortunately, neutropenia and infections may recur despite splenectomy.

34. What other clinical problems occur with increased frequency in RA patients?

Sjögren's syndrome—Up to 20–30% of RA patients develop secondary Sjögren's syndrome with dry eyes and dry mouth. They typically do not have the anti-SS-A or SS-B antibodies commonly seen in primary Sjögren's syndrome.

Amyloidosis—Up to 5% of RA patients develop secondary or AA-associated amyloidosis. This occurs in long-standing, poorly controlled RA and usually presents as nephrotic syndrome.

Osteoporosis—Seen in the majority of RA patients and related to disease activity, immobility, and medications. Insufficiency fractures of the spine, sacrum, and other areas are common in long-standing disease.

Entrapment neuropathy—Median nerve (carpal tunnel), posterior tibial nerve (tarsal tunnel), ulnar nerve (cubital tunnel), and posterior interosseous branch of the radial nerve are most commonly involved.

Laryngeal manifestations—Cricoarytenoid arthritis can present as pain, dysphagia, hoarseness, and rarely, stridor.

Ossicles of ear—Tinnitus and decreased hearing.

Renal and gastrointestinal involvement—Rare. Usually abnormalities are due to NSAIDs causing renal insufficiency or gastric ulcers with hemorrhage. Other medications, such as gold and penicillamine, can cause a membranous nephropathy with significant proteinuria.

35. Are patients with RA at increased risk for joint infections?

Unfortunately, yes. Joint infections tend to occur in abnormal joints, and RA patients have lots of these. Any time an RA patient presents with one or two joints that are swollen, red, and hot, out of proportion to the other joints, the clinician should suspect infection. In addition, following joint replacement surgeries, an infected artificial joint is a constant concern. The most common infecting organism is *Staphylococcus aureus*.

36. Do any markers help predict if an RA patient will have severe disease and a poor prognosis?

1. Generalized polyarthritis involving both small and large joints (>10–20 total joints)
2. Extra-articular disease, especially nodules and vasculitis

3. Persistently elevated ESR or C-reactive protein accompanied by active synovitis
4. RF-positive
5. Radiographic erosions within 2 years of disease onset
6. HLA-DR4 genetic marker
7. Education level <11th grade
8. Health Assessment Questionnaire (HAQ) score >1

37. Discuss the management principles for the initial treatment of RA.

The approach to treatment of RA has changed dramatically over the past decade. It is now recognized that the long-term prognosis for RA patients is poor and warrants the institution of aggressive therapy within the first few months of onset of RA. Clearly, delaying treatment results in a poorer long-term outcome.

Most if not all RA patients should initially receive symptomatic treatment with NSAIDs. Many also receive low-dose ($\leq$5–7.5 mg/day) prednisone. Physical therapy, occupational therapy, rest, patient education, and calcium supplementation to prevent osteoporosis are also part of the initial management (For rehabilitative techniques, see Chapter 90.)

38. What if the patient does not improve on NSAIDs?

Patients with mild RA who do not respond adequately to symptomatic therapy, as well as RA patients with poor prognostic markers, are candidates for disease-modifying antirheumatic drugs (DMARDs). Hydroxychloroquine, minocycline, and sulfasalazine are used for mild RA because they are least toxic, although they are also less potent. Methotrexate, intramuscular gold, and, less often, penicillamine are used for more aggressive disease. Azathioprine, cyclosporine, and combinations of DMARDs (hydroxychloroquine–azulfidine–methotrexate, cyclosporine–methotrexate, or other combinations) are used for the most severe disease or for RA that has failed other therapy. The use of a combination of DMARDs early in the disease course is beginning to be used more commonly.

39. Which clinical and laboratory parameters are most useful to determine response to therapy?

Total number of swollen and tender joints
Patient's perception of how he or she is doing in terms of pain (use visual analogue scales as a measure)
Health assessment measurement — HAQ, AIMS (see Chapter 17)
ESR or C-reactive protein level
Patient's perception of how he or she is doing overall
Physician's assessment of how the patient is doing overall
A meaningful response to therapy is improvement of at least 20% and preferably 50% in the number of tender and swollen joints, plus improvement in at least three of the remaining five categories.

40. What is the long-term prognosis for RA patients?

RA is clearly a disease that shortens survival and produces significant disability. Approximately 50% of patients will be functional Class III or IV within 10 years of disease onset. Over 33% of RA patients who were working at the time of onset of their disease will leave the workforce within 5 years. In addition, the standardized mortality ratio is 2–2.5 to 1 compared to people of same sex and age without RA. Overall, RA shortens the lifespan of patients by 5–10 years. The patients with a poorer long-term outcome can be identified by prognostic markers (see Question 35). Aggressive DMARD therapy can reduce disability by 30% over 10–20 years.

41. What causes the increased mortality in RA patients?

- Cardiovascular — 42%. Frequency, however, is not increased over the general population.
- Infections (especially pneumonias) — 9%. Increased five times over that in the general population.

- Cancer and lymphoproliferative malignancies—14%. Increased five to eight times over the rate in the general population.
- Others, including renal disease due to amyloidosis, gastrointestinal hemorrhage due to NSAIDs (4%), and RA complications (5%).

42. What is "seronegative" RA?

It is one term to identify patients who are thought to have RA but are RF-negative. In general, RA patients who are RF-negative have a better prognosis, fewer extra-articular manifestations, and better survival. Additionally, a number of these patients over time will, in fact, be found to have some other disease. Thus, when dealing with seronegative RA patients, the clinician should always look for the possibility of psoriatic arthritis, lupus arthritis, crystal deposition disease, gout, hemochromatosis, or another form of arthritis other than RA.

43. What is the RS_3PE syndrome?

A syndrome characterized by the acute severe onset of symmetrical synovitis of the small joints of the hands, wrists, and flexor tendon sheaths accompanied by pitting edema of the dorsum of the hand (''boxing-glove'' hand). Other joints may be involved. This syndrome affects mostly elderly (mean age 70) white men (M/F ratio 4:1). All patients are RF-negative. Symptoms do not respond to NSAIDs but are very sensitive to low-dose prednisone and hydroxychloroquine. Bony erosions do not occur. The disease predictably remits in <36 months and, unlike RA, does not recur after withdrawal of medications.

BIBLIOGRAPHY

1. Bacon PA: Extra-articular rheumatoid arthritis. In McCarty DJ, Koopman WJ (eds): Arthritis and Allied Conditions, 12th ed. Philadelphia, Lea & Febiger, 1993, pp 811–840.
2. Felson DT, Anderson JJ, Boers M, et al: American College of Rheumatology preliminary definition of improvement in rheumatoid arthritis. Arthritis Rheum 38:727–735, 1995.
3. Fries JF, Williams CA, Morfeld D, et al: Reduction in long-term disability in patients with rheumatoid arthritis by disease-modifying antirheumatic drug-based treatment strategies. Arthritis Rheum 39:616–622, 1996.
4. Harris ED: Clinical features of rheumatoid arthritis. In Kelley WK, Harris ED, Ruddy S, Sledge CB (eds): Textbook of Rheumatology, 4th ed. Philadelphia, W.B. Saunders, 1993, pp 874–911.
5. Hochberg MC, Chang RW, Dwosh I, et al: The American College of Rheumatology 1991 revised criteria for the classification of global functional status in rheumatoid arthritis. Arthritis Rheum 35:498–502, 1992.
6. Kirwan JR: The effect of glucocorticoids on joint destruction in rheumatoid arthritis. N Engl J Med 333:142–146, 1995.
7. McCarty DJ, O'Duffy JD, Pearson L, Hunter JB: Remitting seronegative symmetrical synovitis with pitting edema (RS_3PE) syndrome. JAMA 254:2763–2767, 1985.
8. O'Dell JR, Haire CE, Erikson N, et al: Treatment of rheumatoid arthritis with methotrexate alone, sulfasalazine and hydroxychloroquine, or a combination of all three medications. N Engl J Med 334:1287–1291, 1996.
9. Pincus T, Brooks RH, Callahan LF: Prediction of long-term mortality in patients with rheumatoid arthritis according to simple questionnaire and joint count measures. Ann Intern Med 120:26–34, 1994.
10. Tilley BC, Alarcon GS, Heyse SP, et al: Minocycline in rheumatoid arthritis. Ann Intern Med 122:81–89, 1995.
11. Tugwell P, Pincus T, Yocum D, et al: Combination therapy with cyclosporin and methotrexate in severe rheumatoid arthritis. N Engl J Med 333:137–141, 1995.
12. Wolfe F, Mitchell DM, Sibley JT, et al: The mortality of rheumatoid arthritis. Arthritis Rheum 37:481–494, 1994.

20. SYSTEMIC LUPUS ERYTHEMATOSUS

Brian L. Kotzin, M.D.

1. Who is the typical patient with systemic lupus erythematosus (SLE)?
The typical patient is a female between the ages of 15 and 45 years. Although SLE can occur at nearly any age, the incidence of disease clearly increases in women of child-bearing age. The female-to-male ratio during these ages may be >8:1, but during childhood or after the menopause, the ratio is closer to 2:1. This pattern strongly suggests that sex hormones influence the probability of developing or expressing SLE, a conclusion that is supported by studies in animal models of lupus. It should be emphasized that although males develop disease less frequently, their illness is not milder than in females. Also, the incidence of SLE is about 2–4 times greater in blacks and hispanics than in whites in the United States.

2. Describe the criteria used in the classification of SLE.
Any person having 4 or more of the following 11 criteria, serially or simultaneously, during any interval of observation is considered to have SLE for the purposes of clinical studies.

CRITERION	DEFINITION
1. Malar rash	Fixed erythema, flat or raised over the malar eminences, tending to spare the nasolabial folds.
2. Discoid rash	Erythematous raised patches with adherent keratotic scaling and follicular plugging; atrophic scarring may occur in older lesions
3. Photosensitivity	Skin rash as a result of unusual reaction to sunlight, by patient history or physician observation
4. Oral ulcers	Oral or nasopharyngeal ulceration, usually painless, observed by a physician
5. Arthritis	Nonerosive arthritis involving two or more peripheral joints, characterized by tenderness, swelling, or effusion
6. Serositis	Pleuritis: convincing history of pleuritic pain or rub heard by physician or evidence of pleural effusion, *or* Pericarditis documented by EKG or rub or evidence of pericardial effusion
7. Renal disorder	Persistent proteinuria >0.5 gm/day or >3+ if quantitation not performed, *or* Cellular casts (red cell, hemoglobin, granular, tubular, or mixed)
8. Neurologic disorder	Seizures in the absence of offending drugs or known metabolic derangements, e.g., uremia, ketoacidosis, or electrolyte imbalance, *or* Psychosis in the absence of offending drugs or known metabolic derangements, e.g., uremia, ketoacidosis, or electrolyte imbalance
9. Hematologic disorder	Hemolytic anemia with reticulocytosis, *or* Leukopenia <4000/μl total on two or more occasions, *or* Lymphopenia <1500/μl on two or more occasions, *or* Thrombocytopenia <100,000/μl in the absence of offending drugs
10. Immunologic disorders	Positive LE cell preparation, *or* Anti-DNA: antibody to native DNA in abnormal titer, *or* Anti-Sm: presence of antibody to Sm nuclear antigen, *or* False-positive serologic test for syphilis known to be positive for at least 6 months and confirmed by TPI or FTA-ABS
11. Antinuclear antibody (ANA)	An abnormal titer of ANA by immunofluorescence or an equivalent assay at any point in time and in the absence of drugs known to be associated with "drug-induced lupus"

Adapted from Tan EM, et al: The 1982 revised criteria for the classification of systemic lupus erythematosus. Arthritis Rheum 25:1271–1277, 1992.
TPI = *Treponema pallidum* immobilization test; FTA-ABS = fluorescent treponemal antibody absorption test.

3. How do the criteria for the classification of SLE relate to making a *diagnosis* of SLE?

Although these criteria are extremely helpful when considering the diagnosis of SLE for an individual patient, it should be emphasized that these criteria were designed for classification and not diagnosis. Especially for mild cases and patients with early disease, the classification criteria may not be sensitive for making the diagnosis. For example, a patient with a classic malar rash and a high positive test for ANA almost certainly has SLE, and yet would not satisfy the classification criteria. Similarly, a patient with glomerulonephritis, elevated anti-DNA antibodies, and a positive ANA almost certainly has SLE.

4. What is the evidence that heredity is important in the development of SLE?

The best evidence that SLE is genetically determined is from studies of familial aggregation (i.e., an increased frequency of persons with SLE in the same family). For example, an identical twin of a patient with SLE may have a 1 in 3 chance (24–60% in different studies) of developing the disease, but this risk is much less if the affected twin was nonidentical (risk~2–5%). Still, this latter risk is much greater than that in the general population (~1 in 1000 for white females).

Population-based studies have also shown that susceptibility to SLE, like other autoimmune diseases in humans, is linked to particular class II genes of the major histocompatibility complex (HLA) in humans. Additional evidence comes from animal models of lupus in which mice can be bred to develop lupus-like autoantibody production and disease.

5. What is the laboratory hallmark of SLE?

ANA. Greater than 99% of patients with SLE demonstrate elevated serum levels of ANA, which is considered to be the laboratory hallmark of this disease. This test, however, is not specific for SLE.

6. How is a screening test for ANA usually performed in a clinical laboratory?

Today, an indirect immunoflourescence test is the most common assay used to detect ANA. The patient's serum is diluted and then layered onto a slide on which either tissue or cells have been fixed. After any unbound antibodies are washed off, a fluorescein-tagged antibody reagent directed to human immunoglobulin is added as a secondary reagent. Any antibodies (from the patient) bound to the nucleus will be stained, and the nucleus will fluoresce when viewed under a fluorescence microscope. The results are registered as positive or negative, and the highest dilution (titer) of serum giving a positive reaction is recorded.

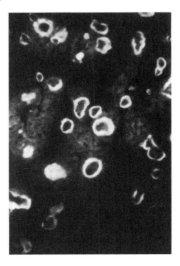

Indirect immunofluorescence test demonstrating a positive rim pattern.

Frequently, serum dilutions begin at about 1:40, and a dilution of at least 1:80 may be required to consider a test significantly positive. The cutoff for a positive test is usually chosen such that <5% of healthy control individuals will be positive. Even using a cutoff of >1:80, <1 in 40 people with a positive test will have SLE. False-positive reactions also increase with age.

The laboratory also reports a pattern of nuclear staining (rim, diffuse, speckled, or nucleolar). The peripheral or rim pattern (corresponding to autoantibodies to deoxynucleoproteins) is the most specific pattern for SLE, whereas a speckled pattern, which is the most common pattern in both SLE and other patients, is the least specific. Patterns have less significance today because a positive test is usually followed up with an ANA profile, which tests for specific types of autoantibodies including those highly specific for SLE.

7. Which ANAs are most specific for the diagnosis of SLE?

The screening ANA test is fairly nonspecific in that patients with other rheumatic diseases or other types of inflammatory disorders may also be positive. Certain ANA are more specific for the diagnosis of SLE, especially antibodies to double-stranded (ds) DNA and to the Sm antigen. The higher the levels of antibodies to these nuclear antigens, the greater the specificity for SLE.

8. List the most common autoantibodies found in SLE and some of their major clinical associations.

Autoantibodies in SLE and Some of Their Clinical Associations

TARGET	CLINICAL ASSOCIATIONS
dsDNA	High diagnostic specificity for SLE
	Correlation with disease activity (esp. activity of lupus nephritis)
ssDNA	Low diagnostic specificity
Histones (H1, H2A, H2B, H3, H4)	SLE and drug-induced lupus
Sm (SnRNP core proteins	High diagnostic specificity for SLE
B, B^1, D, E)	No correlation with disease activity
U1-RNP (SnRNP specific proteins	Mixed connective tissue disease or overlap syndrome (when not
A, C, 70-kD)	accompanied by anti-Sm antibodies)
Ro/SS-A (60-kD and 52-kD proteins)	Neonatal lupus (with anti-SS-B/La)
	Photosensitivity
	Subacute cutaneous lupus
La/SS-B (48-kD protein)	Neonatal lupus (with anti-SS-A/Ro)
	Associated Sjögren's syndrome
Ku	Diagnostic specificity for SLE and related overlap syndromes
Proliferating cell nuclear antigen	High diagnostic specificity for SLE
(PCNA)/cyclin	
Ribosomal P proteins	High diagnostic specificity for SLE
	Cytoplasmic staining
	Psychiatric disease
Phospholipids	Inhibition of in vitro coagulation tests (lupus anticoagulant)
	Thrombosis
	Recurrent abortions/fetal wasting
	Neurologic disease (focal presentations)
	Thrombocytopenia
Cell surface antigens	
Red blood cells	Hemolytic anemia
Platelets	Thrombocytopenia
Neuronal cells	Neurologic disease (diffuse presentations)

RNP = ribonucleoprotein. (Adapted from Kotzin BL, O'Dell JR: Systemic lupus erythematosus. In Frank MM, et al. (eds). Samter's Immunologic Diseases, 5th ed. Boston, Little, Brown and Co., 1995, pp 667–697.)

9. Describe four different types of rash associated with SLE.

1. **Malar or butterfly rash.** The malar rash typifies acute photosensitive rashes in SLE and indicates that the patient has systemic disease. The rash extends from the cheeks over the bridge of the nose and spares the nasiolabial folds. It can be macular but is usually erythematous and raised with papules and/or plaques. These lesions heal without scarring.

2. **Acute photosensitive rashes elsewhere.** Many of the acute rashes in SLE are related to photosensitivity and therefore are more likely to occur in sun-exposed areas. These rashes have similar characteristics to the malar rash, including healing without scarring.

3. **Subacute LE.** These raised erythematous lesions are also commonly related to sun exposure and are frequently associated with antibodies to Ro/SS-A. The lesions are nonfixed and can be annular or serpiginous, sometimes with central areas of scaling. These lesions usually heal without scarring but can leave areas of depigmentation, which can be especially prominent in dark-skinned individuals.

4. **Discoid LE.** These lesions may begin as erythematous papules or plaques and evolve into larger, coin-shaped (discoid), chronic lesions with central areas of epithelial thinning and atrophy and with follicular plugging and damage. Lesions can expand with active erythematous inflammation at the periphery, leaving depressed central scarring, depigmentation, and patches of alopecia. Discoid lesions frequently leave scars after healing. The most affected skin areas include the face, scalp, neck, and extensor surfaces of the arms. Some patients can have prolonged discoid disease and not develop systemic disease. However, about 15–30% of patients with SLE demonstrate discoid disease at some time in their disease course.

Less common rashes include bullous lesions, palpable purpura secondary to small vessel vasculitis, urticaria which may also be related to small vessel vasculitis, panniculitis with subcutaneous nodules, and livedo reticularis frequently associated with anti-phospholipid antibodies.

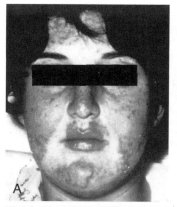

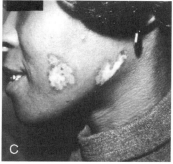

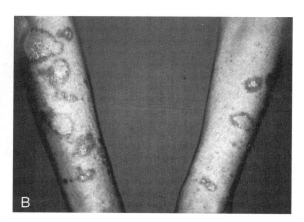

Rashes associated with SLE. *A*, Malar rash; *B*, Subacute cutaneous; *C*, Discoid. (From the Revised Clinical Slide Collection on the Rheumatic Diseases. Atlanta, American College of Rheumatology, 1991; with permission.)

10. **What are the four most common causes of death in patients with SLE?**
    1. Infection
    2. Lupus nephritis, renal failure, and its complications
    3. Cardiovascular disease
    4. CNS lupus

It is of note that infection appears to be more related to the complications of immuno-suppressive therapy, especially to prolonged use of high-dose corticosteroids, than to the activity of disease. Cardiovascular disease, which is mostly a problem late in the disease after years of therapy, appears to be multifactorial in its basis. Thus, atherosclerosis in the setting of SLE may be related to metabolic and lipid abnormalities caused by corticosteroids, the lipid abnormalities related to nephrotic syndrome, hypertension, and/or vascular damage secondary to immune complexes, anti-phospholipid antibodies, and/or platelet abnormalities. The presence and extent of renal disease is probably the most important prognostic factor in SLE. This relates not only to the possibility of developing renal failure but also to the probability of receiving potentially toxic therapy (high-dose prednisone and cytotoxic drugs) required to treat the disease.

11. Which type of hand rash strongly suggests the diagnosis of SLE?

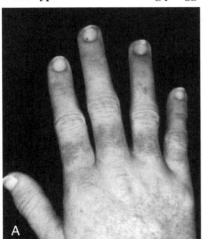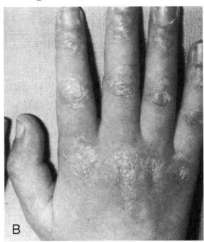

(From the Revised Clinical Slide Collection on the Rheumatic Diseases. Atlanta, American College of Rheumatology, 1991; with permission.)

The rash on the left is almost pathognomonic for SLE. There are erythematous lesions over the dorsum of the hands and fingers, affecting the skin *between* the joints. In contrast, the right panel shows lesions *over* the MCP and PIP joints, and this rash (Gottron's papules) is characteristic of dermatomyositis.

12. Identify five manifestations of lupus that warrant high-dose corticosteroid therapy.
The most common problems that warrant this therapy include:
1. Severe lupus nephritis
2. CNS lupus with severe manifestations
3. Autoimmune thrombocytopenia with extremely low platelet counts (e.g., <30,000/mm^3)
4. Autoimmune hemolytic anemia
5. Acute pneumonitis caused by SLE

Additional problems that may warrant aggressive corticosteroid therapy (with doses ≥60 mg/day in an adult) include severe vasculitis with visceral organ involvement, serious complications that result from serositis (pleuritis, pericarditis, or peritonitis), and sometimes severe systemic disease. It is important to emphasize that several problems in SLE should *not* be treated with high doses of corticosteroids (i.e., lupus arthritis, skin rashes, etc.).

13. How does WHO classify the different pathologic forms of lupus nephritis?

CLASS	DESCRIPTION
I	Normal
II	Mesangial nephritis
III	Focal proliferative glomerulonephritis
IV	Diffuse, proliferative glomerulonephritis
V	Membranous nephropathy

Overall, the World Health Organization's (WHO) histological scheme correlates with clinical severity and prognosis in patients with lupus nephritis. However, it has been emphasized that knowledge of the WHO histologic type of renal disease may add little clinically useful information over and above what is already known from clinical laboratory studies (urinalysis, protein excretion, and especially renal function studies).

When interpreting histologic findings in lupus nephritis, keep in mind that the renal biopsy is only a reflection of what is going on currently in the kidney and that changes from one pathologic stage to another over time are well documented in patients with lupus nephritis. In patients biopsied a second time, up to 40% have undergone a change to another WHO class.

14. Describe the key histologic findings in mesangial nephritis and its clinical implications.
Mesangial nephritis (WHO class II) is characterized by immune deposits in the mesangium that are best seen by immunofluorescence and electron microscopy. Biopsies that are normal on light microscopy are designated as WHO class IIA. Class IIB designates biopsies that show mesangial hypercellularity and/or increased matrix on light microscopy. Deposits in the capillary loops are not apparent in this class of disease. Patients with mesangial nephritis usually demonstrate little clinical evidence of renal involvement, with normal or near-normal urinalysis and renal function, and rarely require any treatment for their renal disease.

15. Describe the key histologic findings in focal proliferative glomerulonephritis and its clinical implications.
Focal proliferative glomerulonephritis (WHO class III) is characterized histologically by hypercellularity due to increases in mesangial, endocapillary, and/or infiltrating cells. These changes result in encroachment of the glomerular capillary space. Active inflammatory lesions are present, often in a segmental pattern (i.e., involving only one area of a glomerulus) and involving <50% of the glomeruli. Patients with this pattern usually demonstrate proteinuria and hematuria, but severe (nephrotic range) proteinuria or progressive loss of renal function is rare.

16. Diffuse proliferative glomerulonephritis (DPGN)?
DPGN (WHO class IV) is seen in almost all SLE patients who progress to renal failure. DPGN is characterized by involvement of >50% of the glomeruli, with generalized hypercellularity of mesangial and endothelial cells. Inflammatory cellular infiltrates and areas of necrosis are common. These changes may ultimately lead to obliteration of the capillary loops and sclerosis. Regions of basement membrane thickening are also usually present. Immunofluorescence microscopy demonstrates extensive deposition of immunoglobulin and complement in the mesangium and capillary loops, and electron microscopy frequently shows immune complex deposits in both subendothelial and subepithelial distributions.

Clinically, patients almost always have proteinuria and hematuria and, not infrequently, decreases in renal function. Hypertension is common.

17. Membranous nephropathy?
Membranous nephropathy (WHO class V) is characterized histologically by diffuse thickening of the basement membrane. Glomeruli usually have normal cellularity. Deposits containing immunoglobulin and complement are apparent along the basement membrane on electron microscopy and immunofluorescence microscopy.

Clinically, patients who have pure membranous disease frequently have extensive protein-uria but only minimal hematuria or renal functional abnormalities. A subset of patients (10–30%) slowly progress to chronic renal failure within a 10-year period. Membranous disease can also be observed as a transition stage after treatment for proliferative glomerulonephritis.

18. In the analysis of a renal biopsy from a patient with SLE, what criteria are used in the "activity" and "chronicity" indices?

Pathologic Indices of Activity and Chronicity

CHRONICITY INDEX	ACTIVITY INDEX
Glomular sclerosis	Cellular proliferation
Fibrous crescents	Fibrinoid necrosis
Tubular atrophy	Cellular crescents
Interstitial fibrosis	Hyaline thrombi
	Leukocyte infiltration in glomerulus
	Mononuclear cell infiltration in interstitium

To obtain a **chronicity score**, each parameter is graded 0–3 depending on severity of in-volvement, and the grades are added. Glomerular sclerosis and fibrous crescents are graded as fol-lows: 0, absent; 1+, <25% of glomeruli involved; 2+, 25–50% of glomeruli involved; 3+, >75% of glomeruli involved. Tubular atrophy and interstitial fibrosis are graded as follows: 0, absent; 1+, mild; 2+, moderate; 3+, severe. The maximal chronicity score is 12.

To obtain an **activity score**, each parameter is graded 0–3 depending on the severity of in-volvement, and the individual grades are added. Fibrinoid necrosis and cellular crescents have been given a "weighting" factor of 2. The maximal activity score is 24.

19. What is the importance of evaluating biopsies for the extent of chronic damage?

The histologic scoring systems for lupus nephritis using chronicity and activity indexes have been developed in an effort to more accurately predict renal outcome and to help determine which patients are most likely to benefit from aggressive therapy. The **chronicity index** measure four histologic components of chronic *irreversible* renal damage, and the **activity index** measures six histologic components of activity of lupus nephritis.

In the last several years, these systems have come into major use, as a number of studies have reported on their predictive associations and usefulness. Most, but not all, studies have found that a higher chronicity index is associated with greater risk for progression to renal failure. Based on its apparent validity as a prognostic indicator as well as the fact that the presence of chronic dam-age identifies disease with destructive potential, several investigators have recommended the use of the chronicity index as a guide to the aggressiveness of therapy. In particular, treatment with agents such as cyclophosphamide was predicted to be most beneficial for patients with interme-diate chronicity index scores.

In contrast to the chronicity index, the validity of the activity index as a predictor of renal outcome is less clear; approximately half of these studies have shown that a higher score corre-lates with increased risk of renal failure. This may relate to the caveat that active lesions are amenable to therapy, whereas chronic lesions represent irreversible destruction.

20. Which serologic tests are most useful when following a patient with lupus nephritis?

Only one ANA has been shown to correlate with the activity of lupus nephritis, antibodies to dsDNA. Therefore, serial monitoring should be limited to tests that specifically quantitate anti-dsDNA antibodies. In addition, patients with active lupus nephritis have decreased levels of com-plement components (e.g., C3 and C4) as well as total hemolytic complement (CH_{50}) which also correlate with the activity of renal disease.

21. What is the evidence that anti-dsDNA antibodies are important in the pathogenesis of lupus nephritis?

IgG antibodies directed to dsDNA appear to play a prominent role in lupus nephritis. The ev-idence for this includes:

(1) Detection of anti-dsDNA antibodies in the glomeruli of patients and animals with active disease

(2) Studies showing enrichment of IgG anti-dsDNA antibodies in glomerular tissues relative to serum and other organs

(3) Longitudinal studies in a subset of SLE patients demonstrating that high levels of circulating anti-dsDNA antibodies frequently precede or coincide with active glomerulonephritis

(4) Demonstration in animals that injection of certain monoclonal IgG anti-dsDNA antibodies or expression of genes that encode pathogenic IgG anti-dsDNA activity can lead to glomerular pathology

It should be emphasized that the correlation of anti-dsDNA autoantibody levels with the extent of renal damage is a general one. For example, numerous studies have shown that glomerulonephritis in SLE can occur in the absence of elevated serum levels of anti-DNA antibodies. Although these cases may represent a failure of the sensitivity of currently available techniques to detect anti-DNA antibodies, it also suggests that in some cases, autoantibodies directed to non-DNA antigens may participate in renal damage in lupus nephritis.

22. What are the proposed mechanisms by which anti-dsDNA antibodies cause glomerulonephritis in SLE?

Anti-DNA antibodies do not appear to mediate renal damage in SLE through the deposition of circulating immune complexes. Even in patients with active glomerulonephritis or animal models with actively increasing amounts of anti-DNA antibodies in the glomerulus, DNA–anti-DNA complexes have been difficult to demonstrate in the circulation. Thus, two alternative theories have been proposed to explain the pathogenic mechanisms of these antibodies:

In the first, anti-DNA–DNA complexes are proposed to form in the glomerulus (in-situ complex formation) rather than being deposited from the blood. Evidence supports a model in which DNA first binds to the glomerulus and is then recognized and bound by anti-DNA antibodies. It is of interest that increased amounts of circulating DNA have been detected in the blood of patients with SLE. The circulating nuclear material could thus become the planted renal target for a subset of pathogenic anti-DNA antibodies.

In an alternative model, the subset of pathogenic anti-DNA antibodies have been hypothesized to cross-react with glomerular antigens which are not DNA in origin. This model is supported by data showing that anti-DNA antibodies do contain other specificities and can bind to different glomerular structures.

The activation of complement components through the classical pathway appears to be involved in the pathogenesis of glomerular damage. Direct damage as well as recruitment of inflammatory cells are likely to be involved. Thus, IgG anti-DNA antibodies that are complement-fixing are more likely to be pathogenic.

23. What is the first-line of therapy for patients with severe lupus nephritis?

Previously untreated patients with active lupus nephritis and severe clinical manifestations (i.e., decreasing renal function and/or high-grade proteinuria) first receive high-doses of corticosteroids. An attempt should be made to control disease activity quickly. The initial dose of the most commonly used drug, **prednisone**, should be approximately 1 mg/kg/day (~60–80 mg/day) in three divided doses. It may take several weeks to achieve control of active nephritis.

24. When are cytotoxic drugs indicated in the treatment of lupus nephritis?

The toxicity of continuous high-dose corticosteroid therapy is cumulative and severe. If a 6–8-week course of high-dose prednisone has not restored serum creatinine levels to normal or the proteinuria continues at >1 gm/day, a renal biopsy can be done to determine whether glomerular sclerosis, fibrous crescents, and irreversible tubulointerstitial changes are present. If these poor prognostic indicators are observed, especially with evidence of continued activity, the addition of cytotoxic drugs or other immunosuppressive modalities should be considered.

The use of cytotoxic drugs in the treatment of lupus nephritis should be reserved for the subgroup of patients with severe, refractory disease. These include (1) patients with evidence of active and severe glomerulonephritis despite treatment with high-dose prednisone; (2) patients who have responded to corticosteroids but who require an unacceptably high dose to maintain a response; and (3) patients with unacceptable side effects from corticosteroids.

25. Which cytotoxic agents are most frequently used?

Oral azathioprine, oral cyclophosphamide, or intermittent intravenous cyclophosphamide. Daily oral chlorambucil has been used occasionally as an alternative to cyclophosphamide. These drugs are given in association with a dose of prednisone (usually 0.5 mg/kg/day) required to control extrarenal manifestations. Cytotoxic drugs in combination with prednisone have been shown to prevent progression to renal failure in some patients more effectively than prednisone alone. However, because of potentially severe toxicity, overall improvements in mortality have been more difficult to demonstrate.

26. Are there any advantages of intermittent intravenous cyclophosphamide compared to daily oral cyclophosphamide therapy in the treatment of lupus nephritis?

There are two major ways to use cyclophosphamide (Cytoxan) in the treatment of SLE patients with severe manifestations such as severe lupus nephritis:

1. Daily oral therapy with doses of ~1.0–2.0 mg/kg/day
2. Monthly boluses of 0.5–1.0 gm/m^2 given intravenously (iv) over about 60 minutes with vigorous hydration

The major advantage of intermittent iv cyclophosphamide relates to a markedly decreased incidence of bladder damage and hemorrhagic cystitis. Theoretically, iv therapy also appears to work more rapidly than continuous oral treatment. There is not much evidence to suggest that the iv regimen is actually more efficacious than oral cyclophosphamide, although trends have been seen in some controlled trials.

27. A 30-year-old woman with severe nephritis and end-stage renal failure is referred for further evaluation and treatment. The patient, who has been on dialysis for nearly 5 years, is being considered for transplantation but is afraid that her lupus will just destroy the donor kidney. She asks for your opinion.

Approximately 30% of patients with severe lupus nephritis will progress over a 10-year follow-up period to end-stage renal disease, and lupus nephritis accounts for up to 3% of cases of end-stage renal failure requiring dialysis or transplantation. For unclear reasons, SLE patients with progressive renal failure and those on dialysis frequently demonstrate a decrease in nonrenal clinical manifestations of active SLE as well as a decrease in serologic markers of active disease. In SLE patients with absent or minimal disease activity, the clinical course and survival on dialysis compare favorably to those of other patient groups. With time, SLE patients appear to be excellent candidates for transplantation, and the recurrence of active lupus nephritis in the transplant is rare. Graft and patient survival for SLE patients after transplantation appear to be similar to those for most other groups.

28. What is the lupus anticoagulant? What are its clinical associations?

Lupus anticoagulant refers to a subset of autoantibodies to phospholipids that interfere with certain clotting tests. It is usually picked up by an abnormally elevated partial thromboplastin time and can be further demonstrated by specific clotting studies. Anti-phospholipid antibodies (APAs) can also be detected by a test for anti-cardiolipin antibodies as well as by a false-positive serologic test for syphilis.

The term lupus anticoagulant is truly a misnomer since the major clinical association of these autoantibodies is thrombosis (not bleeding), and these autoantibodies can occur (and are even more common) in the absence of SLE. Disease from these autoantibodies is referred to as the **primary anti-phospholipid antibody syndrome** (see Chapter 27). Complications associated with APAs include arterial and venous thrombosis, miscarriage and fetal wastage, thrombocytopenia, livedo reticularis, and autoimmune hemolytic anemia. APAs and their complications are a major issue in the care of patients with SLE. The mechanism by which these antibodies cause these complications is unknown.

29. Name three causes of alopecia in the setting of SLE.
1. Active systemic disease can result in diffuse alopecia which is reversible once disease activity is controlled.
2. Discoid disease results in patchy hair loss corresponding to the distribution of discoid skin lesions. This hair loss is permanent.
3. Drugs such as cyclophosphamide can result in diffuse hair loss, which is reversible after therapy is discontinued and disease activity decreases.

30. You are caring for a patient with SLE who has arthritis and complains of severe joint pains. What is the likelihood that this patient will develop severe deformities of her hands?
The arthritis associated with SLE is rarely erosive or destructive of bone and therefore is quite different from rheumatoid arthritis. Joint deformities are unusual and, when they occur, are secondary to ligament loosening rather than cartilage and bone destruction. Occasionally, SLE patients demonstrate ulnar deviation and swan-neck deformities of the hands (called Jaccoud's arthritis).

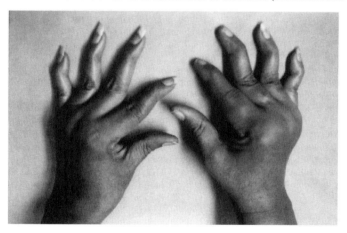

Swan-neck deformities in SLE, which are reversible.

31. What are the best approaches for therapy in an SLE patient with arthritis who has no evidence of internal organ involvement?
The first line of therapy is NSAIDs. Patients can also benefit remarkably from antimalarial drugs, usually given in the form of low doses of daily oral hydroxychloroquine.

32. The hematocrit in a patient with SLE has been dropping over the last several months to a steady level of 31%. RBC indices are otherwise normal, as is the rest of the CBC. Recent medications have included prednisone (5 mg/day) and intermittent low doses of NSAIDs. What is the most likely cause for the anemia in this patient?
The most likely cause is the so-called **anemia of chronic disease**, secondary to the persistent inflammation that occurs in SLE. The mechanisms of this type of anemia mostly relate to decreased production of red blood cells (RBCs) as well as slightly decreased RBC survival. There is an inability for iron to be handled normally by the reticuloendothelial system, and blood tests frequently disclose a low serum iron concentration as well as a low total iron-binding capacity.

The evaluation in this patient should rule out the possibility of an autoimmune hemolytic anemia. This should include a reticulocyte count to determine (in conjunction with a stable hematocrit) whether there is active destruction of RBCs and possibly tests for autoantibodies to RBCs (direct Coombs tests). Remember, however, that many more SLE patients will have a positive Coombs test than a hemolytic anemia. The patient should also be evaluated for the possibility of gastrointestinal blood loss and iron deficiency related to the continued use of NSAIDs.

It is important to determine that the patient has the anemia of chronic disease because it implies ongoing inflammation, prompting careful follow-up of the patient. Patients demonstrating this form of anemia are more likely to demonstrate flares of lupus activity in the near future.

33. A patient with SLE has a low WBC count of 2,500/mm^3 (70% neutrophils, 20% lymphocytes, 8% monocytes, 2% eosinophils). Her prednisone has been tapered to 5 mg/day and there are no clinical manifestations of active disease. A review of systems and the physical exam are negative, except for a mild malar rash. Laboratory tests show no evidence for lupus nephritis or other internal organ involvement. How do you evaluate and treat this leukopenia?
This degree of leukopenia, which includes both a neutropenia and lymphopenia, is not uncommon in SLE and warrants no further evaluation or treatment. It is not associated with an increased risk of infection. It does imply continued disease activity, so the patient needs to be followed carefully.

34. A 25-year-old woman with SLE has had difficulty with severe thrombocytopenia. Previous bone marrow biopsies showed increased numbers of megakaryocytes and no other abnormalities. Past therapy with high doses of corticosteroids has been successful in raising the platelet count to normal levels, but tapering to 20 mg/day has resulted in a progressive decline in platelet counts to <20,000/mm^3. The patient is taking no other medications, and her physical examination is normal. Discuss the options for therapy in this patient.
There are several therapeutic options to consider in this patient with autoimmune thrombocytopenia. One consideration would be **splenectomy**. If the patient had idiopathic thrombocytopenic purpura (ITP) without SLE, this would probably be recommended. However, the value of splenectomy in lupus-related thrombocytopenia has been debated, and its use is controversial. Some studies (retrospective and anecdotal) have suggested a high rate of failure in maintaining adequate platelet counts long-term. Other reports (equally anecdotal) maintain that splenectomy is as valuable a long-term therapy in SLE as it is in ITP. Considering that the patient has no other severe problems from SLE and is a young woman, splenectomy would be a reasonable option.

Another option is **danazol**, an androgen that increases platelet counts and allows the steroid dose to be decreased. Doses of 800 mg/day may be necessary, and the androgenic side effects in a young female may be troubling.

A separate option is the addition of an **immunosuppressive** or **cytotoxic drug** such as azathioprine. This addition will decrease platelet destruction and allow the prednisone dose to be tapered. Azathioprine is less toxic than cyclophosphamide, especially in terms of causing hemorrhagic cystitis, ovarian failure, and probably secondary lymphoma/leukemia, and would certainly be preferred in this setting.

On a separate note, high doses of **intravenous immunoglobulin** (IVIG) have been a very effective therapy to raise platelet counts acutely. For example, this treatment could be used in preparation for splenectomy or if the patient showed signs of bleeding. Because of its cost, however, repeated treatments with IVIG are not a reasonable long-term therapeutic option.

35. List the manifestations of CNS involvement in SLE.
CNS involvement can be either diffuse or focal. Manifestations of diffuse disease include intractable headaches, generalized seizures, aseptic meningitis, organic brain syndrome, psychiatric disease (especially psychosis and severe depression), and coma. Manifestations of focal disease include stroke syndromes such as hemiparesis, focal seizures, movement disorders such as chorea, and transverse myelitis.

36. Name three types of autoantibodies that have been associated with CNS involvement in SLE.

1. Serum anti-phospholipid antibodies—associated with focal neurologic manifestations in CNS lupus.

2. Cerebrospinal fluid anti-neuronal antibodies—associated with diffuse manifestations of CNS lupus.

3. Serum antibodies to ribosomal P proteins (anti-P antibodies)—associated with psychiatric problems (severe depression and psychosis) in SLE.

37. How does SLE cause CNS involvement?

CNS lupus (also referred to as neuropsychiatric lupus erythematosus) with **diffuse** manifestations appears to be caused by autoantibodies directed to neuronal cells or their products. Thus, patients with organic brain syndrome frequently demonstrate elevated levels of anti-neuronal antibodies or other evidence of autoantibody production in the cerebrospinal fluid. As in multiple sclerosis, elevated levels of IgG and oligoclonal bands are markers of abnormal autoantibody production within the CNS and are frequently present in CNS lupus with diffuse manifestations. In patients with diffuse CNS lupus who present with primarily psychiatric disease, serum anti-P antibodies appear to be a helpful diagnostic marker.

CNS lupus with **focal** manifestations is most likely to be related to intravascular occlusion. MRI, which is much more sensitive than CT or brain scanning, almost always shows abnormalities characteristic of ischemic damage in these patients. Furthermore, these patients frequently demonstrate significantly elevated serum levels of anti-phospholipid antibodies (APAs), which are associated with intravascular occlusion. Less commonly, evidence of vasculitis is apparent.

38. A 40-year-old woman with severe lupus nephritis has been treated with 60 mg of prednisone for the last 2 weeks but now seems disoriented and demonstrates bizarre behavior with delusional thinking. Describe the appropriate evaluation and treatment.

The differential diagnosis for the change in behavior in this patient should include CNS lupus, prednisone-induced psychosis, or a separate problem such as infection or metabolic disturbance. First, the patient should be examined carefully, especially for evidence of active lupus, an organic brain syndrome (i.e., decreased intellectual function), and any additional neurologic (especially focal) deficits. Any positive neurologic findings would strongly suggest that the change in behavior was not directly caused by the high doses of prednisone.

Laboratory tests should exclude the possibility of a new metabolic problem and determine the activity of nephritis and/or other organ involvement. Studies directed at the CNS should include MRI, electroencephalogram (which should be normal in steroid-induced psychosis), and lumbar puncture (for standard tests such as cell count, protein level, and culture). In a patient on high doses of steroids, the possibility of infection must be considered and excluded. In addition, analysis of the cerebrospinal fluid should include tests for increased CNS IgG production, oligoclonal bands, and anti-neuronal antibodies. Serologic tests should include anti-P antibodies (which have been associated with psychosis caused by CNS lupus) as well as studies for the systemic activity of disease.

If the evaluation is negative, the most likely cause for the change in behavior is steroid-induced psychosis, and the appropriate treatment would be to decrease its dose. In contrast, evidence for CNS lupus would warrant therapy directed at the pathogenic process. This might include increasing the dose of steroids and/or adding a cytotoxic drug.

39. In what ways can the heart be involved in SLE?

Pericarditis
Myocarditis
Vasculitis
Secondary atherosclerotic coronary artery disease and myocardial infarction
Secondary hypertensive disease
Valvular disease

40. In what ways can the lung be involved in SLE?
Pleuritis
Acute lupus pneumonitis with or without pulmonary hemorrhage
Chronic interstitial lung disease and pulmonary fibrosis (rare)
Pulmonary hypertension
Pulmonary embolism
"Shrinking lung syndrome" (decreased lung volumes without parenchymal disease)
Secondary infection

41. In an SLE patient who is pregnant, which lupus-related autoantibodies can cause problem for the fetus?
Antibodies to **Ro/SSA** in conjunction with antibodies to **La/SS-B** have been associated with the neonatal lupus syndrome. The major manifestation of this complication is congenital heart block, which is frequently severe and abrupt and may require a cardiac pacemaker. A neonatal rash may also be part of this syndrome.

Anti-phospholipid antibodies have been associated with recurrent spontaneous abortion and stillbirths (fetal wastage). One hypothesis for this complication is intravascular thrombosis and placental insufficiency.

Anti-platelet antibodies can occasionally cause autoimmune thrombocytopenia in the fetus with associated hemorrhage, especially at the time of delivery. The management of this complication can be difficult.

42. How often will an SLE patient who has antibodies to Ro/SSA deliver a baby with neonatal lupus syndrome?
SLE patients with anti-Ro/SSA antibodies (especially directed against the 52-kD component) may have up to a 4–5% overall risk of having a baby with the neonatal lupus syndrome. Of these babies, 40% have only rash, 40% have complete heart block (CHB), and 10-20% will have both rash and CHB. Of the babies with CHB, approximately 50% will require a permanent pacemaker, and 10% will die despite the pacemaker. Once an SLE patient with anti-Ro/SSA antibodies has had one child with CHB, there is a 33% overall risk of her next baby having CHB. Patients at risk for having babies with CHB sound have weekly fetal EKGs from the 18th–24th weeks of gestation. If the fetus demonstrates development of heart block, treatment of the mother with dexamethasone and plasmapheresis may occasionally reverse the heart block.

43. A 25-year-old patient with SLE, currently on 5 mg of prednisone per day, and quiescent disease for the last few years wants to become pregnant. What advice can you offer her about potential problems for her or the fetus?
Pregnancy in SLE can be difficult and warrants special consideration. The optimal time for the patient to consider becoming pregnant is when disease activity is quiescent and medications are minimal. Thus, for this patient, this would be a relatively good time to become pregnant. Careful follow-up is essential during pregnancy. Although controversial, some experienced physicians believe that pregnancy increases the risk for disease flares, especially during the third trimester and the immediate post-partum period. Patients need to be followed carefully for blood pressure elevations and evidence of glomerulonephritis. Useful laboratory tests to follow patients include anti-dsDNA antibodies and complement levels. The mainstay of therapy for serious lupus flares during pregnancy is prednisone.

44. A patient with SLE and active lupus nephritis wants to become pregnant. Current medications include prednisone, 20 mg/day. What do you recommend?
In contrast to an SLE patient with quiescent disease, this patient should be counseled *against* becoming pregnant at this time. There is an increased chance of worsening disease activity that could result in renal functional deterioration and increased problems related to hypertension and preeclampsia. It has been estimated that patients with active lupus nephritis have a 50–60%

chance of nephritis exacerbation during pregnancy or immediately post-partum. In contrast, for patients with quiescent disease, the risk of nephritis exacerbation is <10%.

Flares of lupus nephritis during pregnancy can be very severe. In patients with active lupus, there is also a high chance for problems in the fetus. For example, the risk of prematurity may be as high as 60%. Furthermore, if the renal disease should worsen, certain therapies such as cyclophosphamide, are contraindicated. This would limit therapeutic options.

BIBLIOGRAPHY

1. Austin HA, Boumpas DT, Vaughan EM, Balow JE: Predicting renal outcomes in severe lupus nephritis: Contributions of clinical and histologic data. Kidney Int 45:544–550, 1994.
2. Boumpas DT, Austin HA, Vaughan EM, et al: Controlled trial of pulse methylprednisolone versus two regimens of pulse cyclophosphamide in severe lupus nephritis. Lancet 340:741–745, 1992.
3. Canadian Hydroxychloroquine Study Group: A randomized study of the effect of withdrawing hydroxychloroquine sulfate in systemic lupus erythematosus. N Engl J Med 324:150–154, 1991.
4. Ginzler EM, Schorn K. Outcome and prognosis in systemic lupus erythematosus. Rheum Dis Clin North Am 14:67–78, 1988.
5. Hochberg MC: The epidemiology of systemic lupus erythematosus. In Wallace DJ, Hahn BH (eds): Dubois' Lupus Erythematosus, 4th ed. Philadelphia, Lea & Febiger, 1993, pp 49–57.
6. Hochberg MC, Petri M: Clinical features of systemic lupus erythematosus. Curr Opin Rheumatol 5:575–586, 1993.
7. Kotzin BL, O'Dell JR: Systemic lupus erythematosus. In Frank MM, Austen KF, Claman HN, Unanue ER (eds): Samter's Immunologic Diseases, 5th ed. Boston, Little, Brown & Co., 1995, pp 667–697.
8. Kotzin BL, Achenbach GA, West SG: Renal involvement in systemic lupus erythematosus. In Schrier RW, Gottschalk CW (eds): Diseases of the Kidney, 6th. ed. Boston. Little, Brown & Co., 1996.
9. Nossent HC, Swaak TJG, Berden JHM, Dutch Working Party on Systemic Lupus Erythematosus: Systemic lupus erythematosus after renal transplantation: Patient and graft survival and disease activity. Ann Intern Med 114:183–188, 1991.
10. Rubin LA, Urowitz MB, Gladman DD: Mortality in systemic lupus erythematosus: The biomodal pattern revisited. Q J Med 55:87–98, 1985.
11. Steinberg AD, Steinberg SC: Long-term preservation of renal function in patients with lupus nephritis receiving treatment that includes cyclophosphamide versus those treated with prednisone only. Arthritis Rheum 34:945–950, 1991.
12. Tan EM, Cohen AS, Fries JF, et al: The 1982 revised criteria for the classification of systemic lupus erythematosus. Arthritis Rheum 25:1271–1277, 1982.
13. Tan EM: Antinuclear antibodies: Diagnostic markers for autoimmune diseases and probes for cell biology. Adv Immunol 44:93–151, 1989.
14. Wallace DJ, Hahn BH: Dubois' Lupus Erythematosus, 4th ed. Philadelphia, Lea & Febiger, 1993.
15. West SG, Emlen W, Wener MH, Kotzin BL. Neuropsychiatric lupus erythematosus: A 10-year prospective study on the value of diagnostic tests. Am J Med 99:153–163, 1995.

21. DRUG-INDUCED LUPUS

Brian L. Kotzin, M.D.

1. Name five drugs definitely associated with antinuclear antibodies and manifestations of lupus-like disease.
Procainamide, hydralazine, isoniazid, methyldopa, and chlorpromazine.

2. List any other drugs for which there is more than anecdotal evidence for lupus-inducing potential.
Mephenytoin, phenytoin, beta-adrenergic blocking agents, quinidine, and D-penicillamine.

3. How do the clinical manifestations occurring most commonly in procainamide-induced lupus compare with the manifestations of idiopathic systemic lupus erythematosus (SLE)?
Patients with drug-induced lupus have a different distribution of clinical manifestations than those with idiopathic SLE. In procainamide-induced lupus, severe nephritis or manifestations of CNS involvement (e.g., organic brain syndrome, seizures, or psychosis) are very rare; in contrast, nearly 50% of patients with SLE will demonstrate clinical evidence of nephritis during their disease course, and neurologic and/or psychiatric manifestations occur in up to two-thirds of SLE patients. Furthermore, rashes such as a malar rash or discoid lesions are unusual in drug-induced disease but are common in patients with SLE. Frequent problems seen in drug-induced disease include fever, myalgias, arthralgia/arthritis, and pleuritis, with 30–40% of patients having acute pulmonary infiltrates; although pleuritis is also relatively common in SLE, acute infiltrates not related to infection are uncommon and are usually seen only in patients who are acutely ill.

4. How do the clinical manifestations of hydralazine-induced lupus differ from those of procainamide-induced disease?
Like those with procainamide-induced lupus, patients with hydralazine-induced lupus are also likely to have fever, myalgias, and arthritis/arthralgias and rarely manifest either severe lupus nephritis or CNS involvement. Compared to procainamide-induced disease, serositis and pulmonary parenchymal involvement are much less common, and rashes are more likely to be seen, although the classic malar rash and discoid lesions are unusual.

5. Will patients with either drug-induced lupus or SLE usually have a positive test for antinuclear antibodies (ANA)?
Yes. More than 95% of patients with SLE will demonstrate a positive test for ANA. By definition, essentially all patients with drug-induced lupus will demonstrate a positive ANA test.

6. Which autoantibodies are most commonly seen in drug-induced lupus? How do these compare with the autoantibodies seen in idiopathic SLE?
The spectrum of ANAs in drug-induced lupus is much more limited than that seen in SLE. **Anti-histone antibodies** are the most common autoantibody specificity in drug-induced lupus, and nearly all patients with symptomatic drug-induced disease demonstrate elevated levels of IgG anti-histone antibodies. Antibodies to histones are also frequent in SLE, detectable in 50–80% of patients, depending on disease activity. Antibodies to single-stranded DNA are also common in both drug-induced lupus and SLE, but antibodies to double-stranded DNA are highly specific for SLE and rarely found in drug-induced lupus. Antibodies to Sm (~30% of SLE), Ro/SS-A (~60% of SLE), and La/SS-B (~15–20% of SLE) are also rare specificities in drug-induced lupus.

7. Is testing for anti-histone antibodies clinically useful to distinguish drug-induced disease from idiopathic SLE in a patient taking either procainamide or hydralazine?
Testing for anti-histone antibodies can occasionally be useful in situations in which the diagnosis of drug-induced lupus is being considered. As discussed, nearly all patients with symptomatic procainamide- or hydralazine-induced lupus demonstrate elevated serum levels of IgG anti-histone antibodies. Thus, a negative test would make this diagnosis unlikely. However, a positive test for anti-histone antibodies has much less diagnostic value because 50–80% of patients with active SLE also have a positive test. Furthermore, some patients taking either procainamide or hydralazine will have a positive test but not symptoms of lupus-like disease. Remember that in most cases in which drug-induced disease is being considered, performing an ANA test and (if positive) taking the patient off the offending agent may be the most cost-effective approach to the situation.

8. Contrast the type of anti-histone antibodies found in drug-induced lupus versus idiopathic SLE.
In certain specialized research laboratories, the specificity of anti-histone antibodies for individual histones (i.e., H1, H2A, H2B, H3, and H4), histone complexes, or intra-histone epitopes can

be distinguished. Overall, anti-histone antibodies in drug-induced lupus tend to be much more focused on certain histone complexes compared to SLE. For example, in procainamide-induced lupus, the onset of symptomatic disease has been associated with the production of IgG antibodies to the H2A–H2B–DNA complex. Although this complex is also a target in about 15% of patients with SLE, autoantibodies in the idiopathic disease are frequently also directed to other individual histones and other histone complexes. In hydralazine-induced disease, one study has suggested that the major targets are histones H3 and H4 and the H3–H4 complex. In contrast to procainamide-induced lupus and SLE, the autoantibodies induced by hydralazine appear to be directed more to determinants hidden within chromatin rather than exposed on the surface.

9. What percentage of patients taking procainamide or hydralazine develop a positive test for ANA?

Nearly 75% of patients receiving procainamide therapy will develop a positive ANA test within the first year of treatment, and over 90% develop a positive ANA by 2 years. Thirty to 50% of patients taking hydralazine will demonstrate a positive test after a year of drug therapy. For both drugs, the probability of developing a positive ANA test depends on the dose and duration of drug therapy. With long-term drug use, perhaps 10–30% of ANA-positive patients go on to develop symptoms of lupus. It is important to note that many more patients will demonstrate a positive ANA test than develop drug-induced lupus, and the presence of a positive test is not a valid reason for stopping the medication. In drug-induced lupus, the onset of symptoms can be insidious or acute, and an interval of 1–2 months frequently passes before the diagnosis is made and the drug is withdrawn.

10. Do similar genetic factors predispose patients to develop drug-induced lupus and SLE?

The genetic risk factors in drug-induced lupus and idiopathic SLE appear to be quite separate. The major risk for procainamide- or hydralazine-induced lupus appears to be **acetylator phenotype.** Metabolism of these drugs involves the hepatic enzyme N-acetyltransferase, which catalyzes the acetylation of amine or hydrazine groups. The rate at which this reaction takes place is under genetic control. Approximately 50% of the U.S. white population are fast acetylators and the rest are slow acetylators. The slow acetylators, when treated with procainamide or hydralazine, develop ANA earlier and at higher titers and are more likely to develop symptomatic disease compared to fast acetylators. In one study, hydralazine-induced disease developed only in slow acetylators. It should also be noted that N-acetylprocainamide, despite its chemical similarity to procainamide and its similar drug action, has not been associated with drug-induced ANA production or drug-induced lupus.

In SLE, acetylator phenotype does not appear to be involved in genetic susceptibility. Instead, HLA class II genes, complement deficiencies, and multiple other genes are important in the complex genetic basis of SLE (see Chapter 20).

11. What age, sex, and racial groups are most at risk for drug-induced lupus? For idiopathic SLE?

The incidence of SLE increases greatly in women of childbearing age, and the female-to-male ratio overall is about 8:1. In contrast, the usual age of patients with drug-induced lupus is >50 years old, reflecting the age of the population being treated with drugs such as procainamide and hydralazine. The female-to-male ratio in drug-induced lupus is also much closer to unity (procainamide-induced disease may be slightly more frequent in females). The frequency of SLE may be 2–4 times increased in blacks and hispanics compared to whites. In contrast, the frequency of drug-induced lupus may be 6-fold lower in blacks than whites.

12. Will the severity of clinical manifestations of drug-induced lupus frequently progress after the offending drug is discontinued?

No. In nearly all cases, disease manifestations begin to improve within a few days to weeks after the drug is discontinued. If this does not occur, question the diagnosis.

13. A patient is referred to you with fever, arthritis, pleuritis, and a high-titer positive test for ANA. The history reveals that she has been taking procainamide for the last 2 years. Unfortunately, procainamide has been the only medication to control her severe arrhythmias, and the referring cardiologist wants to continue this drug if possible. What laboratory tests might be useful to determine if the patient has drug-induced lupus or idiopathic SLE?

Patients with procainamide-induced lupus usually demonstrate a limited spectrum of ANA specificities. Tests for anti-histone antibodies and anti-ssDNA antibodies are almost always positive. In specialized laboratories, the anti-histone antibodies can be shown to be directed primarily to a complex of histones H2A–H2B with DNA. In idiopathic SLE, anti-histone antibodies (if they are present) may be directed to this epitope but are also likely to be reactive with other individual histones and histone complexes. As noted earlier, patients with SLE may also have antibodies to ds-DNA, Sm, Ro/SS-A, and La/SS-B, which are rare in drug-induced lupus. Hypocomplementemia is also uncommon in drug-induced lupus.

14. Is the use of procainamide or other drugs associated with drug-induced lupus contraindicated in patients with SLE? Can they exacerbate disease activity?

No. The population at risk for developing drug-induced lupus is very different compared with that developing SLE. There is no evidence that drugs capable of causing drug-induced lupus will change or worsen disease activity in a patient with SLE. However, if an alternative drug is available, it may be prudent to use it so that there won't be any confusion if the SLE patient has a disease flare in the future.

15. What is the mainstay of therapy for drug-induced lupus?

The first and most important aspect of treatment is to *discontinue the offending medication*.

16. Describe the management of a patient with procainamide-induced lupus who has fevers, arthritis, and pleuritis as the major manifestations of disease.

First, discontinue procainamide. Many patients with these symptoms can be controlled with NSAIDs, while the symptoms of drug-induced disease gradually resolve after discontinuing the offending drug. A small percentage of patients with severe symptoms may require a short course of prednisone, especially if complications of pleuritis or pericarditis or if pulmonary infiltrates are apparent. If necessary, steroids are usually very effective in reversing the features of drug-induced lupus. More toxic medications, such as azathioprine or cyclophosphamide, are essentially never required in the treatment of drug-induced lupus.

17. A patient returns to your clinic 8 months after being treated for procainamide-induced lupus. Her symptoms resolved about 4 weeks after stopping procainamide and required a short course of prednisone. She has been off prednisone for over 6 months and remains asymptomatic, but a repeat ANA test is still positive in a high titer. What changes in your therapeutic plan are required at this time?

No therapy is required at this time. It is not unusual for the ANA to remain positive for months to years after an episode of drug-induced lupus, despite the rapid resolution of all symptoms of lupus-like disease. As long as the patient is not rechallenged with the offending drug, symptoms should not recur.

18. How do medications such as procainamide and hydralazine induce lupus-like autoantibody production and disease? Is there evidence from animal models of drug-induced lupus?

The failure to metabolize these drugs via *N*-acetyltransferase is likely involved in the induction of disease. Thus, persons who are slow acetylators are more likely to produce ANA and develop symptoms. One study showed that activated neutrophils can convert lupus-inducing drugs to products that are cytotoxic for lymphocytes and other cells. This conversion required the enzymatic action of myeloperoxidase. It was hypothesized that exposure of the immune system to these cytotoxic metabolites is important in the induction of lupus-like disease, perhaps by generating the release of autoantigens or by causing an immune dysregulation.

Despite these interesting clues and the importance of the question in terms of gaining insight into the mechanisms of autoimmunity, nobody truly understands the pathogenesis of drug-induced lupus. There is also no established or reproducible animal model of drug-induced lupus.

BIBLIOGRAPHY

1. Fritzler MJ, Rubin RL: Drug-induced lupus. In Wallace DJ, Hahn BH (eds): Dubois' Lupus Erythematosus, 4th ed. Philadelphia: Lea & Febiger, 1993, pp 442–453.
2. Hess EV, Mongey A-B: Drug-related lupus. Bull Rheum Dis 40(4):1–8, 1991.
3. Jiang X, Khursigara G, Rubin RL: Transformation of lupus-inducing drugs to cytotoxic products by activated neutrophils. Science 266:810–813, 1994.
4. Kotzin BL, O'Dell JR: Systemic lupus erythematosus. In Frank MM, Austen KF, Claman HN, Unanue ER (eds): Samter's Immunologic Diseases, 5th ed. Boston: Little, Brown, & Co, 1995, pp 667–697.
5. Monestier M, Kotzin BL: Antibodies to histones in systemic lupus erythematosus and drug-induced lupus syndromes. Rheum Dis Clin North Am 18:415–436, 1992.
6. Portanova JP, Arndt RE, Tan EM, Kotzin BL: Anti-histone antibodies in idiopathic and drug-induced lupus recognize distinct intrahistone regions. J Immunol 138:446–451, 1987.
7. Rubin RL, Burlingame RW, Arnett JE, et al: IgG but not other classes of anti-(H2A-H2B-DNA) is an early sign of procainamide-induced lupus. J Immunol 154:2483–2493, 1995.
8. Solinger AM: Drug-related lupus: Clinical and etiologic considerations. Rheum Dis Clin North Am 14:187–202, 1988.
9. Tortoritis MC, Tan EM, McNally EM, Rubin RL: Association of antibody to histone complex H2A-H2B with symptomatic procainamide-induced lupus. N Engl J Med 318:1431–1436, 1988.

22. SYSTEMIC SCLEROSIS

David H. Collier, M.D.

1. Define systemic sclerosis.

Systemic sclerosis is an uncommon connective tissue disease with the most prominent feature being thickening or fibrosis of the skin. It is an heterogeneous disorder, both in the involvement of internal organs and joints as well as in the pace and severity of its clinical course. It is a subcategory of scleroderma (*sclero* = thickened, *derma* = skin).

The American College of Rheumatology has proposed preliminary criteria for the diagnosis of this condition:

Major criteria
   Scleroderma proximal to the metacarpophalangeal or
   metatarsophalangeal joints
Minor criteria
   Sclerodactyly
   Digital pitting scars
   Bibasilar pulmonary fibrosis

One major and two minor criteria are needed for diagnosis of definite systemic sclerosis. However, these criteria will not define a significant minority of patients with systemic sclerosis.

2. How is scleroderma classified?

1. **Localized scleroderma:** cutaneous changes consisting of dermal fibrosis without internal organ involvement
   a. **Morphea:** single or multiple (generalized) plaques commonly on the trunk
   b. **Linear scleroderma:** bands of skin thickening commonly on the legs or arms but sometimes on the face (*en coup de sabre*) that typically follow a linear path

2. **Systemic sclerosis**
   a. **Diffuse systemic sclerosis:** fibrotic skin proximal to the elbows or knees excluding the face and neck. This category of patients may have the onset of Raynaud's phenomenon within a year of developing systemic sclerosis and are more likely to have pulmonary, renal, or cardiac involvement. They are more likely to have autoantibodies to topoisomerase-1 (anti-Scl-70) and much less likely to have an anticentromere antibody.
   b. **Limited systemic sclerosis:** fibrotic skin limited to the hands and forearms, feet, neck, and face. This category of patients usually has Raynaud's phenomenon for years and may have telangiectasias, skin calcifications, and a late incidence of pulmonary hypertension. These patients have a high incidence of anticentromere antibody.
3. **Overlap syndromes:** scleroderma associated with other autoimmune diseases

3. **What is the CREST syndrome?**
   This term describes a subgroup of patients with limited systemic sclerosis having:
   C—Calcinosis
   R—Raynaud's phenomenon
   E—Esophageal dysmotility
   S—Sclerodactyly
   T—Telangiectasias
   The term **limited systemic sclerosis** is preferable because the term CREST describes only a narrow part of the spectrum of limited systemic sclerosis.

4. **Who gets systemic sclerosis?**
   Systemic sclerosis is most commonly seen in women (F:M = 3:1) between ages 35–64. Systemic sclerosis is rare in children and men under age 30. It is slightly more common in black women during child-bearing years, but over all ages, there is probably no significant predominance among blacks.

5. **What is the incidence and prevalence of systemic sclerosis?**
   The incidence and prevalence vary considerably among studies depending on the time period and case ascertainment. Studies before 1975 show an **incidence** (new cases detected/population at risk/time period) of 0.6–2.3 cases/million population. Studies after 1975 show an incidence of 6.3–12.0/million population. No period **prevalence** studies have been reported, and prevalence has been derived from incidence studies. Thus, studies before 1975 indicate a prevalence of 4 cases/million, and studies after 1975 suggest a prevalence as high as 126/million. It has been estimated that the average general practitioner sees 1 case of systemic sclerosis in his or her practice during a career.

6. **Describe the cutaneous abnormalities in systemic sclerosis.**
   The hallmark of systemic sclerosis is **thickened skin,** thought to be due to the abnormal production by a subset of fibroblasts of normal type I collagen along with the accumulation of glycosaminoglycan and fibronectin in the extracellular matrix. There is loss of sweat glands and hair loss in areas of tight skin. Although patients seem to have areas of involved and uninvolved skin, as based on the presence of procollagen-1 and adherence molecules, all skin is abnormal. Skin thickening begins on the fingers and hands in virtually *all* cases of systemic sclerosis. When it begins elsewhere, other localized forms of scleroderma or eosinophilic fasciitis should be considered.
   Calcinosis consist of cutaneous deposits of basic calcium phosphate which characteristically occur in the hands (especially over the proximal interphalangeal joints and fingertips), periarticular tissue, and over bony prominences (especially the extensor surface of the elbows and knees) but can occur virtually anywhere on the body. The deposits of calcium are firm, irregular, and generally nontender, ranging in diameter from 1 mm to several centimeters. They can become inflamed, infected, or ulcerated or may discharge a chalky white material.
   Telangiectases are dilated venules, capillaries, and arterioles. In systemic sclerosis, they tend to be *mat* telangiectases, which are oval or polygonal macules 2–7 mm in diameter found on the hands, face, lips, and oral mucosa. They are seen more commonly in limited systemic sclerosis.

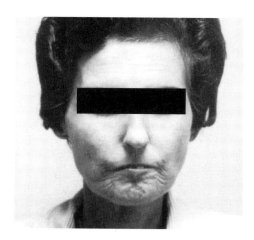

Scleroderma patient demonstrating tightened facial skin. Note exaggerated radial furrowing about the lips (tobacco pouch sign).

7. Discuss the natural history of these cutaneous abnormalities.

The progression of **skin tightening** is quite variable. However, most patients' skin, with no therapy, softens or atrophies over 3–10 years. Internal organ involvement does not mimic the skin improvement and may worsen over time.

Calcinosis can be persistent for years. It is extremely difficult to treat, and no therapy is consistently successful. Therapies used have included warfarin (1–2.5 mg/day, in an attempt to inhibit the Gla matrix protein), aluminum hydroxide, diltiazem, probenecid, and high doses of bisphosphonates.

Telangiectases are usually harmless and a cosmetic problem. They may disappear spontaneously over time. Laser therapy has been used to remove them with some success.

8. What is Raynaud's phenomenon?

Raynaud's phenomenon is an episodic self-limited and reversible vasomotor disturbance manifested as color changes bilaterally in the fingers, toes, and sometimes ears, nose, and lips. The color changes are **pallor, cyanosis,** and then **erythema** (white, blue, and then red) that occur in response to environmental cold and/or emotional stress. There does not need to be a three-color change to diagnose Raynaud's phenomenon; episodic pallor or cyanosis that reverses to erythema or normal skin color may be all that is seen. Patients may describe symptoms of numbness, tingling, or pain on recovery. (*See also* Chapter 78.)

9. How do primary Raynaud's phenomenon and secondary Raynaud's phenomenon differ?

Primary Raynaud's phenomenon is idiopathic, or without an apparent cause. Over time, these patients just complain of color changes in their extremities and develop no internal organ problems. This condition is sometimes referred to as **Raynaud's disease.**

Secondary Raynaud's phenomenon occurs as a manifestation of underlying diseases, such as systemic sclerosis, mixed connective tissue disease, systemic lupus erythematosus, or certain malignancies.

10. Who gets Raynaud's phenomenon?

Typically, young women get primary Raynaud's. The prevalence of Raynaud's in the general population is estimated to be 10%, but the prevalence among young women is as high as 20–30%. Raynaud's phenomenon is found in almost all patients with systemic sclerosis, being the initial complaint in approximately 70% of these patients.

11. In a patient with new-onset Raynaud's phenomenon, what findings would suggest early systemic sclerosis?

- Positive antinuclear antibodies, anti-centromere antibodies, or anti-topoisomerase 1 (Scl-70) antibodies

- Nailfold capillary abnormalities of capillary drop-out
  and/or dilatation (see Chapter 78)
- Tendon friction rubs
- Puffy, swollen fingers or legs
- Associated esophageal reflux

12. How is Raynaud's phenomenon treated?

First, keep hands *and* body warm. Many patients carry gloves at all times. When going to cold places, patients may bring exothermic reaction bags (chemical heat packs), which can be obtained at sporting goods, hardwares, and other fine stores. Repeated soaking in warm water sometimes helps.

The patient should stop smoking. For primary Raynaud's, biofeedback can be very successful if the patient is committed to learning and practicing this technique. Systemic sclerosis patients rarely benefit from biofeedback.

Various prescription vasodilators can be used. Calcium channel blockers are the first choice. The most studied is nifedipine, but diltiazem and the newer calcium channel blockers are used if the patient is having side effects from the nifedipine. The dose of these drugs is increased until the desired effect is obtained or the patient cannot tolerate the side effects. Prazosin and doxazosin and the angiotensin-converting enzyme inhibitors are also used as vasodilators but appear to be less effective than the calcium channel blockers. Topical nitroglycerin ointment applied sparingly over the affected area for 20 minutes three times a day can be helpful, but commonly the patient has an accompanying headache. One-half aspirin a day to inhibit platelet activation is also recommended. The use of intravenous prostacyclin and its analogue (Iloprost) appears promising in severe cases of Raynaud's.

13. Compare and contrast the organ system involvement in diffuse and limited systemic sclerosis.

ORGAN SYSTEM INVOLVEMENT	DIFFUSE	LIMITED
Skin thickening	100%	95%
Telangiectasias	30	80
Calcinosis	5	45
Raynaud's phenomenon	85	95
Arthralgias or arthritis	80	60
Tendon friction rubs	65	5
Myopathy	20	10
Esophageal hypomotility	75	75
Pulmonary fibrosis	35	35
Pulmonary hypertension	<1	10
Congestive heart failure	10	1
Renal crisis	15	1

14. Discuss the pathophysiologic progression of gastrointestinal involvement in systemic sclerosis.

Although no longitudinal studies have been done to document the anatomic progression in the GI system, there is good circumstantial evidence to suggest an orderly series of steps leading to progressive dysfunction. First, there is neural dysfunction thought to be due to arteriolar changes of the vasa nervorum leading to dysmotility. Second, there is smooth muscle atrophy. Third, there is fibrosis of the muscle.

15. How is esophageal dysmotility assessed in patients with systemic sclerosis?

Esophageal dysmotility is documented by manometry, cine-esophagraphy, or by a routine upper GI series with barium swallow. Practically speaking, manometry, although the most sensitive, is so uncomfortable that it is rarely performed. Endoscopy is used to assess reflux esophagitis, candidiasis, Barrett's esophagus, and strictures of the lower esophageal area.

16. How is esophageal dysmotility treated in patients with systemic sclerosis?
Treatment is designed to decrease complications of acid reflux, such as esophagitis, stricture, or nocturnal aspiration of stomach contents. The head of the bed should be elevated 4 inches; adding more pillows to sleep on may only make matters worse by decreasing stomach area. The patient should not eat for 3 hours before bedtime. The acid content in the stomach should be decreased in the evening with antacids, H_2 blockers, or, for progressive problems, omeprazole, or lansoprazole. Motility agents such as metoclopramide or cisapride are sometimes helpful early in the disease, but as the GI smooth muscles fibrose, these agents become ineffective.

17. Patients with systemic sclerosis may have small and large bowel involvement. What symptoms and signs do these patients have?
The major manifestations are due to diminished peristalsis with resulting stasis and dilatation. The diminished peristalsis can lead to bacterial overgrowth. Later, malabsorption can be a major problem. Patients may complain of abdominal distension and pain due to dilated bowel, obstructive symptoms from intestinal pseudo-obstruction, or diarrhea from bacterial overgrowth or malabsorption. If the malabsorption becomes severe, the patient may have signs of vitamin deficiencies or electrolyte abnormalities.

Patients with large bowel involvement may demonstrate wide mouth diverticulae on barium enema. It should be emphasized that barium studies are relatively contraindicated in systemic sclerosis patients with poor GI motility due to the risk of barium impaction.

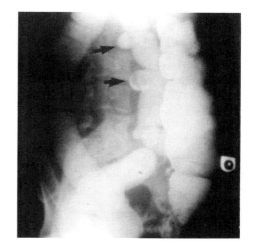

Barium enema in a systemic sclerosis patient, demonstrating wide-mouth diverticulae (*arrows*).

18. How are small and large bowel problems managed in these patients?
Stimulation of gut motility with metoclopramide or cisapride is tried initially. Erythromycin, a motilin agonist, can be given one-half hour before meals to stimulate gut motility. There is limited evidence that daily injectable octreotide may help in severe cases. Fiber may help colonic dysmotility but may make small bowel problems worse. Fiber is worth an empiric trial.

Diarrhea is treated initially as if it were due to bacterial overgrowth. An antibiotic is given that can partially decrease gut flora, such as metronidazole, tetracycline, or amoxicillin. In most cases, this stops the diarrhea. Agents that slow intestinal motility, such as paregoric or loperamide should be avoided. If the diarrhea persists, then a malabsorption work-up should be pursued. Most patients with malabsorption can be treated with supplemental vitamins, minerals, and predigested liquid food supplements. A rare patient will need total parenteral nutrition.

19. Which scleroderma patients get interstitial lung disease? Which get pulmonary hypertension?

CLASSIFICATION	INTERSTITIAL LUNG DISEASE	PULMONARY HYPERTENSION
Localized	None	None
Limited systemic	Typically bibasilar (20%) and	8–28%
sclerosis (LSSc)	usually nonprogressive	Poor prognosis
Diffuse systemic	More common than LSSc (31%–59%)	Very rare
sclerosis	and can be progressive	
	leading to death	
Overlap	Common (19–85%, average 38%)	21–29%
	can progress	

20. Describe the clinical characteristics of lung disease associated with systemic sclerosis.

Many patients with laboratory evidence of **interstitial lung disease** are asymptomatic. Clinical symptoms can be insidious and include exertional dyspnea, easy fatigability, and exertional nonproductive cough, but later may progress to dyspnea at rest. Clinical signs are typically early inspiratory fine or Velcro crackles. Pleuritic chest pains are rare in systemic sclerosis.

Patients with **pulmonary hypertension** usually have an insidious onset of exertional dyspnea, which can rapidly become dyspnea at rest with pedal edema. Physical exam can reveal an increased pulmonic component of the second heart sound (P_2), right ventricular gallops, pulmonic or tricuspid insufficiency murmur, jugular venous distention, and pedal edema. Chest radiographs and CT scans demonstrate interstitial fibrosis predominantly of the lower lobes.

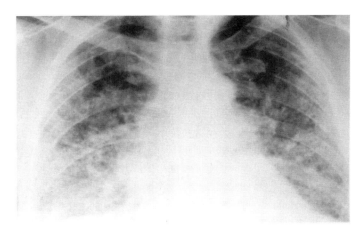

Interstitial lung disease in a systemic sclerosis patient.

21. Describe the cardiac involvement in systemic sclerosis.

Autopsy studies find cardiac involvement unrelated to lung or renal disease relatively common (50%). However, clinically significant heart problems are rare. Pericardial effusion is common at autopsy, but symptomatic pericarditis is rarely seen. Similarly, endocardial involvement is described but clinically insignificant. The most common manifestation of scleroderma heart disease is myocardial fibrosis, usually focal but equally distributed throughout the right and left heart myocardium. Premature coronary artery disease has also been noted in many patients, probably as part of the diffuse vasculopathy occurring in these patients. The use of high-dose corticosteroids is also thought to enhance coronary artery disease. Patients may present with conduction defects and congestive heart failure. The conduction defects, unless showing significant ventricular arrhythmias, are usually not treated. Congestive heart failure is treated in standard ways.

22. Renal failure is one of the most feared complications of systemic sclerosis. What is the presentation of this complication?

Renal failure may present as acute renal crisis, after prolonged hypertension, and less commonly as normotensive renal failure.

Renal crisis is the abrupt onset of arterial hypertension, appearance of grade III (flame-shaped hemorrhages and/or cotton-wool exudates) or grade IV (papilledema) retinopathy, and the rapid deterioration of renal function (within a month). Abnormal laboratory tests include elevated renal function tests, consumptive thrombocytopenia, microangiopathic hemolysis, and elevated renin levels (twice the ULN or greater). Renal crisis usually occurs in the patient with **diffuse** systemic sclerosis. Generally, renal crisis occurs early in the course of the disease, with a mean onset of 3.2 years, and more often in the fall and winter months. Prognosis for recovery is poor.

Prolonged hypertension seems to predispose to renal failure. There is a minority of patients who develop normotensive renal failure with no evidence of renal crisis. The use of high-dose corticosteroids probably increases the risk for renal failure in systemic sclerosis.

23. Which therapeutic intervention has helped avoid renal failure in patients with systemic sclerosis?

The use of **angiotensin-converting enzyme (ACE) inhibitors** have dramatically changed the incidence and outcome of renal involvement in systemic sclerosis. The diastolic blood pressure should be kept below 90 mm Hg in all patients with systemic sclerosis. Captopril and enalapril are the most studied ACE inhibitors in scleroderma, but probably any of the ACE inhibitors are effective.

24. Describe the bone and articular involvement in systemic sclerosis.

Bone involvement is usually demonstrated by resorption of bone. Acrosclerosis with osteolysis is common. Resorption of ribs, mandible, acromion, radius, and ulna have been reported. Arthralgias and morning stiffness are relatively common, but erosive arthritis is rare. Hand deformities and ankylosis are seen, but these are attributed to the tethering effects of skin thickening instead of joint involvement. Tendon sheaths can become inflamed and fibrinous, mimicking arthritis. Tendon friction rubs can be palpated typically over the wrists, ankles, and knees. Mainly, the diffuse systemic sclerosis patients develop tendon friction rubs.

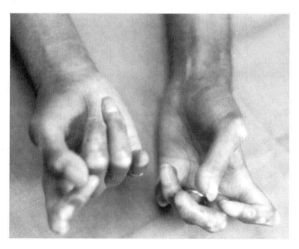

Articular and cutaneous involvement in systemic sclerosis. The skin is taut and thickened, leading to deformity and limited motility of the fingers. Note sclerodactyly and digital ulcerations.

25. Discuss the three types of muscle abnormalities seen in systemic sclerosis.

1. Mild proximal weakness due to a noninflammatory benign myopathy. On histology, this myopathy looks normal or shows muscle fiber type 2 atrophy. This pattern of fiber loss is seen with inactivity and corticosteroid use. The muscle enzymes are typically normal.

2. Mild elevation of muscles enzymes with waxing and waning of symptoms. Muscle biopsy reveals interstitial fibrosis and fiber atrophy. Minimal inflammatory cell infiltration is noted.

3. Inflammatory type of myopathy with elevated muscle enzymes (as seen with polymyositis). These patients are considered to have an overlap syndrome, and many fit the definition of mixed connective tissue disease.

26. Which autoantibodies are seen in diffuse and limited systemic sclerosis?

ANTIBODIES	DIFFUSE SYSTEMIC SCLEROSIS	LIMITED SYSTEMIC SCLEROSIS
Antinuclear antibody	90–95%	90–95%
Anti-topoisomerase I (Scl-70)	20–30	10–15
Anti-centromere antibody	5	50–90
Anti-RNA polymerase III	45	6

27. Which chemicals have been implicated in inducing a scleroderma-like condition?
Vinyl chloride—a number of reports
Silica dust—noted first in gold miners
Rapeseed oil contaminated with aniline dye—toxic oil syndrome noted in Spain in 1981
Contaminated L-tryptophan—implicated in an epidemic of eosinophilia myalgia syndrome
Organic solvents
  Aromatic hydrocarbons—toluene, benzene
  Aliphatic hydrocarbons
    Chlorinated—trichloroethylene, perchloroethylene
    Nonchlorinated—naphtha-*n*-hexane, hexachloroethane
Epoxy resins
Drugs
  Bleomycin
Appetite suppressants
Silicone—breast implants (controversial)

28. What medicines have been used to treat the skin involvement in systemic sclerosis?
No treatment has been shown definitively to be successful in treating scleroderma. The following treatments have been tried in small studies:
- Colchicine (0.6 mg bid)—relatively safe but usually ineffective
- *p*-Aminobenzoic acid (3 gm qid)—safe; used to treat keloid formation; all studies in systemic sclerosis are uncontrolled
- D-Penicillamine (increase slowly to 1,000 mg/day)—the most studied drug in systemic sclerosis; a number of retrospective and uncontrolled studies have demonstrated help with tight skin and possibly interstital lung disease; a relatively toxic drug
- Chlorambucil—showed no help in a good prospective study
- Corticosteroids—thought to increase the incidence of renal crisis and probably should be avoided
- Experimental drugs with limited experience:
  Methotrexate
  Extracorporeal photochemotherapy (photophoresis)
  Plasmapheresis
  5-Fluorouracil
  Gamma-interferon
  Cyclosporine

BIBLIOGRAPHY

1. Althan RD, Medsger TA, Bloch DA, Michel BA: Predictors of survival in systemic sclerosis (scleroderma). Arthritis Rheum 34:403–413, 1991.

2. Borg EJT, Piersma-Wichers G, Smit AJ, et al: Serial nailfold capillary microscopy in primary Raynaud's phenomenon and scleroderma. Semin Arthritis Rheum 24:40–47, 1994.
3. Claman HN, Giorno RC, Seibold JR: Endothelial and fibroblastic activation in scleroderma: The myth of the "uninvolved skin." Arthritis Rheum 34:1495–1501, 1991.
4. Clements PJ, Furst DE (eds): Systemic Sclerosis. Baltimore, Williams and Wilkins, 1996.
5. Donohoe JF: Scleroderma and the kidney. Kidney Int 41:462–477, 1992.
6. Janosik DL, Osborn TG, Moore TL, et al: Heart disease in systemic sclerosis. Semin Arthritis Rheum 19:191–200, 1989.
7. LeRoy EC, Black C, Fleischmajer R, et al: Scleroderma (systemic sclerosis): Classification, subsets and pathogenesis. J Rheumatol 15:202–205, 1988.
8. Medsger TA: Treatment of systemic sclerosis. Ann Rheum Dis 50:877–886, 1991.
9. Meehan R, Spencer R: Systemic sclerosis. Immunol Allergy Clin North Am 13:313–334, 1993.
10. Sjogren RW: Gastrointestinal motility disorders in scleroderma. Arthritis Rheum 37:1265–1282, 1994.
11. Steeh VD, Costantino JP, Shapiro AP, et al: Outcome of renal crisis in systemic sclerosis: Relation to availability of angiotensin converting enzyme (ACE) inhibitors. Ann Intern Med 113:352–357, 1990.
12. Steen VD, Lanz JK, Conte C, et al: Therapy for severe interstitial lung disease in systemic sclerosis: A retrospective study. Arthritis Rheum 37:1290–1296, 1994.
13. Steen VD, Medsger TA: Epidemiology and natural history of systemic sclerosis. Rheum Dis Clin North Am 16:641–654, 1990.
14. Steen VD, Owens GR, Fino GJ, et al: Pulmonary involvement in systemic sclerosis (scleroderma). Arthritis Rheum 28:759–767, 1985.
15. Weiner ES, Hildebrandt S, Senecal JL, et al: Prognostic significance of anticentromere antibodies and anti-topoisomerase 1 antibodies in Raynaud's disease: A prospective study. Arthritis Rheum 34:68–77, 1991.

23. EOSINOPHILIA-MYALGIA SYNDROME, DIFFUSE FASCIITIS WITH EOSINOPHILIA, AND RHEUMATIC DISEASE ASSOCIATED WITH SILICONE BREAST IMPLANTS

Gregory J. Dennis, M.D.

EOSINOPHILIA-MYALGIA SYNDROME

1. List the characteristic clinical features of the eosinophilia-myalgia syndrome (EMS) seen at onset of the disease.

Myalgias	Fever
Maculopapular erythematous skin rashes	Fatigue
Peripheral edema	Weight loss

2. What are some typical findings that occur later in the disease process in EMS?

Scleroderma-like skin thickening	Proximal myopathy
Xerostomia	Perpheral neuropathy
Alopecia	

3. Is EMS recognized as a New or Old World disease?

EMS was recognized during 1989, when it presented in epidemic fashion. Although the initial cases were recognized in Los Alamos, New Mexico, the outbreak was nationwide. Relatively few cases have occurred outside of the United States where the highest rates occurred in the western United States. Since its recognition, a broad spectrum of clinical manifestations have been appreciated with subsequent evolution in afflicted individuals.

4. With which chemical product is EMS associated?

L-tryptophan. EMS is somewhat similar to the toxic oil syndrome that occurred in Spain in 1981, which developed in association with ingestion of denatured rapeseed oil.

5. What three essential features of the disease were established by the Centers for Disease Control (CDC) as the surveillance case definition?

1. Blood eosinophil count $> 10^9$/liter
2. Generalized myalgia of sufficient severity to limit a patient's usual activities
3. Exclusion of neoplasm of infection to account for symptoms

6. Approximately how many cases of EMS were reported in the United States that fulfilled the CDC criteria?

More than 1,500 cases, with 38 deaths, were reported to the CDC criteria. Many more were probably affected but were not reported as they did not fulfill the criteria.

7. Name the most potentially disabling sequelae of the EMS.

Sclerodermatous skin thickening	Neuropathy
Hyperpigmentation	Myopathy
Myalgia	Dyspnea
Muscle cramping	Subjective cognitive impairment
Arthralgia	Fatigue

8. The cutaneous findings in EMS are similar to those of what other disease processes?

Eosinophilic fasciitis and systemic sclerosis

9. When in relation to the onset of disease do the cutaneous manifestations of EMS appear?

The cutaneous findings in EMS have their onset during the initial 3–6 months of disease. Pre-existing edema is not uniformly present, but skin changes often are associated with the presence of papular mucinosis. The distribution of sclerodermatous thickening is similar to that of the sub-classes of skin involvement in idiopathic systemic sclerosis—i.e., diffuse, limited, or localized. There is a wide range of sclerodermatous involvement, increasing from 44% to 82% after 14 to 36 months from disease onset in several series. Hyperpigmentation is also seen in EMS patients.

10. What features of idiopathic systemic sclerosis have *not* been characteristic of patients with EMS?

Patients with EMS generally lack Raynaud's phenomenon, digital ischemic lesions, tendon friction rubs, and acral sclerosis.

11. How do EMS and eosinophilic fasciitis (EF) differ?

1. EMS patients were more likely to require hospitalization, develop fever, and have systemic involvement.
2. Inflammation in EMS is characteristically cutaneous and subcutaneous, whereas the inflammation in EF is primarily subcutaneous.
3. Perineural inflammatory infiltrates are more common in EMS.
4. More immunoglobulin and complement deposition in EF biopsies.

12. List the various manifestations of muscle involvement in EMS.

- The abrupt onset of myalgia is considered one of the hallmarks of EMS and persists in >50% of individuals after 1 year of disease.
- Severe muscle cramps occur in 43–90% of patients with chronic EMS.
- Myopathy may be present in early or late disease, most commonly due to perimyositis. Rarely, myonecrosis or microangiopathy may be responsible for the myopathic process.

13. What types of peripheral neurologic abnormalities have been reported in patients with EMS?

An axonal sensorimotor polyneuropathy has been the most common peripheral neuropathy reported. Others include mononeuritis multiplex, demyelinating neuropathy, and postural tremor.

14. Do clinical manifestations of neuropathy in EMS correlate with findings on electrodiagnostic testing?

Clinical findings of a sensory neuropathy are common, but there may be discordant findings when the patient undergoes electrodiagnostic tests. This discrepancy may be related to the inability of standard nerve conduction velocities to detect involvement of small dermal nerves.

15. How significant is fatigue in patients with EMS?

Fatigue is a significant problem in most patients from the onset. It is one of the principal disabling aspects of chronic EMS, being present in as many as 95% of afflicted individuals.

16. Describe the pathognomonic signs of EMS.

There are no pathognomonic signs. Initially, patients show few abnormal findings. Palpable muscle tenderness and skin rash may be all that is present. A flu-like prodrome is often present, including muscle aches, cough, shortness of breath, and fatigue. Nonspecific symptoms and constitutional symptoms may also be present.

17. What manifestation is considered to be the hallmark of EMS?

A high eosinophil count is considered to be the hallmark of the disease. The eosinophil count, however, is often transient and is found only early in the disease process. The absence of eosinophilia should not preclude a diagnosis of EMS. Eosinophil degranulation in tissue samples has been shown to occur.

18. Describe the principal pathologic lesions found in muscle biopsy specimens.

Fibroplasia

Interstitial inflammatory infiltrate with rare eosinophils. The inflammatory infiltrates have been detected more in the perimysium and fascia but have also been found in the endomysium and perivascular areas.

Occlusive microangiopathy

19. How is EMS treated?

Discontinuation of L-tryptophan-containing products is a necessity, but does not always lead to improvement. There is variable responsiveness to glucocorticoid medications, but long-term efficacy has not demonstrated with their use. Additional immunomodulating therapies have resulted in inconsistent responses.

EOSINOPHILIC FASCIITIS (DIFFUSE FASCIITIS WITH EOSINOPHILIA)

20. Is eosinophilic fasciitis (EF) also associated with ingestion of chemicals?

No. EF is a connective tissue disorder of uncertain etiology, first described in 1974, that has not been associated with the ingestion of chemicals. It is classified in association with scleroderma and scleroderma-like syndromes, but in contrast to scleroderma, individuals with EF generally do not have Raynaud's phenomenon and have normal nailfold capillaries. Strenuous physical exertion may precede its development in some patients.

21. What are some common early clinical manifestations of EF?

Diffuse swelling

Stiffness

Tenderness of the involved areas

22. Is there a characteristic distribution of involvement in EF?

There is usually simultaneous involvement in all areas affected. The most frequent pattern includes involvement of both the arms and legs in a symmetrical fashion. The proximal areas of the extremities are generally more affected than the distal.

The initial manifestations of EF are often followed by the development of severe induration of the skin and subcutaneous tissues of the affected areas. There is a coarse orange-peel appearance to the skin (*peau d'orange*). Although the induration often remains confined to the extremities, it may variably affect extensive areas of the trunk and face.

23. Which common musculoskeletal problem may afflict individuals with EF?
Because of involvement of the fascia, **carpal tunnel syndrome** is an early feature in many patients. Flexion contractures of the digits may occur as a consequence of the fascial involvement.

24. Is eosinophilia uniformly present throughout the course of an EF patient's illness?
Eosinophilia is often present during the early stages of the patient's illness but tends to decline later in the illness. The degree of eosinophilia does not closely parallel disease activity.

25. Are there any hematologic associations with EF?
A variety of hematologic complications have been appreciated. Those described in a small number of patients include thrombocytopenia, aplastic anemia, and myelodysplastic syndromes. The pathogenesis of these conditions is thought to involve autoimmune mechanisms. These complications may occur at any time in the course of EF and do not correlate with the severity of disease.

26. How is the diagnosis of EF confirmed histologically?
Histologically, the diagnosis is best confirmed by performing a deep wedge en-bloc biopsy of an involved area. The biopsy should be deep enough acquire skin, subcutis, fascia, and muscle for study. Although inflammation and fibrosis are generally found in all layers, they are usually most intense in the fascia. The inflammatory infiltrate consists of abundant lymphocytes, plasma cells, and histiocytes. Eosinophilic infiltration may be particularly striking, especially early in the disease process.

27. What laboratory abnormality other than eosinophilia is commonly found in patients with EF?
Other than eosinophilia, the only other commonly reported laboratory abnormality that is generally present is **hypergammaglobulinemia.** The IgG fraction appears to be primarily responsible for the elevation in the total gammaglobulin pool.

28. Describe the course of illness in patients with EF.
In many patients, the illness is self-limited with spontaneous improvement and occasionally complete remission after 2 or more years. Some patients are less fortunate, having persistent or recurrent disease. Fixed joint contractures may be responsible for permanent disability in some patients.

29. Are any therapies effective in patients with EF?
Corticosteroids often result in marked and rapid improvement in both the eosinopilia and presence of fasciitis. Other medications, such as cimetidine, hydroxychloroquine, penicillamine, and immunosuppressive medications, have been used with variable success.

30. Without therapy, what percentage of individuals will develop progressive disease?
If untreated, fascial inflammation will lead to joint contractures in 85%. In addition, the skin that is initially indurated frequently may become bound down and develop a *peau d'orange* appearance.

31. Does the inflammatory process in EF ever extend beyond the fascia?
Deeper layers of the dermis have been involved with cellular infiltration in over 30% of cases. The inflammatory infiltrate has been noted to extend to the epi- and perimysial connective tissue. However, muscle fiber nerosis and phagocytosis are rare.

32. When should the diagnosis of EF be considered?
The diagnosis should be considered in an individual with:
- Scleroderma-like skin tightening
- Skin thickening that spares the digits
- Peripheral eosinophilia
- No Raynaud's phenomenon

RHEUMATIC DISEASE ASSOCIATED WITH SILICONE BREAST IMPLANTS (CONTROVERSIAL)

33. What are some of the recognized complications of augmentation mammoplasty?
- Infection
- Hemorrhage
- Local skin necrosis
- Capsule formation
- Implant rupture

34. When were the first reports of connective tissue diseases in patients with breast implants?
The first report of a connective tissue disease after breast augmentation appeared in the Japanese literature in 1964. One of these patients had dramatic improvement after removal of the foreign substance. The first report in the English literature was in 1979. These early reports were mostly in women receiving breast augmentation with injections of non-medical-grade silicone or paraffin.

The connective tissue diseases reported in patients with breast implants have included systemic sclerosis, mixed connective tissue disease, rheumatoid arthritis, SLE, and sicca syndrome (Sjögren's). Many patients have had complaints of chronic fatigue, arthralgias, and myalgias that defy classification into a specific category of connective tissue disease.

35. Which types of medical-grade polymers are under consideration in the association of silicone with connective tissue disease?
Polydimethylsiloxane (PDMS) polymers are widely used in application ranging from the manufacture of food-processing materials to the production of cosmetics and medical devices. Gels used in breast implants that have been implicated with connective tissue disease are generally produced by the addition of vinyl to PDMS.

36. For which connective tissue disease does there appear to be the greatest concern? Does its clinical expression differ from that considered to be idiopathic in origin?
While a number of connective tissue disease syndromes are thought perhaps to be increased in individuals with silicone breast implants, the one that has received the most notoriety has been **systemic sclerosis** (scleroderma). Thus far, the clinical expression of systemic sclerosis in patients with silicone breast implants does not appear to be any different from that in individuals without implants.

37. Do patient's symptoms resolve or improve when the silicone breast implants are removed?
Improvement and resolution of the patient's problems on removal of the implants have been reported in multiple cases, but only this occurs in a minority of patients. These patients have usually had rheumatoid arthritis or SLE and not scleroderma. The reversibility of illnesses after removal of the implants has increased suspicion that there may be a link between silicone implants and connective tissue disease.

38. Does the silicone act as an adjuvant in connective tissue disease?
There is presently no scientific evidence to support the theory that silicone acts as an adjuvant. Consequently, use of the term *human adjuvant disease* to refer to this group of individuals seems inappropriate. Potential mechanisms that could be involved in silicone-induced disease includes the following:
1. Medical-grade silicone contains 25–33% silica, which has been shown to have an adjuvant effect on antibody production.
2. A cellular response to silicone may be induced, resulting in granulomatous reactions.

39. In patients having silicone breast implants with connective tissue disease, can laboratory variables be used to identify this group?
To date, there are no laboratory markers that exist to allow differentiation of those who have problems with implants from those without problems. Likewise, those with problems cannot be distinguished serologically or otherwise from those with idiopathic disease. Antinuclear antibodies have been commonly detected in those with silicone breast implants, but acute-phase reactants primarily correlate with objective evidence of inflammatory disease.

40. Are imaging studies helpful in the evaluation of patients with possible connective tissue disease (controversial)?
Imaging studies such as mammography or breast MRI may be helpful in detecting implant rupture prior to operative intervention. However, breast implant imaging studies are not helpful in predicting which individuals are at risk for developing a connective tissue disease.

41. Does breast implant rupture increase the risk of connective tissue disease occurrence?
The presence of objective implant rupture thus far has not been shown to correlate with the risk of developing connective tissue disease. Fragmentation of the surface of most breast implants occurs over time, resulting in leakage, migration, or transport of implant contents into surrounding tissue. In the absence of rupture, it is hypothesized that silicone gel may migrate through the elastomeric envelope.

42. What specific recommendations have been made regarding silicone breast implants in the United States?
Silicone gel-filled breast implants are currently not authorized for use in the United States. Controlled prospective studies to investigate the relationship between silicone-containing implants and connective tissue diseases are necessary to reach definitive conclusions.

43. Have any controlled, prospective studies shown a relationship between silicone breast implants and connective tissue disease?
All controlled studies to date have been retrospective. The largest and best done studies have not shown a statistical association between silicone breast implants and classical connective tissue disease. No study has investigated whether nonspecific musculoskeletal complaints are associated with breast implants. These studies have resulted in the American College of Rheumatology's issuing a statement that there is no relationship between silicone breast implants and connective tissue disease. There has been considerable debate and controversy over this issue, but a definitive prospective, controlled study involving a sufficient number of patients is unlikely ever to be done.

44. What other implants have been reported to cause connective tissue diseases or musculoskeletal symptoms?

Temporomandibular joint prostheses	Dermal collagen injection
Silicone joint implants	Breast augmentation with paraffin

BIBLIOGRAPHY

1. Angell M: Do breast implants cause systemic disease?: Science in the courtroom. N Engl J Med 330:1748–1749, 1994.
2. Bridges AJ, Conley C, Wang G, et al: A clinical and immunologic evaluation of women with silicone breast implants and symptoms of rheumatic disease. Ann Intern Med 118:929–936, 1993.
3. Fock KM, Feng PH, Tey BH: Autoimmune disease developing after augmentation mammoplasty: Report of 3 cases. J Rheumatol 11:98–100, 1984.
4. Gabriel SE, O'Fallon WM, Kurland LT, et al: Risk of connective tissue diseases and other disorders after breast implantation. N Engl J Med 330:1697–1702, 1994.
5. Kaufman LD: The evolving spectrum of eosinophilia myalgia syndrome. Rheum Dis Clin North Am 20:973–995, 1994.

6. Lakhanpal S, Ginsberg WW, Michet CJ, et al: Eosinophilic fasciitis: Clinical spectrum and therapeutic responses in 52 cases. Semin Arthritis Rheum 17:221–319, 1988.
7. Martin RW, Duffy J, Engel AG, et al: The clinical spectrum of the eosinophilia-myalgia syndrome associated with L-tryptophan ingestion. Ann Intern Med 113:124–134, 1990.
8. Michet CJ, Doyle JA, Ginsburg WW: Eosinophilic fasciitis: Report of 15 cases. Mayo Clin Proc 56:27–34, 1981.
9. Philen RM, Posada M: Toxic oil and eosinophilia-myalgia syndrome: May 8–10 1991, World Health Organization meeting report. Semin Arthritis Rheum 23:104–124, 1993.
10. Rodnan GP, Di Bartolomeo AG, Medsger TA: Eosinophilic fasciitis: Report of seven cases of a newly recognized scleroderma-like syndrome. Arthritis Rheum 18:422–423, 1975.
11. Sánchez-Guerrero J, Colditz GA, Karlson EW, et al: Silicone breast implants and the risk of connective-tissue diseases and symptoms. N Engl J Med 332:1666–1670, 1995.
12. Shulman LE: Diffuse fasciitis with hypergammaglobulinemia and eosinophilia: A new syndrome. J Rheumatol 1(Suppl 1):46, 1974.
13. Shulman LE: Diffuse fasciitis with eosinophilia: A new syndrome. Arthritis Rheum 20:133, 1977.
14. Varga J, Schumacher HR, Jimenez SA: Systemic sclerosis after augmentation mammoplasty with silicone implants. Ann Intern Med 111:377–383, 1989.
15. Varga J, Uitto J, Jimenez SA: The cause and pathogenesis of the eosinophilia-myalgia syndrome. Ann Intern Med 116:140–147, 1992.

24. INFLAMMATORY MUSCLE DISEASE

Robert T. Spencer, M.D.

1. Idiopathic inflammatory myopathies comprise which disorders?

Polymyositis (PM) and **dermatomyositis** (DM) are the most common of these uncommon disorders which cause nonsuppurative muscle inflammation. Other disorders in this classification include inclusion body myositis, eosinophilic myositis, giant cell myositis, and focal or localized myositis.

2. How are PM and DM classified?

Although several classification schemes have been devised, the system described by Bohan and Peter appears to be most popular:

1. Adult polymyositis
2. Adult dermatomyositis
3. PM/DM associated with malignancy
4. Childhod DM (less often PM)
5. PM/DM associated with other connective tissue disorders

3. What are some of the epidemiologic features of these disorders?

- Annual incidence of 2–10 cases/million
- Peak age of onset is bimodal in distribution: one peak at 10–15 years of age, and the other at 45–55 years
- Female to male ratio is 2–3:1 overall, but 1:1 ratio in childhood DM and 8–10:1 in PM/DM associated with other connective tissue disorders
- In the United States, African-Americans are affected more commonly than whites at a ratio of 3–4:1

4. What are the major diagnostic criteria for PM/DM?

- **Proximal motor weakness:** Weakness occurs earliest and most severely around the shoulder/pelvic girdles and neck flexors. Ocular and facial motor weakness is strikingly unusual. Pain is typically absent or minimal.
- **Elevated serum muscle enzymes:** Creatine kinase (CK) is elevated in almost all patients

at some time during the course of active disease. Other markers of muscle damage include aldolase, myoglobinemia, myoglobinuria, aspartate and alanine aminotransferase, and lactate dehydrogenase.

- **Abnormal neurodiagnostic studies:** The electromyogram (EMG) in PM/DM reveals polyphasic motor unit action potentials (MUAPs) with short duration and low amplitude. This pattern is in contrast to those seen in neuropathic disorders, which are characterized by large-amplitude, long-duration, polyphasic MUAPs (see Chapter 13). Nerve conduction velocity (NCV) studies are abnormal in neuropathic diseases. They are normal in the idiopathic inflammatory myopathies, with the exception of inclusion-body myositis in which neuropathic disease can develop along with the myopathy.
- **Muscle biopsy:** Muscle biopsy should be performed in all cases to confirm the suspected diagnosis. Typical findings are perivascular and endomysial inflammation with accompanying muscle fiber necrosis and muscle fiber regeneration. In PM, endomysial infiltration by chronic inflammatory cells is seen; most of these cells are cytotoxic CD8+ Tcells. In DM, a somewhat different picture is seen in that the chronic inflammatory cell infiltration develops in perivascular as well as endomysial regions and consists of predominantly CD8+ T cells, but with a higher proportion of CD4+ T cells and B cells
- **Characteristic rash of dermatomyositis (see below).**

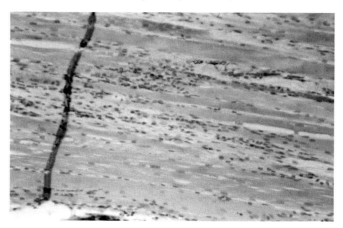

Muscle biopsy demonstrating inflammatory infiltrate and muscle fiber necrosis in a patient with polymyositis.

5. Describe the dermatologic manifestations of dermatomyositis.

Heliotrope (lilac-colored) **rash:** Purple to erythematous rash affecting the eyelids, malar region, forehead, and nasolabial folds. (Eyelids and nasolabial folds are typically spared in the rash of SLE).

Gottron's papules: Purple to erythematous raised lesions over the interphalangeal regions of the fingers (i.e., knuckles). (See Chapter 20, question 10.)

V-sign rash: Confluent erythematous rash over the anterior chest and neck.

Shawl-sign rash: Erythematous rash over the shoulders and proximal arms.

Mechanic's hands: Characterized by cracking and fissuring of the skin of the finger pads.

Nailfold abnormalities: Periungal erythema, cuticular overgrowth, dilated capillary loops (see Chapter 78).

Subcutaneous calcification: Seen nearly exclusively in the juvenile form of DM; Can be very extensive.

6. What measures can be taken to maximize muscle biopsy yield?

- Biopsy a muscle that is clearly weak, but not severely so.
- Biopsy the muscle contralateral to one that is abnormal by EMG (i.e., perform neurodiag-

nostic studies unilaterally, and biopsy the contralateral side based on EMG results). Do not biopsy a muscle that has undergone recent EMG evaluation to avoid spurious results (i.e., EMG artifact).

- MRI scanning can be helpful to direct muscle biopsy in difficult cases. Areas of inflamed muscle demonstrate increased signal on T2-weighted images (i.e., denoting an area of edema/inflammation).

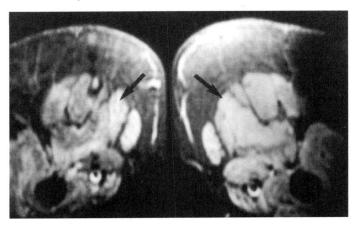

MRI scan of muscles of a patient with myositis. T2-weighted images demonstrate increased signal intensity *(arrows)*.

7. How do the motor manifestations of PM/DM typically present?
Most patients experience an insidious onset of muscle weakness over 3–6 months. Weakness is greatest and most severe in the proximal musculature (hip and shoulder girdles, neck flexors).

8. List some of the extramuscular or extradermatologic manifestations of PM/DM.
Constitutional symptoms: fatigue, low-grade fever, weight loss
Musculoskeletal: arthralgias/arthritis (20–70%)
Pulmonary: interstitial lung disease (5–10%); aspiration pneumonia; respiratory muscle weakness; pulmonary hypertension
Gastrointestinal: esophageal dysmotility (10–30%); intestinal perforation due to vasculitis (juvenile DM)
Cardiac: ECG abnormalities (dysrhythmias, conduction blocks); myocarditis
Vascular: vasculitis causing livedo reticularis, skin ulcerations (juvenile DM); Raynaud's phenomenon (20–40%)
Other: manifestations of other connective tissue diseases when PM/DM occurs in "overlap" syndromes or in association with mixed connective tissue disease (MCTD)

9. Is there an association between PM/DM and underlying neoplastic disease?
Associated cancers are present at diagnosis or at some point during follow-up (usually within first 1–2 years) in about 10% of adult patients with PM and in about 15% of adult patients with DM. Cancers reported in association with PM/DM include, among others, lung, stomach, ovary, breast, pancreas, and Hodgkin's lymphoma. This association has long been controversial, but the association with DM does appear to be significant. Therefore, it is generally advised that patients with PM, and especially those with DM, be screened for underlying neoplastic disease. This screen should at least include a complete history and exam (including breast, pelvis, prostate), stool occult blood testing, chest x-ray, mammogram, and routine laboratory tests.

10. Which laboratory abnormalities are seen in PM/DM?
- **Nonspecific abnormalities**
  Elevated muscle enzymes
  Erythrocyte sedimentation rate (elevated in 50%)
- **Non-myositis-specific autoantibodies**
  ANA (50–80%)
  Anti-RNP antibody (MCTD and "overlap" syndromes)
  Anti-PM-Scl antibody (PM-scleroderma overlap)
  Anti-Ku antibody (PM-scleroderma overlap)
- **Myositis-specific autoantibodies**

11. What are some of the more common myositis-specific autoantibodies?

AUTOANTIBODY	ANTIGEN	PREVALENCE IN PM/DM	CLINICAL ASSOCIATION	HLA ASSOCIATION
Antisynthetase (e.g., anti-Jo-1)	Aminoacyl-tRNA synthetase	20–50%	Antisynthetase syndrome	DRw52, DR3
Anti-SRP	Signal recognition particle	<5%	Severe, resistant PM	DRw52, DR5
Anti-Mi-2	?	5–10%	Classic DM	DRw53, DR7

12. What is the clinical significance of myositis-specific autoantibodies?
   Presence of these autoantibodies helps to predict clinical manifestations and prognosis. For example, the presence of anti-Jo-1 antibody is associated with an increased risk for interstitial lung disease (ILD), among other somewhat unique problems.

	ANTI-SYNTHETASE	ANTI-SRP	ANTI-MI-2
Onset	Acute; spring	Very acute; winter	Acute
Clinical manifestations	PM>>DM	Severe PM	Classic DM
	ILD (40–60%)	Cardiac involvement	V-sign and shawl-sign rashes
	Arthritis (deforming, nonerosive)		Periungal erythema
	Mechanic's hands		Cuticular overgrowth
	Raynaud's phenomenon		
Steroid response	Moderate	Poor	Good

13. Which conditions should be considered in the differential diagnosis of inflammatory myopathies?
Drug and toxin induced myopathies
Neuromuscular disorders
  Muscular dystrophies (e.g., Duchenne's)
  Neuromuscular junction disorders (e.g., myasthenia gravis, Eaton-Lambert syndrome)
  Denervating conditions (e.g., amyotrophic lateral sclerosis)
Endocrine disorders
  Hypothyroidism (may see CK as high as 3000)
  Hyperthyroidism
  Acromegaly
  Cushing's disease
  Addison's disease

Infectious myositis
  Bacterial (*Staphylococcus, Streptococcus, Borrelia burgdorferi*)
  Viral (e.g., HIV, adenovirus, influenza)
  Parasitic (e.g., *Toxoplasma, Trichinella, Taenia*)
Metabolic myopathies
  Glycogen storage diseases (e.g., McArdle's or myophosphorylase deficiency, acid maltase deficiency)
  Abnormalities of lipid metabolism (e.g., carnitine deficiency, carnitine palmitoyl transferase deficiency)
  Mitochondrial myopathies

Miscellaneous
  Other rheumatic disorders (e.g., polymyalgia
    rheumatica, fibromyalgia syndrome,
    inflammatory arthritides, systemic
    vasculitis)
  Carcinomatous neuromyopathy
  Acute rhabdomyolysis
  Organ failure (uremia, liver failure)

Nutritional disorders (malabsorption,
  vitamin D and E deficiencies)
Electrolyte disorders (hypo- and hypercalcemia, hypokalemia, hypophosphatemia)
Sarcoidosis

14. What is the approach to treatment of PM/DM?

Corticosteroids are the mainstay of therapy for PM/DM. Commonly, prednisone is started at a dose of 1–1.5 mg/kg/day in divided doses, and the dose is maintained until remission is achieved (improved strength and normalization of muscle enzymes). Subsequently, the dose is slowly tapered while monitoring for recurrence of disease activity.

Immunosuppressive agents are used in life-threatening disease and in disease resistant to corticosteroids alone. Methotrexate and azathioprine are used most often. Cyclophosphamide and cyclosporine are used rarely but have been reported to be of possible benefit.

Of **experimental therapies,** intravenous immunoglobulin (IVIG) has been reported to be effective in severe, refractory disease. Plasmapheresis has been tried in small numbers of patients and is of questionable benefit.

In the initial stages of disease, when muscle inflammation is most severe and when the patient is most weak, **rehabilitation** is recommended to involve only passive/active assisted range of motion exercises. Later, as strength returns and muscle inflammation subsides, exercise for strengthening can slowly be added to the physical therapy regimen.

15. What is the overall prognosis for these disorders?

Clinical subgroups: Similar 5–year survivals are seen in idiopathic PM/DM and in those cases with associated connective tissue diseases ($\geq$ 85%). In patients with associated neoplastic disease, a much poorer survival rate is observed.

Serologic subgroups: Patients with the anti-Mi-2 antibody appear to have a very favorable prognosis, with a 5–year survival of > 90%. Patients who are myositis-specific antibody negative and those with anti-synthetase antibodies have a less favorable prognosis, but still have 5-year survivals > 65%. The worst prognosis is seen in patients with an associated anti-SRP antibody in whom 5–year survival is approximately 30%.

16. What is inclusion body myositis?

Inclusion body myositis (IBM) predominantly affects white males over age 50. Onset of weakness is slow and insidious. Proximal muscles are involved, but distal muscles are also affected early in the disease course. Weakness is usually bilateral, but asymmetry is common. The legs, especially the anterior thigh, are typically affected more than the arms, and muscle atrophy can be prominent.

Some patients have a mild peripheral neuropathy with loss of deep tendon reflexes. EMG usually shows both myopathic and neuropathic changes. Extraskeletal muscle involvement of the lungs, joints, and heart rarely occurs in these patients. Antinuclear antibodies can be present, but myositis-specific autoantibodies (e.g., anti-Jo-1) do not occur. Muscle biopsy shows foci of chronic inflammatory cells without perifascicular atrophy. The inflammatory infiltrate is predominantly CD8$^+$ T cells. The characteristic findings in IBM on muscle biopsy are red-rimmed vacuoles containing beta-amyloid. Patients respond poorly to immunosuppressive therapy, and the course is slowly progressive, requiring supportive care.

17. How does inclusion body myositis differ from polymyositis?

Despite IBM and polymyositis both being inflammatory myopathies, there are several clinical and immunologic differences that distinguish between them.

	IBM	POLYMYOSITIS
Demographics	M > F	F > M
	Age > 50	All ages
Muscle involvement	Proximal and distal	Proximal
	Asymmetric	Symmetric
Other organ involvement	Neuropathy	Interstitial lung disease, arthritis, heart involvement
Antinuclear antibodies	Sometimes	Frequent
Myositis-specific antibodies	No	Yes
EMG	Myopathic and neuropathic	Myopathic
Muscle biopsy	$CD8^+$ T–cell infiltrate Red-rimmed vacuoles with beta-amyloid	$CD8^+$ T–cell infiltrate
Response to immunosuppressive therapy	No	Frequent

BIBLIOGRAPHY

1. Bernard P, Bonnetblanc JM: Dermatomyositis and malignancy. J. Invest Dermatol 100:128S, 1993.
2. Bunch TW: Polymyositis: A case history approach to the differential diagnosis and treatment. Mayo Clin Proc 65:1480, 1990.
3. Dalakas MC: Medical progress: Polymyositis, dermatomyositis, and inclusion-body myositis. N Engl J Med 325:1487, 1991.
4. Kagen LJ: Inflammatory muscle disease: Management. In Klippel JH, Dieppe PA (eds): Rheumatology. London, Mosby, 1994.
5. Medsger TA, Oddis CV: Inflammatory muscle disease: Clinical features. In Klippel JH, Dieppe PA (eds): Rheumatology. London, Mosby, 1994.
6. Miller FW: Humoral immunity and immunogenetics in the idiopathic inflammatory myopathies. Curr Opin Rheumatol 3:902, 1991.
7. Plotz PH: Not myositis: A series of chance encounters. JAMA 268:2074, 1992.
8. Plotz PH, Dalakas MC, Leff RL, et al: Current concepts in the idiopathic inflammatory myopathies: Polymyositis, dermatomyositis, and related disorders. Ann Intern Med 111:143, 1989.
9. Plotz PH, Rider LG, Targoff IN, et al: Myositis: Immunologic contributions to understanding cause, pathogenesis, and therapy. Ann Intern Med 122:715, 1995.
10. Sigurgeirsson B, Lindelöf B, Edhag O, et al: Risk of cancer in patients with dermatomyositis or polymyositis: A population-based study. N Engl J Med 326:363, 1992.
11. Wortmann RL: Inflammatory diseases of muscle. In Kelley WN, Harris ED, Ruddy S, Sledge CB (eds): Textbook of Rheumatology. Philadelphia, W.B. Saunders, 1993.
12. Wortmann RL: Proximal weakness of unknown etiology. In Klippel JH, Dieppe PA (eds): Rheumatology. London, Mosby, 1994.

25. OVERLAP SYNDROMES AND MIXED CONNECTIVE TISSUE DISEASE

Vance J. Bray, M.D.

1. What is the difference between mixed connective tissue disease (MCTD), undifferentiated connective tissue disease (UCTD), and overlap syndromes?
Mixed connective tissue disease, first described by Sharp et al. in 1972, is characterized by a combination of manifestations similar to those seen in systemic lupus erythematosus (SLE), scleroderma (PSS), and myositis (PM); it requires the presence of high-titer anti-RNP antibodies. These

patients lack other autoantibodies such as anti-Sm, anti–SS-A, anti–SS-B, and anti–double-stranded DNA. Undifferentiated connective tissue disease describes a syndrome in which a patient develops clinical features of an autoimmune disease and nonspecific autoantibodies without developing enough manifestations to meet criteria for a more specific diagnosis (e.g., a patient with inflammatory arthritis and a positive antinuclear antibody). Overlap syndromes occur when patients develop enough clinical and serologic manifestations to meet criteria for the diagnosis of one connective tissue disease, in addition to manifestations of another distinct entity (e.g., patients with SLE may develop a positive rheumatoid factor and an erosive arthritis in a distribution similar to rheumatoid arthritis [RA]; the overlap of SLE and RA is known as rhupus). It is estimated that up to 25% of patients with one connective tissue disease will develop an overlap syndrome. Although the features of both diseases may occur concurrently, usually one syndrome gradually takes on the features of another.

2. What is the most common disease in overlap syndromes and with which other diseases is it associated?
Sjögren's syndrome is the most common overlap and is seen with RA, SLE, PSS, PM, MCTD, primary biliary cirrhosis (PBC), necrotizing vasculitis, autoimmune thyroiditis, chronic active hepatitis, mixed cryoglobulinemia, and hypergammaglobulinemic purpura.

3. What are the early clinical manifestations of MCTD and how do they change over time?
The onset of MCTD is characterized by features of scleroderma, SLE and myositis that occur in concert or sequentially (see following table). The most common lupus-like manifestation at onset is arthralgia or nondeforming arthritis. Skin changes seen in the early stages of scleroderma are usually limited to edematous hands; only a minority of patients have more widespread skin changes. Raynaud's phenomenon occurs in over 90% of patients. Esophageal dysmotility is common. Myositis is present in up to 75% of the patients early in the disease course. It is unusual to have renal disease. These patients generally respond to therapy with corticosteroids. Over time, the manifestations of MCTD tend to become less severe and less frequent. Inflammatory symptoms become much less common. Persistent problems are most often those associated with scleroderma, such as sclerodactyly, Raynaud's phenomenon, and esophageal dysmotility. These patients have fewer problems with arthralgias, arthritis, serositis, fever, hepatomegaly, and splenomegaly. Lymphadenopathy and symptomatic muscle disease also become less frequent with time. Renal disease continues to be unusual.

Clinical Features of Patients with Mixed Connective Tissue Disease at Onset and at Follow-up (Average Follow-up Duration of 12 Years)

CLINICAL MANIFESTATION	PRESENCE %	
	AT ONSET	AT FOLLOW-UP
Joint symptoms	93	64
Swelling or sclerodermatous changes of the hands	71	43
Raynaud's phenomenon	93	71
Esophageal dysmotility	57	43
Muscle involvement	50	29
Lymphadenopathy	71	21
Fever	36	0
Hepatomegaly	21	0
Serositis	29	0
Splenomegaly	21	0
Renal disease	7	7
Anemia	64	14
Leukopenia	57	57
Hypergammaglobulinemia	79	64

4. What other autoimmune syndrome is classically associated with PBC?
Approximately 4% of patients with PBC have an overlap syndrome with the CREST variant of scleroderma (**c**alcinosis, **R**aynaud, **e**sophageal dysmotility, **s**clerodactyly, **t**elangiectasias). CREST

usually antedates PBC by an average of 14 years, although occasionally PBC may develop first. The anticentromere antibody, usually associated with CREST, is present in 10–29% of PBC patients; likewise, the antimitochondrial antibody that is usually associated with PBC is found in 18–27% of CREST patients.

5. Describe the typical MCTD patient.

Mixed connective tissue disease is diagnosed in women at least 15 times more often than in men. The mean age at diagnosis is 37 years, with a range of 5–80 years. There are no apparent racial or ethnic predispositions. Although the exact prevalence is not known, MCTD is thought to be more common than PSS and PM but not as common as SLE.

6. What are the common gastrointestinal manifestations of MCTD?

Gastrointestinal (GI) symptoms and their frequencies were recorded in 61 patients with MCTD and are listed in the following table. The most common manifestations are similar to those of scleroderma: upper and lower esophageal sphincter hypotension, esophageal body hypomotility, gastroesophageal reflux disease with its complications, and pulmonary aspiration. Esophageal function is abnormal in up to 85% of patients, although it may be asymptomatic. In some patients, esophageal pressures improve with corticosteroid therapy. Small bowel and colonic disease is less common in MCTD than in scleroderma. Other less common GI complications include intestinal vasculitis, acute pancreatitis, and chronic active hepatitis.

Gastrointestinal Symptoms in Patients with Mixed Connective Tissue Disease

SYMPTOM	FREQUENCY (%)
Heartburn or regurgitation	48
Dysphagia	38
Dyspepsia	20
Diarrhea	8
Constipation	5
Vomiting	3

7. What are the pulmonary manifestations of MCTD and how are they managed?

Involvement of the lungs is common in MCTD; two-thirds to three-fourths of patients evaluated have some abnormality. The typical manifestations and their frequencies are detailed below.

Pulmonary Manifestations of Mixed Connective Tissue Disease

Symptoms	
Dyspnea	16%
Chest pain and tightness	7%
Cough	5%
Chest x-ray findings	
Interstitial changes	19%
Small pleural effusions	6%
Nonspecific pneumonitis	4%
Pleural thickening	2%
Segmental atelectasis	1%
Pulmonary function studies	
Restrictive pattern	69%
Decreased carbon monoxide diffusion	66%
Pulmonary hypertension	23%

Management involves identifying the specific abnormalities and directing therapy appropriately. Manifestations caused by active inflammation, such as interstitial inflammation or pleuritis, may respond to nonsteroidal anti-inflammatory drugs or corticosteroids. Other medications such as azathioprine or cyclophosphamide may be used to treat interstitial lung disease, although the data is not adequate to assess their efficacy. Pulmonary hypertension may result from vascular intimal proliferation; however, it is likely that pulmonary vasculature vasospasm, which can be treated with vasodilators such as the calcium channel blockers, is also a component. Aspiration secondary to esophageal disease may also contribute to pulmonary compromise, so treatment with antacids, even in the absence of reflux symptoms, is indicated.

8. What are the common nervous system manifestations of MCTD?
Severe central nervous system involvement is unusual with MCTD. Trigeminal neuralgia is the most common problem, as it is in PSS. Headaches are also relatively common, but convulsions and psychosis rarely occur.

9. What are the typical laboratory findings in a patient with MCTD?
The typical findings are detailed below.

Laboratory Findings in Patients with MCTD

ABNORMALITY	FREQUENCY (%)
Anemia	75
Leukopenia	75
False-positive VDRL	10
Rheumatoid factor	50
Antinuclear antibody	100
Anti-RNP	100
Hypocomplementemia	25

Anemia is usually that of chronic disease. Coombs' positivity is detected in 60% of patients, although overt hemolytic anemia is uncommon. Thrombocytopenia is uncommon. The sedimentation rate is usually elevated and can be related to disease activity. Hypocomplementemia is not associated with any particular clinical manifestation.

10. What is RNP?
RNP is an extractable nuclear antigen that consists mainly of protein and ribonucleic acid. It belongs to a group of small nuclear ribonuclearproteins (snRNPs) that are important mediators of gene expression. It is, by definition, present in high titer (e.g., > 1:600 by hemagglutination method) in MCTD. The titer of anti-RNP antibody can fluctuate over time but does not correlate with disease activity or severity. The presence of high-titer anti-RNP results in a high-titer antinuclear antibody with a speckled pattern. In MCTD the anti-RNP is the only specific antinuclear antibody present. This antibody is also present in other rheumatic diseases such as SLE, but in those cases it is generally present in low titer and in association with other antibodies, such as anti-DNA and/or anti-Sm.

11. What is the course and prognosis of MCTD?
There is a low incidence of life-threatening renal disease and neurologic disease in MCTD. The major mortality results from progressive pulmonary hypertension and its cardiac sequelae. The general consensus is that patients with MCTD have a better prognosis than those with SLE, but because there is tremendous variability in disease severity and manifestations, it is misleading to tell an individual that he or she has an excellent prognosis. The development of end-organ involvement dictates the morbidity and mortality.

As a general rule, the SLE-like features of arthritis and pleurisy are treated with NSAIDs, antimalarials, low-dose prednisone (less than 20 mg/day), and occasionally methotrexate. Inflammatory myositis is treated with high doses of prednisone (60 mg/day) and rarely methotrexate or azathioprine. PSS-like features of Raynaud's phenomenon, dysphagia, and reflux esophagitis are treated as described in Chapter 22. Vigorous therapy of myocarditis and/or early pulmonary hypertension with corticosteroids and cyclophosphamide can be beneficial. Symptomatic and progressive pulmonary hypertension is treated with trials of intravenous prostacycline, ACE inhibitors, and/or calcium channel blockers, usually with limited success. Lung transplantation may be the only option in severe cases, although experience with this procedure in MCTD is limited.

BIBLIOGRAPHY

1. Bennett RM: Scleroderma overlap syndromes. Rheum Dis Clin North Am 16:185–198, 1990.
1. Cervera R, Khamashta MA, Hughes GRV: "Overlap" syndromes. Ann Rheum Dis 49:947–948, 1990.
3. Doria A, Bonavina L, Anselmino M, et al: Esophageal involvement in mixed connective tissue disease. J Rheumatol 18:685–690, 1991.
4. Lundberg I, Hedfors E: Clinical course of patients with anti-RNP antibodies: A prospective study of 32 patients. J Rheumatol 18:1511–1519, 1991.
5. Lundberg I, Nyman U, Pettersson I, Hedfors E: Clinical manifestations and anti-(U1)snRNP antibodies: A prospective study of 19 anti-RNP antibody positive patients. Br J Rheumatol 31:811–817, 1992.
6. Marshall JB, Kretschmar JM, Gerhardt DC, et al: Gastrointestinal manifestations of mixed connective tissue disease. Gastroenterology 98:1232–1238, 1990.
7. Mukerji B, Hardin JG: Undifferentiated, overlapping and mixed connective tissue diseases. Am J Med Sci 305:114–119, 1993.
8. Nimelstein SH, Brody S, McShane D, et al: Mixed connective tissue disease: A subsequent evaluation of the original 25 patients. Medicine 59:239–248, 1990.
9. Prakash UBS, Luthra HS, Divertie MB: Intrathoracic manifestations in mixed connective tissue disease. Mayo Clin Proc 60:813–821, 1985.
10. Sharp GC, Irvin WS, Tan EM, et al: Mixed connective tissue disease—an apparently distinct rheumatic disease syndrome associated with a specific antibody to an extractable nuclear antigen (ENA). Am J Med 52:148–159, 1972.

26. SJÖGREN'S SYNDROME

Vance J. Bray, M.D.

1. Who was Sjögren and what is his syndrome?

Henrich Sjögren was born in 1899 in Stockholm and received his M.D. from the Karolinska Institut in 1927. In 1933 he published a monograph associating dry eyes with arthritis. He also introduced rose Bengal staining to identify corneal lesions and introduced the term *keratoconjunctivitis sicca* to describe the ocular manifestations. Sjögren's syndrome refers to a systemic disease most frequently manifested by dry eyes, dry mouth, and arthritis.

2. What are the alternative names for Sjögren's syndrome?

Sjögren's syndrome has also been known as Mikulicz's disease, Gougerot's syndrome, sicca syndrome, and autoimmune exocrinopathy. Hadden, Leber, and Mikulicz initially described the association of dry eyes, dry mouth, and glandular enlargement in the late 1800s. Gougerot in 1925 and Sjögren in 1933 associated these findings with polyarthritis and systemic disease.

3. Who typically develops Sjögren's syndrome?

The typical patient is a middle-aged female. The female to male ratio is 9:1, and the usual age is 30–50 years. Sjögren's has rarely been reported in children.

4. What is the difference between primary and secondary Sjögren's syndrome?

The clinical manifestations of primary and secondary Sjögren's syndrome are the same. **Primary** Sjögren's is diagnosed in the absence of another underlying rheumatic disease, is immunogenetically associated with HLA–B8–DR3, and is associated with antinuclear antibodies to Ro/SS-A and La/SS-B. **Secondary** Sjögren's is diagnosed when there is accompanying evidence of another connective tissue disease, most frequently rheumatoid arthritis. The immunogenetic and serologic findings are usually those of the accompanying disease (e.g., HLA-DR4-positive if associated with rheumatoid arthritis).

5. How common is Sjögren's syndrome?
An estimated 1–2 million people in the United States have Sjögren's, and most are undiagnosed. Primary Sjögren's occurs at a rate of 1/1000 individuals, which is equal to the frequency of systemic lupus erythematosus. Secondary Sjögren's accounts for the remainder of cases. Approximately 30% of patients with rheumatoid arthritis have secondary Sjögren's syndrome.

6. What are the common initial manifestations of primary Sjögren's syndrome?
Xerophthalmia	47%
Xerostomia	42%
Arthralgias/arthritis	28%
Parotid gland enlargement	24%
Raynaud's phenomenon	21%
Fever/fatigue	10%
Dyspareunia	5%

7. What is the underlying pathology of Sjögren's syndrome?
The manifestations of Sjögren's syndrome result from lymphocytic infiltration of glandular and nonglandular organs. Lymphocytic infiltration of the lacrimal glands and salivary glands interferes with the production of tears and saliva, respectively. Lymphocytic infiltration of other organs, such as the lungs and GI tract, results in a variety of major organ manifestations. The lymphocytes are predominantly CD4+ helper T cells. B cells account for 20% of the lymphocytes and are responsible for increased immunoglobulin production.

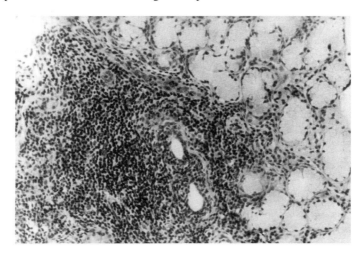

Minor salivary gland biopsy demonstrating mononuclear cell infiltration and salivary gland destruction. (From the Clinical Slide Collection on the Rheumatic Diseases. Atlanta, American College of Rheumatology, 1991; with permission.)

8. What are the most common ocular symptoms of Sjögren's syndrome?
Patients most often complain of dry eyes or painful eyes, which is also known as **keratoconjunctivitis sicca** or **xerophthalmia.** These patients may experience a foreign-body or gritty sen-

sation, a burning sensation, itchiness, blurred vision, redness, and/or photophobia. Symptoms worsen as the day progresses, presumably because of evaporation of ocular moisture during the time that the eyes are open. This pattern contrasts with blepharitis in which, as a result of inflammation of the eyelids, there is crusting and discomfort most pronounced in the morning on awakening.

9. What are other causes of dry eyes besides Sjögren's?
Blepharitis, viral infections, contact lens irritation, and medications such as antihistamines, diuretics, and psychotropic drugs.

10. What tests are used to document dry eyes in a patient with suspected Sjögren's syndrome?
The two most common tests of tear production and adequacy are the Schirmer's test and rose bengal staining. The **Schirmer's test** involves placing a piece of filter paper under the inferior eyelid and measuring the amount of wetness over a specified time. Wetting of < 5 mm in 5 minutes is a strong indication of diminished tear production. There is a 15% false-positive and false-negative rate with Schirmer's testing.

Rose bengal stain is applied topically and is taken up by devitalized or damaged epithelium of the cornea and conjunctiva, thus documenting dryness of enough severity to injure corneal tissue. The area of maximum uptake is along the palpebral fissure, where the maximum exposure to the environment and evaporation of tears occur. There is a 5% false-positive and false-negative rate with rose bengal staining.

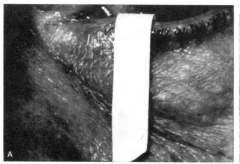 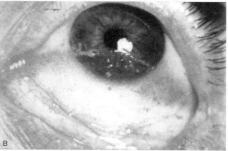

A, Schirmer's test demonstrating decreased tear production. *B*, Rose bengal test with increased dye uptake in areas of devitalized epithelium. (From the Clinical Slide Collection on the Rheumatic Diseases. Atlanta, American College of Rheumatology, 1991; with permission.)

11. What are the common symptoms of decreased production of saliva?
Decreased saliva production is known as **xerostomia.** It may result in a variety of problems, including:

Difficulty swallowing dry food
Inability to speak continuously
Change in taste
Burning sensation
Increase in dental caries
Problems in wearing dentures
Gastroesophageal reflux symptoms (due to lack of salivary buffering)
Disturbed sleep (due to dry mouth and/or nocturia)
Predisposition to oral candidiasis

12. How can salivary gland involvement be determined?

A variety of methods are used to determine salivary function. **Lashley cups** can be used to quantitate saliva production. Alternatively, a patient can place a dry **sponge** in his or her mouth; the difference between dry and wet weights indicates the amount of saliva produced. **Sialography** will outline the salivary duct anatomy but may be painful, predispose to infections, or cause obstruction. **Scintigraphy** utilizes the uptake and secretion of ^{99m}Tc pertechnetate during a 60-minute period following intravenous injection to quantitate salivary flow rates.

Finally, **minor salivary gland** involvement will demonstrate lymphocytic infiltration. An incisional **biopsy** through the lower labial mucosa yielding 5–10 minor glands is adequate for assessment. An area of $\geq$50 lymphocytes is defined as a focus, with $>$ 1 focus/4 mm^2 supporting the diagnosis of the salivary component of Sjögren's. The findings in the minor salivary glands generally parallel involvement of other organs, so biopsy of the parotid glands or major salivary glands is generally not necessary. The minor salivary gland biopsy also may be abnormal before decreased salivary flow can be documented with scintigraphy, because it takes time for the infiltrate to destroy enough salivary gland tissue to cause decreased saliva production.

13. What are the common causes of decreased salivary secretion?

Temporary
Short-term drug use (e.g., antihistamines)
Viral and bacterial infections (especially mumps)
Dehydration
Psychogenic causes (fear, depression)
Chronic
Chronically administered drugs (antidepressants, anticholinergics,
   neuroleptics, clonidine, diuretics)
Systemic diseases
   Sjögren's syndrome
   Granulomatous diseases (sarcoid, tuberculosis, leprosy)
   Amyloidosis
   HIV infection
   Graft-versus-host disease
   Cystic fibrosis
   Diabetes mellitus (uncontrolled)
Other
Therapeutic radiation to the head and neck
Trauma or surgery to the head and neck
Absent or malformed glands (rare)

14. What is the differential diagnosis of salivary gland enlargement?

Usually unilateral
Primary salivary gland neoplasms
Bacterial infection
Chronic sialadenitis
Obstruction
Usually bilateral (asymmetric, with hypofunction)
Viral infection (mumps, cytomegalovirus, influenza, coxsackie A)
Sjögren's syndrome
Granulomatous diseases (sarcoid, tuberculosis, leprosy)
Recurrent parotitis of childhood
HIV infection
Bilateral, symmetric (soft, nontender)

Idiopathic	Hepatic cirrhosis	Acromegaly
Diabetes mellitus	Anorexia/bulimia	Gonadal hypofunction
Hyperlipoproteinemia	Chronic pancreatitis	Phenylbutazone ingestion

15. What is DILS?
Diffuse infiltrative lymphocytosis syndrome is a disorder that mimics Sjögren's and is seen in patients infected with the human immunodeficiency virus (HIV). Common clinical features include fever, lymphadenopathy, weight loss, and bilateral parotid gland enlargement. In contrast to most patients with primary Sjögren's, patients with DILS experience more xerostomia than xerophthalmia and keratoconjunctivitis sicca. DILS patients may also experience recurrent sinus and middle ear infections, lymphocytic interstitial pneumonitis, lymphocytic hepatitis, infiltration of the gastric mucosa (which can mimic linitus plastica), lymphocytic interstitial nephritis, aseptic meningitis, sensorimotor neuropathies, uveitis, and cranial nerve palsies.

DILS differs from Sjögren's syndrome in that the infiltrating lymphocytes in DILS are CD8+ cells, not CD4+ as seen in Sjögren's. DILS patients also lack antibodies to Ro/SS-A and La/SS-B. In contrast to other patients infected with HIV, DILS patients maintain their CD4 counts in the range of asymptomatic HIV-infected individuals and tend not to develop opportunistic infections or Kaposi's sarcoma. However, they are four times more likely to develop a high-grade non-Hodgkin's B-cell lymphoma in the salivary or lacrimal glands and elsewhere.

16. List the common extraglandular manifestations of primary Sjögren's syndrome.

Arthralgias/arthritis	60–70%
Raynaud's phenomenon	35–40%
Esophageal dysfunction	30–35%
Lymphadenopathy	15–20%
Vasculitis	5–10%
Lung involvement	10–20%
Kidney involvement	10–15%
Liver involvement	5–10%
Peripheral neuropathy	2–5%
Myositis	1–2%
Lymphoma	5–8%

17. Describe the arthritis of primary Sjögren's.
The distribution of Sjögren's arthritis is similar to that of rheumatoid arthritis. The patient experiences symmetric arthralgias and/or arthritis of the wrists, metacarpophalangeal and proximal interphalangeal joints, frequently associated with morning stiffness and fatigue. In contrast to rheumatoid arthritis, Sjögren's arthritis is nonerosive and tends to be mild. It usually responds to mild medications such as NSAIDs, antimalarials (hydroxychloroquine), and/or low doses of prednisone (≤5 mg).

18. Are there typical laboratory and autoantibody findings in patients with primary Sjögren's syndrome?

↑ Erythrocyte sedimentation rate	80–90%
Hypergammaglobulinemia	80%
Anemia of chronic disease	25%
Leukopenia	10%
Thrombocytopenia	Rare
Autoantibodies	
Rheumatoid factor	80–95%
Antinuclear antibody (ANA)	90%
anti-SS-A antibody	70–90%
anti-SS-B antibody	40–50%

19. What is the risk of cancer in Sjögren's syndrome patients?
Sjögren's patients are at a 44-fold greater risk of developing lymphoma than age-matched controls, with an overall frequency of lymphoma of 5–8%. The onset of lymphoma may be preceded by the development of a monoclonal gammopathy. Alternatively, concern for lymphoma is raised by the loss of a previously positive rheumatoid factor, the loss of the monoclonal gammopathy, or the development of hypogammaglobulinemia. Other clues of excessive lymphoproliferation

include regional or generalized lymphadenopathy, hepatosplenomegaly, pulmonary infiltrates, renal insufficiency, purpura, or leukopenia.

20. Which criteria have been proposed to diagnose Sjögren's syndrome?

Primary Sjögren's

Dry eyes with keratoconjunctivitis sicca documented by an abnormal Schirmer's or positive rose bengal test

Dry mouth documented by abnormal salivary scintigraphy or positive minor salivary gland biopsy

Abnormal serologies manifested by a positive rheumatoid factor, positive ANA, and/or positive anti-SSA or anti-SSB (or both)

Secondary Sjögren's

Dry eyes (as documented above)

Dry mouth (as documented above)

Associated autoimmune disease (usually rheumatoid arthritis)

21. How is the xerophthalmia of Sjögren's syndrome treated?

Dry eyes are treated with eye drops. Many preparations with differing degrees of viscosity are available. Those with a watery consistency may require frequent applications; more viscous preparations may provide longer benefit but may blur vision in some patients. Lubricant ointments are available and may be especially useful during the night. Slow-release artificial tears are also available but require a small amount of residual tear production to be effective. Recently, oral pilocarpine has been released for stimulation of tear and saliva production. Humidifiers are useful in arid climates and at high altitudes. Evaporation of tears may be slowed by the use of glasses with side shields; but swim goggles are an inexpensive means of obtaining occlusive eyewear. Punctal occlusion, performed by the ophthalmologist, will obstruct the normal lacrimal drainage system, allowing tears to last longer. Temporary plugs are generally inserted before permanent obstruction is considered.

22. Describe the management for other mucosal dryness in Sjögren's.

The complications of xerostomia are best prevented by good dental care, with frequent use of fluoridated toothpaste and mouthwash as well as regular professional dental attention. Sugarless mints or candies may stimulate salivary flow without increasing the risk of dental caries. Saliva substitutes and pilocarpine are also available. Oral candidiasis is best treated with oral application of nystatin vaginal tablets. Dentures must be removed while the mouth is being treated and may also need to be treated in order to cure and prevent recurrence of oral candidiasis. Oral fluconazole for 2 weeks can be used in resistant cases.

Vaginal dryness is treated with topical lubricants. Dry skin usually improves with lotions and creams.

23. How are the other manifestations of Sjögren's managed?

Fatigue is a common symptom that may be difficult to alleviate. If associated with poor sleep, treatment similar to that recommended for fibromyalgia may be of benefit, although tricyclic antidepressants are likely to aggravate dryness of the mucous membranes. If there are associated inflammatory parameters, such as an elevated sedimentation rate and/or hypergammaglobulinemia, the patient may benefit from treatment with an antimalarial or a low dose of prednisone (controversial).

Arthritis generally responds to NSAIDs, antimalarials, and low doses of prednisone. Severe extraglandular disease may require higher doses of systemic corticosteroids, azathioprine, or cyclophosphamide. Lymphoma should be treated in consultation with an oncologist and based on the type and stage of disease.

BIBLIOGRAPHY

1. Alexander E: Central nervous system disease in Sjögren's syndrome. Rheum Dis Clin 18:637–672, 1992.
2. Chan EKL, Andrade LEC: Antinuclear antibodies in Sjögren's syndrome. Rheum Dis Clin 18:551–570, 1992.

3. Constantopoulous SH, Tsianos EV, Moutsopoulos HM: Pulmonary and gastrointestinal manifestations of Sjögren's syndrome. Rheum Dis Clin 18:617–635, 1992.
4. Daniels TE, Fox PC: Salivary and oral components of Sjögren's syndrome. Rheum Dis Clin 18:571–589, 1992.
5. Fox RI: Treatment of the patient with Sjögren's syndrome. Rheum Dis Clin 18:699–709, 1992.
6. Fox RI, Kang H: Pathogenesis of Sjögren's syndrome. Rheum Dis Clin 18:517–538, 1992.
7. Friedlaender MH: Ocular manifestations of Sjögren's syndrome: Keratoconjunctivitis sicca. Rheum Dis Clin 18:591–608, 1992.
8. Itescu S, Winchester R: Diffuse infiltrative lymphocytosis syndrome: A disorder occurring in human immunodeficiency virus-1 infection that may present as sicca syndrome. Rheum Dis Clin 18:683–697, 1992.
9. Moutsopoulos HM, Tzioufas AG: Sjögren's syndrome. In Klippel JH, Dieppe PA (eds): Rheumatology. London, Mosby-Year Book Europe Ltd., 1994.
10. Provost TT, Watson R: Cutaneous manifestations of Sjögren's syndrome. Rheum Dis Clin 18:609–616, 1992.
11. Reveille JD, Arnett FC: The immunogenetics of Sjögren's syndrome. Rheum Dis Clin 18:539–550, 1992.
12. Talal N: Sjögren's syndrome: Historical overview and clinical spectrum of disease. Rheum Dis Clin 18:507–515, 1992.
13. Waltuck J, Buyon JP: Autoantibody-associated congenital heart block: Outcome in mothers and children. Ann Intern Med 120:544–551, 1994.

27. ANTIPHOSPHOLIPID ANTIBODY SYNDROME

Woodruff Emlen, M.D.

1. What are antiphospholipid antibodies?

Antiphospholipid antibodies (aPL) are a heterogeneous group of antibodies that bind to negatively charged phospholipids, including cardiolipin, phosphatidylserine, phosphatidylinositol, and phosphatidic acid. Low levels of aPL may be found in normal individuals ("natural" autoantibodies), but when levels of aPL are increased, they are associated with a specific clinical syndrome.

2. How are aPL measured?

aPL are measured in the clinical laboratory by three assays:

Anti-cardiolipin enzyme-linked immunosorbent assay (ELISA)

Lupus anticoagulant (functional clotting assays)

False-positive VDRL (Venereal Disease Research Laboratory) test

3. Do each of the assays measure the same antibodies?

No. Although some aPL are detected by all three assays, others are detected by only one assay. The term **aPL** refers to the group of antibodies detected by any of these assays. The term **lupus anticoagulant** refers to those antibodies detected by functional clotting assays, and the term **anti-cardiolipin antibodies** (aCL) refers to those aPL detected by the anti-cardiolipin ELISA.

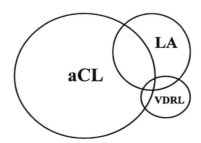

Venn diagram showing approximate distribution of aPL detected by anti-cardiolipin ELISA (aCL), lupus anticoagulant (LA), and false-positive VDRL tests.

4. What is lupus anticoagulant, and how is it detected?

The term lupus anticoagulant describes aPL that are detected by functional clotting assays. The most common method for detecting lupus anticoagulant is measuring the activated partial thromboplastin time (aPTT), although different laboratories may employ different clotting tests, such as the kaolin clotting time. In tests measuring the aPTT (or KCT), the intrinsic clotting system is activated, and for a clot to form, activated factor X must interact with factor V and prothrombin on a negatively charged phospholipid surface. aPL, by binding to the phospholipid surface, prevents the formation of the factor Va/Xa/prothrombin complex, thereby prolonging the aPTT (see figure).

The aPTT can also be prolonged by a deficiency in any of the intrinsic clotting factors. To exclude clotting factor deficiencies as a cause for prolonged aPTT, the patient's plasma is mixed in a 1:1 ratio with normal plasma, which contains the necessary clotting factors. If the original aPTT was prolonged because of clotting factor deficiency, the aPTT will correct; if the aPTT was prolonged because of the presence of an inhibitor such as aPL, the aPTT will not correct and will remain prolonged. Thus, detection of lupus anticoagulant in the laboratory requires the presence of a prolonged aPTT which does not correct with a 1:1 mix with normal plasma. Inhibitors of specific clotting factors may also prolong the aPTT, although unlike the lupus anticoagulant, when specific factor inhibitors are present, correction of the aPTT with a 1:1 mix with normal plasma is time-dependent. Since some factor inhibitors are associated with excessive bleeding, the clinician must be aware of this possibility and ensure that the coagulation laboratory excludes factor inhibitors before identifying a lupus anticoagulant.

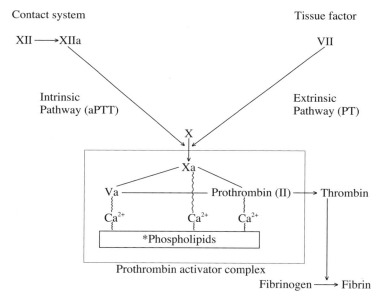

Coagulation pathways, showing interactions of clotting factors in determining clotting time (PT for extrinsic pathway and aPTT for intrinsic pathway). aPL react with phospholipids (*asterisk*) to prevent formation of Va/Xa/prothrombin complex and prolong aPTT.

5. In a plasma that contains lupus anticoagulant, why isn't the prothrombin time (PT) prolonged as well as the aPTT?

To test the extrinsic system of coagulation (measured by the PT), coagulation is initiated by the addition of tissue factor which contains large amounts of phospholipids. The phospholipids present in tissue factor absorb the aPL and thereby prevent the aPL from inhibiting the clotting reaction. Initiation of the intrinsic pathway (to measure aPTT) utilizes only small amounts of phospholipids, and therefore the aPTT is much more sensitive to aPL inhibition than the PT.

6. What is the Russell viper venom time (RVVT)?

The RVVT is a confirmatory test for the lupus anticoagulant. Russell's viper venom directly activates factor X and thereby bypasses the factors required in the intrinsic pathway of coagulation. RVVT is performed like the aPTT, except intrinsic coagulation factors proximal to factor X are not required and less phospholipids are present in the reaction. Therefore, the RVVT is not affected by factor deficiencies and is more sensitive in the detection of lupus anticoagulant than prolongation of the aPTT.

7. What does the platelet neutralization procedure indicate?

Frozen platelets provide a rich source of surface phospholipids. When frozen platelets are added to the aPTT reaction, the aPL bind to the frozen platelets and are therefore removed from the system, resulting in correction of the prolonged aPTT. Correction of the aPTT with the addition of frozen platelets confirms that a phospholipid-binding inhibitor (lupus anticoagulant) is present in the system.

8. What is the significance of a prolonged PT in a patient who also has the lupus anticoagulant?

A prolonged PT might indicate an extremely high level of lupus anticoagulant, but more often it indicates the presence of a prothrombin (factor II) deficiency. This condition can be caused by liver disease, vitamin K deficiency, or anticoagulation with warfarin. In addition, isolated factor II deficiency is rarely associated with autoimmune disorders, including systemic lupus erythematosus. It is extremely important to detect factor II deficiency since it is associated with excessive bleeding rather than hypercoagulability. If both aPTT and PT are prolonged, a prothrombin level should be measured directly to exclude a deficiency.

9. Why can patients with aPL have a false-positive VDRL?

The VDRL (Venereal Disease Research Laboratory) test measures agglutination (flocculation) of lipid particles which contain cholesterol and the negatively charged phospholipid cardiolipin. aPL bind to the cardiolipin in these particles and cause flocculation, indistinguishable from that seen in patients with syphilis. False-positivity of the VDRL must be confirmed by obtaining negative results for direct tests of treponemal antibodies.

10. Which clinical syndrome is associated with elevated levels of aPL?

aPL are associated with a hypercoagulable state characterized by:

    C—Clot: recurrent arterial and/or venous thromboses (clots).

    L—Livedo reticularis: lace-like rash over the extremities and trunk exaggerated by cold.

    O—Obstetrical loss: recurrent fetal loss.

    T—Thrombocytopenia

11. How is the antiphospholipid antibody syndrome (APS) defined?

An individual is said to have the antiphospholipid antibody syndrome if he or she has elevated levels of aPL (as measured by any one of the aPL tests) and the presence of one of the following: thrombosis, recurrent fetal loss, or thrombocytopenia.

12. Where do thromboses occur in the antiphospholipid antibody syndrome?

Thromboses can occur in either the venous or arterial system. Deep venous thromboses (DVT) can occur anywhere and may be associated with pulmonary emboli. Arterial thromboses can result in strokes, retinal artery thrombosis, or occasional peripheral artery thrombosis. Recurrent thromboses usually (70–80%) occur in the same system (venous or arterial) as the initial event.

13. Does the thrombocytopenia associated with antiphospholipid antibody syndrome lead to bleeding?

Only rarely. The thrombocytopenia is usually mild (>50,000 platelets/μl) and almost never associated with bleeding. A fall in platelet count below 50,000/μl or episodes of bleeding should prompt an investigation for other etiologies of thrombocytopenia, including disseminated intravascular coagulation, autoimmune thrombocytopenia, or thrombotic thrombocytopenic purpura.

14. How great is the risk of an initial thrombotic event in a patient with elevated levels of aPL?

In answering this question, one must distinguish between absolute risk (risk of an event occurring) and relative risk (risk of an event occurring in a patient with aPL compared to an individual without aPL). The **relative risk** of a stroke, fetal loss, or deep venous thrombosis occurring in an individual with aPL compared to an individual without aPL is in the range of 2–4. However, the **absolute risk** of these events may be low. Good data on these issues are scarce, but an example of relative and absolute risks of first strokes is given in the following table.

Relative and Absolute Risks of First Stroke

RISK FACTOR	AGE (YRS)	RELATIVE RISK	ABSOLUTE RISK
Atrial fibrillation	>50	3.6	16.3
Hypertension	>50	2.6	6.6
aPL (by aCL ELISA)	>50	2.2	9.9
aPL (by aCL ELISA)	<50	8.3	0.5

In the table, relative risk is defined as the frequency of strokes compared to the frequency in an individual without the given risk factor. Absolute risk is defined as the frequency of strokes per 1,000 patient-years in individuals with the risk factor present.

15. What is the risk of a recurrent thrombotic event in a patient with elevated levels of aPL?

The risk of thrombosis recurrence is clearly **increased** in patients with aPL compared to individuals without aPL. While controlled studies are rare, estimates are that without treatment, 0.15–0.19 thrombotic events will occur per patient-year after the initial event. Stroke data indicate a recurrence rate of 18.7% per year after an initial event in an aPL-positive individual.

16. Among patients with recurrent thromboses or fetal loss, how frequently can aPL be implicated as a cause?

Coagulopathies of some type are present in 10–30% of all patients with recurrent thromboses. Of the coagulopathies, activated protein C resistance, protein C and protein S deficiencies (or abnormalities) and elevated aPL are the most common. aPL have been implicated as a cause in approximately 5–20% of unselected patients with recurrent fetal loss and 5–10% of patients with recurrent thromboses.

17. Is the level of aPL stable over time?

No. aPL levels may fluctuate widely over time spontaneously or in response to clinical events such as a flare of systemic lupus erythematosus disease activity, change in pregnancy status, or thrombosis. aPL levels may or may not change with therapy for antiphospholipid antibody syndrome.

18. What are the characteristics of fetal loss associated with aPL?

aPL-associated fetal loss can occur at any time during pregnancy, but most often it occurs during the second or third trimester. Examination of the placentas from these aborted fetuses shows thrombosis of multiple small placental vessels. This observation has led to the proposal that fetal loss may occur as a result of placental insufficiency.

19. List the *main* types of diseases associated with increased aPL production.

Increased aPL production is frequently associated with chronic immune stimulation. The primary conditions can be remembered by the mnemonic **MAIN:**

   M—Medications
   A—Autoimmune
   I—Infectious diseases
   N—Neoplasms

20. What medications are associated with elevated levels of aPL?
Although many drugs have been associated with elevated aPL, the most common are the phenothiazines and other drugs associated with drug-induced lupus: chlorpromazine (phenothiazines), hydralazine, phenytoin, procainamide, and quinidine.

21. Which infectious diseases are associated with elevated levels of aPL?
Many acute infections, both bacterial and viral, have been associated with transiently elevated levels of aPL. Chronic infections, and in particular HIV, are also associated with increased aPL; 60–80% of patients who are HIV-positive have elevated levels of aPL. aPL in these patients are most often detected by the anti-cardiolipin ELISA (aCL). aPL levels do not correlate with stage or severity of HIV infection.

22. Do the aPL associated with these clinical conditions carry a high risk of thrombosis?
Probably not. While it is clear that the aPL produced in patients with autoimmune diseases, such as systemic lupus erythematosus, are strongly associated with thrombosis, the aPL produced in infections such as HIV do not appear to be associated with thrombosis to the same extent. However, episodes of thrombosis have been reported in patients who have had drug-induced aPL or virally induced aPL. Reliable laboratory distinction between thrombogenic aPL and nonthrombogenic aPL is not yet possible.

23. What is the difference between primary and secondary antiphospholipid antibody syndrome?
Secondary antiphospholipid antibody syndrome (APS) is defined as the presence of APS in association with a defined cause of increased aPL production. Examples include the APS associated with systemic lupus erythematosus, drugs, or infection. **Primary** APS is present when no underlying cause for the production of aPL can be identified. Other than the presence or absence of an underlying disease, the primary and secondary APSs are clinically similar. Patient management is also similar, although in the secondary APS, attention should also be directed toward removing the possible source of aPL production (e.g., drugs) and in treating the underlying condition (e.g., lupus).

24. How do elevated levels of aPL cause thrombosis in vivo?
It is still not clear whether elevated aPL are directly causative of thrombosis or are simply associated with thrombosis in a noncausative manner. Histologic examination of vessels of patients with APS shows thrombus formation with no surrounding inflammation ("bland" vasculopathy), indicating that the pathology of APS represents a fundamentally different process from that seen in vasculitis. Multiple mechanisms have been proposed by which aPL might induce a hypercoagulable state, including disruption of the protein C/protein S anticoagulant system as well as direct interaction with platelets or endothelial cells. However, to date, no mechanism has been described that can adequately account for the thrombotic complications in most patients.

25. How should you treat an individual with elevated levels of aPL but with *no* history of thromboses or recurrent fetal loss?
This patient should be treated conservatively. While there is evidence that this patient has an increased relative risk for thrombotic events, the absolute risk of these events occurring is extremely low and may not be as great as the risks associated with aggressive treatment. Current recommendations are that these individuals be treated only with one aspirin a day.

26. What is the treatment for a patient who has had one or more thrombotic complications and has elevated levels of aPL?
Patients with significant thrombotic events should be anticoagulated long-term (possibly lifetime) with warfarin. Data suggest that thromboses can recur on treatment with aspirin alone or with low-dose warfarin. Therefore, it is recommended that adequate warfarin be given to maintain the INR between 3–4. In two studies, this level of anticoagulation was associated with an extremely low rate of thrombosis recurrence. However, this high level of anticoagulation is associated with a sig-

nificant rate of major bleeding complications, and these patients should therefore be monitored carefully. Because of the high levels of anticoagulation required to prevent recurrent thromboses, the issue of whether minor thromboses (simple deep venous thrombosis) require life-long anticoagulation is controversial, whereas there is general agreement that major thromboses (pulmonary emboli, stroke) require life-long anticoagulation.

27. What is the best treatment for the pregnant patient with elevated aPL who has had prior fetal loss?
These patients should be followed closely as high-risk obstetric patients and treated with subcutaneous heparin, 7,500–12,000 units twice daily. At these doses, coagulation parameters do not need to be routinely monitored. These patients are also routinely given one baby aspirin per day. There is no controlled evidence that corticosteroids improve fetal survival.

28. How can aPL be detected in a patient who is already anticoagulated?
Measurement of aPL by the anti-cardiolipin ELISA or VDRL is not affected by anticoagulation and can therefore be used to determine aPL levels in a patient on heparin or warfarin. However, coagulation tests to detect the lupus anticoagulant are affected by heparin and warfarin, and care must be taken in determining lupus anticoagulants in these situations. In the patient on heparin, plasma can be treated with heparinase to remove the heparin prior to the coagulation tests. In a patient on warfarin, it is the PT that is primarily affected, and the aPTT is usually not prolonged. Thus, prolongation of aPTT in a patient on warfarin is still suggestive of the presence of a lupus anticoagulant. Because warfarin depletes vitamin K-dependent factors, a 1:1 mix of the patient's plasma with normal plasma should correct the factor deficiencies induced by warfarin. Thus, if the alterations of clotting parameters are due to warfarin, the PT as well as aPTT will correct. However, as discussed earlier, a prolonged aPTT that does not correct in this situation is indicative of a lupus anticoagulant.

29. How should heparinization be monitored in patients who already have a prolonged PTT from the lupus anticoagulant?
In patients who are heparinized, heparin levels can be monitored directly to give an indication of anticoagulant effect. In addition, the thrombin time which measures the clotting system distal to the effects of aPL can be used as a good indicator of heparinization. In a patient on warfarin, the PT is primarily affected and, as discussed, is not usually profoundly affected by the lupus anticoagulant. Therefore, the PT is an adequate measure of warfarin anticoagulation, even in a patient who has the lupus anticoagulant.

30. When should tests for aPL be ordered?
Measurement (with all three tests) should be considered as part of the standard hypercoagulation work-up—specifically, in patients with deep venous thrombosis, pulmonary emboli, or unusual or early onset of major thrombotic events, including stroke and myocardial infarction. In addition, women with recurrent spontaneous abortions (≥ 2) should be examined for aPL. It is not cost-effective to screen all pregnancies for aPL.

31. Does the level or type of aPL affect the risk of developing thrombosis?
This issue is controversial and unresolved. However, most data indicate that high levels of aPL are associated with a higher thrombosis risk and that IgG antibodies (as measured by aCL ELISA) are more thrombogenic than IgM or IgA antibodies. The presence of a lupus anticoagulant (aPL detected by functional clotting assay) is associated with a higher risk of thrombosis than aPL detected by aCL. Patients with only a false-positive VDRL do not have an increased risk of thrombosis. However, these generalizations are not strong enough to alter therapy; in a patient with clinical thrombosis and elevated aPL, treatment should not be altered based on the level or isotype of aPL.

BIBLIOGRAPHY

1. Branch DW, Silver RM, Blackwell JL, et al: Outcome of treated pregnancies in women with antiphospholipid syndrome: An update of the Utah experience. Obstet Gynecol 80:614–620, 1992.

2. Brey RL: Stroke prevention in patients with antiphospholipid antibodies. Lupus 3:299–302, 1994.
3. Cowchock FS, Reece EA, Balaban D, et al: Repeated fetal losses associated with antiphospholipid antibodies: A collaborative randomized trial comparing prednisone with low-dose heparin treatment. Am J Obstet Gynecol 166:1318–1323, 1992.
4. Inbar O, Blank M, Faden D, et al: Prevention of fetal loss in experimental antiphospholipid syndrome by low-molecular-weight heparin. Am J Obstet Gynecol 169:423–426, 1993.
5. Khamashta MA, Cuadrado MJ, Mujie F, et al: The management of thrombosis in the antiphospholipid-antibody syndrome. N Engl J Med 332:993–997, 1995.
6. Kittner SJ, Gorelick PB: Antiphospholipid antibodies and stroke: An epidemiological perspective. Stroke 23(suppl I):I19–I-22, 1992.
7. Levine SR, Brey RL, Joseph CLM, Havstad S: Risk of recurrent thromboembolic events in patients with focal cerebral ischemia and antiphospholipid antibodies. Stroke 23(suppl I):I-29–I-32, 1992.
8. Lockshin MD: Antiphospholipid antibody syndrome. Rheum Dis Clin North Am 20:45–59, 1994.
9. Lockshin MD: Which patients with antiphospholipid antibody should be treated and how? Rheum Dis Clin North Am 19:235–247, 1993.
10. McNeil HP, Chesterman CN, Krilis SA: Immunology and clinical importance of antiphospholipid antibodies. Adv Immunol 49:193–280, 1991.
11. Rosove MH, Brewer PMC: Antiphospholipid thrombosis: Clinical course after the first thrombotic event in 70 patients. Ann Intern Med 117:303–308, 1992.
12. Sammaritano LR, Gharavi AE, Lockshin MD: Antiphospholipid antibody syndrome: Immunologic and clinical aspects. Semin Arthritis Rheum 20:81–96, 1990.
13. Triplett DA: Antiphospholipid antibodies and thrombosis: A consequence, coincidence, or cause? Arch Pathol Lab Med 117:78–88, 1993.

28. ADULT-ONSET STILL'S DISEASE

Vance J. Bray, M.D.

1. What is Still's disease?

Still's disease is a variant of juvenile rheumatoid arthritis that is characterized by seronegative chronic polyarthritis in association with a systemic inflammatory illness. It was initially described in 1897 by George F. Still, a pathologist. The characteristic features of this illness have subsequently been reported in adults, as detailed by Eric Bywaters in 1971.

2. How do adults with Still's disease generally present?

Patients are usually young adults who present with a prolonged course of nonspecific signs and symptoms. The most striking manifestations are severe arthralgias, myalgias, malaise, weight loss, fever, and sore throat. These patients appear severely ill and have often received numerous courses of antibiotics for presumed sepsis, although cultures are negative. As many as 5% of patients being evaluated for "fever of unknown origin" may be diagnosed eventually with Still's disease. A few patients may have had similar episodes of illness as children.

3. Describe the characteristic fever of Still's disease.

The fever in Still's disease generally occurs only once or twice a day, usually in the early morning and/or late afternoon. The temperature elevation is marked, although between fever spikes the patient's temperature is normal or below normal. This pattern is known as either **quotidian** or **diquotidian.** Patients with Still's disease generally feel very ill when febrile but feel well when their body temperature is normal. This poses a dilemma for physicians, because hospital rounds and clinic visits may not occur during the times when the patients are febrile. The fever pattern in Still's disease contrasts with the pattern seen in the setting of infection, in that infections generally cause a baseline elevation in body temperature in addition to episodic fever spikes.

4. What are the common signs and symptoms seen in Still's disease?

Signs and Symptoms of Adult-Onset Still's Disease

MANIFESTATION	FREQUENCY
Arthralgias	98–100%
Fever	83–100%
Myalgias	84–98%
Arthritis	88–94%
Sore throat	50–92%
Rash	87–90%
Weight loss	19–76%
Lymphadenopathy	48–74%
Splenomegaly	45–55%
Pleuritis	23–53%
Abdominal pain	9–48%
Hepatomegaly	29–44%
Pericarditis	24–37%
Pneumonitis	9–31%

Unusual manifestations include alopecia, Sjögren's syndrome, subcutaneous nodules, necrotizing lymphadenitis (Kikuchi's), amyotrophy, acute liver failure, pulmonary fibrosis, cardiac tamponade, CNS involvement, peripheral neuropathy, proteinuria, microscopic hematuria, amyloidosis, hemolytic anemia, disseminated intravascular coagulation, thrombotic thrombocytopenic purpura, inflammatory eye disease, and cataracts.

5. Describe the rash associated with Still's disease.

Although the rash is said to occur in the vast majority of patients with Still's disease, it is often unappreciated unless specifically sought. The characteristic appearance is that of an evanescent, salmon-colored, macular or maculopapular lesion that is nonpruritic. It is usually seen on the trunk, arms, legs, or areas of mechanical irritation. Often, it is only seen when the patient is febrile. The rash can sometimes be elicited with heat, such as that produced by applying a hot towel or taking a hot bath or shower. Koebner phenomenon (i.e., the rash can be induced by rubbing the skin) is reported in approximately 40% of patients.

6. Describe the arthritis associated with Still's disease.

The arthritis associated with Still's disease may be overshadowed by the systemic features of the illness. It may not be present at the time of disease onset, may involve only one or a few joints, or be fleeting. The joints involved are those typical for other forms of rheumatoid arthritis: knees, wrists, ankles, proximal interphalangeals (PIPs), elbows, shoulders, metacarpophalangeals (MCPs), metatarsophalangeals (MTPs), hips, distal interphalangeals (DIPs), and temporomandibular joints (TMJ). Arthrocentesis generally yields class II inflammatory synovial fluid, and radiographs usually reveal soft-tissue swelling, effusions, and occasionally periarticular osteoporosis. Joint erosions and/or fusion of the carpal bones may be seen.

7. What are the characteristic laboratory features of Still's disease?

Laboratory Findings in Adult-onset Still's Disease

	FREQUENCY
Elevated erythrocyte sedimentation rate	96–100%
Leukocytosis	71–97%
Anemia	59–92%
Neutrophils ≥80%	55–88%
Hypoalbuminemia	44–85%
Elevated hepatic enzymes	35–85%
Thrombocytosis	52–62%
Positive antinuclear antibodies	0–11%
Positive rheumatoid factor	2– 8%

There are no diagnostic tests for Still's disease. Rather, the diagnosis is one of exclusion, made in the setting of the proper clinical features and laboratory abnormalities and the absence of another explanation (such as infection or malignancy).

An elevated ferritin has been reported in most patients. Some believe that an extremely elevated ferritin level is suggestive of Still's disease, with a value of $\geq 1,000$ mg/dl in the proper clinical setting being confirmatory of the diagnosis. The reason for this elevation is not known, although ferritin is an acute phase reactant and reflects inflammation.

8. How is Still's disease treated?

In 20% of cases, aspirin or other nonsteroidal anti-inflammatory drugs (NSAIDs) adequately control Still's disease. However, most patients require corticosteroid therapy. Approximately one-third of patients require at least 60 mg of prednisone daily. When the prednisone cannot be tapered to a low dose without disease recurrence, one of the slow-acting antirheumatic drugs or immunosuppressive agents (methotrexate) may be used.

9. What is the clinical course and prognosis of Still's disease?

The median time to achieve clinical and laboratory remission while receiving therapy is 10 months. The median time to enter remission requiring no therapy is 32 months.

The course of illness generally follows one of three patterns, with approximately one-third of patients pursuing each: self-limited illness, intermittent flares of disease activity, or chronic Still's disease. The patients who experience a self-limited course undergo remission within 6–9 months. Of those with intermittent flares, two-thirds will only have one recurrence, occurring from 10–136 months after the original illness. The minority of patients in this group will experience multiple flares, with up to 10 flares being reported at intervals of 3–48 months. The recurrent episodes are generally milder than the original illness and respond to lower doses of medications. In the group that experiences a chronic course, arthritis and loss of joint range of motion become the most problematic manifestations and may result in the need for joint arthroplasty, especially of the hip. The systemic manifestations tend to become less severe.

The presence of polyarthritis or large-joint (shoulder, hip) involvement at onset are poor prognostic signs and are associated with the development of chronic disease. The 5-year survival rate in adult-onset Still's disease is 90–95%, which is similar to the survival rate for lupus. Deaths occurring in Still's disease have been attributed to infections, liver failure, amyloidosis, adult respiratory distress syndrome, heart failure, carcinoma of the lung, status epilepticus, and hematologic manifestations including disseminated intravascular coagulation and thrombotic thrombocytopenic purpura.

BIBLIOGRAPHY

1. Bray VJ, Singleton JD: Disseminated intravascular coagulation in Still's disease. Semin Arthritis Rheum 24:222–229, 1994.
2. Bywaters EGL: Still's disease in the adult. Ann Rheum Dis 30:121–133, 1971.
3. Cush JJ, Medsger TA, Christy WC, et al: Adult-onset Still's disease: Clinical course and outcome. Arthritis Rheum 30:186–194, 1987.
4. Elkon KB, Hughes GRV, Bywaters EGL, et al: Adult-onset Still's disease: Twenty-year follow-up and further studies of patients with active disease. Arthritis Rheum 25:647–654, 1982.
5. Esdaile JM, Tannenbaum H, Hawkins D: Adult Still's disease. Am J Med 68:825–830, 1980.
6. Ohta A, Yamaguchi M, Tsunematsu T, et al: Adult Still's disease: A multicenter survey of Japanese patients. J Rheumatol 17:1058–1063, 1990.
7. Ota T, Higashi S, Suzuki H, et al: Increased serum ferritin levels in adult Still's disease. Lancet 1:562–563, 1987.
8. Pouchot J, Sampalis JS, Beaudet F, et al: Adult Still's disease: Manifestations, disease course, and outcome in 62 patients. Medicine 70:118–136, 1991.
9. Reginato AJ, Schumacher HR, Baker DG, et al: Adult onset Still's disease: Experience in 23 patients and literature review with emphasis on organ failure. Semin Arthritis Rheum 17:39–57, 1987.
10. Still GF: On a form of chronic joint disease in children. Med Chir Trans 80:47–49, 1987. [Reprinted in Arch Dis Child 16:156–65, 1941.]

29. POLYMYALGIA RHEUMATICA

James D. Singleton, M.D.

1. How does "SECRET" describe the clinical features of polymyalgia rheumatica?

S = Stiffness and pain
E = Elderly individuals
C = Constitutional symptoms, caucasians
R = Arthritis (rheumatism)
E = Elevated erythrocyte sedimentation rate (ESR)
T = Temporal arteritis

2. Where did the term polymyalgia rheumatica originate?

Reports of this syndrome appeared in the medical literature for years under a variety of designations. The name polymyalgia rheumatica (PMR) was introduced by Barber in 1957 in a report of 12 cases.

3. Define polymyalgia rheumatica.

PMR is an inflammatory syndrome of older individuals that is characterized by pain and stiffness in the shoulder and/or pelvic girdles. Formal criteria have included:

- Patient age > 50 years
- Bilateral symptoms involving two of three areas (neck, shoulder girdle, or hip girdle) for at least 1 month
- ESR > 40 mm/hr
- Exclusion of other diagnoses except temporal arteritis

Constitutional symptoms and arthritis are common. Some definitions have included a rapid response to glucocorticoid therapy (prednisone equivalent of 10–15 mg daily).

4. Who is affected by PMR?

PMR rarely affects those under age 50 and becomes more common with increasing age. Most patients are > 60 years of age, with the mean age of onset being approximately 70 years. Women are affected twice as often as men. PMR, like temporal arteritis, largely affects whites and is uncommon in black, Hispanic, Asian, and native American individuals. Whites in the southern United States appear to be less frequently affected than those in northern areas.

5. How common is PMR?

PMR is a relatively common syndrome in the elderly white population and is more common than temporal arteritis. In a study from Olmstead County, Minnesota, the annual incidence of PMR was 53.7 cases/100,000 persons aged ≥ 50 years, and the prevalence was approximately 500/100,000 persons aged ≥ 50. This rate compares with an annual incidence of 28.6/100,000 in Göteborg, Sweden.

6. Describe the typical stiffness and pain of PMR.

- Stiffness and pain are usually insidious in onset, symmetric, and profound, and they involve more than one area (neck, shoulders, pelvic girdle). However, at times, the onset is abrupt or the initial symptoms are unilateral and then progress to symmetric involvement.
- The shoulder is often the first area to be affected, and a single area may be the predominant source of pain.
- The magnitude of the pain limits mobility; stiffness and gelling phenomena are dramatic. Pain at night is common and may awaken the patient.
- Patients may complain of a sensation of muscle weakness due to the pain and stiffness.

7. Describe the arthritis of PMR.

Clinically detectable synovitis has been reported by many authors. In one series of patients followed over 16 years, 31% had clinical manifestations of synovitis. Effusions of the knees, wrist synovitis (often with carpal tunnel syndrome), and sternoclavicular synovitis are detected most frequently. Knee effusions can be large (30–150 ml). Synovitis is often transient and relatively mild. It is likely to be present either at disease onset or with rapid tapering of the glucocorticoid dose, and it is readily controlled by glucocorticoids.

8. What are the findings on physical examination in patients with PMR?

Physical findings are less striking than the history would lead one to believe. Patients may appear chronically ill due to the presence of weight loss, fatigue, depression, and low-grade fever. High, spiking fevers are unusual unless temporal arteritis is present. The neck and shoulders are often tender, and active shoulder motion may be limited by pain. With longer duration of illness, capsular contracture of the shoulder (limiting passive motion) and muscle atrophy may occur. Joint movement increases the pain, which is often felt in the proximal extremities, not the joints. Clinical synovitis is most frequently noted in the knees, wrists, and sternoclavicular joints. Carpal tunnel syndrome may be present. Muscle strength testing is often confounded by the presence of pain. However, strength is normal unless disuse atrophy has occurred.

9. What is the etiology of PMR?

The cause of PMR is unknown, but there is no evidence of an infectious agent or toxin. Clues are presumably provided by the epidemiology of the disease, yet the association of PMR with aging is without clear explanation. The preponderance of whites has suggested a genetic predisposition, and an association with HLA-DR4 has been reported. The immune system is implicated in the pathogenesis, but no persistent immune defects or characteristic antibodies have been identified.

10. Explain the source of the symptoms of PMR.

PMR is a systemic inflammatory syndrome, accounting for the frequent constitutional symptoms. **Synovitis** of the hips and shoulders is difficult to detect clinically but is believed by many authors to be the cause of the proximal stiffness and pain. This is supported by scintigraphic evidence of axial synovitis, documentation of synovitis by clinical observation, synovial fluid analysis, and synovial biopsy. Other authors contend that PMR is an expression of underlying **arteritis** and that synovitis has little to do with the clinical symptoms. Muscle biopsies are usually normal and, when abnormal, have shown nonspecific changes and no inflammation.

11. What is the most characteristic laboratory finding? Is it always present?

An elevated erthyrocyte sedimentation rate (ESR), often > 100 mm/hr, is the characteristic lab finding. PMR may occasionally occur with a normal or only mildly elevated ESR.

12. Are there other commonly encountered laboratory abnormalities?

Findings reflecting the systemic inflammatory process (normochromic normocytic anemia, thrombocytosis, increased gamma globulins, elevated acute phase reactants) are common. Liver-associated enzyme abnormalities may be seen in up to one-third of patients; an increased alkaline phosphatase level is most common. Renal function, urinalysis, and serum creatine kinase level are normal. Tests for antinuclear antibodies and rheumatoid factor are negative.

13. Describe the results of synovial fluid analysis.

Synovial fluid is typically inflammatory with a poor mucin clot. However, leukocyte counts have varied from 1,000–20,000 cell/mm^3 with 40–50% polymorphonuclear leukocytes. Culture and crystal examinations are negative.

14. How are PMR and temporal arteritis (TA) related?

These two disorders frequently occur synchronously or sequentially in individual patients. PMR has been noted in 40–60% of patients with TA and may be the initial symptom complex in

20–40%. Conversely, TA may occur in patients with PMR. In 1963, Alestig and Barr reported the presence of histologic TA in patients with PMR who had no clinical evidence of arteritis. Although studies from Scandinavia have shown TA to occur in almost 50% of PMR patients, only 15–20% of PMR patients in North America have coexistent TA.

15. When should a temporal artery biopsy be performed on a patient with PMR? (*Controversial*)
Temporal artery biopsy is not necessary unless symptoms or signs suggest the presence of TA. The patient should be queried regarding current or recent headache, jaw claudication, visual disturbance, scalp tenderness, and other features of TA. The arteries of the head, neck, torso, and extremities should be examined for tenderness, enlargement, bruits, and decreased pulsation. Constitutional symptoms and laboratory values in PMR and TA are similar and therefore are not of discriminatory value. However, the failure of prednisone to significantly improve symptoms or to normalize the ESR should suggest the presence of TA and prompt temporal artery biopsy.

16. How is the diagnosis of PMR established?
The diagnosis of PMR is a clinical one, relying on the features in the clinical definition.

17. Should other diagnoses be considered? How are they differentiated?

Differential Diagnoses in Polymyalgia Rheumatica/Temporal Arteritis

DIAGNOSIS	DISTINGUISHING FEATURES
Fibromyalgia syndrome	Tender points, normal ESR
Hypothyroidism	Elevated thyroid-stimulating hormone, normal ESR
Depression	Normal ESR
Polymyositis	Weakness predominates; elevated creatine kinase; abnormal electromyography
Malignancy	Clinical evidence of neoplasm (there is no association of cancer with PMR)
Infection	Clinical suspicion of infection; cultures
Rheumatoid arthritis	Positive rheumatoid factor, small joint involvement

18. How is PMR distinguished from rheumatoid arthritis?
It is often difficult to distinguish PMR from the onset of rheumatoid arthritis in older patients, in whom constitutional symptoms and morning stiffness often surpass joint manifestations. Features that support the diagnosis of PMR are:
    Absence of rheumatoid factor
    Lack of involvement of small joints of hands and feet
    Lack of development of joint damage
    Absence of erosive disease during follow-up
The response to glucocorticoids is *not* a reliable distinguishing feature.

19. How are NSAIDs used in the treatment of PMR?
NSAIDs are an effective therapy in only 10–20% of patients and are best used in those with mild symptoms. As with other diseases, no individual NSAID is necessarily more effective than another, and selection is based on perception of tolerability and safety for the patient. NSAIDs may be added to glucocorticoid therapy to facilitate steroid tapering. However, the toxicities of NSAIDs need to be kept in mind, particularly given the age of these patients and the duration of therapy.

20. Describe the initial use of glucocorticoids in PMR.
Prednisone in a dose of 10–20 mg/day usually evokes a dramatic and rapid response. Most patients are significantly better within 1–2 days, though others may take a few more days to respond

completely. A single daily dose is more effective than alternate-day dosing, and initial dosage selection is determined largely by the severity of symptoms (doses > 20 mg/day are unnecessary). The dose is reduced every 2–4 weeks, using the patient's response as the most reliable parameter to follow. The ESR should steadily decline, although normalization may take several weeks. Dosage is decreased by 2.5-mg increments until a dose of 10 mg/day is attained. Further tapering is by 1-mg increments as the patient and ESR are monitored.

21. What is the course of PMR?
The course of PMR is longer and recurrences more frequent than once believed. In one study, 70% of 246 patients were still taking prednisone after 2 years of treatment; some patients required glucocorticoids for up to 10 years. Relapses of PMR after therapy has been stopped are seen in about 20% and may occur months or years later. The ESR may not be as high as with the original presentation.

22. Given the course of PMR, how long should prednisone be continued?
Optimally, prednisone should be tapered and discontinued as quickly as possible. However, since too rapid a taper results in relapse, observe the patient for about 1 year after a prednisone dose of about 5 mg/day is attained. Side effects and toxicities are usually minimal at this dose and relapses unusual. If there is then no evidence of disease recurrence, prednisone is tapered by 1 mg every 1–2 months until discontinued.

If relapse occurs, control is often regained by only a small increase in dosage ($\leq$ 5 mg). A slow taper can again be done, halting at a dose just above that at which relapse occurred. Further tapering is attempted again after a period of 6 months to a year. In this way, patients are not relegated to indefinite prednisone therapy, yet therapy can be continued for those with longer courses of disease.

23. Other than medication, what should be included in the treatment plan of PMR?
Reassurance
Patient education
Regular physician monitoring
Range of motion exercises, especially where muscle atrophy and/or contracture have occurred
Attention to glucocorticoid side effects, especially osteoporosis

BIBLIOGRAPHY

1. Barber HS: Myalgic syndrome with constitutional effects: Polymyalgia rheumatica. Ann Rheum Dis 16:230–237, 1957.
2. Cohen MD, Ginsburg WW: Polymyalgia rheumatica. Rheum Dis Clin North Am 16:325–338, 1990.
3. Hunder GG: Giant cell arteritis and polymyalgia rheumatica. In Kelley WK, Harris ED, Ruddy S, Sledge CB (eds): Textbook of Rheumatology, 4th ed. Philadelphia, W.B. Saunders, 1993, pp 1103–1112.
4. Healey LA: On the epidemiology of polymyalgia rheumatica and temporal arteritis. J Rheumatol 20:1639–1640, 1993.
5. Healey LA: Polymyalgia rheumatica and the American Rheumatism Association criteria for rheumatoid arthritis. Arthritis Rheum 26:1417–1418, 1983.
6. Healey LA: Polymyalgia rheumatica. In Schumacher HR (ed): Primer on the Rheumatic Diseases, 10th ed. Atlanta, Arthritis Foundation, 1993, pp 148–149.

V. The Vasculitides and Related Disorders

We are too much accustomed to attribute to a single cause that which is the product of several, and the majority of our controversies come from that.
Baron Justus Von Liegig (1803–1873)
German chemist

30. APPROACH TO THE PATIENT WITH SUSPECTED VASCULITIS

Steven A. Older, M.D.

1. In simple terms, what is the definition of vasculitis?
Inflammation and necrosis of a blood vessel with subsequent impairment of the circulation.

2. What two vascular consequences of vasculitis result in clinical signs and symptoms?
- Vessel wall destruction leading to perforation and hemorrhage into adjacent tissues
- Endothelial injury leading to thrombosis and ischemia/infarction of dependent tissues

3. What are the characteristic histologic features of vasculitis?
- Infiltration of the vessel wall by neutrophils, mononuclear cells, and/or giant cells
- Fibrinoid necrosis (panmural destruction of the vessel wall)
- Leukocytoclasis (dissolution of leukocytes, yielding "nuclear dust")

Note: Perivascular infiltration is a nonspecific histologic finding observed in a variety of disease processes. It is not considered diagnostic of vasculitis, even though it may coexist in vasculitic tissues.

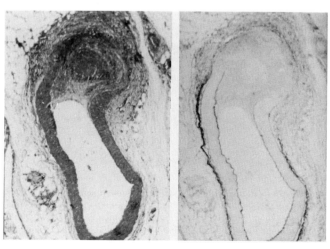

Necrotizing vasculitis in a bowel specimen from a patient with polyarteritis nodosa. The arterial lumen is partially occluded by thrombus. Adjacent arterial wall is necrotic, resulting in destruction of the elastic laminae. (*Left,* hematoxylin-eosin; *right,* elastic tissue stain; low power.) (From the Revised Clinical Slide Collection on the Rheumatic Diseases. Atlanta, American College of Rheumatology, 1991; with permission.)

4. Through which immune mechanisms does vasculitis occur?
Depending on the type of vasculitis, either **cell-mediated** (granulomatous) or **humoral** (immune complex) mechanisms are involved.

Granulomatous	Immune Complex
Giant cell arteritis	Polyarteritis nodosa
Takayasu's arteritis	Microscopic polyangiitis
Wegener's granulomatosis	Kawasaki's disease (controversial)
Churg-Strauss syndrome	Hypersensitivity vasculitis
Isolated CNS vasculitis	Henoch-Schönlein purpura

5. How is vasculitis categorized when classified according to the size of the vessel involved (pathologic classification)?

VESSEL SIZE	VASCULITIS
Large	Takayasu's arteritis
	Giant cell arteritis
Medium	Polyarteritis nodosa
	Kawasaki's disease
Small	Hypersensitivity vasculitis
	Churg-Strauss vasculitis
	Wegener's granulomatosis
	Microscopic polyangiitis

Each of the types of vasculitis can involve more than one size of vessel. For example, polyarteritis nodosa can involve both medium and small vessels.

6. Using the more commonly accepted clinical classification, categorize the vasculitides.

Clinical Classification of Vasculitis

Systemic necrotizing vasculitis
  Classic polyarteritis nodosa
  Churg-Strauss vasculitis
  Polyangiitis overlap
Hypersensitivity vasculitis
  Exogenous stimuli proved or suspected:
    Henoch-Schönlein purpura
    Serum sickness and serum sickness-like reactions
    Other drug-related vasculitides
    Vasculitis associated with infectious disease
  Endogenous antigens likely involved; vasculitis associated with:
  Neoplasms
  Systemic connective tissue diseases
  Other underlying diseases
  Congenital complement deficiencies

Wegener's granulomatosis
Giant cell arteritis
  Temporal arteritis
  Takayasu's arteritis
Other vasculitic syndromes
  Mucocutaneous lymph node syndrome
    (Kawasaki's disease)
  Isolated CNS vasculitis
  Thromboangiitis obliterans (Buerger's disease)
  Miscellaneous vasculitides

Adapted from Fauci AS: Vasculitis syndromes. In Braunwald E, et al (eds): Harrison's Principles of Internal Medicine, 12th ed. New York, McGraw-Hill, 1991.

7. In general, how does one approach the diagnosis of vasculitis?
1. Suspect the disease
2. Rule out the vasculitis mimickers
3. Define the extent of disease
4. Confirm the diagnosis

8. How does vasculitis typically present?
There is no single presentation typical of vasculitis. Vasculitis may present as a rash, headache, foot-drop, vague constitutional symptoms, or a major visceral event such as stroke, bowel infarction, or alveolar hemorrhage. Because of its protean manifestations, vasculitis can easily be confused with other diseases. "Mimickers" of vasculitis must be excluded early in the evaluation, since treatment varies dramatically, and misdiagnosis may result in morbidity and/or mortality.

9. What disorders can mimic vasculitis?

Large arteries: fibromuscular dysplasia, radiation fibrosis, neurofibromatosis, congenital coarctation of aorta

Medium arteries: ergotism, *cholesterol emboli syndrome, atrial myxoma,* lymphomatoid granulomatosis, *thromboembolic disease,* type IV Ehlers-Danlos

Small arteries: *mycotic aneurysm with emboli, anti-phospholipid antibody syndrome, sepsis (gonococcal, meningococcal),* ecthyma gangrenosum (pseudomonal), *infectious endocarditis,* thrombocytopenia

Note: Common clinical entities are in italic.

10. What clinical situations should provoke the consideration of vasculitis as a primary diagnosis?

Multisystem disease; fever of unknown origin or unexplained constitutional symptoms; ischemic signs or symptoms, especially in a young person; mononeuritis multiplex; and suspicious skin lesions.

11. Which skin lesions are suggestive of vasculitis?

Palpable purpura, livedo reticularis, subcutaneous nodules, "punched-out" ulcers, digital infarction, splinter hemorrhages, hemorrhagic macules, and urticaria lasting >24 hrs.

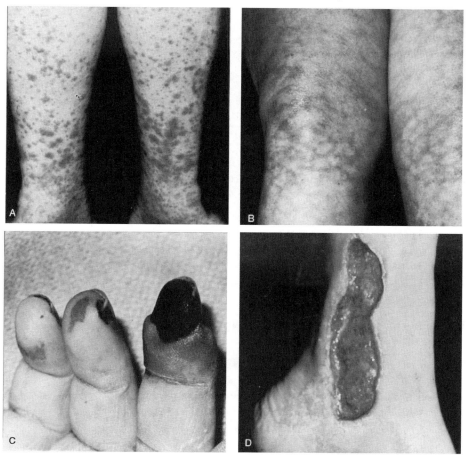

A, Palpable purpura; *B,* livedo reticularis; *C,* digital infarction; *D,* "punched-out" ulcer. (From the Revised Clinical Slide Collection on the Rheumatic Diseases. Atlanta, American College of Rheumatology, 1991; with permission.)

12. Which laboratory tests are useful in the evaluation of suspected vasculitis?

Screening

Complete blood count	BUN/creatinine
Westergren ESR	Liver-associated enzymes
C-reactive protein	Viral hepatitis panel (hepatitis B/C)
Urinalysis	Stool for occult blood

Directed

Blood cultures	Infectious serologies
CSF studies	Cryoglobulins
ANA, rheumatoid factor	Creatine kinase
Anti-phospholipid antibodies	Antineutrophil cytoplasmic antibody (ANCA)
C3/C4/CH$_{50}$	Serum protein electrophoresis

13. Which other diagnostic studies are commonly used in the evaluation of suspected vasculitis?

Chest x-ray	Echocardiography
Sinus x-rays or CT scan	Angiography
Electromyography and nerve conduction studies	Tissue biopsy

14. Tissue biopsy is unquestionably the procedure of choice in the diagnosis of vasculitis. List some of the frequently approached biopsy sites.

Common	Less common
Skin	Testicle
Sural nerve	Rectum
Temporal artery	Liver
Muscle	Heart
Kidney	Brain
Lung	

15. If tissue biopsy is not feasible, which alternative procedure can yield a diagnosis?
Angiography.

SITE	DIAGNOSIS
Abdomen (celiac trunk, superior mesenteric, and renal arteries)	Polyarteritis nodosa
Aortic arch	Takayasu's arteritis
Extremity	Buerger's disease
Brain	Isolated CNS angiitis

16. List two characteristic angiographic features of vasculitis.

    Irregular tapering and narrowing
    Aneurysms ("rosary beading")
See figure on next page.

17. Describe the general approach to the treatment of a vasculitis.

- Identify and remove inciting agents (i.e., medications, etc.)
- Treat primary underlying disease associated with the vasculitis (i.e., antibiotics for endocarditis; interferon for hepatitis B or C).
- Anti-inflammatory and/or immunosuppressive therapy tailored to the extent of vasculitis. Small-vessel vasculitis confined to the skin usually needs less-aggressive treatment than systemic vasculitis involving large and/or medium-sized arteries.

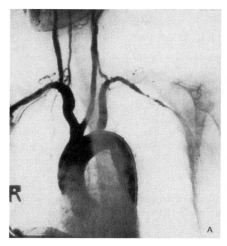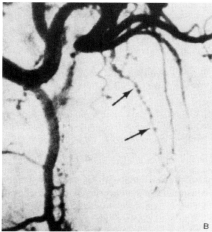

Angiography in vasculitis. *A,* Irregular tapering and narrowing of the left subclavian artery in Takayasu's arteritis. *B,* Typical "rosary beading" aneurysm formation in a patient with isolated CNS vasculitis.

BIBLIOGRAPHY

1. Conn DL: Update on systemic necrotizing vasculitis. Mayo Clin Proc 64:535–543, 1989.
2. Dahlberg PJ, Lockhart JM, Overholt EL: Diagnostic studies for systemic necrotizing vasculitis: Sensitivity, specificity, and predictive value in patients with multisystem disease. Arch Intern Med 149:161–165, 1989.
3. Fauci AS, Leavitt RY: Vasculitis. In: McCarthy DJ, Koopman WJ (eds): Arthritis and Allied Conditions, 12th ed. Philadelphia, Lea & Febiger, 1993.
4. Gibson LE, Su WPD: Cutaneous vasculitis. Rheum Dis Clin North Am 16:309–324, 1990.
5. Jennette JC, Falk RJ: Disease associations and pathogenic role of antineutrophil cytoplasmic autoantibodies in vasculitis. Curr Opin Rheumatol 4:9–15, 1992.
6. Jennette JC, Falk RJ, Andrassy K, et al: Nomenclature of systemic vasculitides: Proposal of an international consensus conference. Arthritis Rheum 37:187–192, 1994.
7. Kallenberg CGM, Mulder AHL, Tervaert JWC: Antineutrophil cytoplasmic antibodies: A still growing class of autoantibodies in inflammatory disorders. Am J Med 93:675–682, 1992.
8. Lie JT: Diagnostic histopathology of major systemic and pulmonary vasculitic syndromes. Rheum Dis Clin North Am 16:269–292, 1990.
9. Lie JT: Vasculitis simulators and vasculitis look-alikes. Curr Opin Rheumatol 4:47–55, 1992.
10. Mandell BF, Hoffman GS: Differentiating the vasculitides. Rheum Dis Clin North Am 20:409–442, 1994.

31. LARGE-VESSEL VASCULITIS: GIANT CELL ARTERITIS AND TAKAYASU'S ARTERITIS

Gregory J. Dennis, M.D.

1. List the primary large-vessel vasculitides and the rheumatic diseases associated with large-vessel vasculitis.

Giant cell arteritis, Takayasu's arteritis, and other rheumatic diseases associated with aortitis such as seronegative spondyloarthropathies, relapsing polychondritis, and Behçet's disease.

GIANT CELL ARTERITIS

2. What are some other names for giant cell arteritis (GCA)?
Cranial arteritis, temporal arteritis, and Horton's headache.

3. Discuss the typical demographic characteristics of a patient with GCA.
GCA occurs primarily in patients over age 50 years. The incidence increases with age, with GCA being almost 10 times more common among patients in their 80s than in patients aged 50–60 years. GCA is twice as common among women than men. Siblings of a patient with GCA are at increased risk (10-fold) of getting the disease.

GCA has been most commonly reported in whites of Northern European descent. Recent reports suggest that the incidence of GCA in blacks, Hispanics, and Asians is not as rare as once thought.

4. How do patients with GCA present clinically?
Most patients will present with one of four presentations:
1. Cranial symptoms with superficial headache, scalp tenderness, jaw and tongue claudication, and rarely scalp necrosis, diplopia, or blindness.
2. Polymyalgia rheumatica (PMR) with pain and stiffness of proximal muscle groups, such as neck, shoulders, hips, and thighs. Muscle symptoms are usually symmetric.
3. Both cranial and PMR symptoms. About 20–50% of patients with GCA have PMR symptoms.
4. Fever and systemic symptoms without any localized symptoms. Patients can present with a fever of unknown origin.

Onset of symptoms may be acute or insidious. Most patients have fever, weight loss, fatigue, and malaise as nonspecific symptoms.

5. Are there any physical findings that may be helpful in suggesting a diagnosis of GCA?
Several physical abnormalities are highly specific for temporal arteritis, but unfortunately, most have a low or only moderate degree of sensitivity for the diagnosis. **Scalp tenderness** and **temporal artery abnormalities**, such as a reduction in the pulse in conjunction with palpable tenderness, yield the greatest sensitivity for diagnosis. The presence of a visual abnormality (diplopia, amaurosis fugax, unilateral loss of vision, optic neuritis, and optic atrophy) may lend additional support for the diagnosis but are relatively less sensitive.

6. When should GCA be suspected?
GCA should be suspected in individuals over age 50 who develop a new type of headache, jaw claudication, unexplained fever, or polymyalgia rheumatica.

7. What is the most dreaded complication of GCA? How commonly does it occur?
Sudden blindness occurs in 15% of patients, can be an early symptom, and is most commonly due to ischemic optic neuritis. Anatomic lesions that produce ischemic optic neuritis in these patients result from arteritis involving the posterior ciliary branches of the ophthalmic arteries, resulting in ischemia of the optic nerve. The blindness is abrupt and painless. Retinal artery involvement appears to be a relatively uncommon cause of blindness.

8. The clinical manifestations of GCA might also include what other ocular problems.
Blurring of vision, transient visual loss (amaurosis fugax), iritis, conjunctivitis, scintillating scotomata, photophobia, glaucoma, and ophthalmoplegia due to ischemia of extraocular muscles may also be manifestations of GCA. Visual blurring and/or amaurosis fugax usually occur as warning signs for months before sudden blindness occurs.

9. Does GCA only involve the cranial circulation?
Although cranial involvement is the most frequently recognized and characteristic manifestations of GCA, the process is a generalized vascular disease not limited to the cranial vessels. Extracranial GCA usually involves the aorta and its major branches and is clinically detectable in 10–15% of patients.

10. Name some common clinical presentations of GCA involving the extracranial circulation.
GCA involving the extracranial circulation may present as the **aortic arch syndrome** when involving the aorta and subclavian arteries, as **aneurysms** of major arteries such as the carotids, or as **claudication** of the extremities when involving the distal aorta, iliac, or femoral vessels.

11. What neurologic complications can occur in patients with GCA?
Neurologic complications are relatively rare in GCA. The internal carotid and vertebral arteries may be involved, leading to strokes, seizures, acute hearing loss, vertigo, cerebral dysfunction, and depression. Involvement of the intracranial arteries is unusual since these vessels lack an internal elastic lamina.

12. List the resulting manifestation when GCA involves a particular vascular distribution.

VASCULATURE	COMPLICATION
Ophthalmic	Blindness
Subclavian	Absent pulses
Renal	Hypertension
Coronary	Angina pectoris
Carotid	Stroke
Vertebral	Dizziness, stroke
Iliac	Claudication
Mesenteric	Abdominal ischemia

Note that GCA can involve both large- and medium-sized arteries. Pulmonary artery involvement is unusual. Small-artery involvement is much less common, so skin manifestations are rare.

13. What other symptoms can occur in patients with GCA?
- **Synovitis**—Arthralgias are common, but objective swelling of joints occurs in <10% of patients.
- **Cough**—GCA can present as a nonproductive cough.
- **Hypothyroidism**—There is an increased incidence of hypothyroidism (5%) in patients with GCA.

14. Is the erythrocyte sedimentation rate (ESR) helpful in the diagnosis of GCA?
The ESR is the most consistently abnormal laboratory test, and it tends to be higher in GCA than in other vasculitides. It is almost always >50 mm/hr, averaging 80–100 mm/hr by the Westergren method. Rarely, it may be normal. Although in the appropriate clinical setting, the ESR is a sensitive indicator of GCA, its specificity is <50%. Indeed, other diseases, particularly infections and multiple myeloma, can give systemic symptoms associated a ESR >100 mm/hr.

15. Are any other laboratory abnormalities frequently seen in patients with GCA?
Anemia thrombocytosis, abnormal liver function tests (especially alkaline phosphatase), and increased C-reactive protein (frequently to very high levels, >10 mg/dl).

16. How often do patients with GCA have liver enzyme abnormalities?
They occur in 20–30% of patients. The particular enzymes that may be abnormal includes AST, ALT, and alkaline phosphatase. Not uncommonly, the hepatic enzymes are elevated 3–5-fold but normalize rapidly with corticosteroid therapy.

17. Is the anemia typical for iron deficiency?
No, the anemia is most often mild to moderate, with hemoglobin values in the 9–11-gm/dl range. Ordinarily, it is a hypochromic or normochromic anemia. The iron studies are usually not indicative of iron deficiency and instead are consistent with the anemia of chronic disease (low iron, low total iron-binding capacity normal or high ferritin).

18. Which test, if any, is used for confirmation of the clinical diagnosis of GCA?
Biopsy of the most abnormal segment of the temporal artery should be performed to confirm the diagnosis, since other diseases may present with similar manifestations. Patients with arteritis of extracranial vessels can have a characteristic **angiogram.**

19. What characteristic of the disease process may hamper the ability to demonstrate vasculitis on biopsy?
GCA is characterized by patchy or segmental arterial involvement. Consequently, a 3–6-cm segment should be obtained when the physical findings are indeterminate. The arterial biopsy specimen should be sliced like a salami at 1–2 mm intervals and examined histologically at multiple levels.

20. How often does a properly performed temporal artery biopsy define the need for therapy?
The properly performed biopsy will define the need for therapy in approximately 80–90% of cases. However, if the biopsy is negative and the clinical suspicion for disease remains high, consideration should be given toward biopsy of the opposite side, which will be positive in an additional 10–15% of cases.

21. Describe the characteristic histologic findings on temporal artery biopsy in GCA.
More than 90% of positive biopsies show a granulomatous inflammatory reaction concentrated around the inner half of the media and centering on a disrupted internal elastic lamina.

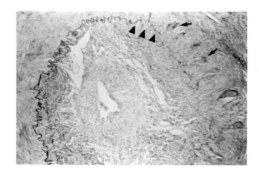

Temporal artery biopsy in a patient with GCA, showing the disrupted internal elastic lamina (*arrowheads*) and Langhans' giant cells (*arrows*).

22. Is GCA a genetic disease? How does heredity relate to its pathogenesis?
The cause of GCA is unknown and its pathogenesis is poorly understood. The localization of the inflammatory reaction around the fragmented internal elastic lamina suggests that GCA may result from an autoimmune reaction to elastin or other macromolecules, although this is unproven. The inflammatory infiltrate is primarily macrophages and CD4+ T lymphocytes of Th1 type, with approximately 25% being activated T cells. Recently, it has been discovered that the majority of GCA and PMR patients express the HLA-DR4 allele (60–70%). These patients have a common sequence motif of amino acids of the HLA-DR β-1 chain with localization to the second hypervariable region of the antigen-binding site of the HLA-DR molecule.

23. Is there a standard therapy in the management of GCA?
Currently, high-dose corticosteroids (prednisone, 20 mg three times a day) remain the treatment of choice. Alternate-day corticosteroid regimens are not effective. Several investigations, however, are underway to assess the role and efficacy of other medications (i.e., methotrexate) in the management of this disease.

24. Should one implement therapy before obtaining a temporal artery biopsy?
It depends on the assessed risk for a serious complication and how soon the biopsy can be obtained. Symptoms for which corticosteroid therapy might be instituted sooner are complications

such as sudden blindness, stroke, and angina. In general, clinicians should have a low threshold for starting corticosteroids early in patients who have a clinical syndrome compatible with GCA.

25. Does treatment with corticosteroids influence the biopsy findings?

While it is possible that corticosteroid therapy may influence temporal artery biopsy findings, recent studies have shown that biopsies may show arteritis even after >14 days of corticosteroid therapy in the presence of clinical indications of active disease. In general, the biopsy should be obtained within 7 days of starting corticosteroid therapy if possible.

26. Do patients respond rapidly to the initiation of appropriate therapy?

Corticosteroids usually are dramatically effective in suppressing the systemic symptoms of GCA within 72 hours after initiation of therapy. Localized manifestations of arteritis, such as headaches, scalp tenderness, and jaw or tongue claudication, steadily improve over a longer period of time.

27. Does the initiation of corticosteroid therapy prevent catastrophic events such as blindness and strokes?

There have been many instances that support the prevention of catastrophic events by corticosteroids in patients with temporal arteritis. Sudden blindness and other stroke-like events have occasionally been reversed in patients by the institution of high-dose corticosteroid therapy.

28. Is it possible for patients with GCA to present with a normal ESR?

Yes. Although the vast majority of patients present with ESRs >50 mm/hr, there have been case reports and small series describing the association of biopsy-proven GCA with rates <40 mm/hr. One series consisting of five such individuals emphasized an increased frequency of polymyalgia rheumatica or prior treatment with corticosteroid medications for other conditions as perhaps being responsible for this occurrence. In these patients, an elevated C-reactive protein may be helpful.

29. How common is it for untreated patients with GCA to develop blindness?

In absence of the initiation of appropriate therapy, blindness occurs in 36–55% of patients at some time during their clinical course.

30. When should the level of corticosteroid medications be reduced?

Patients should receive close periodic observation to identify potential harbingers of complications and to allow the gradual discontinuation of corticosteroid therapy. When clinical evidence of the inflammatory process, including symptoms and laboratory evidence of inflammation, have subsided, the corticosteroid dosage can be lowered gradually. A good rule of thumb is to begin tapering 1 month after clinical and laboratory parameters, particularly the ESR, have normalized.

If patients do not achieve complete remission or are not able to be tapered to low doses of corticosteroids (<10–20 mg prednisone a day), cytotoxic or other immunosuppressive should be considered. Some clinicians are starting low-dose weekly pulse methotrexate simultaneously with corticosteroids in an effort to taper patients off corticosteroids more quickly. This, however, is still an investigational approach.

31. How long do patients with GCA usually receive corticosteroid therapy?

Treatment usually continues for at least 6 months, and often low-dose prednisone is needed for years. It has been well-documented that discontinuation of corticosteroid medications too early is associated with worsening of disease activity, and recurrences of disease are known to occur several years after the completion of an appropriate therapeutic regimen. Every effort should be made to limit side effects of corticosteroids such as osteoporosis (calcium and vitamin D therapy).

32. Is mortality increased in GCA patients compared to the general elderly population?

Risk of death from GCA appears to be increased within the first 4 months of starting therapy. Patients typically die of vascular complications, such as stroke, myocardial infarction, ruptured aneurysm, or dissecting aneurysm. After 4 months, the mortality is similar to that of an aged-matched general population.

TAKAYASU'S ARTERITIS

33. What are some other names of Takayasu's arteritis (TA)?
Pulseless disease
Aortic arch syndrome
Occlusive thromboaortopathy

34. Discuss the typical demographic characteristics of a patient with TA.
TA occurs most commonly in young women. The average age is 10–30 years, but it can occur in younger and much older individuals. TA is eight times more common among women then men. TA occurs most commonly in Asian females but has been reported worldwide in all racial groups.

35. What are the major clinical presentations of TA?
A triphasic pattern of progression of disease has been described:
- **Phase I** — Pre-pulseless, inflammatory period characterized by nonspecific systemic complaints such as fever, arthralgias, and weight loss. These patients are often diagnosed as a prolonged viral syndrome. Patients under age 20 frequently present with disease in this phase.
- **Phase II** — Vessel inflammation dominated by vessel pain and tenderness.
- **Phase III** — Fibrotic stage when bruits and ischemia predominate.

Patients can present in any phase or combination of phases since TA is a chronic, recurrent disease. Up to 10% present with no symptoms, and the incidental finding of unequal pulses/blood pressures, bruits, or hypertension prompts further evaluation.

36. List some of the more common clinical features occurring in TA.

Bruits	80%
Claudication	70%
Decreased pulses	60%
Arthralgias	50%
Asymmetric blood pressure	50%
Constitutional symptoms	40%
Headache	40%
Hypertension	30%
Dizziness	30%
Pulmonary	25%
Cardiac	10%
Erythema nodosum	8%

Symptoms occur primarily due to stenoses of the aorta and its branches. The aortic arch and abdominal aorta are most commonly affected. Upper-extremity and thoracic vessels (subclavian, carotid, vertebral) are more commonly involved than iliac arteries. Pulmonary artery involvement can occur in up to 70% of patients, with <25% having symptoms of pulmonary hypertension. Cardiac involvement with angina, myocardial infarction, heart failure, sudden death, and aortic valvular regurgitation occurs in up to 15% of patients.

37. Are there any specific laboratory tests useful for the diagnosis of TA?
No. Nonspecific laboratory studies indicate active inflammation such as anemia of chronic disease, thrombocytosis, and an elevated ESR, and C-reactive protein. The ESR does not always follow the degree of active, ongoing inflammation and may be normal in up to 33% of patients with active disease.

38. How is the diagnosis of TA made?
Angiography is the old standard for detecting arterial involvement in TA. Full aortography should be performed. The lesions of TA are most often long-segment stenoses or arterial occlu-

sions of aorta and visceral vessels at their aortic origins. Aneurysms can occur but are uncommon (see Chapter 30).

Noninvasive imaging studies such as MRI are gaining popularity. With MRI, there is no radiation risk, and it is useful in detecting vessel wall thickness and inflammation as well as mural thrombus. It can also detect pulmonary artery involvement. Overall, MRI will miss some lesions, particularly in the proximal aortic arch or distal aortic branches, which are best detected by angiography.

39. Is the histopathologic description of TA the same as that for GCA?
The histologic appearance of TA is a focal panarteritis which can be very similar to GCA. Like GCA, focal "skip lesions" are common. One point that helps separate TA from GCA is that the cellular infiltrate in TA tends to localize in the adventitia and outer parts of the media including vasa vasorum, whereas the inflammation of GCA concentrates around the inner half of the media. Biopsy of a vessel is not necessary to establish the diagnosis of TA if the angiogram and clinical symptoms are characteristic.

40. Is TA a genetic disease?
The etiology and pathogenesis of TA are unknown. Studies linking TA to HLA Class I and II genes have provided controversial results. There is no link to HLA-DR4 as is seen in GCA.

41. What is the treatment for TA?
High-dose corticosteroids (prednisone, 20 mg three times a day) are the initial therapy for active inflammatory TA. Alternate-day regimens are not successful. Corticosteroids are maintained at high doses until symptoms and laboratory evidence (ESR) of inflammation normalize. Unfortunately, the ESR does not always reflect the degree of inflammation observed if a blood vessel is biopsied. With control of inflammation, corticosteroids are tapered.

Relapses do occur, and up to 40% of TA patients will require cytotoxic therapy. Methotrexate is preferred due to its limited toxicity and its ability to induce remission in 80% of patients. However, up to 20% of TA patients never achieve remission.

Other medical therapy includes antihypertensive therapy (vasodilators should be avoided unless the patient has heart failure), antiplatelet therapy to prevent thrombis, calcium therapy to prevent osteoporosis, and control of hyperlipidemia. Surgery is used to bypass stenotic lesions that fail to improve with medical management. Percutaneous transluminal angioplasty has been used in some patients to treat stenotic vessels once inflammation is controlled.

42. What is the prognosis for patients with TA?
Sudden death may occur due to myocardial infarction, stroke, or aneurysmal rupture or dissection. Cardiac and renal failure can occur. Long-term survival rates are 80–90%.

BIBLIOGRAPHY

1. Achkar AA, Lie JT, Hunder GG, et al: How does previous corticosteroid treatment affect the biopsy findings in giant cell (temporal) arteritis? Ann Intern Med 120:987–992, 1994.
2. Arend WP, Michel BA, Bloch DA, et al: The American College of Rheumatology 1990 criteria for the classification of Takayasu's arteritis. Arthritis Rheum 33:1122–1128, 1990.
3. Arend WP, Michael BA, Bloch DA, et al: The American College of Rheumatology 1990 criteria for the classification of giant cell arteritis. Arthritis Rheum 33:1129–1136, 1990.
4. Hoffman GS, Leavitt RY, Kerr GS: Treatment of gluococorticoid-resistant or relapsing Takayasu arteritis with methotrexate. Arthritis Rheum 37:578–582, 1994.
5. Kerr GS, Hallahan CW, Giordano J, et al: Takayasu's arteritis. Ann Intern Med 120:919–929, 1994.
6. Nesher G, Sonnenblick M, Friendlander Y: Analysis of steroid related complications and mortality in temporal arteritis: A 15 year survey of 43 patients. J Rheumatol 21:1283–1286, 1994.
7. Ninet JP, Bachet P, Dumontet CM, et al: Subclavian and axillary involvement in temporal arteritis and polymyalgia rheumatica. Am J Med 88:13–20, 1990.
8. Nordborg E, Nordborg C, Malmvall BE, et al: Giant cell arteritis. Rheumatic Dis Clin North Am 21:1013–1026, 1995.

32. MEDIUM-VESSEL VASCULITIDES: POLYARTERITIS NODOSA, ALLERGIC ANGIITIS AND GRANULOMATOSIS OF CHURG-STRAUSS, AND THROMBOANGIITIS OBLITERANS

Ramon A. Arroyo, M.D.

1. What is a medium-vessel vasculitis?
It is a clinical and pathologic process caused by inflammation of medium-sized blood vessels. The inflammation can involve arteries and veins. A number of different clinical and pathologic types have been described.

2. Are there other size vessels involved in the medium-vessel vasculitides?
Yes, pathologic changes are not restricted to medium-size vessels alone. Large and, more frequently, small vessel changes are often found.

3. What conditions are grouped under medium-vessel vasculitis?
Because of the overlap of size and organ distribution and the similar histologic and clinical picture among the various vasculitides, classification methods have not been entirely satisfactory. The conditions considered under medium-vessel vasculitis include (controversial):
Polyarteritis nodosa
Churg-Strauss syndrome
Wegener's granulomatosis (see Chapter 33)

4. What is polyarteritis nodosa (PAN)?
PAN is a multisystem condition characterized by inflammation of small- and medium-sized arteries. It most commonly involves the vessels of the skin, kidney, peripheral nerves, muscle, and gut. Involvement of other organs is rare.

5. How common is PAN?
It's uncommon. PAN has an annual incidence of 5–10 cases per 1,000,000 population. It is more common in males by a ratio of 2:1. It affects all racial groups, with an average age at diagnosis ranging from the mid-40s to mid-60s.

6. What are the clinical features of this condition?
The disease presents in a variety of ways. Typically, the patient experiences constitutional features of fever, malaise, and weight loss along with the following manifestations of multisystem involvement. However, PAN can be limited to one organ without detectable systemic involvement. This usually is seen as cutaneous PAN, which may represent 10% of cases.

ORGAN	MANIFESTATION	ESTIMATED PREVALENCE
Peripheral nerves	Mononeuritis multiplex	50–70%
Kidney	Focal necrotizing glomerulonephritis	70%
Skin	Palpable purpura, infarction, livedo	50%
Joint	Arthralgias	50%
	Arthritis	20%
Muscle	Myalgias	50%
Gut	Abdominal pain, liver function abnormalities	30%
Heart	Congestive heart failure, myocardial infarction	Low
CNS	Seizures, stroke	Low
Lung	Interstitial pneumonitis	Low
Temporal artery	Jaw claudication	Low
Testis	Pain	Low
Eye	Retinal hemorrhage	Low

7. Are any specific laboratory tests helpful in the diagnosis of PAN?
No, most tests are nonspecific and reflect the systemic inflammatory nature of this condition. Elevated ESR, normocytic normochromic anemia, thrombocytosis, and diminished levels of albumin are usually present. Decreased complement occurs in about 25% of cases during active disease. Hepatitis B surface antigen is present in 10–50%, depending on the series.

8. Then how do you make the diagnosis of PAN?
It's often difficult. You should suspect PAN in any patient who presents with constitutional symptoms and multisystem involvement. Key **clinical features** suggestive of PAN include skin lesions (e.g., palpable purpura, livedo, necrotic lesions, infarct of the finger tips), peripheral neuropathy (most frequently mononeuritis multiplex), and renal sediment abnormalities. Once you suspect PAN, the diagnosis should be determined by **biopsying** accessible tissues. If clinically involved tissues are not amenable to biopsy, a visceral **angiogram** should be considered.

9. Which tissue should be sampled to diagnose PAN?
The likelihood of finding arteritis is greatest when symptomatic sites are examined. The most accessible tissues are skin, sural nerve, skeletal muscle, liver, rectum, and testicle.

10. Can a kidney biopsy be diagnostic of PAN?
No. In cases with abnormalities of urinary sediment or proteinuria, renal biopsy will usually reveal a focal necrotizing glomerulonephritis. This can be seen in almost all the vasculitides, so renal biopsy is not helpful in differentiating between medium-vessel vasculitides, but it could be useful if no other tissues are involved or available for diagnosis.

11. Describe the histologic features in PAN.
The pathologic lesion defining classic PAN is a **focal segmental necrotizing vasculitis** of medium-sized and small arteries (see figure), less commonly arterioles, and rarely, venules. Involvement of large vessels such as the aorta is virtually unknown.

The lesions occur in all parts of the body, but usually less so in the pulmonary and splenic arteries. The inflammation is characterized by fibrinoid necrosis and pleomorphic cellular infiltration of the vessel wall, predominantly PMNs and variable numbers of lymphocytes and eosinophils. The normal architecture of the vessel wall, including the elastic laminae, is disrupted. Thrombosis or aneurysmal dilation may occur at the site of the lesion. Healed areas of arteritis show proliferation of fibrous tissue and endothelial cells, which may lead to vessel occlusion. Remember, the lesions are focal and sectorial, involving only parts of the arterial circumference.

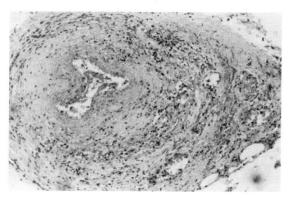

PAN involving a medium-sized artery.

12. When do you perform an angiogram for the diagnosis of PAN?
When clinically involved tissue is not available for biopsy (i.e., a patient who presents with constitutional symptoms and digital ischemia). Angiographic evaluation for PAN usually requires study of the abdominal viscera. The best plan is to study the kidney, liver, spleen, stomach, and small bowel. In rare cases, hand or foot arteriography is necessary.

13. Describe the angiographic findings in PAN.
Small aneurysms (microaneurysm), occlusion, and stenoses of the small and medium-sized vessels of the viscera (see figure).

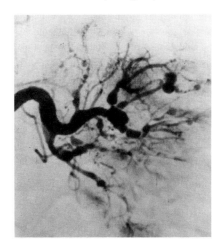

Angiogram of the kidney in a patient with PAN demonstrating multiple aneurysmal dilatations.

14. What causes PAN?
Unknown. An immune complex-mediated mechanism is frequently considered, but immune complex deposits or complement components are seldom found in involved vessels. Direct endothelial injury with subsequent release of cytokines and mediators of inflammatory reaction is another theory, but the triggering factor or antigen has not been found. Several conditions have been associated with PAN or PAN-like vasculitis, including:

       Viral infections (e.g., hepatitis B, CMV, HTLV-1, HIV, parvovirus)

       Autoimmune disorders (e.g., SLE, rheumatoid arthritis, dermatomyositis, Cogan's
         syndrome)

       Medications (e.g., allopurinol, sulfa)

       Hairy cell leukemia

15. How is PAN treated?
Decisions regarding the initial management of PAN without HBV infection depends on the extent of disease, rate of disease progression, and organs involved. Treatment of this systemic vasculitis should include high doses of corticosteroids. If severe, intravenous pulse methylprednisolone (15 mg/kg) given over 1–2 hours daily for 1–3 days is frequently used. Corticosteroids are then given at doses of 1–2 mg/kg/day in divided doses (usually three doses). Cytotoxic medications such as cyclophosphamide (2 mg/kg daily oral or 500–1000 mg/m^2 iv each month) are added to the corticosteroids in most cases with systemic involvement.

16. How does the therapy for hepatitis B virus (HBV) associated with PAN differ from that for PAN not associated with hepatitis B?
In HBV-associated PAN, the traditional treatment with corticosteroids and cyclophosphamide jeopardizes the patient's outcome by allowing the virus to persist and cause further liver damage

and ongoing antigenemia. Consequently, patients who are HBeAg-positive are treated with a combination of prednisone (30 mg/day) to control systemic symptoms, plasmapheresis to remove circulating immune complexes, and antiviral agents (vidarabine or interferon α-2b) to eliminate the virus. Successful therapy will be accompanied by seroconversion from HBeAg to anti-HBe antibodies.

17. What is the prognosis of PAN?
The outcome of PAN depends on the presence and extent of visceral and CNS involvement. Most deaths occur within the first year, usually due to uncontrolled vasculitis, delay in diagnosis, or complications of treatment. Death occurring after the first year are usually due to complications of treatment, infections, or a vascular event such as myocardial infarction or stroke. The overall 5-year survival rate is 65–75% with aggressive treatment.

18. What is microscopic polyarteritis (MPA)? How does it differ from classic PAN?
MPA is defined as a systemic necrotizing vasculitis that clinically and histologically affects small vessels (i.e., capillaries, venules, or arterioles) associated with focal segmental necrotizing glomerulonephritis. It can be separated from classic PAN primarily because it does not cause microaneurysm formation of abdominal or renal vessels. It can be differentiated from Wegener's granulomatosis in that it does not cause granuloma formation or a granulomatous vasculitis.

CLINICAL FEATURES	PAN	MPA
Kidney involvement		
Renal vasculitis with infarcts and microaneurysms	Yes	No
Rapidly progressive glomerulonephritis with crescents	No	Yes
Lung involvement		
Lung hemorrhage	No	Yes
Laboratory data		
HBV-infection	Yes (50%)	No
P-ANCA	<20%	50–80%
Abnormal angiogram with microaneurysms	Yes	No
Histology	Necrotizing vasculitis	Necrotizing vasculitis (no granulomas)
Relapses	Rare	Common

Adapted from Llotte F, Guillevin L: Polyarteritis nodosa, microscopic polyangiitis, and Churg-Strauss syndrome: Clinical aspects and treatment. Rheum Dis Clin North Am 21:911–948, 1995.

19. What is Churg-Strauss syndrome (CSS)?
CSS, also known as allergic angiitis and granulomatosis of Churg-Strauss, is a granulomatous inflammation of small- and medium-sized vessels, frequently involving the skin, peripheral nerves, and lungs, which is associated with peripheral eosinophilia. It occurs primarily in patients with a previous history of allergic manifestations, such as rhinitis and asthma. There is controversy about whether CSS should be classified as a medium, small, or ANCA-associated vasculitis.

20. Describe the three clinical phases of CSS.
These phases may appear simultaneously and do not have to follow one another in the order presented here.

1. **Prodromal phase.** This phase may persist for years and consists of allergic manifestations of rhinitis, polyposis, and asthma.

2. **Peripheral blood and tissue eosinophilia,** frequently causing a picture resembling Löffler's syndrome (shifting pulmonary infiltrates and eosinophilia), chronic eosinophilic pneumonia, or eosinophilic gastroenteritis. This second phase may remit or recur over years before the third phase.

3. **Life-threatening systemic vasculitis**

21. What are the major clinical features of Churg-Strauss syndrome?

ORGAN	CLINICAL MANIFESTATIONS
Paranasal sinus	Acute or chronic paranasal sinus pain or tenderness, rhinitis, polyposis, opacifications of paranasal sinus on radiographs
Lungs	Asthma, patchy and shifting pulmonary infiltrates, nodular infiltrates without cavitations, and diffuse interstitial lung disease seen on chest radiograph
Skin	Subcutaneous nodules, petechiae, purpura, skin infarction
Cardiac	Congestive heart failure
Joints	Arthralgias and arthritis (rare)
Gastrointestinal	Abdominal pain, bloody diarrhea, abdominal masses
Miscellaneous	Renal failure, corneal ulcerations, seizures, etc.

22. What laboratory abnormalities are seen in CSS?

The characteristic laboratory abnormality is **eosinophilia.** Anemia, elevated ESR, and elevated IgE may be found. Antineutrophil cytoplasmic antibodies (ANCA) are present in 67% of patients. These are directed primarily against myeloperoxidase and give a P-ANCA pattern.

23. How do you diagnose CSS?

On the basis of its clinical and pathologic features. The diagnosis should be suspected in a patient with a previous history of allergy or asthma who presents with eosinophilia and systemic illness involving pulmonary infiltrates or multisystemic disease. The diagnosis is corroborated by biopsy of involved tissue.

24. Describe the histopathologic findings in CSS.

The characteristic pathologic changes in CSS include **small necrotizing granulomas** as well as **necrotizing vasculitis of small arteries and veins.** Granulomas are usually extravascular near small arteries and veins. They are composed of a central eosinophilic core surrounded radially by macrophages and giant cells. Inflammatory cells are also present, with eosinophils predominating and smaller numbers of PMNs and lymphocytes.

25. How is CSS differentiated from Wegener's granulomatosis?

	CSS	WEGENER'S GRANULOMATOSIS
ENT	Rhinitis, polyposis	Necrotizing lesions
Allergy, bronchial asthma	Frequent	No more frequent than in general population
Renal involvement	Uncommon	Common
Eosinophilia	>10% of peripheral leukocytes	Minimally elevated
Histology	Eosinophilic necrotizing granuloma	Necrotizing epithelioid granuloma
Prognosis (major cause of death)	Cardiac	Pulmonary and renal
ANCA	P-ANCA 67%	C-ANCA 90%

26. How do you treat CSS? What is its prognosis?

The treatment of choice is glucocorticoids. Prednisone at high doses (60 mg/day) is usually sufficient to control the disease. In severe cases with life-threatening organ involvement, cytotoxics should be considered.

The 5-year survival rate for CSS is 75%. The major cause of death is cardiac involvement (50%) with myocardial infarction and congestive heart failure.

27. Is thromboangiitis obliterans (TO) a true vasculitis?

TO is an inflammatory, obliterative, nonatheromatous vascular disease that most commonly affects the small- and medium-sized arteries, veins, and nerves. In the acute phase of this condition, a highly inflammatory thrombus will form, and although there is some inflammation in the blood vessel wall itself, the inflammatory changes are not nearly as prominent as in other forms of vasculitis. But, because of the associated mild inflammatory changes within the blood vessel, TO is pathologically considered as a vasculitis.

28. What is the etiology of TO?
There is no clear etiologic mechanism. There is an extremely strong association with tobacco use. Other etiologic factors may be important as well, such as genetic predisposition and possibly autoimmune mechanisms.

29. Who is affected by TO?
Typically young smokers aged 18–50 years, and rarely beyond. The average age at diagnosis is the mid-30s. Most reports describe heavy smokers, but TO has been reported in smokers using 3–6 cigarettes a day for a few years. The disease has also been reported in pipe smokers and tobacco chewers.

TO is predominantly a disease of males but is seen in women as well. The recent increase in incidence of this disease in women appears to relate to improvements in the recognition of this condition and the increased use of tobacco in this group.

30. What are the clinical features of this condition?
Usually TO's initial manifestation is ischemia or claudication of both legs, and sometimes hands, which begins distally and progresses cephalad. Two or more limbs are commonly involved. Superficial thrombophlebitis is described in one-third to one-half of patients, and Raynaud's phenomenon in about 10%.

31. What are some of the presenting symptoms that prompt the patient to seek medical attention?
1. Claudication, pain at rest, and digital ulceration are the primary manifestations. Because the disease starts distally, dysesthesias, sensitivity to cold, rubor, or cyanosis prompts the patient to seek medical attention in one-third of cases.

2. Pedal (instep) claudication is characteristic of TO, and patients often seek special shoes or orthopedic or podiatry care before the process is fully appreciated.

3. Gangrene and ulceration or rest pain is the presenting complaint in one-third of the patients. This occurs predominantly in the toes and fingers. It may occur spontaneously but more often follows trauma, such as nail trimming or pressure from tight shoes.

32. How is TO diagnosed?
To confirm your clinical diagnosis, you need to exclude conditions that mimic TO. The most important and common of these are atherosclerosis and emboli. All patients suspected of having TO should undergo an echocardiogram to rule out cardiac thrombi and an arteriogram to rule out atherosclerosis. The arteriogram will also help confirm your clinical diagnosis of TO, as arteriographic findings are suggestive (though not pathognomonic) of the disease.

33. Describe the arteriographic findings in TO.
Although no single arteriographic feature is specific for TO, the radiographic constellation in conjunction with the clinical picture *is* diagnostic. On arteriograms, there is involvement of the small- and medium-sized blood vessels, most commonly the digital arteries of the fingers and toes as well as the palmar, plantar, tibial, peroneal, radial, and ulnar arteries (see figure). The angiographic appearance is bilateral focal segments of stenosis or occlusion with normal proximal or intervening vessels. An increase in collateral vessels often occurs around areas of occlusion, giving a tree root, spider web, or corkscrew appearance. Note that in the arteriographic description, the affected arteries may have normal segments, but most important is that the proximal arteries are normal without evidence of atherosclerosis or emboli.

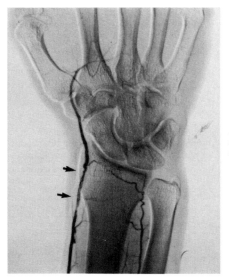

Angiogram of hand in TO. Note irregularity of radial artery (*arrows*) and cutoff of palmar arch vessels with no digital vessels.

34. Is a biopsy needed to make the diagnosis?

Pathologic specimens are not commonly obtained during the acute phase of TO. Reluctance to obtain biopsy specimens of these vessels is because the distal extremity is usually ischemic and biopsy may lead to new ulceration. Therefore, most pathologic specimens come from amputated limbs. In the acute phase, a panvasculitis with a highly cellular thrombus is found. In the subacute phase, the thrombus is less cellular and recanalization of the thrombus is apparent. There may be perivascular fibrosis during this phase. In the late phase, there is often organized and recanalized thrombus and perivascular fibrosis. Unlike other medium-vessel vasculitides, venulitis is frequently prominent in pathologic specimens obtained from patients with TO.

35. What conditions should be included in the differential diagnosis of TO?

Systemic lupus erythematosus	Small-vessel vasculitides
Rheumatoid arthritis	Various blood dyscrasias
Scleroderma	Occupational hazards
PAN	Hypothenar hammer syndrome
Anti-phospholipid antibody syndrome	Thrombosed aneurysm
Giant cell or Takayasu's arteritis	

36. How do you treat TO?

1. *Cessation* of smoking or tobacco use in any form. (Many patients continue to smoke despite disease severe enough to result in amputation.)
2. Treatment of local ischemic ulceration.
    Foot care (lubricate skin with lanolin-based cream, place lamb's wool between toes, avoid trauma)
    Trial of calcium channel blockers and/or pentoxifylline
    Iloprost (not currently available in the United States)
    Sympathectomy
3. Treat cellulitis with antibiotics
4. Treat superficial phlebitis with NSAIDs
5. Amputate limb when all else fails

37. Is surgical recanalization an option in the treatment of TO?

Usually not. Because vascular involvement is distal, appropriate sites for bypass graft insertion are generally not present. In the few patients who have undergone arterial bypass, long-term results are poor.

BIBLIOGRAPHY

1. Calabrese LH: Vasculitis of the central nervous system. Rheum Dis Clin North Am 21:1059–1076, 1995.
2. Conn DL: Polyarteritis. Rheum Dis Clin North Am 16:341–362, 1990.
3. Fauci AS, Haynes BF, Katz P: The spectrum of vasculitis: Clinical, pathologic, immunologic, and therapeutic considerations. Ann Intern Med 89:660–676, 1978.
4. Gross WL: New developments in the treatment of systemic vasculitis. Curr Opin Rheumatol 6:11–19, 1994.
5. Joyce JW: Buerger's disease (thromboangiitis obliterans). Rheum Dis Clin North Am 16:463–470, 1990.
6. Llotte F, Guillevin L: Polyarteritis nodosa, microscopic polyangiitis and Churg-Strauss syndrome: Clinical aspects and treatment. Rheum Dis Clin North Am 21:911–948, 1995.
7. Lightfoot RW, Michel BA, Block DA, et al: The American College of Rheumatology 1990 criteria for the classification of polyarteritis nodosa. Arthritis Rheum 33:1088–1093, 1990.
8. Masi AT, Hunder GG, Lie JT, et al: The American College of Rheumatology 1990 criteria for the classification of Churg-Strauss syndrome (allergic granulomatosis angiitis). Arthritis Rheum 33:1094–1110, 1990.
9. Olin JW: Thromboangiitis obliterans. Curr Opin Rheumatol 6:44–50, 1994.

33. WEGENER'S GRANULOMATOSIS AND OTHER ANCA-ASSOCIATED DISEASES

Mark Malyak, M.D.

1. Define Wegener's granulomatosis.
Wegener's granulomatosis (WG) is a clinicopathologic syndrome of unknown etiology characterized by:
- Extravascular granulomatous inflammation, granulomatous vasculitis of predominantly small-sized vessels, and necrosis of the **upper and lower respiratory tracts**
- **Glomerulonephritis,** usually pauci-immune, focal and segmental, and necrotizing
- Variable involvement of **other organ systems** with granulomatous vasculitis of mostly small-sized vessels, extravascular granulomatous inflammation, and necrosis
- Strong association with cytoplasmic anti-neutrophil cytoplasmic antibodies (C-ANCA)

Though WG is considered a primary vasculitis syndrome, the inflammatory changes in it, including granulomas, often occur in parenchymal sites outside vessel walls. Indeed, extravascular granulomatous infiltration may be the predominant lesion in WG.

2. How does the American College of Rheumatology define WG?
The College has proposed the following criteria for WG. Patients meeting 2 or more of these 4 criteria can be classified (? diagnosed) as having WG with a sensitivity of 88% and a specificity of 92%
- Nasal or oral inflammation characterized as oral ulcers or purulent or bloody nasal discharge
- Abnormal chest radiograph showing nodules, fixed infiltrates, or cavities
- Abnormal urinary sediment showing microhematuria or RBC casts
- Characteristic granulomatous inflammation in the wall of an artery or in perivascular/extravascular areas

3. How is the upper respiratory tract affected clinically by WG?
Chronic inflammation of the mucosa of the upper respiratory tract characterized by granulomatous inflammation, vasculitis, and necrosis may lead to clinical manifestations in the following locations:
Paranasal sinuses—Chronic sinusitis is a common presenting manifestation (50%) that ultimately affects 80% of patients with WG.

Nasal mucosa—Chronic inflammation occurs in approximately 70% of patients, resulting in chronic purulent nasal discharge, epistaxis, mucosal ulcerations, and, less commonly, perforation of the nasal septum and disruption of the supporting cartilage of the nose (saddle-nose deformity).

Oral mucosa—Chronic inflammation may lead to oral ulcers that may or may not be painful.

Pharyngeal mucosa—Chronic inflammation may lead to obstruction of the auditory canal, resulting in acute suppurative otitis media or chronic serous otitis media.

Laryngeal and tracheal mucosa—Chronic inflammation may lead to subglottic stenosis which, in severe cases, may result in stridor and respiratory insufficiency.

4. Describe the pathologic findings in the lower respiratory tract in WG.

Lower Respiratory Tract Pathology in WG

Extravascular inflammation
  Chronic: granulomatous
  Acute: with neutrophilic infiltration
Vasculitis
  Chronic: granulomatous
  Acute: neutrophilic infiltration and fibrinoid necrosis
Fibrosis

Pulmonary disease in WG is characterized by variable degrees of chronic (granulomatous) and acute (neutrophilic) inflammation and necrosis of the alveolar septa and small blood vessels. Airways and larger blood vessels are involved less commonly.

Chronic inflammation results in the characteristic lesion of WG, the granuloma, typically occurring in the extravascular interstitium of the alveolar septa, but also within vessel and airway walls. **Acute inflammation** results in infiltration of neutrophils and other inflammatory cells in vessel walls, extravascular interstitium, and alveolar spaces.

If acute or chronic inflammation resolves, it may be characterized by resolution (healing) or organization (collagen deposition and scar formation). Also, acute inflammation may evolve into a chronic inflammatory process with granulomatous infiltration. Many patients with WG have variable degrees of both acute and chronic inflammation on pathologic examination, often with one type predominating. When inflammation occurs adjacent to the serosal surface of the lung, chronic fibrinous pleuritis may result.

5. How does lower respiratory tract involvement manifest clinically?

Lower Respiratory Tract Involvement in WG

CLINICAL SYNDROME	PATHOLOGY	RADIOGRAPHIC FINDINGS
Asymptomatic (common)	Predominantly chronic inflammation	Fixed, focal infiltrates and/or nodules
Subacute/chronic cough, without other symptoms of pulmonary involvement (common)	Predominantly chronic inflammation	Fixed, focal infiltrates and/or nodules
Alveolar hemorrhage syndrome (uncommon)	Capillaritis within alveolar septa (acute inflamation)	Fleeting, focal alveolar infiltrates (intra-alveolar hemorrhage)
Acute/subacute pneumonitis with acute respiratory failure (uncommon)	Predominantly acute inflammation	Transient focal or diffuse interstitial/alveolar infiltrates
Chronic respiratory insufficiency (uncommon)	Chronic inflammation and/or fibrosis	Fixed diffuse infiltrates
Pleuritis (uncommon)	Chronic fibrinous pleuritis	± Pleural effusion

Clinical evidence of pulmonary disease is common on presentation (50%) in WG, ultimately affecting 85% of patients. Approximately one-third of these patients, despite having radiographically evident pulmonary disease, do not have lower respiratory tract symptoms. The clinical manifestations of pulmonary involvement are variable, including subacute or chronic nonproductive cough without other symptoms of pulmonary involvement, mild to severe hemoptysis, and acute or chronic respiratory insufficiency/failure.

Chronic inflammation with granuloma infiltration of the alveolar septa and small blood vessels may lead to the formation of nodules and/or fixed infiltrates on chest radiographs (see figure). If this process is extensive, subacute or chronic respiratory insufficiency may result. Chronic respiratory insufficiency may also be caused by diffuse fibrosis resulting from organization of previous chronic or acute inflammation.

Acute inflammation with necrotizing vasculitis of small blood vessels and neutrophilic infiltration of extravascular sites (alveolar septa and intra-alveolar spaces) may lead to a diffuse acute pneumonitis and consequent acute respiratory insufficiency/failure. It may also lead to capillaritis of alveolar septa, which may result in an alveolar hemorrhage syndrome with hemoptysis and variable degrees of acute respiratory insufficiency/failure.

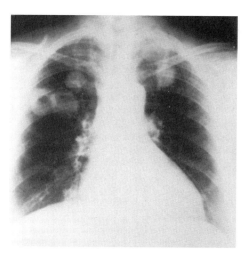

Chest radiograph demonstrating nodules (some cavitating) in a patient with WG. (From the Clinical Slide Collection on the Rheumatic Diseases. Atlanta, American College of Rheumatology, 1991; with permission.)

6. Besides direct involvement, how else may the upper and lower respiratory tracts be affected in WG?

Bacterial sinusitis, most often due to *Staphylococcus aureus,* is common in patients with upper respiratory tract involvement in WG. Obstruction of the paranasal sinus ostia by the inflammatory process is the usual cause. Similarly, obstruction of bronchi by nodules or intrabronchial lesions may lead to postobstructive suppurative bacterial pneumonia.

Infections may also result as a complication of treatment-induced immunosuppression. The two agents most commonly used, glucocorticoids and cyclophosphamide, can suppress both humoral and cellular immunity. Thus, patients are predisposed to pulmonary infections with opportunistic organisms such as *Pneumocystis carinii,* herpesviruses, mycobacteria, fungi, and *Legionella,* as well as the common suppurative bacteria such as *Streptococcus pneumoniae.*

Finally, medications may have direct toxic effects on the lungs. Cyclophosphamide, even in the relatively low doses used to treat WG, may rarely lead to pulmonary fibrosis.

7. How does involvement of the kidney by WG manifest clinically and pathologically?

Clinical evidence of renal disease occurs in approximately 15% of patients with WG on presentation, ultimately affecting 50%. Most patients remain asymptomatic.

The typical renal lesion is a pauci-immune, focal and segmental, necrotizing **glomerulonephritis.** In more severe cases, diffuse proliferative and crescentic glomerulonephritis occurs. Immunofluorescent studies often reveal little or no deposition of immunoglobulin, immune complexes, or complement, thus the designation pauci-immune. Renal vasculitis is less common and may be characterized as necrotizing vasculitis with or without granulomatous infiltration.

Most patients with glomerulonephritis have asymptomatic renal disease, manifesting as an "active" urinary sediment (hematuria, pyuria, proteinuria, and cellular casts) with variable degrees of disturbance of renal function (characterized by an elevated serum creatinine). Patients with more severe renal involvement may develop progressive renal disease leading to acute or chronic renal failure.

8. Besides the upper and lower respiratory tracts and kidney, what other organ systems may be affected?

All organ systems may be affected to variable degrees by WG. Additionally, "constitutional symptoms," such as anorexia, weight loss, fatigue, malaise, and fever, are common and likely result from circulating cytokines, particularly interleukins (IL) 1 and 6 and tumor necrosis factor-α (TNF-α), elaborated by the inflammatory process.

The **eye** is commonly involved, eventually affecting 50% of patients. Proptosis due to inflammatory and fibrotic infiltration of the retro-orbital space (retro-orbital pseudotumor) eventually affects 15% of patients with WG. This process may result in loss of visual acuity due to impingement on the optic nerve and loss of conjugate gaze due to impingement and infiltration of the extra-ocular muscles. Other less-specific ocular abnormalities include scleritis, episcleritis, uveitis, conjunctivitis, optic neuritis, and retinal artery thrombosis.

The **skin** is evenually involved in 50% of patients with WG. Lesions include palpable purpura, ulcers, subcutaneous nodules, and vesicles. Pathologic examination may reveal necrotizing vasculitis with or without granulomatous infiltration of the vessel walls, in addition to extravascular granulomatous infiltration and necrosis. Children with WG may present with and be misdiagnosed as having Henoch-Schönlein purpura.

Involvement of the **musculoskeletal systems** commonly manifests as arthralgias and myalgias, eventually affecting 67% of patients. Arthritis is less common and, when it does occur, does not result in deformities or destruction of articular cartilage.

Involvement of the peripheral and central **nervous systems** occurs in 15% and 8% of patients, respectively. The most common peripheral neuropathy is mononeuritis multiplex. CNS syndromes include cranial neuropathy, infarctions, seizures, and cerebritis.

Approximately 5% of patients develop **pericarditis,** which rarely results in interference with ventricular filling. Involvement of the myocardium, endocardium, and coronary vasculature is unusual. Involvement of other organ systems may occur but is distinctly unusual.

9. Discuss the epidemiology of WG.

The true prevalence and incidence of WG are unknown, but it is a rare disorder. It is much less common than other rheumatologic disorders such as rheumatoid arthritis, systemic lupus erythematosus (SLE), polymyalgia rheumatica, and giant cell arteritis. The mean age at diagnosis is 41 years. Although the age range is 5–78 years, only 16% of patients are <18 years old. The male:female ratio is 1:1. Approximately 97% of patients are white; only 2% are African-American.

10. Define ANCA.

ANCA (anti-neutrophil cytoplasmic antibodies) are antibodies directed against specific proteins in the cytoplasm of neutrophils and are present in the sera of patients having several underlying diseases. When alcohol-fixed neutrophils are used as a source of antigen in the indirect immunofluorescence test, three categories of ANCA may be detected by their resulting pattern: C-ANCA, P-ANCA, and atypical patterns (see figure). The **cytoplasmic,** or C-ANCA, is characterized by diffuse staining of the neutrophil cytoplasm; the **perinuclear,** or P-ANCA, results in perinuclear cytoplasmic staining; patterns not clearly C-ANCA or P-ANCA are labeled **atypical.** The protein actually recognized by C-ANCA is nearly always proteinase-3, a serine proteinase present in the primary granules of the neutrophil. The protein recognized by P-ANCA is often myeloperoxidase and, less commonly, elastase and other proteins within the granules of neutrophils. The protein target of the atypical ANCA is usually unclear, but in some cases it is common to P-ANCA.

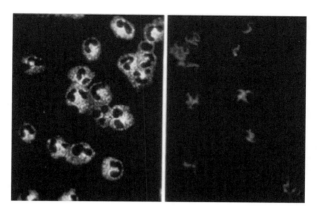

C-ANCA (*left*) and P-ANCA (*right*) immunofluorescence pattern using alcohol-fixed neutrophils as antigen source.

11. What is the clinical association of ANCA and WG?

C-ANCA, due to the presence of anti-proteinase 3 antibodies, is strongly associated with WG. The sensitivity and specificity of C-ANCA for WG are 30–90% and 98%, respectively. The wide range of sensitivity is due to the fact that the presence and titer of C-ANCA depend upon the extent of the disease and disease activity. Thus, patients with active WG clinically limited to the upper and lower respiratory tracts have lower C-ANCA titers and more false-negative tests than patients with clinical involvement of the upper and lower respiratory tracts and kidneys. Regardless of the extent of disease, disease activity as assessed clinically is an important factor determining the presence and titer of C-ANCA. Overall, C-ANCA correlates with WG disease activity in 60% of cases. Furthermore, some studies suggest that a rise in the C-ANCA titer of patients with clinically inactive WG heralds an exacerbation of disease. Additionally, since the ANCA titers tend to rise in exacerbations of WG whereas they usually do not in acute infection, the ANCA may aid in distinguishing an exacerbation of WG from an infectious process in patients with previously quiescent disease. Some patients with WG also have detectable P-ANCA.

12. What other disorders are associated with C-ANCA?

DISEASE ENTITY	SENSITIVITY OF	
	ANTI-PROTEINASE 3	ANTI-MYELOPEROXIDASE
WG	85%	10%
Microscopic polyangiitis	15–45%	45–80%
Idiopathic crescentic glomerulonephritis	25%	65%
Churg-Strauss syndrome	10%	60%
Polyarteritis nodosa	5%	15%

Adapted from Kallenberg CGM, et al: Anti-neutrophil cytoplasmic antibodies: Current diagnostic and pathophysiological potential. Kidney Int 46:1–15, 1994.

Although the presence of C-ANCA, and thus anti-proteinase 3 antibodies, is quite specific (98%) for WG, there are a number of other disease associations, particularly microscopic polyangiitis and idiopathic crescentic glomerulonephritis. Interestingly, the glomerular lesions of these three disorders are indistinguishable and are characterized by the absence of scant deposition of immune complexes (pauci-immune). Thus, these C-ANCA-associated pauci-immune disorders are a distinct category of autoimmune disease and can be distinguished from immune complex disease, such as SLE and anti-basement membrane antibody disease (Goodpasture's disease).

13. Which disorders are assoicated with P-ANCA and atypical ANCA?

Whereas C-ANCA represents the presence of anti-proteinase 3 antibodies and is associated with a small number of diseases, P-ANCA and atypical ANCA may be due to a variety of different antibodies and may be present in a wide range of diseases. Specific antibodies that may result in a positive P-ANCA or atypical ANCA include antibodies directed against myeloperoxidase, elastase, cathepsin G, lactoferrin and β-glucuronidase. P-ANCA in the setting of idiopathic crescentic glomerulonephritis, Churg-Strauss syndrome, microscopic polyangiitis, polyarteritis nodosa, or WG is usually due to anti-myeloperoxidase antibodies. P-ANCA present in other disorders is less well characterized but is usually not due to antibodies directed against myeloperoxidase.

Disease Associations of P-ANCA and Atypical ANCA

DISEASE CATEGORY/EXAMPLE	CHARACTERISTICS
Primary vasculitis syndrome	
WG	P-ANCA due to anti-MPO (10%)
	C-ANCA due to anti-P3 (85%)
Microscopic polyangiitis	P-ANCA due to anti-MPO (45–80%)
	C-ANCA due to anti-P3 (15–45%)
Idiopathic crescentic glomeru-lonephritis	P-ANCA due to anti-MPO (65%)
	C-ANCA due to anti-P3 (25%)
Churg-Strauss syndrome	P-ANCA due to anti-MPO (60%)
	C-ANCA due to anti-P3 (10%)
Polyarteritis nodosa	P-ANCA due to anti-MPO (15%)
	C-ANCA due to anti-P3 (5%)
Diffuse connective tissue disease	
SLE	P-ANCA and atypical ANCA (20%) due to anti-elastase, lactoferrin, MPO, other
Rheumatoid arthritis	P-ANCA and atypical ANCA (25%) due to anti-elastase, lactoferrin, MPO, other
Inflammatory bowel disease	
Ulcerative colitis	P-ANCA and atypical ANCA (70%) due to anti-lactoferrin, cathepsin G, other
Crohn's disease	P-ANCA and atypical ANCA (30%) due to anti-lactoferrin, cathepsin G, other
Autoimmune liver disease	
Primary sclerosing cholangitis	P-ANCA and atypical ANCA (70%) due to anti-lactoferrin, cathepsin G, other
Chronic active hepatitis	P-ANCA and atypical ANCA not characterized
Primary biliary cirrhosis	P-ANCA and atypical ANCA not characterized
Infection	
HIV	ANCA not characterized
Cystic fibrosis with infection	ANCA not characterized
Bacterial endocarditis	ANCA not characterized

MPO, myeloperoxidase; P3, proteinase 3. Adapted from Kallenberg et al: Anti-neutrophil cytoplasmic antibodies: Current diagnostic and pathophysiological potential. Kidney Int 46:1–15, 1994; and Savige et al: Antineutrophil cytoplasmic antibodies (ANCA): Their detection and significance: Report from workshops. Pathology 26:186–193, 1994.

14.   Besides the ANCA, what other laboratory tests may be abnormal in WG?

Abnormal laboratory tests in WG reflect the presence of systemic inflammation and end-organ involvement. Other than the ANCA, there are no specific laboratory tests for WG.

The systemic inflammatory nature of WG often results in anemia of chronic inflammation, leukocytosis, thrombocytosis, and elevation of the ESR. Low serum albumin and elevated globulin levels may also be present. These abnormalities are likely due to circulating cytokines, such as IL-1, IL-6, and TNF-α, elaborated by the inflammatory process. Importantly, leukopenia and thrombocytopenia are unusual, often helping to distinguish WG from other autoimmune disorders.

Evidence of glomerulonephritis is suggested by the presence of hematuria, pyuria, cellular casts, and proteinuria. If renal function is compromised by the inflammatory process, elevated serum creatinine is expected. Other laboratory tests may be helpful in the investigation of specific end-organ damage, such as electrocardiography and echocardiography for pericarditis, nerve conduction velocity for mononeuritis multiplex, and MRI for retro-orbital infiltration.

15. The prototypic pulmonary–renal syndromes are WG, Goodpasture's disease, and SLE. Since routine hematoxylin and eosin staining of these kidney biopsies is nonspecific, what other studies performed on renal tissue may aid in distinguishing these three disorders?

Immunofluorescence studies. **Goodpasture's disease** results from the presence of circulating anti-basement membrane antibodies, which bind to epitopes in the basement membranes of glomeruli and alveoli. The resultant antibody–antigen interaction leads to fixation of complement and initiation of the inflammatory process, causing glomerulonephritis and alveolar hemorrhage. Immunofluorescence staining with antibodies against immunoglobulin (Ig) detects the **linear** deposition of Ig in the glomerular basement membranes.

Glomerulonephritis due to **SLE** results from immune complex deposition in the glomerulus. Immunofluorescence studies detect **granular** (lumpy) deposition of Ig, characteristic of immune complex deposition, within the glomerulus.

The pathophysiology of glomerulonephritis in **WG** is unclear, but the disease does not appear to be due to immune complexes or detectable direct antibody binding to epitopes within the glomerular tissue. Thus, immunofluorescence studies usually are negative or reveal only scant Ig deposition, usually in areas of necrosis.

16. Discuss the differential diagnosis of WG.

Differential Diagnosis of WG

SYNDROME	EXAMPLE	DISTINGUISHING FEATURES
Primary vasculitis syndromes	Churg-Strauss syndrome Microscopic polyangiitis	Atopic history Marked eosinophilia Destructive upper airway disease unusual Cavitary pulmonary nodules unusual Absence of granuloma
Angiocentric immunoproliferative lesions	Lymphomatoid granulomatosis	Glomerulonephritis unusual
Pulmonary renal syndromes	Goodpasture's disease Immune complex disease (e.g., SLE)	Anti-basement membrane antibodies Immunofluorescence: linear deposition ANA* Anti-dsDNA, Sm antibodies Immunofluorescence: granular deposition
Granulomatous infections	Mycobacterium Fungi Actinomycosis Syphilis	Proper stains and cultures
Intranasal drug abuse	Cocaine	History Predominantly nasal septal pathology
Pseudovasculitis syndromes	Atrial myxoma Subacute bacterial endocarditis Cholesterol emboli syndrome	Echocardiography Blood cultures Echocardiography Transesophageal echocardiography Angiography Biopsy

* ANA = antinuclear antibody

17. What causes WG?

The etiology is unknown. The clinical disease frequently begins within the upper respiratory tract, followed by the lower respiratory tract and later the kidneys, which suggests that the etiologic agent may be airborne and inhaled. Despite vigorous study of various tissues from affected patients, no infectious or noninfectious agent has been identified. Specifically, agents demonstrated to cause granulomatous disease have not been found.

18. Describe its pathophysiology.

The pathophysiology of WG is also unknown. Because of the absence of significant Ig deposition in affected tissue, WG does not appear to be due to typical immune complex disease, such as SLE, or to autoantibodies against structural components, such as Goodpasture's disease. The presence of granulomata and numerous CD4+ T cells suggests the possibility of cell-mediated immunopathology. Additionally, anti-proteinase 3 antibodies conceivably may play a pathologic role. Under certain conditions, such as a typical viral or bacterial infection, neutrophils and endothelial cells produce and express proteinase 3 on their surfaces. Anti-proteinase 3 antibodies may bind to surface proteinase 3 on endothelial cells, fix complement, and initiate an inflammatory event within vessel walls, resulting in vasculitis. Anti-proteinase 3 antibody binding to surface proteinase 3 on neutrophils may activate these cells, amplifying the inflammatory response. These possibilities are being studied and remain controversial.

19. What is the natural history of WG?

Untreated WG, particularly when the lower respiratory tract and kidneys are involved, is a uniformly fatal disorder with a mean survival time of <1 year. Death may result from respiratory failure, renal failure, infection, other end-organ involvement, or as a complication of treatment.

Because of greater awareness and the availability of the ANCA test, WG is now often diagnosed early in the disease course, sometimes with involvement limited to the upper respiratory tract. Study of these cases will determine if some WG patients have a benign course that does not evolve into fatal multisystem disease.

20. How do you treat WG?

Standard treatment is oral cyclophosphamide (2 mg/kg/day) and oral prednisone (1 mg/kg/day). After 4 weeks and if a substantial clinical response has occurred, prednisone may be converted to an alternate-day regimen over a period of 1–2 months, followed by gradual and complete tapering as tolerated. Cyclophosphamide should be continued for approximately 1 year after complete clinical response, followed by tapering by 25-mg amounts every 2–3 months as tolerated. A major acute complication of this regimen is leukopenia, so often the cyclophosphamide dose must be adjusted to maintain the total WBC level above 3000–3500/µl and the neutrophil level above 1000–1500/µl. This regimen has resulted in complete remission in 75% of patients, with marked improvement in an additional 16%. In patients attaining complete remission, approximately half will experience a relapse of WG up to 16 years later.

In patients who present with fulminant life-threatening WG, initially more aggressive therapy may be warranted. Cyclophosphamide may be started at 3–5 mg/kg/day as tolerated. Glucocorticoids may be administered parenterally at prednisone-equivalent doses of 2–15 mg/kg/day.

Because the standard therapy for WG is associated with substantial morbidity and occasional mortality, less rigorous regimens are being studied for patients who have limited or less active WG. These regimens include intermittent low-dose oral methotrexate, oral trimethoprim/sulfamethoxazole, intermittent pulse intravenous cyclophosphamide, cyclosporine, and intravenous immunoglobulin. Oral trimethoprim/sulfamethoxazole is frequently used as adjunctive therapy in patients with WG who are receiving standard treatment with oral cyclophosphamide and prednisone.

BIBLIOGRAPHY

1. Hoffman GS, Fauci AS: Wegener's granulomatosis. In Klippel JH, Dieppe PA (eds): Rheumatology. London, Mosby, 1994, pp 6:19.1–10.
2. Hoffman GS, Kerr GS, Leavitt RY, et al: Wegener granulomatosis: An analysis of 158 patients. Ann Intern Med 116:488–498, 1992.
3. Kallenberg CGM, Brouwer E, Weening JJ, Tervaert JWC: Anti-neutrophil cytoplasmic antibodies: Current diagnostic and pathophysiological potential. Kidney Int 46:1–15, 1994.
4. Mark EJ, Matsubara O, Tan-Liu NS, Fienberg R: The pulmonary biopsy in the early diagnosis of Wegener's (pathergic) granulomatosis: A study based on 35 open lung biopsies. Hum Pathol 19:1065– 1071, 1988.
5. Savige JA, Davies DJ, Gatenby PA: Anti-neutrophil cytoplasmic antibodies (ANCA): Their detection and significance: Report from workshops. Pathology 26:186–193, 1994.
6. Yoshikawa Y, Watanabe T: Pulmonary lesions in Wegener's granulomatosis: A clinicopathologic study of 22 autopsy cases. Hum Pathol 17:401–410, 1986.

34. SMALL-VESSEL VASCULITIDES, INCLUDING HENOCH-SCHÖNLEIN PURPURA AND URTICARIAL VASCULITIS

Ramon A. Arroyo, M.D.

1. What is small-vessel vasculitis?

Small-vessel vasculitis includes a variety of conditions that are grouped together because of involvement of small blood vessels of the skin, especially arterioles and venules. **Leukocytoclastic vasculitis** (LCV) or **necrotizing vasculitis** are terms used to describe the usual histopathology, in which small blood vessels are infiltrated with polymorphonuclear neutrophils (PMNs). As the process evolves, fibrinoid necrosis of the vessel wall with leukocytes fragments (leukocytoclasis) and destruction of the blood vessel wall is seen.

Various other names have been used for small-vessel necrotizing vasculitis, including **allergic angiitis** and **hypersensitivity vasculitis.** These terms may not be appropriate because they imply that the vasculitis is due to an allergic reaction, and to this day, the exact etiology of many types of LCV is not known.

2. How are the small-vessel vasculitides classified?

- According to the predominant infiltrating cell (neutrophilic, lymphocytic, or granulomatous)
- According to the clinical pattern of skin involvement (e.g., LCV with palpable purpura, LCV without palpable purpura, or urticarial vasculitis)
- According to the proposed etiologic agent (those secondary to an exogenous or endogenous antigen)

3. Which conditions are considered small-vessel vasculitides?

When classified according to the proposed etiologic mechanism, there are two major categories:

- Those secondary to an **exogenous** antigen
    Drugs (any: esp. penicillins, sulfas, quinidine, allopurinol, propylthiouracil, etc.)
    Infections (any: esp. strep, hepatitis B, influenza, mononucleosis, HIV, *Neisseria*)
    Henoch-Schönlein purpura (possibly viral)
- Those secondary to **endogenous** or **unknown** antigen
    Autoimmune disorders (SLE, RA, Sjögren's, other vasculitides, etc.)
    Malignancy (leukemia, lymphoma, myeloma, solid tumors)
    Essential mixed cryoglobulinemia
    Urticarial vasculitis

4. What causes small-vessel vasculitis?

The cause of cutaneous vasculitis is not a single factor and is dependent on the underlying associated condition(s). The vascular injury is believed to be triggered by the deposition of immune complexes in the vessel wall with activation of complement, leading to migration of PMNs to the area, release of lysosomal enzymes, and damage to the vessel wall.

5. What is the major clinical manifestation in small-vessel vasculitis?

Palpable purpura is the most common primary lesion in cutaneous vasculitis. Typically, hundreds of discrete, subtly palpable, purpuric spots suddenly appear on the feet and lower extremities (see figure). The hands, arms, and other body sites also may be affected. In addition to the palpability, the presence of a central necrotic punctum is helpful in distinguishing a purpura of vasculitis from purpuras of other causes. These lesions are dynamic, often beginning as asymptomatic, nonpalpable, purpuric mascules and eventually becoming palpable. Some may become nodular, bullous, infarctive, and ulcerative.

Urticarial lesions are the second most common cutaneous presentation. Other cutaneous manifestations include livedo reitcularis and erythema multiforme-like lesions.

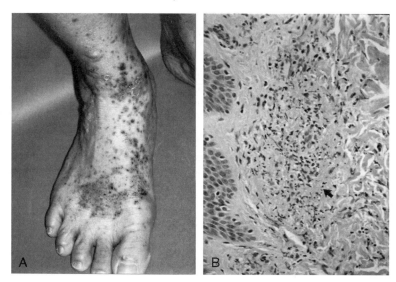

Small-vessel vasculitis. *A*, Palpable purpura. *B*, Histopathology of cutaneous blood vessel, demonstrating leukocytoclastic vasculitis with nuclear dust (*arrow*).

6. Are there systemic manifestations of small-vessel vasculitis?

Yes. Constitutional symptoms, including fever, frequently accompany the appearance of the skin lesions. Arthralgias are present in most patients; arthritis is less common. Proteinuria, hematuria, and occasional renal insufficiency can occur. Gastrointestinal manifestations include abdominal pain and GI bleeding, which can be severe and life-threatening. Other organ involvement is less common.

7. Are any laboratory findings specific for small-vessel vasculitis?

The laboratory abnormalities are usually nonspecific. Normocytic, normochromic anemia, elevated ESR, or eosinophilia are seen in approximately two-thirds of the patients. In those patients with renal involvement, hematuria and proteinuria may be present, as well as an increase in serum creatinine. The ANA is positive in 10%, and rheumatoid factor is present in 20%. The clinical significance of these serologic findings is uncertain. Hypocomplementemia (low C3 and C4) is infrequent. Hepatitis B surface antigenemia and hepatitis C antigenemia with cryoglobulinemia have been associated with LCV in some patients.

8. How does one make the diagnosis of small-vessel vasculitis?

The evaluation of these patients requires a full medical evaluation and appropriate lab tests depending on the clinical situation. Diagnosis is made by **skin biopsy,** identifying the presence of cutaneous vasculitis and, less commonly, a potential inciting agent as well.

9. How is small-vessel vasculitis treated?

Treatment has to be determined individually. If the associated disorder can be identified, then treating this problem may suffice. Any potential drug or antigen should be discontinued or removed. Mild cases without internal organ involvement may be self-limited, requiring no specific treatment. If systemic symptoms are present and skin lesions are diffuse, or if internal organ involvement is present, glucocorticoids are usually the treatment of choice.

10. What are the histopathologic features of Henoch-Schönlein purpura (HSP)?

The histopathologic features of HSP are leukocytoclastic vasculitis or necrotizing small-vessel vasculitis. The characteristic direct immunofluorescence finding is **IgA deposition** in affected blood vessels. IgA can also be found in the glomerular mesangium. The skin biopsy finding of IgA deposition is what makes this syndrome pathologically different from the other forms of small-vessel vasculitis.

11. Why is HSP classified as a small-vessel vasculitis secondary to an exogenous antigen?

There is circumstantial evidence implicating a hypersensitivity reaction to bacteria or viruses as a possible cause. HSP occurs most often in the spring, often following an upper respiratory tract infection.

12. Describe the clinical manifestation of this syndrome.

The classic triad of palpable purpura, arthritis, and abdominal pain occurs in up to 80% of cases. The rash may begin as a macular erythema, urticarial lesions, but may progress rapidly to purpura. The lower extremities and buttocks are the most common sites for the rash. The joints are involved in 60–80% of patients. The involvement is symmetrical and most commonly involves the ankles and knees; usually they are swollen, warm, and tender. Gastrointestinal lesions may cause severe cramping, abdominal pain, intussusception, hemorrhage, and, rarely, perforation. Renal involvement is seen in 50% of patients and is usually manifest by asymptomatic proteinuria and hematuria.

HSP is often acute in onset, and resolution is rapid and complete, except in a minority of patients who develop chronic renal disease. Persons of any age can be affected, but it occurs primarily in children between ages 2–10 years old.

13. How is HSP treated?

The disease is generally self-limited, lasting from 6–16 weeks. For mild cases, supportive treatment alone may be adequate. Systemic glucocorticoids may be used in patients with GI involvement or bleeding. Progressive renal disease is difficult to treat and usually does not respond to glucocorticoids or cytotic agents.

14. What is urticarial vasculitis?

Urticarial vasculitis is a small-vessel vasculitis presenting with an urticarial lesion instead of the more typical palpable purpura. Because of this unusual presentation, urticarial vasculitis was separated from the other types of necrotizing small-vessel vasculitis.

15. How is urticarial vasculitis differentiated from typical urticaria?

- The individual lesions are more often long-lived, lasting between 24–72 hours. Allergic urticarial lesions typically last 4–8 hours.
- The lesions may resolve with some residual pigmentation or ecchymosis.
- The lesions are often characterized by pain and burning rather than pruritus.
- Symptoms or signs of systemic disease, such as fever, arthralgias, abdominal pain, lymphadenopathy, or abnormal urine sediment, tend to occur.

16. Is there other organ involvement in urticarial vasculitis?

Other clinical features include arthralgias and arthritis. There appears to be an increased incidence of obstructive pulmonary disease in patients who also are cigarette smokers. Other less common associations include uveitis, episcleritis, fever, angioedema, and seizures.

17. What are the major laboratory abnormalities in urticarial vasculitis?

An increased ESR in two-thirds of the patients, and hypocomplementemia in approximately 38%. ANA and rheumatoid factor are usually negative, unless the vasculitis is associated with another connective tissue disease such as SLE.

18. Which are some of the conditions associated with urticarial vasculitis?
Although in most cases no etiologic factor or disease association is found, urticarial vasculitis has been described in association with SLE, Sjögren's syndrome, hepatitis B antigenemia, drug reactions, and sun exposure. The etiology is thought to be related to immune complex deposition. Some patients have serum IgG antibodies that react with C1q, leading to deposition and activation of complement in vasculitic lesions.

19. How is urticarial vasculitis treated?
Therapy consists of supportive measures and treatment of any associated or underlying disorder. Assuming that there is no internal organ involvement, a conservative treatment is reasonable. Both H_1 and H_2 antihistamines are used. NSAIDs (typically indomethacin) help with arthralgias and arthritis. In addition, prednisone in doses from 10–60 mg may be required. Dapsone has been reported to benefit some patients. For those patients with severe disease, use of azathioprine and cyclophosphamide has been reported in individual case reports.

BIBLIOGRAPHY

1. Calabrese LH, Michel BA, Bloch DA, et al: The American College of Rheumatology 1990 criteria for the classification of hypersensitivity vasculitis. Arthritis Rheum 33:1108–1113, 1990.
2. Callen JP: Cutaneous vasculitis. In Klippel JH, Dieppe PA (eds): Rheumatology, London, Mosby, 1994, sec. 6, 25. 1–8.
3. Gibson LE, Su WPD: Cutaneous vasculitis. Rheum Dis Clin North Am 21:1079–1114, 1995.
4. Ilan Y, Naparstek Y: Henoch-Schönlein syndrome in adults and children. Semin Arthritis Rheum 21:103–109, 1991.
5. Mills JA, Michel BA, Bloch DA, et al: The American College of Rheumatology 1990 criteria for the classification of Henoch-Schönlein purpura. Arthritis Rheum 33:1114–1121, 1990.
6. Szer IS: Henoch-Schönlein purpura. Curr Opin Rheumatol 6:25–31, 1994.
7. Wisnieski J, Baer A, Christensen J, et al: Hypocomplementemia urticarial vasculitis syndrome. Medicine 74:24–41, 1995.

35. CRYOGLOBULINEMIA
Raymond J. Enzenauer, M.D.

1. Define cryoglobulins.
Cryoglobulins are immunoglobulins or immunoglobulin-containing complexes that spontaneously precipitate and form a gel at low temperatures. They become soluble again when the temperature rises.

2. What are the three major types of cryoglobulins?
Brouet et al. studied 86 patients with cryoglobulinemia and, from them, identified three groups of cryoglobulins:

Type I is a single homogeneous monoclonal immunoglobulin with only one class or subclass of heavy or light chain. In type I cryoglobulinemia, serum levels are usually high (5–30 mg/ml), and the immunoglobulin readily precipitates in the cold.

Type II comprises mixed cryoglobulins with a monoclonal component that acts as an antibody against polyclonal IgG (i.e., rheumatoid factor activity). Most are IgM-IgG, although IgG-IgG and IgA-IgG can also occur. Serum levels of type II cryoglobulins are usually high, with 40% at a level of 1–5 mg/ml and 40% with levels > 5 mg/ml.

Type III includes mixed polyclonal cryoglobulins that are consistently heterogeneous; they are composed of one or more classes of polyclonal immunoglobulins and sometimes nonimmunoglobulin molecules, such as complement proteins or lipoproteins. Most are also im-munoglobulin–antiimmunoglobulin cryoglobulins. Type III cryoglobulins are usually more difficult to detect because they precipitate slowly and tend to be present in small quantities (0.1–1 mg/ml).

3. Describe the requirements for collection of cryoglobulin specimens.
1. Specimens must be collected at body temperature; otherwise, significant quantities of cryoglobulins may be lost.
2. Blood is drawn into a warmed syringe and immediately allowed to clot for 1–2 hours at 37°C.
3. After clotting, the serum is harvested at the warm temperature and then incubated at 4°C for 5–7 days.
4. Quantitation is accomplished by direct measurement of packed volume of precipitate after centrifugation (cryocrit) or spectrophotometric determination of protein concentration.

4. What is the overall incidence of each cryoglobulin type?
25% of patients have type I, 25% type II, and 50% type III.

5. Which infection(s) is most commonly associated with mixed cryoglobulinemia?
Hepatitis B virus (HBV). Mixed cryoglobulinemia was first reported in 1977 as an extrahe-patic manifestation of HBV infection. Recent studies document HBV and hepatitis C virus (HCV) in 50% of cases of mixed cryoglobulinemia, with 70% of patients having HCV and/or HBV in-fection. HCV positivity is more common in mixed cryoglobulinemia patients with biopsy-proven hepatitis or with increased levels of serum transaminases.

Various other infections have been reported in association with cryoglobulinemia, including that with other viruses (Epstein-Barr virus, cytomegalovirus, adenovirus, HIV), bacteria (suba-cute bacterial endocarditis, leprosy, post-streptococcal syndrome, syphilis, Q fever), fungi (coc-cidiodomycosis), and parasites (kala-azar, toxoplasmosis, echinococcosis, schistosomiasis, malaria).

6. List the reported causes of cryoglobulinemia.
Infection
    Viral

Viral	Bacterial
Fungal	Parasitic

Autoimmune disease

Systemic lupus erythematosus	Sarcoidosis
Rheumatoid arthritis	Henoch-Schönlein purpura
Polyarteritis nodosa	Behçet's disease
Sjögren's syndrome	Polymyositis
Scleroderma	Thyroiditis

Lymphoproliferative disease

Macroglobulinemia	Chronic lymphocytic leukemia
Lymphoma	Angioimmunoblastic lymphadenopathy

Renal disease (proliferative glomerulonephritis)
Liver disease
Familial
Essential
Experimental (post-vaccination)

7. Which type of cryoglobulins are most commonly seen in association with autoimmune disease?
Mixed cryoglobulins are a frequent finding in patients with connective tissue diseases, with two-thirds of cases having type III mixed cryoglobulinemia. Systemic lupus erythematosus and rheumatoid arthritis are the most common connective tissue diseases associated, with cryoglob-ulins seen in 50% and 25% of cases, respectively. Rheumatoid arthritis patients with cryoglobu-lins more often have rheumatoid vasculitis or Felty's syndrome. Other autoimmune diseases as-sociated with cryoglobulinemia include polyarteritis nodosa, Sjögren's syndrome, scleroderma,

sarcoidosis, thyroiditis, Henoch-Schönlein purpura, Behçet's disease, polymyositis, celiac disease, pulmonary fibrosis, and pemphigus vulgaris.

8. What is the most common presenting symptoms of cryoglobulinemia?
Cutaneous manifestations are the most common complaint of patients with cryoglobulinemia. Palpable purpura may be seen in 60–70% of patients with mixed cryoglobulinemia (types II and III), although this condition is seen in only 15% of patients with type I monoclonal cryoglobulins. Patients with monoclonal cryoglobulins more often present with distal ulceration/necrosis (40%). Other symptoms include Raynaud's phenomenon in 40%–60% and arthralgias/arthritis in 35% (especially in low-level mixed cryoglobulinemias). Renal disease is seen in 20–25% of patients and peripheral neuropathy in 25%.

9. What two main mechanisms are responsible for the clinical findings in cryoglobulinemia (*Controversial*)?
    1. **Intravascular deposits of cryoglobulin** were first suggested on clinical (cold-induced symptoms of vascular insufficiency) as well as histologic (occlusion of various sized vessels) grounds. These symptoms are more commonly seen in patients with type I or type II cryoglobulins.
    2. **Immunoglobulins** found in the cryoprecipitate have been demonstrated in blood vessel walls of patients with cryoglobulinemia. In addition, circulating immune complexes have been demonstrated in the serum of patients with mixed cryoglobulinemia. The cutaneous vasculitis and glomerulonephritis are consistent with an immune-complex-mediated disease, most frequently in patients with type II and type III mixed cryoglobulinemia.

10. Summarize the major clinical and laboratory features of cryoglobulinemia.

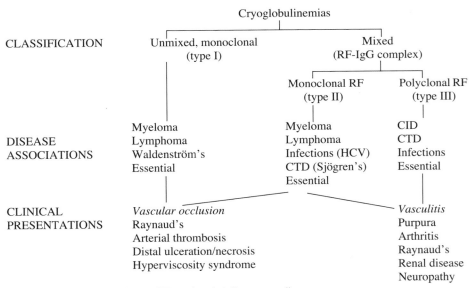

CTD = connective tissue disease; CID = chronic inflammatory disease.

11. Renal complications are more common with which cryoglobulin type?
Renal complications are more common in type II than in type III mixed cryoglobulinemia and range from isolated proteinuria with microscopic hematuria to an acute nephritic syndrome. Nephrotic syndrome and a more insidious progression to chronic renal failure also occur.

12. Does any clinical parameter correlate with prognosis in mixed cryoglobulinemia?
Prognosis is very much influenced by the presence of **renal disease**. In a 7-year followup period, 70% of patients with renal disease will die compared to 31% without renal involvement.

13. What are the three leading causes of death in patients with mixed cryoglobulinemia?
Renal disease, systemic vasculitis, and infection.

14. List the common signs and symptoms of cryoglobulinemia.

Cutaneous	80%
Liver disease	70%
Arthralgia/arthritis	35–50%
Renal disease	55%
Raynaud's phenomenon	10–50%
Neurologic	7–17%
Acrocyanosis	10%
Hemorrhage	7%
Abdominal pain	2%
Arterial thrombosis	1%

15. Cutaneous manifestations are virtually universal in patients with cryoglobulinemia and are a frequent presenting complaint. List the various cutaneous manifestations of cryoglobulinemia.

Palpable purpura	60–97%
Pigmentary changes	40%
Petechiae	31%
Distal necrosis	14%
Telangiectasias	11%
Urticaria	4–10%
Livedo	10–19%
Leg ulcers	10–25%

16. Explain the pathogenesis of articular disease in cryoglobulinemia.
The pathogenesis of the articular lesions is unknown. Their occurrence as a prominent feature during the early phase of disease, as well as the lack of frank arthritis or deforming disease even after years of symptoms, suggests that symptoms are related to circulating immune complex deposition.

17. What laboratory abnormalities are commonly seen in mixed cryoglobulinemia?

Serum protein electrophoresis	
Hypergammaglobulinemia	60%
Hypogammaglobulinemia	5%
Monoclonal gammopathy	5%
Rheumatoid factor positive	92%
>1:640	45%
>1:160 <1:640	24%
<1:160	32%
Elevated ESR	70%
Hypocomplementemia	
Low CH_{50}	82%
Low C3	58%
Low C4	63–80%
Abnormal urinalysis	
Hematuria	64%
Pyuria	64%
Proteinuria	73%
Anemia (hematocrit < 35%)	70%
Azotemia	46%
Elevated transaminases	50%

18. Pulmonary involvement is a frequent, often overlooked finding in mixed cryoglobulinemia. Describe the pulmonary abnormalities seen.
Dyspnea is the most frequent pulmonary complaint, seen in 39% of patients. Less frequent complaints include cough (13%), asthma (9%), pleurisy (4%), and hemoptysis (4%). Roentgenographic findings show moderate interstitial involvement in 74% of patients. Pulmonary function testing is frequently abnormal and indicative of small airways disease.

19. Is there liver involvement in mixed cryoglobulinemia?
Clinical or biochemical evidence of liver dysfunction is seen in 84% of patients with mixed cryoglobulinemia. Hepatomegaly is detected in 77%, with splenomegaly detected in 54%. Abnormalities in bilirubin, alkaline phosphatase, or serum aspartate aminotransferase (AST, SGOT) are seen in 77%. Only a minority of patients (11%) have overt liver disease. Up to 70% of patients will have serologic evidence of HBV and/or HCV infection.

20. Describe the treatment approach to patients with cryoglobulinemia (*Controversial*).
Treatment regimens for cryoglobulinemia vary since there have been no controlled studies. The patient's clinical condition is the main factor affecting treatment decisions. Patients without major organ involvement but who have complaints of arthralgia, mild purpura, and fatigue should be treated with protective measures against cold, bedrest, and NSAIDs. Antimalarial drugs may be of some benefit.

Patients with severe vasculitis involving the kidneys, CNS, skin, or liver require more aggressive immunosuppressive therapy. Corticosteroids are the most widely used drugs in the treatment of severe cryoglobulinemia. They may also be used in combination with other immunosuppressive/cytotoxic therapy, such as chlorambucil, azathioprine, and cyclophosphamide.

Patients with cryoglobulinemia associated with hepatitis C (and probably B) may benefit from treatment with alfa-interferon.

21. What are the indications for plasmapheresis in cryoglobulinemia?
Plasmapheresis should be saved for patients with acute, life-threatening forms of disease, including vasculitis, nephritis, malignant hypertension, severe CNS involvement, vascular insufficiency (distal necrosis), and hyperviscosity syndrome. Concominant immunosuppressive therapy must be instituted to prevent rebound antibody production after pheresis.

BIBLIOGRAPHY

 1. Abel G, Zhang Q-X, Agnello V: Hepatitis C virus infection in type II mixed cryoglobulinemia. Arthritis Rheum 36:1341–1349, 1993.
 2. Bombardieri S, Paoletti P, Ferri C, et al: Lung involvement in essential mixed cryoglobulinemia. Am J Med 66:748–756, 1979.
 3. Bonomo L, Casato M, Afeltra A, Caccavo D: Treatment of idiopathic mixed cryoglobulinemia with alpha interferon. Am J Med 83:726–730, 1987.
 4. Brouet J-C, Clauvel J-P, Danon F, et al: Biologic and clinical significance of cryoglobulins: A report of 86 cases. Am J Med 57:775–788, 1984.
 5. Cohen SJ, Pittelkow MR, Su WPD: Cutaneous manifestations of cryoglobulinemia: Clinical and histopathologic study of seventy-two patients. J Am Acad Dermatol 25:21–27, 1991.
 6. Ferri C, Greco F, Longombardo G, et al: Antibodies to hepatitis C virus in patients with mixed cryoglobulinemia. Arthritis Rheum 34:1606–1610, 1991.
 7. Frankel AH, Singer DRJ, Winearls CG, et al: Type II essential mixed cryoglobulinemia: Presentation, treatment and outcome in 13 patients. Q J Med 82:101–124, 1992.
 8. Geltner D: Therapeutic approaches in mixed cryoglobulinemia. Semin Immunopathol 10:103–113, 1988.
 9. Gorevic PD, Kassab HJ, Levo Y, et al: Mixed cryoglobulinemia: Clinical aspects and long-term follow-up of 40 patients. Am J Med 69:287–308, 1980.
10. Levo Y, Gorevic PD, Kassab HJ, et al: Liver involvement in the syndrome of mixed cryoglobulinemia. Ann Intern Med 87:287–292, 1976.
11. Lightfoot RW: Palpable purpura: Identifying the cause. Hosp Pract (Dec):39–47, 1992.
12. Malchesky PS, Clough JD: Cryoimmunoglobulins: Properties, prevalence in disease, and removal. Cleve Clin Q 52:175–192, 1985.
13. Winfield JB: Cryoglobulinemia. Hum Pathol 14:350–354, 1983.

36. BEHÇET'S SYNDROME

Raymond J. Enzenauer, M.D.

1. What are the criteria for Behçet's disease?

Recurrent oral ulceration: Minor aphthous, major aphthous, or herpetiform ulceration observed by a physician or patient, which occurred at least 3 times in one 12-month period

Plus 2 of the following:

Recurrent genital ulceration: Aphthous ulceration or scarring observed by a physician or patient

Eye lesions: Anterior uveitis, posterior uveitis, or cells in vitreous on slit lamp examination; or retinal vasculitis observed by an ophthalmologist

Skin lesions: Erythema nodosum observed by physician or patient, pseudofolliculitis, or papulopustular lesions; or acneiform nodules observed by physician in postadolescent patients not on corticosteroid treatment

Positive pathergy test: 2 mm erythema 24–48 hrs after #25 needleprick to depth of 5mm

Prior to publication in 1990 of the criteria of the International Study Group (ISG) for Behçet's Disease, five sets of criteria for the diagnosis of Behçet's disease had been in use, which hindered interpretation of different studies and collaborative research. Sensitivity and specificity of the ISG crtitera are 95% and 98%, respectively, with more specificity and little loss of sensitivity compared to the other five sets of previously used criteria.

2. Behçet's disease is a clinical diagnosis. What other diseases must be considered and ruled out in a patient presenting with possible Behçet's disease?

Virtually all the features of Behçet's disease can be seen in Crohn's colitis. Inflammatory bowel disease must be considered particularly in patients with iron deficiency, markedly elevated ESR (>100 mm/hr), or even minor bowel complaints. Other collagen vascular diseases with oral ulcers, ocular disease, and arthritis need to be considered, including systemic lupus erythematosus, Reiter's syndrome, and systemic vasculitis.

3. Describe "pathergy."

Pathergy is the hyperreactivity of the skin to any intracutaneous injection or needlestick (pathergy test). Originally described in 1935, this reaction is felt by some to be pathognomonic for Behçet's disease. The mechanism of pathergy in Behçet's is unknown, but it is thought to be related to increased neutrophil chemotaxis. The rate of a positive reactions varies in different populations, being more common in Japan and Turkey and less common in England and the United States.

4. Who gets Behçet's disease?

The disease occurs in both males and females equally, with the mean age of patients being about 40 years.

5. What is the relationship between this disease and the old Silk Route of Marco Polo?

Although Behçet's disease occurs worldwide, it is much more prevalent in individuals living along the old Silk Route (trade trail of Marco Polo), extending from the Orient (Japan) through Turkey and into the Mediterranean basin. The Japanese and eastern Mediterranean peoples have a 3–6 times increased incidence of HLA-B5, and subtype B51, in Behçet's disease patients compared to controls. The presence of HLA-B51 appears to be associated with a more complete expression of manifestations and a more severe clinical course of disease. HLA-B5 and B51 are not increased in frequency in Behçet's patients in the United States.

6. Describe the aphthous ulcers associated with Behçet's disease.

Aphthous-like stomatitis is the initial manifestation in 25–75% of patients with Behçet's disease. Preferential sites of ulceration are the mucous membranes of the lips, gingiva, cheeks (buccal mucosa), and tongue. The palate, tonsils, and pharynx are rarely involved (unlike Reiter's or Stevens-Johnson syndrome). Most oral ulcers occur in crops and heal without scarring within 10 days.

7. List a differential diagnosis of aphthous stomatitis.
Underlying conditions may be identified in as many as 30% of patients with severe aphthous stomatitis. Most cases remain idiopathic, however.

CONDITION	% OF AFFECTED POPULATION
Idiopathic	70%
B12/folate/iron deficiency	22%
Gluten-sensitive enteropathy	2%
Menstrually related	2%
Severe aphthosis	2%
Inflammatory bowel disease	1%
Behçet's disease	1%

8. What is complex aphthosis?
This recently described entity describes patients without systemic manifestations of Behçet's disease who have recurrent oral and genital aphthous ulcers or almost constant multiple (>3) oral aphthae. Differentiation from complex aphthosis may be difficult because the initial clinical presentation or Behçet's disease is often confined to oral and genital ulceration.

9. How frequently do the various clinical symptoms of Behçet's disease occur?
Oral aphthous ulcers	93–100%
Genital ulcers	69–100%
Ocular symptoms	50–79%
Arthritis	30–50%
Skin lesions	35–65%
CNS disease	10–30%
Major vessel occlusion/aneurysm	10–37%

10. Describe the genital ulcers of Behçet's disease.
Aphthous ulcers similar to those in the mouth also occur on the genitalia, most frequently the scrotum and vulva. The penis and the perianal and vaginal mucosa may also be involved. Lesions in men tend to be more painful than those in women. The genital ulcers are usually deeper than oral lesions and may leave scars after healing. Vulvar ulcers often develop during the premenstrual stage of the cycle.

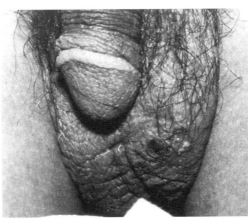

Scrotal ulcer in a patient with Behçet's disease. Oral aphthous ulcers have a similar appearance.

11. Are nonvenereal genital ulcers commonly due to Behçets?
No. Although genital ulcers are virtually universal in Behçet's disease, Behçet's is a rare cause of genital ulceration. Venereal ulcers are the most common type of genital ulceration and include herpes simplex, syphilis, chancroid, lymphogranuloma venereum (LGV), and granuloma inguinale (donovanosis). Nonvenereal causes of genital ulceration include trauma (mechanical, chemical), adverse drug reactions, nonvenereal infections (nonsyphylitic spirochetes, pyogenic, yeast), vesiculobullous skin diseases, and various neoplasms such as precarcinoma (Bowen's disease) and carcinoma (basal cell carcinoma and squamous cell carcinoma). More common rheumatic causes of genital ulceration include Reiter's syndrome and Crohn's disease.

12. What are the ophthalmologic manifestations of Behçet's disease?
Anterior/posterior uveitis, conjunctivitis, corneal ulceration, papillitis, and arteritis. Blindness is limited mostly to patients with posterior uvetiis, and occurs on average 4 years after onset of Behçet's disease.

13. What is a hypopyon?
The presence of inflammatory cells in the anterior chamber of the eye. While initially felt to be pathognomonic of ocular Behçet's disease, hypopyon is more commonly seen with severe B27-associated uveitis (*see* Chapter 79).

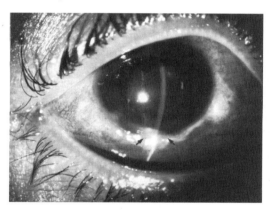

Hypopyon iritis (*arrows*).

14. Behçet's disease is a leading cause of acquired blindness in Japan. True or false?
True. Between 11–12% of all acquired blindness in or before middle-age in Japan develops as a result of ocular involvement of Behçet's syndrome.

15. Describe the arthritis associated with Behçet's disease.
Slightly more than one-half of patients will develop signs or symptoms of joint involvement. The arthritis is usually migratory, mono- or oligoarticular, and asymmetric, principally affecting the knees, ankles, elbows, and wrists. Shoulders, spine, hips, and small joints of the hands and feet are infrequently involved. The arthritis may be polyarticular and occasionally resemble rheumatoid arthritis. Erosive changes are rare. Synovial fluid cell counts average 5000–10,000/mm^3 and neutrophils predominate. Note that **arthralgia** is more common but lacks diagnostic value.

16. What are the cutaneous manifestations of Behçet's disease?
Erythema nodosum
Thrombophlebitis
Acneiform skin eruption
Hyperirritability of skin (pathergy)

17. A thrombotic tendency is a feature of Behçet's disease. Describe the vascular involvement in Behçet's disease.
Thrombosis of the large veins and arteries may occur, as can arterial aneurysms. Vascular thrombosis may be seen in one-fourth of all patients and include thrombosis of the superior or inferior vena cava or the portal or hepatic veins. Behçet's disease is virtually alone among the vasculitides as a frequent cause of fatal aneurysms of the pulmonary arterial tree.

18. How often do neurologic manifestations occur in Behçet's disease?

Headaches (52%)	Cerebellar ataxia
Menigoencephalitis (28%)	Hemiplegia/paraparesis
Cranial nerve palsies (16%)	Pseudobulbar palsy
Seizures (13%)	Extrapyramidal signs

Neurologic symptoms tend to recur during flares of oral, genital, and joint lesions. CNS involvement, which may be life-threatening, is usually a late manifestation occurring from 1–7 years after the initial onset of disease. Mortality of CNS Behçet's disease may be 41%.

19. What are the common laboratory findings in Behçet's disease?
Laboratory parameters are nonspecific in Behçet's. Some of the common findings include increased serum levels of IgG, IgA, and IgM; increased C-reactive protein and α_2-globulin; elevated CSF protein and cell count (in patients with neurologic involvement); leukocytosis; and an elevated ESR. These findings most often occur during disease exacerbation and often return to normal during remission.

20. What are the major causes of mortality in Behçet's disease?
> CNS involvement
> Vascular disease
> Bowel disease (perforation)
> Pulmonary disease (hemoptysis)
> Serious cardiac disease

Mortality may be 16% in 5 years.

21. What is the drug-of-choice for severe meningoencephalitis or uveitis associated with Behçet's disease?
Chlorambucil is the drug-of-choice for severe ocular or CNS disease. More recent studies, however, suggest that blindness (visual acuity of ≤20/200) results in 75% of patients despite chlorambucil treatment, with universal gonadal toxicity in treated patients. These findings suggest that the risks of long-term chlorambucil treatment may outweigh its benefits.

22. Which drugs are reported to be successful in treating the mucocutaneous lesions of Behçet's syndrome?
> Oral colchicine, 0.5–0.6 mg 2–3 times a day
> Dapsone, 100 mg/day
> Thalidomide, 100–400 mg/day
> Levamisole, 150 mg/day for 3 days every 2 wks

23. Which immunosuppressive agents are reported to be successful in treating severe ocular/CNS Behçet's disease?
> Systemic corticosteroids
>> Oral, 1–2 mg/kg/day
>> IV, 1 gm/day for 3 days
> Chlorambucil, 0.1–0.2 mg/kg/day
> Azathioprine, 2.5 mg/kg/day orally
> Cyclophosphamide
>> IV, 0.5–1.0 gm/m^2 per month
>> Oral, 1–2 mg/kg/day

Cyclosporine, 5–10 mg/kg/day
Levamisole, 150 mg po 2–3 times weekly
Methotrexate, 7.5–15 mg/wk po
FK506, 0.1 mg/kg/day

24. Who was Behçet?
Hulusi Behçet, a Turkish dermatologist, in 1937 described a chronic relapsing syndrome of oral ulceration, genital ulceration, and uveitis that now bears his name.

25. Describe the MAGIC syndrome.
Although chondritis has been noted in association with many other rheumatic diseases, the relationship between idiopathic relapsing polychondritis and Behçet's disease is particularly close. In 1985, Firestein and colleagues proposed the name "Mouth And Genital ulceration with Inflamed Cartilage" (MAGIC) syndrome in an attempt to encompass both clinical entities.

BIBLIOGRAPHY

1. Chajek T, Fainaru M: Behçet's disease: Report of 41 cases and a review of the literature. Medicine 54:179–196, 1975.
2. Engelkens HJH, Stolz E: Genital ulcer disease. Int J Dermatol 32:169–181, 1993.
3. Firestein GS, Gruber HE, Weisman MH, et al: Mouth and genital ulcers with inflamed cartilage: MAGIC syndrome: Five patients with features of relapsing polychondritis and Behçet's disease. Am J Med 79:65–72, 1985.
4. Friedman-Birnbaum R, Bergman R, Aizen E: Sensitivity and specificity of pathergy test results in Israeli patients with Behçet's disease. Curtis 45:261–264, 1990.
5. Hutton KP, Rogers RS: Recurrent aphthous stomatitis. Dermatol Clin 5:761–768, 1987.
6. International Study Group for Behçet's Disease: Criteria for diagnosis of Behçet's disease. Lancet 335:1078–1080, 1990.
7. Jorizzo JL: Behçet's disease. Neurol Clin 5:427–440, 1987.
8. Nussenblatt RB, Palestine AG, Chan C-C, et al: Effectiveness of cyclosporin therapy for Behçet's disease. Arthritis Rheum 28:671–679, 1985.
9. O'Duffy JD, Robertson DM, Goldstein NP: Chlorambucil in the treatment of uveitis and menigoencephalitis of Behçet's disease. Am J Med 76:75–84, 1984.
10. Sandler HM, Randle HW: Use of colchicine in Behçet's syndrome. Cutis 37:344–348, 1986.
11. Schreiner DT, Jorizzo JL: Behçet's disease and complex aphthosis. Dermatol Clin 5:769–778, 1987.
12. Shimizu T, Ehrlich GE, Inaba G, Hayashi K: Behçet's disease (Behçet syndrome). Semin Arthritis Rheum 8:223–260, 1979.
13. Tabbara KF: Chlorambucil in Behçet's disease: A reappraisal. Ophthalmology 90:906–908, 1983.

37. RELAPSING POLYCHONDRITIS

Steven A. Older, M.D.

1. Define relapsing polychondritis (RPC).
Relapsing polychondritis is an uncommon episodic systemic disease, probably autoimmune in nature, characterized by recurrent inflammation and destruction of cartilaginous tissues.

2. Who gets RPC?

Race:	Predominantly caucasian
Sex:	Male:female ≈1:1
Age at onset:	Range 20–60 years, peak in fourth decade
Genetics:	No clear hereditary predisposition or HLA association

3. Briefly discuss the etiopathogenetic hypotheses of RPC.

The etiology of RPC is unknown. It is thought to be an autoimmune process for the following reasons: (1) lymphocytes of RPC patients, when confronted with cartilage mucopolysaccharide, induce lymphoblast transformation and macrophage migration responses indicative of cell-mediated immunity; and (2) antibodies to native type 2 collagen and circulating immune complexes have been identified in RPC patients, suggestive of humoral immunity. In both cases, the degree of immune response correlates with clinical disease activity.

An inciting agent (infectious, toxic, immunologic) has not yet been indentified. However, once stimulated, activated lymphocytes and macrophages are thought to secrete mediators that induce the release of lysosomal enzymes, especially proteases. The resulting inflammatory destruction of cartilage generates an attempt at repair by local fibroblasts and chondrocytes, leading to the formation of granulation tissue and fibrosis.

4. Describe the histopathology of RPC.

The histopathology of involved cartilage, regardless of location, is similar and highly characteristic:
- The cartilage matrix, which is normally basophilic (blue), becomes acidophilic (pink) when examined by routine hematoxylin and eosin staining.
- Inflammatory cell infiltrates (initially polymorphonuclear cells and later lymphocytes and plasma cells) are seen invading the cartilage from the periphery inward.
- Granulation tissue and fibrosis develop adjacent to inflammatory infiltrates, occasionally resulting in sequestration of cartilage segments.
- Increased lipids and lysosomes in chondrocytes are demonstrated by electron microscopy.

5. Define the diagnostic criteria for RPC set forth by McAdam in 1976.
- Recurrent chondritis of both auricles
- Nonerosive inflammatory polyarthritis
- Chondritis of nasal cartilages
- Inflammation of ocular structures, including conjunctivitis, keratitis, scleritis/episcleritis, and/or uveitis
- Chondritis of the respiratory tract involving laryngeal and/or tracheal cartilages
- Cochlear and/or vestibular damage manifested by neurosensory hearing loss, tinnitus, and/or vertigo

The presence of three or more clinical features is considered diagnostic of RPC.

6. Which target organs are most commonly involved in the clinical presentation and eventual course of RPC?

Clinical Manifestations of Relapsing Polychondritis*

MANIFESTATION	PRESENTING SYMPTOM %	EVENTUAL INVOLVEMENT %
Auricular chondritis	26	89
Arthritis	23	81
Nasal chondritis	13	72
Ocular inflammation	14	65
Respiratory tract	14	56
Audiovestibular	6	46
Miscellaneous	6	—
Cardiovascular	—	24
Skin	—	17

*Data from McAdam LP, O'Hanlan MA, Bluestone R, et al: Relapsing polychondritis: Survival and predictive role of early disease manifestations. Ann Intern Med 104:74–76, 1986.

7. Discuss the clinical features and potential complications of the auricular and nasal chondritis of RPC.

Auricular chondritis is the most frequent and characteristic clinical feature of RPC. It typically presents as the sudden onset of burning pain, warmth, swelling, and purplish-red discoloration of the pinnas of both ears (see figure, *A*). Because only the cartilaginous portion is affected, the earlobes are always spared. Attacks may last from a few days to several weeks. After one or more attacks, the external ear loses its structural integrity owing to inflammatory dissolution of cartilage. This results in a drooping, floppy ear that has been termed "cauliflower ear" (see figure, *B*).

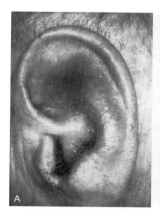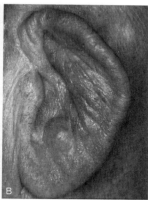

A, The ear in early inflammatory RPC. *B*, Chronic collapse of the cartilaginous pinna in a patient with RPC. (Reprinted from the Revised Clinical Slide Collection on the Rheumatic Diseases, copyright 1991. Used by permission of the American College of Rheumatology.)

Nasal chondritis develops suddenly as a painful fullness of the nasal bridge. Epistaxis occasionally accompanies the inflammation. It is less recurrent than auricular chondritis; however, even in the absence of clinical inflammation, cartilage collapse may occur, resulting in a "saddle nose" deformity (see figure below).

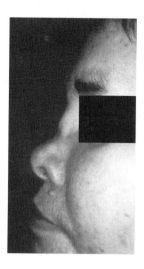

Saddle nose deformity due to nasal septal collapse. (Reprinted from the Revised Clinical Slide Collection on the Rheumatic Diseases, copyright 1991. Used by permission of the American College of Rheumatology.)

8. Describe the arthritis of RPC.
The arthritis of RPC is usually an oligo- or polyarticular asymmetric nonerosive inflammatory arthritis with a predilection for the large joints of the extremities and the sternoclavicular, costochondral, and sternomanubrial joints. When the small joints of the hands and feet are affected, the

disease may mimic seronegative rheumatoid arthritis. Flail chest has been described secondary to inflammatory lysis of the costosternal cartilage.

9. Describe the ocular involvement of RPC.

Virtually every structure of the eye and surrounding tissues may be affected. Episcleritis, conjunctivitis, and uveitis are most common. Complications may include cataracts, optic neuritis, keratitis, proptosis, corneal ulcerations and thinning, and extraocular muscle palsies. Loss of visual acuity and even blindness have been reported.

10. Discuss the distribution of disease, clinical symptoms, and potential complications of the respiratory tract in RPC.

Cartilage inflammation may occur early in the larynx and trachea, and eventually in the first- and second-order bronchi. In mild cases, symptoms might consist of throat tenderness, hoarseness, and a nonproductive cough. In severe cases, laryngeal and epiglottal edema may cause choking, stridor, dyspnea, or respiratory failure requiring emergency tracheostomy. Repeated or persistent inflammation of the airways can lead to either tracheal stenosis or dynamic airway collapse caused by dissolution of the tracheal and bronchial cartilaginous rings. Flail chest can interfere with ventilatory efforts. In addition, respiratory tract infections may complicate (and confuse) the clinical course of these patients.

11. What about audiovestibular damage in RPC?

Audiovestibular involvement presents as hearing loss, tinnitus, vertigo, and fullness in the ear (due to serous otitis media). Conductive hearing loss results form inflammatory edema or cartilage collapse of the auricle, external auditory canal, and/or eustachian tubes. Sensorineural hearing loss can be caused by inflammation of the internal auditory artery.

12. Describe the cardiac manifestations of RPC.

Aortic insufficiency is the most common cardiac manifestation and, after respiratory involvement, is the most serious complication of RPC. It is usually due to progressive dilatation of the aortic root, which distinguishes it from the aortic insufficiency of other common rheumatic diseases (see following table). Less frequent cardiac complications include pericarditis, arrhythmias, and conduction defects.

Aortic Insufficiency: Patterns of Disease Association

PATHOLOGY	UNDERLYING CONDITION
Valvulitis	Rheumatic fever
	Rheumatoid arthritis
	Ankylosing spondylitis*
	Endocarditis
	Reiter's syndrome*
	Behçet's syndrome*
Congenital	Bicuspid aortic valve
Dilatation of valve ring	Marfan's syndrome
	Syphilis
	Relapsing polychondritis
	Dissecting aneurysm
	Idiopathic

*Also dilatation of valve ring
From Trentham DE: Arthritis and Allied Conditions, 12th ed. Philadelphia, Lea & Febiger, 1993; with permission.

13. What other clinical manifestations occur in RPC?

Vasculitis may occur in up to 30% of cases. Involved vessels range in size from capillaries (leukocytoclastic vasculitis) to large arteries (aortitis).

Neurologic manifestations may include cranial neuropathies (second, sixth, seventh, eighth), headaches, seizures, encephalopathy, hemiplegia, and ataxia.

Dermatologic features range from alopecia, abnormal nail growth, and postinflammatory hyperpigmentary changes to leukocytoclastic vasculitis.

14. What laboratory data support the diagnosis of RPC?

Laboratory abnormalities in RPC are nonspecific and generally reflective of an inflammatory state: elevated erythrocyte sedimentation rate, leukocytosis, thrombocytosis, chronic anemia, and increased alpha and gamma globulins. Low titers of rheumatoid factor and antinuclear antibody may be seen.

15. Describe the radiographic abnormalities of RPC.

Soft-tissue radiographs of the neck may demonstrate narrowing of the tracheal air column, suggestive of tracheal stenosis. Tomography or computerized axial tomography can more accurately define the degree of tracheal narrowing (see figure below). Repeated inflammation may lead to cartilaginous calcification of the pinnas. This radiographic feature has been seen in other conditions, especially frostbite. Radiographs of the joints may occasionally demonstrate periarticular osteopenia, joint space narrowing, and erosions suggestive of rheumatoid arthritis.

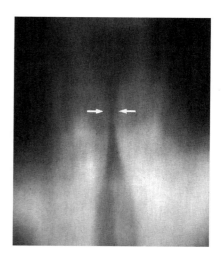

Tracheal tomogram demonstrating subglottic edema and tracheal narrowing (*arrows*) in a patient with RPC. This "steeple sign" is also seen in children with croup. (Reprinted from the Revised Clinical Slide Collection on the Rheumatic Diseases, copyright 1991. Used by permission of the American College of Rheumatology.)

16. What is the differential diagnosis of RPC?

Like RPC, syphilis and Wegener's granulomatosis also cause saddle nose deformities. Other disorders that destroy cartilage, such as infectious perichondritis, frostbite, and midline granuloma, do not present as multifocal chondritis. Inherited degenerative chondropathy is a recently described autosomal dominant disease caused by myxoid degeneration of thyroid and cricoid cartilage and characterized by saddle nose deformity at birth and laryngeal stenosis at 9 to 12 years of age.

17. Which diseases commonly coexist in patients with RPC?

Several collagen vascular diseases are seen in association with RPC, including systemic lupus erythematosus, rheumatoid arthritis, Sjögren's syndrome, spondyloarthropathy, and systemic vasculitis (most common). Usually the collagen vascular disease precedes the onset of RPC. Manifestations of these diseases may mimic or overlap those of RPC, and suggest similar mechanisms of pathogenesis.

18. Which diagnostic modalities are useful in detecting disease activity and cartilage damage in patients with RPC?
The erythrocyte sedimentation rate is an accurate predictor of disease activity in most patients. Functional complications may be demonstrated by radiographic imaging as outlined previously and by the use of pulmonary function testing with flow volume loops. Echocardiography is useful in the diagnosis and follow-up of valvular heart disease.

19. What medications are used in the treatment of RPC?
Glucocorticoids are the pharmacologic mainstay of therapy in RPC. During active disease, doses of 20–60 mg/day are used until control is obtained. Continued inflammation or an inability to taper glucocorticoids to safe maintenance doses warrants the addition of a steroid-sparing agent. Medications that have been useful in this regard include methotrexate, azathioprine, hydroxychloroquine, and cyclophosphamide. Dapsone, a drug that blocks polymorphonuclear lysosomal activity, has also been used successfully in RPC.

20. When does surgery play a role in the management of RPC?
Surgical intervention is indicated for complications involving the respiratory tract or heart. Tracheostomy may be required in patients with airway collapse. Airway obstruction caused by tracheal stenosis or tracheomalacia may require surgical resection. Intrabronchial stent placement has been reported as a potential remedy for dynamic airway collapse. Aortic insufficiency may require valve replacement, and aortic aneurysm formation may necessitate surgical grafting.
Surgical reconstruction of nasal septal collapse is *not* recommended because further collapse and deformity frequently occur postoperatively.

21. What is the prognosis in patients with RPC?
In a large Mayo clinic study,[7] the 5- and 10-year survival of 112 patients with RPC was 74% and 55%, respectively. Infection and systemic vasculitis were the major causes of death. Fifteen percent died as a direct consequence of cardiovascular or respiratory tract RPC. Poor prognostic indicators included coexistent vasculitis and early saddle nose deformity in younger patients, and the presence of anemia in older patients.

BIBLIOGRAPHY

1. Cohen PR, Rapini RP: Relapsing polychondritis. Int J Dermatol 25:280–285, 1986.
2. Eng J, Sabanathan S: Airway complications in relapsing polychondritis. Ann Thorac Surg 51:686–692, 1991.
3. Herman JH: Polychondritis. Curr Opin Rheumatol 3:28–31, 1991.
4. Isaak BL, Liesegang TJ, Michet CJ: Ocular and systemic findings in relapsing polychondritis. Ophthalmology 93:681–689, 1986.
5. McAdam LP, O'Hanlan MA, Bluestone R, Pearson CM: Relapsing polychondritis: Prospective study of 23 patients and a review of the literature. Medicine 55:193–215, 1976.
6. Michet CJ, McKenna CH, Luthra HS, O'Fallon WM: Relapsing polychondritis: Survival and predictive role of early disease manifestations. Ann Intern Med 104:74–76, 1986.
7. Michet CJ: Vasculitis and relapsing polychondritis. Rheum Dis Clin 16:441–444, 1990.
8. Trentham DE: Relapsing polychondritis. In McCarty DJ, Koopman WJ (eds): Arthritis and Allied Conditions, 12th ed. Philadelphia, Lea & Febiger, 1993.

VI. Seronegative Spondyloarthropathies

Which of your hips has the most profound sciatica?
William Shakespeare (1564–1616)
Measure for Measure, I

38. ANKYLOSING SPONDYLITIS

Robert W. Janson, M.D.

1. What is ankylosing spondylitis? How was the term derived?
Ankylosing spondylitis (AS) is a chronic systemic inflammatory disease affecting the sacroiliac joints, spine, and, not infrequently, peripheral joints. Sacroiliitis is its hallmark. The name is derived from the Greek roots *ankylos,* meaning "bent" (*ankylosis* means joint fusion), and *spondylos,* meaning spinal vertebra.

2. Ankylosing spondylitis is also known by what eponyms?
Marie-Strümpell's or von Bechterew's disease, after physicians who contributed to the clinical description of the disease in the late 19th century.

3. Describe the clinical characteristics of AS.
The clinical manifestations of AS usually begin in late adolescence or early adulthood, with onset after age 40 being uncommon. It occurs more commonly in males than females (3:1), but AS is often more difficult to diagnose in females due to less-pronounced clinical features and possibly slower development of radiographic changes. Patients complain of back pain with prolonged morning and, often, nocturnal stiffness. This stiffness improves with movement and exercise. Physical examination reveals sacroiliac joint tenderness, decreased spinal mobility, and sometimes reduced chest expansion due to costovertebral joint involvement.

4. What features in the history and physical examination are helpful in differentiating inflammatory low back pain (LBP) in AS from mechanical low back pain?

Differentiation of Low Back Pain

	INFLAMMATORY LBP	MECHANICAL LBP
Age of onset	<40 yrs of age	Any age
Type of onset	Insidious	Acute
Symptom duration	>3 mos	<4 wks
Morning stiffness	>60 min	<30 min
Nocturnal pain	Frequent	Absent
Effect of exercise	Improvement	Exacerbation
Sacroiliac joint tenderness	Frequent	Absent
Back mobility	Loss in all planes	Abnormal flexion
Chest expansion	Often decreased	Normal
Neurologic deficits	Unusual	Possible

5. Describe six physical examination tests used to assess sacroiliac joint tenderness or progression of spinal disease in AS.
- **Occiput-to-wall test.** Assesses loss of cervical range of motion.

- **Chest expansion.** Measured at the fourth intercostal space, normal chest expansion is approximately 5 cm.
- **Schober test.** Detects limitation of forward flexion of the lumbar spine. Place a mark at the level of the posterior superior iliac spine and another 10 cm above in the midline. With maximal forward spinal flexion with locked knees, the measured distance should increase from 10 cm to at least 15 cm (see figure).

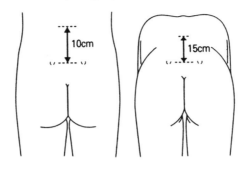

Schober test.

- **Pelvic compression.** With the patient lying on one side, compression of the pelvis should elicit sacroiliac joint pain.
- **Gaenslen test.** With the patient supine, a leg is allowed to drop over the side of the exam table while the patient draws the other leg toward the chest. This test should elicit sacroiliac joint pain on the side of the dropped leg (see figure).
- **Patrick's test.** With the patient's heel placed on the opposite knee, downward pressure on the flexed knee with the hip now in *f*lexion, *ab*duction, and *e*xternal *r*otation (FABER) should elicit contralateral sacroiliac joint tenderness (see figure).

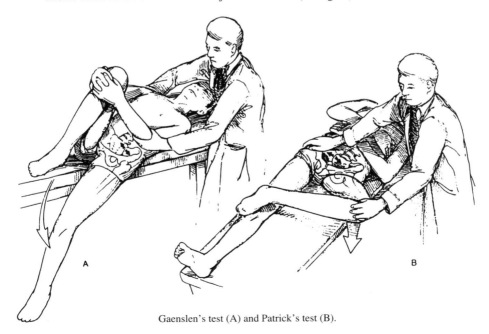

Gaenslen's test (A) and Patrick's test (B).

6. What is an enthesis? How does it relate to the disease process in AS?
An enthesis is a site of insertion of a ligament, tendon, or articular capsule into bone. In AS, the initial inflammatory process involves the enthesis, followed by a process which results in new bone formation or fibrosis. Sites of enthesopathy in AS include the sacroiliac joints; ligamentous structures of the intervertebral discs, manubriosternal joints, and symphysis pubis; ligamentous attachments in the spinous processes, the iliac crests (whiskering), trochanters, patellae, clavicles, and calcanei (Achilles tendonitis or plantar fasciitis); and capsules and intracapsular ligaments of large synovial joints.

7. Which peripheral joints are most commonly involved in AS?
The hips and shoulders. Rarely, arthritis of the sternoclavicular, temporomandibular, cricoarytenoid, or symphysis pubis occurs. Approximately 30% of patients with AS develop a peripheral arthritis.

8. What are the extraskeletal manifestations of AS?
Remembering the first few letters of the disease's name will help in recalling these.

A Aortic insufficiency, ascending aortitis, and other cardiac manifestations, such as conduction abnormalities, diastolic dysfunction, and pericarditis (10% of patients)
N Neurologic: atlantoaxial subluxations and cauda equina syndrome
K Kidney: secondary amyloidosis and chronic prostatitis

S Spine: cervical fracture, spinal stenosis
P Pulmonary: upper lobe fibrosis, restrictive changes
O Ocular: anterior uveitis (25–30% of patients)
N Nephropathy (IgA)
D Discitis or spondylodiscitis (Andersson lesions)

In addition, 30–60% of patients have asymptomatic microscopic colitis in their terminal ileum and colon.

9. Which human leukocyte antigen (HLA) shows a strong association with AS? Does this association vary among different racial groups?
HLA-B27 is present in at least 90% of white patients with AS and in a lower percentage of nonwhite patients with AS. This difference is due in part to a decreased prevalence of HLA-B27 in these nonwhite populations (1% in healthy African black and Asian populations, 3% in healthy North American blacks, but in 8% of healthy whites). Thus, the prevalence of AS is much lower in nonwhite populations.

10. How prevalent is AS among individuals who are HLA-B27-positive? Among individuals who are HLA-B27-positive with a relative with AS?
Two percent of HLA-B27-positive persons develop AS. Among those HLA-B27-positive persons with an affected relative, the rate rises to 15–20%.

11. When should an HLA-B27 test be ordered?
Most patients with AS can be diagnosed on the basis of history, physical exam, and the finding of sacroiliitis on radiographs, obviating the need for HLA testing. Knowing the HLA-B27 status of a patient with back pain of an inflammatory nature with negative radiographic findings might be helpful.

12. How is HLA-B27 hypothesized to play a role in the pathogenesis of AS?
Infection with an unknown organism or exposure to an unknown antigen in a genetically susceptible individual (HLA-B27+) is hypothesized to result in the clinical expression of AS.

- The arthritogenic response might involve specific microbial peptides that bind to HLA-B27 and then are presented to CD8$^+$ (cytotoxic) T cells.
- The induction of autoreactivity to self-antigens might develop due to "molecular mimicry" between sequences or epitopes on the infecting organism or antigen and a portion of the HLA-B27 molecule.
- Endogenous HLA-B27 itself could be the source of the antigenic peptide resulting in the induction of an autoimmune response.
- HLA-B27 could function at the level of the thymus to select a repertoire of specific CD8$^+$ T cells that are involved in an arthritogenic response when exposed to certain microbial antigens.
- HLA-B27 might only be a marker for a disease susceptibility gene in linkage disequilibrium with HLA-B27.

The potential role of HLA-B27 in the pathogenesis of AS is further supported by the finding that transgenic rats expressing the HLA-B27 gene develop an inflammatory disease that resembles a spondyloarthropathy with axial and peripheral arthritis.

13. Describe the typical radiographic features of AS.

The radiographic changes of AS are predominantly seen in the axial skeleton (sacroiliac, apophyseal, discovertebral, and costovertebral) as well as at sites of enthesopathy ("whiskering" of the iliac crest, ischial tuberosities, femoral trochanters, calcaneus, and vertebral spinous processes). Sacroiliitis is usually bilateral and symmetric, and initially it involves the synovial-lined lower two-thirds of the sacroiliac joint (see figure). Progression of the erosive process results in an initial "pseudo-widening" of the sacroiliac joint space with bony sclerosis eventually followed by complete bony ankylosis or fusion of the joint. In cases of early sacroiliitis where plain radiographs may be normal, magnetic resonance imaging (MRI) will demonstrate inflammation and edema.

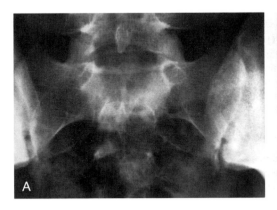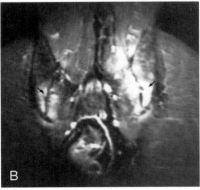

A, Radiograph of the pelvis demonstrating bilateral sacroiliitis. *B*, MRI of the sacroiliac joints demonstrating edema (*arrows*) due to inflammation of these joints.

Inflammatory disease of the spine involves the insertion of the annulus fibrosis to the corners of the vertebral bodies, resulting in initial "shiny corners" followed by "squaring" of the vertebral bodies (see figure). Gradual ossification of the superficial layers of the annulus fibrosis forms intervertebral bony bridges called **syndesmophytes.** Fusion of the apophyseal joints and calcification of the spinal ligaments along with bilateral syndesmophyte formation can result in complete fusion of the vertebral column, giving the appearance of a "bamboo" spine.

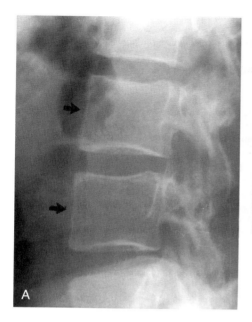

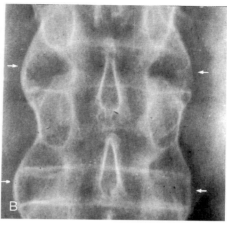

A, Lateral radiograph of the lumbar spine demonstrating anterior squaring of vertebrae (*arrows*). *B*, Anteroposterior radiograph of the spine demonstrating bilateral, thin, marginal syndesmophytes (*arrows*).

14. What is osteitis condensans ilii (OCI)?

An asymptomatic disorder of multiparous young women, OCI is characterized by radiographic findings of a triangular area of dense sclerotic bone only on the iliac side and adjacent to the lower half of the sacroiliac joints. This benign condition is not a form of AS and is not associated with HLA-B27 status.

15. How are AS and diffuse idiopathic skeletal hyperostosis different?

Diffuse idiopathic skeletal hyperostosis (DISH, Forestier's disease) is a noninflammatory disease occurring in males aged >50 years. It is characterized by flowing hyperostosis (bone formation), calcification of the anterior longitudinal ligament of at least four contiguous vertebral bodies, and nonerosive enthesopathies (whiskerings). The disease is not associated with sacroiliitis, apophyseal joint ankylosis, or HLA-B27. The flowing osteophytes in DISH typically occur on the right side of the spine, contralateral to the heart. On a lateral spine radiograph, a linear area of radiolucency exists between the calcified anterior longitudinal ligament and the anterior surface of the vertebra.

16. What are other causes of radiographic sacroiliac joint abnormalities?

Inflammatory: spondyloarthropathies, infection (bacterial, fungal, mycobacterial)
Traumatic: fracture, osteoarthritis, osteitis condensans ilii
Generalized disease: gout, hyperparathyroidism, Paget's disease, paraplegia, neoplastic metastases

17. Name the radiographic view used to specifically visualize the sacroiliac joints.

An **anteroposterior** projection of the pelvis (AP pelvis) is often sufficient to evaluate the inferior aspects of the sacroiliac joints. The **Ferguson** view (AP with the tube angled 25–30° cephalad) counteracts the overlap of the sacrum with the ilium, enabling a full view of the sacroiliac joint. This view is recognized because the symphysis pubis overlaps the sacrum.

18. Describe the natural course of AS.

Although the course is variable, most patients have a satisfactory functional outcome and maintain the ability to work. Factors that may influence overall prognosis include cervical spine ankylosis, hip joint involvement, uveitis, pulmonary fibrosis, and a persistent elevation of the sedimentation rate. It is likely that patients with mild AS have a normal life expectancy.

19. Which medications are helpful in the management of AS?

Although there is no cure for AS, most patients can be managed by controlling inflammatory symptoms and participating in an exercise program to minimize deformity and disability. The following modalities are helpful:

NSAIDs. Indomethacin is the most widely used NSAID for AS. Other NSAIDs may also be beneficial, and the choice is balanced by tolerance and effectiveness. Simple analgesics can be added for additional pain relief but should not be used as primary therapy.

Second-line treatment. Sulfasalazine (3 gm/day) may be beneficial in patients with early progressive disease with peripheral arthritis. Although not well studied, low-dose weekly methotrexate therapy may benefit patients with prominent peripheral joint involvement.

Corticosteroids. Oral corticosteroids have *no* value in the treatment of the musculoskeletal aspects of AS. Local corticosteroid injections are useful in the treatment of enthesopathies and recalcitrant peripheral synovitis.

20. How is physiotherapy used in AS?

Daily exercises need to be performed to maintain good posture and chest expansion and to minimize deformities. Hydrotherapy (swimming) provides the best environment to maximize the exercise program. Patients should sleep on a firm mattress on their back or in the prone position without a pillow in order to prevent progressive deformity. Cigarette smoking should be avoided in light of potential diminished chest expansion and apical lobe fibrosis.

21. When is surgery indicated in AS?

Total hip replacement is indicated in the setting of severe pain and limitation of motion. Vertebral wedge osteotomy to correct severe kyphotic deformities in some patients may be warranted, but it carries the risk of operative neurologic damage. Cardiac manifestations of AS may require aortic valve replacement or pacemaker insertion.

BIBLIOGRAPHY

1. Boushea DK, Sundstrom WR: The pleuropulmonary manifestations of ankylosing spondylitis. Semin Arthritis Rheum 18:277–281, 1989.
2. Cohen MD, Ginsburg WW: Late-onset peripheral joint disease in ankylosing spondylitis. Ann Rheum Dis 41:574–578, 1982.
3. Dihlmann W, Delling G: Disco-vertebral destructive lesions (so-called Andersson lesions) associated with ankylosing spondylitis. Skeletal Radiol 3:10–16, 1978.
4. Escalante A: Ankylosing spondylitis. A common cause of low back pain. Postgrad Med 94(1):153–160, 1993.
5. Forrester DM: Imaging of the sacroiliac joints. Radiol Clin North Am 28:1055–1072, 1990.
6. Gran JT, Husby G: Ankylosing spondylitis in women. Semin Arthritis Rheum 19:303–312, 1990.
7. Gran JT, Husby G: The epidemiology of ankylosing spondylitis. Semin Arthritis Rheum 22:319–334, 1993.
8. Hunter T: The spinal complications of ankylosing spondylitis. Semin Arthritis Rheum 19:172–182, 1989.
9. Khan MA: Ankylosing spondylitis. In Schumacher HR (ed): Primer on the Rheumatic Diseases, 10th ed. Atlanta, Arthritis Foundation, 1993, pp 154–158.
10. Khan MA: Spondyloarthropathies: Ankylosing spondylitis: clincial features. In Klippel JH, Dieppe PA (eds): Rheumatology. London, Mosby, 1994, pp 3.25.1–3.25.10.
11. Lipsky PE: Spondyloarthropathies: Etiology and pathogenesis. In Klippel JH, Dieppe PA (eds): Rheumatology. London, Mosby, 1994, pp 3.26.1–3.26.6.
12. O'Neill TW, Breshnihan B: The heart in ankylosing spondylitis. Ann Rheum Dis 51:705–706, 1992.

39. ENTEROPATHIC ARTHRITIDES

Sterling West, M.D.

1. What bowel diseases are associated with inflammatory arthritis?
- Idiopathic, inflammatory bowel disease (ulcerative colitis, Crohn's disease) and pouchitis
- Microscopic colitis and collagenous colitis
- Infectious gastroenteritis
- Whipple's disease
- Gluten-sensitive enteropathy (celiac disease)
- Intestinal bypass arthritis

2. How often does an inflammatory peripheral and/or spinal arthritis occur in patients with idiopathic inflammatory bowel disease?

	ULCERATIVE COLITIS	CROHN'S DISEASE
Peripheral arthritis	10%	20%
Sacroiliitis	15%	15%
Sacroiliitis/spondylitis	5%	5%

3. What are the most common joints involved in ulcerative colitis (UC) and Crohn's disease?

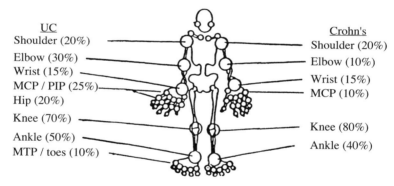

UC
Shoulder (20%)
Elbow (30%)
Wrist (15%)
MCP / PIP (25%)
Hip (20%)
Knee (70%)
Ankle (50%)
MTP / toes (10%)

Crohn's
Shoulder (20%)
Elbow (10%)
Wrist (15%)
MCP (10%)
Knee (80%)
Ankle (40%)

Upper extremity and small joint involvement are more common in UC than in Crohn's disease. Both UC and Crohn's-related arthritis affect the knee and ankle predominantly.

4. Describe the clinical characteristics of the inflammatory peripheral arthritis associated with idiopathic inflammatory bowel disease (IBD).
The arthritis occurs equally in males and females, and children are affected as commonly as adults. The arthritis is typically acute in onset, migratory, asymmetric, and pauciarticular (usually involves < 5 joints). Synovial fluid analysis reveals an inflammatory fluid with up to 50,000 white blood cells/mm^3 (predominantly neutrophils) and negative crystal examination and cultures. Most arthritic episodes resolve in 1–2 months and do not result in radiographic changes or deformities.

5. What other extraintestinal manifestations commonly occur with idiopathic IBD and inflammatory peripheral arthritis?
P Pyoderma gangrenosum (< 5%)
A Aphthous stomatitis (< 10%)
I Inflammatory eye disease (acute anterior uveitis) (5–15%)
N Nodosum (erythema) (< 10%)

6. Do the extent and activity of the IBD and the activity of the peripheral inflammatory arthritis show any correlation?

Ulcerative colitis and Crohn's disease patients are more likely to develop a peripheral arthritis if the colon is extensively involved. Most arthritic attacks occur during the first few years following onset of the bowel disease. The episodes coincide with flares of bowel disease in 60–70% of patients. Occasionally, the arthritis may precede symptoms of IBD, especially in children with Crohn's disease. Consequently, lack of gastrointestinal symptoms or even a negative stool quaiac test does not exclude the possibility of occult Crohn's disease in a patient who presents with a characteristic arthritis!

7. What are the clinical characteristics of the inflammatory spinal arthritis occurring in idiopathic IBD?

The clinical characteristics and course of spinal arthritis in IBD is similar to those for ankylosing spondylitis.

- Inflammatory spinal arthritis occurs more commonly in males than females (3:1).
- Patients complain of back pain and prolonged stiffness, particularly at night and upon awakening. This improves with exercise and movement.
- Physical examination reveals sacroiliac joint tenderness, global loss of spinal motion, and sometimes reduced chest expansion.

8. Does the activity of inflammatory spinal arthritis correlate with the activity of the IBD?

No. The onset of sacroiliitis/spondylitis can precede by years, occur concurrently, or follow by years the onset of IBD. Furthermore, the course of the spinal arthritis is completely independent of the course of the IBD.

9. What human leukocyte antigen (HLA) occurs more commonly than expected with inflammatory arthritis secondary to IBD?

HLA-B27. Eight percent of a normal healthy Caucasian population has the HLA-B27 gene, but a patient with IBD who possesses the HLA-B27 gene has a 7–10 times increased risk of developing an inflammatory sacroiliitis/spondylitis compared to IBD patients who are HLA-B27 negative.

Frequency of HLA-B27 in IBD

	CROHN'S	UC
Sacroiliitis/spondylitis	55%	70%
Peripheral arthritis	Same as normal healthy control population	

10. What are the typical radiographic features of inflammatory sacroiliitis and spondylitis in IBD patients?

They are similar to those of ankylosing spondylitis. (See Chapter 38.)

11. What other rheumatic problems occur with increased frequency in IBD patients?

Achilles tendinitis/plantar fasciitis
Clubbing (5%)
Hypertrophic osteoarthropathy
Psoas abscess or septic hip from fistula formation (Crohn's disease)
Osteoporosis secondary to medications (i.e., prednisone)
Vasculitis
Amyloidosis

12. Which treatments are effective for alleviating symptoms of inflammatory peripheral arthritis and/or sacroiliitis/spondylitis in IBD patients?

Treatment of IBD-related Inflammatory Peripheral or Spinal Arthritis

	PERIPHERAL ARTHRITIS	SACROILIITIS/SPONDYLITIS
NSAIDs*	Yes	Yes
Intra-articular corticosteroids	Yes	Yes (sacroiliitis)
Sulfasalazine	Yes	Maybe
Immunosuppressive medication	Yes	No
Bowel resection		
UC	Yes	No
Crohn's	No	No

*NSAIDs may exacerbate the IBD.

13. What rheumatic disorders have been associated with pouchitis, microscopic (lymphocytic) colitis (MC), and collagenous colitis (CC)?

	POUCHITIS	MC	CC
IBD-like peripheral inflammatory arthritis	Yes	Yes	Yes (10%)
Rheumatoid arthritis	No	Yes	Yes
Ankylosing spondylitis	No	Yes*	No
Thyroiditis/other autoimmune disease	No	Yes	Yes

*Up to 50% of ankylosing spondylitis patients have asymptomatic microscopic colitis/Crohn's like lesions on right-sided colon biopsies.

14. Why are patients with IBD prone to develop an inflammatory arthritis?
One theory is that environmental antigens capable of inciting rheumatic disorders gain entry to the body's circulation by traversing the respiratory mucosa, skin, or gastrointestinal (GI) mucosa. The human GI tract has an estimated surface area of 1000 m^2 and functions not only to absorb nutrients but to exclude potentially harmful antigens. The gut-associated lymphoid tissue (GALT), which includes Peyer's patches, the lamina propria, and intraepithelial T cells, constitutes 25% of the GI mucosa and helps to prevent entry of bacteria and other foreign antigens. Although the upper GI tract is normally not exposed to microbes, the lower GI tract is constantly in contact with millions of bacteria (up to 10^{12}/g of feces). Inflammation, whether from idiopathic IBD or infection with pathogenic microorganisms, can disrupt the normal integrity and function of the bowel, leading to increased gut permeability. This increased permeability may allow **nonviable** bacterial antigens in the gut lumen to enter the circulation more easily. These microbial antigens could then either deposit directly in the joint synovia, leading to a local inflammatory reaction, or cause a systemic immune response, resulting in immune complexes that could then deposit in joints and other tissues.

15. What rheumatic manifestations have been described in patients with celiac disease (gluten-sensitive enteropathy)?
- Arthritis—symmetric polyarthritis involving predominantly large joints (knees and ankles > hips and shoulders). May precede enteropathic symptoms in 50% of cases.
- Osteomalacia due to steatorrhea from severe enteropathy
- Dermatitis herpetiformis

16. What human leukocyte antigen (HLA) is more common in celiac disease patients than in normal healthy controls?
HLA-DR3, frequently in association with HLA-B8, is seen in 95% of celiac disease patients compared to 12% of the normal population.

17. How is the arthritis occurring in celiac disease treated?
The arthritis responds dramatically to a **gluten-free diet.**

18. What is the intestinal bypass arthritis–dermatitis syndrome?
This syndrome occurs in 20–80% of patients who have undergone intestinal bypass surgery for morbid obesity. The arthritis is inflammatory, polyarticular, symmetric, and frequently migratory, and it affects both upper and lower extremity joints. Radiographs usually remain normal despite 25% of patients having chronic recurring episodes of arthritis. Up to 80% develop dermatologic abnormalities, the most characteristic of which is a maculopapular or vesiculopustular rash. The pathogenesis involves bacterial overgrowth in the blind loop, resulting in antigenic stimulation causing immune complex formation (frequently cryoprecipitates containing bacterial antigens) which may deposit in the joints and skin. Treatment includes NSAIDs and oral antibiotics which usually improve symptoms. Only surgical reanastomosis of the blind loop can result in complete elimination of symptoms.

BIBLIOGRAPHY

1. Chakravarty K, Scott DGI: Oligoarthritis—a presenting feature of occult coeliac disease. Br J Rheumatol 31:349–350, 1992.
2. DeVos M, Cuvelier C, Mielants H, et al: Ileocolonoscopy in seronegative spondyloarthropathy. Gastroenterology 96:339–344, 1989.
3. Mielants H, Veys EM, Goemaere S, et al: A prospective study of patients with spondyloarthropathy with special reference to HLA-B27 and to gut histology. J Rheumatol 20:1353–1358, 1993.
4. Roubenoff R, Ratain J, Giardiello I, et al: Collagenous colitis, enteropathic arthritis, and autoimmune diseases: Results of a patient survey. J Rheumatol 16:1229–1232, 1989.
5. Wands JR, LaMont TJ, Mann BS, et al. Arthritis associated with intestinal bypass procedure for morbid obesity: complement activation and characterization of circulatory cryoproteins. N Engl J Med 294:121– 124, 1976.
6. Weiner SR, Clarke J, Taggart NA, et al: Rheumatic manifestations of inflammatory bowel disease. Semin Arthritis Rheum 20:353–366, 1991.
7. Wollheim FA: Enteropathic arthritis. In Kelley WK, Harris ED, Ruddy S, Sledge CB (eds): Textbook of Rheumatology, 4th ed. Philadelphia, W.B. Saunders, 1993, pp 985–997.

40. REITER'S SYNDROME AND REACTIVE ARTHRITIDES

Danny C. Williams, M.D.

1. What is Reiter's syndrome?
As originally described in 1916, Reiter's syndrome is the clinical triad of urethritis, conjunctivitis, and arthritis following an infectious dysentery. Reiter's syndrome is now considered to be a form of reactive arthritis.

2. Define "reactive" arthritis.
Reactive arthritis is an infection-induced systemic illness characterized primarily by an inflammatory synovitis from which viable microorganisms *cannot* be cultured. With few exceptions, the clinical features of reactive arthritis are similar to those found in other seronegative spondyloarthropathies.

3. How is reactive arthritis acquired?
Susceptibility to reactive arthritis is conferred by specific Class I major histocompatibility antigens (e.g., HLA-B27). However, its acquisition is strictly dependent on infection with certain gastrointestinal (enterogenic) or genitourinary (urogenital) pathogens.

HLA-B27 + Infection = Reactive Arthritis

4. What infectious agents "cause" classic reactive arthritis?

Urogenital	***Chlamydia*** *trachomatis*
Enterogenic	***Salmonella*** *typhimurium, S. enteritidis,*
	S. heidelberg, S. cholerae-suis
	Shigella *flexneri* serotype 2a, *S. sonnei*
	Yersinia *enterocolitica* serotype 3,
	Y. pseudotuberculosis
	Campylobacter *jejuni*
Others	*Ureaplasma urealyticum*
	Clostridium difficile
	Vibrio parahaemolyticus
	Borrelia burgdorferi
	Neisseria gonorrhoeae

5. Who gets reactive arthritis?
Primarily young adults, aged 20–40 years. Patients with enterogenic reactive arthritis exhibit equal sex distribution, while those with the urogenital form are predominantly male. Reactive arthritis is rare in children and uncommon in blacks. Reiter's syndrome is the most common type of inflammatory arthritis affecting young, adult males.

6. After the initial infection, when do symptoms of reactive arthritis first appear?
Though the initial infection may be mild or inapparent (10%), most patients will develop systemic symptoms within 1–4 weeks.

7. List the extra-articular features associated with reactive arthritis.

Constitutional
Low-grade fever
Weight loss

Ocular
Sterile conjunctivitis (60%)
Anterior uveitis (unilateral) (20%)

Gastrointestinal
Infectious ileitis/colitis
Sterile ileitis/colitis

Cardiac
Heart block (1%)
Aortic regurgitation
Aortitis (1%)
Pericarditis

Genitourinary
Infectious urethritis
Sterile urethritis
Prostatitis
Cystitis
Salpingitis

Mucocutaneous
Circinate balanitis (30%)
Keratoderma blennorrhagicum (20%)
Hyperkeratotic nails (10%)
Painless oral ulcers (25%)

Other
Neuropathy
IgA nephropathy
Renal amyloidosis
Thrombophlebitis
Erythema nodosum (*Yersinia*)

8. What two cutaneous lesions are characteristic of Reiter's syndrome?
Circinate balanitis and **keratoderma blennorrhagicum** are relatively specific for Reiter's syndrome. Circinate balanitis is a **painless,** serpiginous ulceration of the glans penis. Similarly, keratoderma blennorrhagicum refers to psoriasiform lesions occurring primarily on the plantar surface of the heel and metatarsal heads. Both lesions are predominantly associated with urogenital reactive arthritis and resolve spontaneously.

9. Describe the musculoskeletal manifestations of reactive arthritis.
Arthritis. In reactive arthritis, the joints tend to be moderately inflamed and characterized by prolonged stiffness. Joint involvement is typically asymmetric, oligoarticular (<5 joints), and

confined to the knees, ankles, and/or feet. Upper limb arthritis (e.g., wrist and digits) may also occur. Joint erosions may result from chronic disease.

Enthesitis is inflammation of the tendon-bone junction (enthesis). In reactive arthritis, enthesitis commonly causes heel pain (Achilles tendon and plantar fascia), metatarsalgia (plantar fascia), and "sausage" digits (dactylitis).

Spondylitis. Forty percent of patients with reactive arthritis may have axial skeleton disease. The risk of developing sacroiliitis and/or spondylitis is enhanced by disease chronicity and HLA-B27.

10. What is the differential diagnosis for reactive arthritis?

MOST LIKELY	LESS LIKELY
Acute septic arthritis	Ankylosing spondylitis
Gonococcal arthritis	Rheumatic fever
Psoriatic arthritis	Gout/pseudogout
Inflammatory bowel disease arthritis	Lyme disease
Rheumatoid arthritis	Behçet's syndrome

In addition, reactive arthritis must always be considered as a possible complication of HIV infection.

11. Compare Reiter's syndrome with gonococcal arthritis.

Clinical Features of Reiter's Syndrome and Gonococcal Arthritis

FEATURE	REITER'S	GONOCOCCAL
Sex ratio	> Male	> Female
Age	20–40 yrs	All ages, most 20–40 yrs
Migratory arthralgias	No	Yes
Arthritis	Lower limbs	Upper limbs, knees
Enthesitis	Yes	No
Spondylitis	Yes	No
Tenosynovitis	Yes	Yes
Urethritis	Yes	Yes
Uveitis	Yes	No
Oral ulcers	Yes	No
Cutaneous lesions	Keratoderma, balanitis	Pustules
Culture positive	No	Yes (<50%)
HLA-B27 positive	Yes (80%)	Same as rest of population (7%)
Penicillin responsive	No	Yes

12. Compare Reiter's syndrome with rheumatoid arthritis.

Clinical Features of Reiter's Syndrome and Rheumatoid Arthritis

FEATURE	REITER'S SYNDROME	RA
Sex ratio	> Male	> Female
Age	20–40 yrs	All ages
Arthritis	Oligoarticular (asymmetric)	Polyarticular (symmetric)
Enthesitis	Yes	No
Spondylitis	Yes	No
Ocular disease	Conjunctivitis, uveitis	Keratitis, scleromalacia
Lung disease	No	Yes
Urethritis	Yes	No
Cutaneous lesions	Keratoderma, balanitis	Subcutaneous nodules, vasculitis
Rheumatoid factor positive	No	Yes (85%)
HLA association	HLA-B27 (80%)	HLA-DR4 (70%)

13. Which laboratory investigations are useful in confirming the diagnosis of reactive arthritis?

The diagnosis of reactive arthritis is clinical, and *no* laboratory investigation can substitute for a proper history and physical exam. However, they can be used in confirming the clinical diagnosis.

		EXPECTED RESULT
Primary (essential)		
	Erythrocyte sedimentation rate	Elevation
	Complete blood count and differential	Polymorphonuclear leukocytosis
		Thrombocytosis and anemia
	Rheumatoid factor	Negative
	Urinalysis	Pyuria, $+/-$ bacteria
	Synovial fluid analysis	Moderate leukocytosis
		$(-)$ Gram stain, $(-)$ crystals
	Cultures	
	Throat	$(+/-)$ culture
	Urine	$(+/-)$ culture
	Stool	$(+/-)$ culture
	Synovial fluid	$(-)$ culture
	Urethra/cervix	$(+/-)$ culture
Secondary (optional)		
	C-reactive protein	Elevation
	Antinuclear antibody	Negative
	Antibody serology	Positive (e.g., *Yersinia* and *Chlamydia*)
	Blood cultures	Negative, unless septic
	Radiographs	
	Peripheral joints	Arthritis, enthesitis
	Axial joints	Spondylitis, enthesitis
	Anteroposterior pelvis	Sacroiliitis
	Electrocardiogram	Heart block
	Ileocolonoscopy	Ileitis/colitis

14. What are the usual synovial fluid findings from a patient with reactive arthritis?

The synovial fluid typically reveals a predominance of leukocytes, ranging from 5,000–50,000 cells/mm^3. In acute reactive arthritis, most of these cells are neutrophils, but in chronic disease, either lymphocytes or monocytes are prevalent.

Other synovial fluid characteristics include decreased viscosity, normal glucose level, increased protein, and, in contrast to rheumatoid effusions, increased complement. Large, vacuolar macrophages (Reiter's cells), containing intact lymphocytes or fragmented nuclei, are occasionally seen. Reiter's cells are not specific for reactive arthritis.

The synovial fluid of reactive arthritis is nondiagnostic. Arthrocentesis is primarily performed to exclude septic and/or crystalline arthritis.

15. Describe the radiographic features seen in patients with reactive arthritis.

Remember your **ABCDE'S.** These radiographic features are typical of all seronegative spondyloarthropathies.

A—Ankylosis of the spine occurs in up to 20% of patients. There are large, nonmarginal syndesmophytes, called "jug-handle" syndesmophytes, which usually occur in an asymmetric distribution. These syndesmophytes can also occur in psoriatic spondylitis but differ from the thin, marginal, bilateral syndesmophytes seen in ankylosing spondylitis (see figure top of next page).

B—Bony reactivity at sites of enthesitis (Achilles tendon and plantar fascia insertions) and periostitis are common. **Bone osteoporosis** is seen in a periarticular distribution compatible with an inflammatory arthritis.

C—Cartilage-space narrowing occurs uniformly across the joint space of weight-bearing joints compatible with an inflammatory arthritis. No abnormal cartilage or soft tissue **calcifications** are seen.

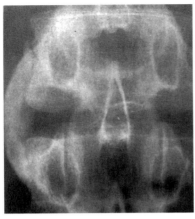

Radiograph of spine showing a large "jug-handle" syndesmophyte.

D—**Distribution** of arthritis is primarily in the lower extremity, whereas psoriatic arthritis usually affects the upper extremity. The sentinel joint involved is the interphalangeal joint of the great toe (see figure below).

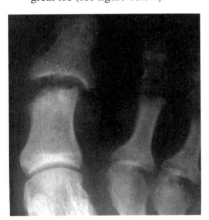

Radiograph of foot in a patient with Reiter's syndrome showing erosions of the interphalangeal joint of the great toe and second and third MTP joints.

E—**Erosions** are common in the metatarsophalangeal joints (MTPs). Sacroiliac joint erosions tend to involve one sacroiliac joint more than the other (asymmetric), which contrasts to the symmetric involvement of ankylosing spondylitis (see figure below).

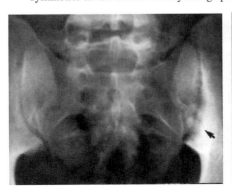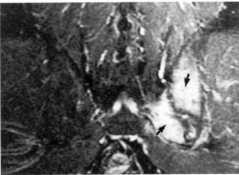

Radiograph (*left*) and MRI (*right*) of pelvis showing left sacroiliitis (*arrows*).

S—Soft tissue swelling and dactylitis (diffuse swelling of toes). Psoriatic arthritis causes dactylitis of the fingers more than toes.

16. How do the radiographic features of sacroiliac and spine involvement in reactive arthritis compare with those in ankylosing spondylitis?

	ANKYLOSING SPONDYLITIS	REACTIVE ARTHRITIS
Sacroiliitis	Bilateral, symmetric	Unilateral or asymmetric
Spondylitis	Bilateral, thin, marginal syndesmophytes	Asymmetric, nonmarginal, "jug-handle" syndesmophytes

Note that 100% of patients with ankylosing spondylitis develop radiographic changes in the sacroiliac joints, compared to only 25% of reactive arthritis patients. Patients with inflammatory bowel disease also develop radiographic changes of their spine similar in appearance to those of ankylosing spondylitis, whereas psoriatic arthritis produces changes similar to reactive arthritis.

17. Is HLA-B27 determination useful?
A sufficient number of patients with reactive arthritis will *not* be HLA-B27-positive, thus rendering HLA-B27 determination useless as a screening test. Most patients with reactive arthritis can be successfully diagnosed and managed without HLA-B27 determination. However, HLA-B27 determination may be useful when the clinical picture is incomplete, such as absence of an antecedent infection or lack of extra-articular features.

18. Describe the nonpharmacologic management of reactive arthritis.
Initial management begins with bedrest and splinting of the affected joints. Transient relief of joint inflammation may be obtained by use of ice packs and/or warm compresses. Once inflammation subsides (1–2 weeks), **passive** strengthening and range of motion exercises should be initiated. Progression to **active** exercises reduces the likelihood of muscle atrophy. Avoidance of behavior promoting reinfection is critical.

19. Describe the pharmacologic management of reactive arthritis.
    Infectious disease. Elimination of the "triggering" infection with appropriate antibiotics is the first therapeutic goal in reactive arthritis.
    Extra-articular disease. The mucocutaneous features of reactive arthritis are usually self-limited and require no specific therapy. The one exception is uveitis, for which ophthalmologic evaluation is mandatory.
    Articular disease. In most patients, reduction of inflammation and restoration of function can be achieved with NSAIDs alone. Indomethacin (150–200 mg/day) is the prototypic NSAID for treatment of reactive arthritis. Alternative NSAIDs (e.g., diclofenac) may be necessary due to patient intolerance and lack of efficacy. Aspirin and propionic acid derivatives (e.g., ibuprofen) seem less effective and are not recommended for initial therapy.
    Some patients with recurrent or chronic symptoms may require additional therapeutic measures for disease control. Intra-articular corticosteroids may be used judiciously to alleviate NSAID-resistant synovitis. Obviously, joint sepsis must be excluded prior to corticosteroid injection. Systemic corticosteroids are usually ineffective in reactive arthritis, but a therapeutic trial may be warranted in patients having resistant disease and disorders (e.g., AIDS) in which cytotoxic therapy is contraindicated. There is no cure for reactive arthritis.

20. How do you treat refractory reactive arthritis?
In most patients, remission of symptoms usually occurs within 2–6 months after disease inception. Patients experiencing symptoms recurrence, persistence, and/or flare, despite adequate anti-inflammatory therapy, may require a disease-modifying agent. Sulfasalazine (2–3 gm/day) is the drug of choice for refractory reactive arthritis and may also be safely used in patients with HIV infection. Other disease-modifying agents, such as methotrexate, azathioprine, and cyclophosphamide, also have been used with variable success. In contrast, intra-muscular gold, antimalarials and D-penicillamine seem ineffective.

21. Should antibiotics be used in reactive arthritis? If so, for how long? (*Controversial*)
Once an antecedent infection has triggered reactive arthritis, it is unlikely that antibiotics will affect the course of illness. Some rheumatologists advocate the empiric use of antibiotics, although there is insufficient evidence to support this practice. The demonstration of bacterial cell wall antigens in synovial tissue suggests that antigens alone, *not* viable microorganisms, may perpetuate reactive arthritis. Therefore, antibiotics should only be used for treatment of recovered pathogens.

In a recent study, patients with *Chlamydia, Yersinia,* or *Campylobacter*-associated reactive arthritis were given three months of lymecycline (a tetracycline derivative) in a double-blind, placebo-controlled trial. Lymecycline therapy significantly reduced the duration of illness only in patients with *Chlamydia*-associated disease. This study suggests that certain pathogens may reside in hidden reservoirs and persistently induce chronic reactive arthritis. Thus, in *Chlamydia*-associated urogenital disease, a trial of prolonged antibiotic therapy seems reasonable.

22. When should you suspect that reactive arthritis may be a complication of HIV infection?
Reactive arthritis may be the first manifestation of HIV infection. Therefore, HIV antibody status should be determined when the appropriate risk factors and/or clinical features are present. Furthermore, patients with refractory reactive arthritis and risk factors for HIV should have antibody determination prior to the use of immunosuppressive agents.

23. What is the prognosis for patients with reactive arthritis?
Though the prognosis of reactive arthritis is variable, most patients fully recover from their initial illness. However, a significant number (15–70%) will have one or more recurrences of ocular disease, mucocutaneous lesions, and/or arthritis. Twenty percent of patients will manifest some form of chronic peripheral arthritis and/or axial skeleton disease. The spondylitis of reactive arthritis is prevalent (40%) but typically mild. Factors such as reinfection, stress, genetic susceptibility (HLA-B27), and heel pain are associated with a poorer prognosis. In general, disability due to articular disease is uncommon.

BIBLIOGRAPHY

 1. Amor B, Dougados M, Khan MA: Management of refractory ankylosing spondylitis and related spondyloarthropathies. Rheum Dis Clin North Am 21:117, 1995.
 2. Arnett FC: Seronegative spondylarthropathies. Bull Rheum Dis 37:1, 1987.
 3. Butler MJ, Russell AS, Percy JS, Lentle BC: A follow-up study of 48 patients with Reiter's syndrome. Am J Med 67:808, 1979.
 4. Calin A: How to characterize and manage Reiter's syndrome and reactive arthritis. J Musculoskel Med 3(4):21, 1986
 5. Catterall RD: Clinical aspects of Reiter's disease. Br J Rheumatol 22(suppl 2):151, 1983.
 6. Dougados M, van der Linden S, Juhlin R, et al: The European Spondlyarthropathy Study Group preliminary criteria for the classification of spondylarthropathy. Arthritis Rheum 34:1218, 1991.
 7. Fan PT, Yu DTY: Reiter's syndrome. In Kelly WN, Harris ED, Ruddy S, Sledge CB (eds): Textbook of Rheumatology, 4th ed. Philadelphia, W.B. Saunders, 1993, p 961.
 8. Ford DK: Reiter's syndrome: Reactive arthritis. In McCarty DJ (ed): Arthritis and Allied Conditions, 11th ed. Philadelphia, Lea & Febiger, 1989, p 944.
 9. Fox R, Calin A, Gerber RC, Gibson D: The chronicity of symptoms and disability in Reiter's syndrome. Ann Intern Med 91:190, 1979.
10. Inman RD, Scofield RH: Etiopathogenesis of ankylosing spondylitis and reactive arthritis. Curr Opin Rheumatol 6:360, 1994.
11. Keat A: Reiter's syndrome and reactive arthritis in perspective. N Engl J Med 309:1606, 1983.
12. Lauhio A, Leirisalo-Repo M, Lahdevirta J, et al: Double-blind, placebo-controlled study of three-month treatment with lymecycline in reactive arthritis, with special reference to *Chlamydia* arthritis. Arthritis Rheum 34:6, 1991.
13. McGuigan LE, Hart HH, Gow PJ, et al: The functional significance of sacroiliitis and ankylosing spondylitis in Reiter's syndrome. Clin Exp Rheumatol 3:311, 1985.
14. Scopelitis E, Martinez-Osuna P: Gonococcal arthritis. Rheum Dis Clin North Am 19:363, 1993.
15. Toivanen A: Reactive arthritis. In Klippel JH, Dieppe PA (eds): Rheumatology. London, Mosby, 1994, p 4–9.1.

41. ARTHRITIS ASSOCIATED WITH PSORIASIS AND OTHER SKIN DISEASES

William R. Gilliland, M.D.

1. How prevalent is psoriasis and psoriatic arthritis in the general population?
Epidemiologic studies suggest the prevalence of psoriasis is approximately 1.2%. While estimates of polyarthritis accompanying psoriasis range from 5–50%, major textbooks estimate the prevalence to be 5–7%. The prevalence of axial involvement is 2%.

2. Do genetic factors play a role in psoriatic arthritis?
Yes. Both family studies and HLA typing suggest a genetic predisposition to psoriatic arthritis. Moll and Wright found that first-degree relatives of psoriatic arthritis patients may be 50 times more likely to develop arthritis.

Certain HLA haplotypes are associated with psoriasis as well as peripheral arthritis. The specific associations are not important. On the other hand, between 50–75% of psoriatic arthritis patients with sacroiliitis and spondylitis are HLA-B27 positive.

3. Does gender play a role in its prevalence?
Unlike the classic connective tissue disorders such as systemic lupus erythematosus or rheumatoid arthritis, the sexual distribution is equal in peripheral arthritis. However, in spinal involvement, the male to female ratio is almost 3:1.

4. How old is the typical patient?
Most patients present between the ages of 35 and 50. However, juvenile psoriatic arthritis is also well-recognized and usually presents between ages 9–12.

5. Is there a relationship between the onset of psoriasis and the onset of arthritis?

Psoriasis precedes arthritis	67%
Arthritis precedes psoriasis or occurs simultaneously	33%

6. If psoriasis is not obvious, what areas should be closely examined?
Umbilicus, scalp, anus, and ears.

7. Is there a relationship between the extent of skin involvement and arthritis?
No particular pattern or extent of psoriasis is associated with arthritis. However, some suggest that arthritis is more deforming and widespread with extensive skin involvement.

8. What are the characteristic patterns of joint involvement in psoriatic arthritis?
Approximately 95% of patients with psoriatic arthritis have peripheral joint disease. Another 5% have axial spine involvement exclusively. In 1973, Moll and Wright divided psoriatic arthritis into five broad categories. In reality, they overlap, creating a heterogeneous combination of joint disease.

Classification of Joint Involvement in Psoriatic Arthritis

SUBTYPE	PERCENTAGE	TYPICAL JOINTS
1. Asymmetric oligoarticular disease	>50%	DIPs and PIPs of hands and feet, MCPs, MTPs, knees, hips, and ankles
2. Predominant DIP involvement	5–10%	DIPs
3. Arthritis mutilans	5%	DIPs, PIPs
4. Polyarthritis "rheumatoid-like"	15–25%	MCPs, PIPs, and wrists
5. Axial involvement	20–40%	Sacroiliac, vertebral

9. What other features are associated with certain subtypes?

Asymmetric oligoarthritis—Dactylitis
Predominant DIP involvement—Nail changes
Arthritis mutilans—Osteolysis of involved joints, "telescoping" of digits
"Rheumatoid-like" disease—Fusion of wrists
Axial involvement—Asymmetric sacroiliitis and syndesmophytes

10. Which is the most "classic" pattern of psoriatic arthritis?

Predominant DIP involvement. It is also the least common pattern.

11. How does the axial involvement in psoriatic arthritis differ from that in other seronegative spondyloarthropathies?

Asymmetric sacroiliac involvement is typical of psoriatic arthritis and Reiter's syndrome. The other major seronegative spondyloarthropathies, ankylosing spondylitis and inflammatory bowel disease, tend to be more **symmetric.** Additionally, syndesmophytes are characteristically large, nonmarginal (''jug handle''-like) as opposed to the thin, marginal, symmetric syndesmophytes that occur in ankylosing spondylitis.

12. What clinical features suggest psoriatic arthritis rather than other polyarthritic diseases such as rheumatoid arthritis?

Asymmetric joint involvement
Absence of rheumatoid factor
Significant nail pits
Involvement of the DIPs in the absence of osteoarthritis
"Sausage digits"
Family history of psoriasis or psoriatic arthritis
Axial radiographic evidence of sacroiliitis, paravertebral ossification, and syndesmophytes
Peripheral radiographic evidence of erosive arthritis with relative lack of osteopenia

13. Are there any extra-articular features associated with psoriatic arthritis?

Unlike rheumatoid arthritis, psoriatic arthritis has only two major extra-articular features: nail changes and eye disease. **Nail changes** are seen in 80% of patients with arthritis, as opposed to only 30% with psoriasis only. These changes include pitting, transverse ridging, onycholysis, hyperkeratosis, and yellowing. **Eye disease** includes conjunctivitis in 20% and iritis in 7%. Iritis is more commonly associated with axial involvement.

14. Are there additional concerns when someone presents acutely with severe psoriasis or psoriatic arthritis?

Especially in young or middle-aged men, one needs to consider concurrent HIV infection. Clinically, psoriasis or psoriatic arthritis associated with HIV infection is more severe and less responsive to medical therapy. Some authors suggest it is a poor prognostic factor because it is associated with recurrent and life-threatening infections. The detection of HIV is also important therapeutically, because drugs such as methotrexate have been associated with worsening immunodeficiency and death. Therefore, methotrexate is contraindicated in most HIV patients.

15. Can laboratory tests help in diagnosing psoriatic arthritis?

By definition, psoriatic arthritis is classified as a "seronegative" arthritis, meaning that the rheumatoid factor is typically negative. (When psoriatic patients have erosive disease and a positive rheumatoid factor, it most likely represents coexistent rheumatoid arthritis.) Antinuclear antibodies are no more prevalent in psoriatic patients than in the general population (5%). As in other inflammatory diseases, erythrocyte sedimentation rates, C-reactive protein, and anemia may vary with disease activity. Analysis of synovial fluid reveals inflammatory fluid with a neutrophilic predominance.

16. What radiographic features help to differentiate psoriatic arthritis from other inflammatory diseases?
Asymmetric involvement
Relative absence of juxta-articular osteopenia
Involvement of the DIPs
Erosion of the terminal tufts (acro-osteolysis)
Whittling of the phalanges
Cupping of the proximal portion of the phalanges (pencil-in-cup deformity)
Bony ankylosis
Osteolysis of bones (arthritis mutilans)
Sacroiliac and spondylitic changes (usually asymmetric)

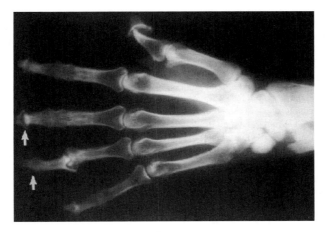

Psoriatic arthritis, showing erosions and ankylosis of DIP (arrows) and PIP joints. (From the Perlman SG, Barth WF: Psoriatic arthritis: Diagnosis and management. Compr Ther 5:60–66, 1979, with permission.)

17. How do you treat psoriatic arthritis?
Most patients can be managed with NSAIDs alone. Intra-articular steroid injections are also helpful in joints that are resistant to NSAIDs and proven not to be infected. When NSAIDs fail to control the inflammation, disease-modifying agents should be considered. Parental gold, auranofin, D-penicillamine, sulfasalazine, methotrexate, and other immunosuppressive agents have all been shown to be effective in some studies. Methotrexate is especially popular because of its efficacy in treating both the skin and arthritis.

The role of antimalarials is controversial. Exacerbation of the psoriasis and erythroderma can occur with antimalarials, and consequently some consider them to be contraindicated. Systemic glucocorticoids should also be used cautiously because of the risk of inducing a flare of skin disease if tapered too rapidly.

18. How does the prognosis of psoriatic arthritis compare with that of rheumatoid arthritis?
Unlike those with rheumatoid arthritis, most patients with psoriatic arthritis do not experience persistent dysfunction. One large follow-up study found that only 5% developed a significantly disabling arthritis. Of the various patterns, oligoarticular disease has the best prognosis.

19. What other dermatologic conditions have been associated with arthritis?
Palmoplantar pustulosis, acne conglobata, acne fulminans, and hidradenitis suppurativa. Note that acne vulgaris is not included.

20. What musculoskeletal symptoms are associated with these cutaneous pustular lesions?
- Anterior chest wall—pain and swelling in the sternoclavicular, manubrosternal, and sternocostal joints
- Axial skeleton—chronic cervical or lumbar pain
- Peripheral arthritis—least common type; usually involves <3 joints (wrist, PIP, elbow, acromioclavicular, and MTPs are the most common)

21. What is SAPHO syndrome?

    S Synovitis
    A Acne
    P Pustulosis
    H Hyperostosis
    O Osteitis

The name was proposed in 1987 by Chamot et al. because they were impressed by the association of a sterile arthritis (frequently involving the anterior chest) and various skin conditions.

BIBLIOGRAPHY

1. Arnett FC, Reveille JD, Duvuc M: Psoriasis and psoriatic arthritis associated with human immunodeficiency virus infection. Rheum Dis Clin North Am 17:59–78, 1991.
2. Bennett RM: Psoriatic arthritis. In McCarty DJ, Koopman WJ (eds): Arthritis and Allied Conditions, 12th ed. Philadelphia, Lea & Febiger, 1993, pp 1079–1094.
3. Cuellar ML, Silveira LH, Espinoza LR: Recent developments in psoriatic arthritis. Curr Opin Rheum 6:378–384, 1994.
4. Duvic M, Johnson T, Rapini RP, et al: Acquired immunodeficiency-associated psoriasis and Reiter's syndrome. Arch Dermatol 123:1622–1632, 1987.
5. Espinoza LR, Zakraoui L, Espinoza CG, et al: Psoriatic arthritis: Clinical response and side effects to methotrexate therapy. J Rheumatol 17:872–877, 1992.
6. Goupille P, Soutif D, Valat J: Treatment of psoriatic arthritis. Semin Arthritic Rheum 21:355–367, 1992.
7. Kahn M, Chamot A: SAPHO syndrome. Rheum Dis Clin North Am 18:225–246, 1992.
8. Michet CJ: Psoriatic arthritis. In Kelley WK, Harris ED, Ruddy S, Sledge CB (eds): Textbook of Rheumatology, 4th ed. Philadelphia, W.B. Saunders, 1993, pp 974–984.
9. Moll JMH, Wright V: Psoriatic arthritis. Semin Arthritis Rheum 3:55–78, 1973.
10. Olafsson S, Kahn MA: Musculoskeletal features of acne, hidradenitis suppurativa and dissecting cellulitis of the scalp. Rheum Dis Clin North Am 18:215–224, 1992.
11. Stern RS: The epidemiology of joint complaints in patients with psoriasis. J Rheumatol 12:315–320, 1985.
12. Suarez-Almazor ME, Russell AS: Sacroiliitis in psoriasis: Relationship to peripheral arthritis and HLA-B27. J Rheumatol 17:804–808, 1990.

VII. Arthritis Associated with Infectious Agents

As it takes two to make a quarrel, so it takes two to make a disease, the microbe and its host.

Charles V. Chapin
(1856–1941)

42. BACTERIAL SEPTIC ARTHRITIS

William R. Gilliland, M.D.

1. How do nongonococcal and gonococcal septic arthritis differ?

	GONOCOCCAL	NONGONOCOCCAL
Host	Young, healthy adults	Small children, elderly, immunocompromised
Pattern	Migratory polyarthralgias/arthritis	Monarthritis
Tenosynovitis	Common	Rare
Dermatitis	Common	Rare
Positive joint cultures	<25%	>95%
Positive blood cultures	Rare	40–50%
Outcome	Good in >95%	Poor in 30–50%

2. What clinical manifestations are typical of nongonococcal septic arthritis?
An abrupt onset of swelling and pain involving one joint is the classic presentation. Many patients have serious underlying illnesses and are febrile. Shaking chills may occur in bacteremic patients.

3. How do organisms reach the synovium to cause septic arthritis?
- Hematogenously from a remote infection
- Dissemination from adjacent osteomyelitis (especially in children)
- Lymphatic spread from infection near the joint
- Iatrogenic infections from arthrocentesis or arthroscopy
- Penetrating trauma from plant thorns or other contaminated objects

4. What factors predispose an individual to develop septic arthritis?
Impaired host defense
    Neoplastic disease
    Elderly
    Chronic, severe illness (i.e., diabetes, cirrhosis, chronic renal disease)
    Immunosuppressive agents (i.e., glucocorticoids, chemotherapy)
Direct penetration
    Intravenous drug abuse; puncture wounds; invasive procedures
Joint damage
    Prosthetic joints
    Chronic arthritis (i.e., rheumatoid arthritis, hemarthrosis, osteoarthritis)
Host phagocytic defects
    Complement deficiencies; impaired chemotaxis

5. Which joints are most commonly involved in nongonococcal septic arthritis?

Knee	55%
Hip	11%
Ankle	8%
Shoulder	8%
Wrist	7%
Elbow	6%
Others	5%
Polyarticular	12%

6. Which bacteria are usually responsible for nongonococcal septic arthritis?

Staphylococcus aureus	61%
Beta-hemolytic streptococci	15%
Gram-negative bacilli	17%
Streptococcus pneumoniae	3%
Polymicrobial	4%

7. Describe the trend in the bacteriology of septic arthritis over the past several decades.
Gram-negative bacilli, non-group A streptococci, and anaerobes are being recovered more frequently. Pneumococci are recovered less frequently.

8. Which organisms are commonly involved in septic arthritis in children?
Considerable institutional variation exists, but the most common organisms in various age groups are as follows:

Neonates	**Age < 2 yrs**
Staphylococcus aureus	*Hemophilus influenzae*
(hospital-acquired)	*Staphylococcus aureus*
Streptococci (community-acquired)	
Gram-negative bacilli	
Age 2–15 yrs	
Staphylococcus aureus	
Streptococcus pyogenes	

9. Name the organisms that are associated with underlying disorders in septic arthritis.

Rheumatoid arthritis	*Staphylococcus aureus*
Alcoholism/cirrhosis	Gram-negative bacilli
	Streptococcus pneumoniae
Malignancies	Gram-negative bacilli
Diabetes mellitus	Gram-negative bacilli
	Gram-positive cocci
Drug abuse	*Pseudomonas aeruginosa*
	Serratia marcescens
	Staphylococcus aureus
Dog/cat bites	*Pasteurella multocida*
Hemoglobinopathies	*Streptococcus pneumoniae*
	Salmonella spp
Raw milk/dairy products	*Brucella* spp

10. How helpful are synovial fluid analysis and culture in nongonococcal septic arthritis?
Arthrocentesis with demonstration of the bacteria on Gram stain or culture establishes the diagnosis of septic arthritis. Of the tests that can be run on the synovial fluid, culture, Gram stain, and leukocyte (WBC) counts are the most helpful.

Laboratory Tests in Nongonococcal Septic Arthritis

PROCEDURE	TECHNICAL ASPECTS	DIAGNOSTIC YIELD
Culture	Plate or inoculate culture bottles immediately	Nearly 100% positive in nongono-coccal arthritis
Gram stain	May increase yield by centrifuging synovial fluid	75% in gram-positive cocci, 50% in gram-negative bacilli
WBC count	Usually >50,000 cells/mm^3 but often 100,000 cells/mm^3 (>85% PMNs)	Counts often overlap other inflammatory disease (gout, RA, Reiter's)
Glucose	<50% of serum glucose	Helpful if present
Cell wall antigens	CIE or similar test	Only helpful in *H. influenzae* and *S. pneumoniae*

CIE = counterimmunoelectrophoresis; RA = rheumatoid arthritis; PMN = polymorphonuclear leukocytes.

Pearl: Only 40–50% of all patients with septic arthritis have synovial fluid WBC counts >100,000 cells/mm^3. So even if the synovial fluid WBC is not "classic" for septic arthritis, there can still be an infection.

11. Are any blood tests useful in septic arthritis?
Blood cultures are probably the most useful, as 50% of patients with nongonococcal septic arthritis have positive cultures. **Leukocytosis** and **elevated sedimentation rates** are seen in most individuals but are not usually helpful diagnostically.

12. Do plain radiographs play a role in diagnosing septic arthritis?
Initial radiographs should be obtained to rule out adjacent osteomyelitis and to establish a baseline. However, definitive changes of septic arthritis may take several days to 2 weeks to develop.

13. How can I remember these radiologic and/or pathologic changes in septic arthritis?
Remember A-B-C-D-E-S.

	RADIOGRAPHIC SIGN	PATHOLOGIC CORRELATE
A	Bony **ankylosis**	Fibrous or bony ankylosis
B	Osteoporosis	Increased **blood** flow
C	Joint space loss	Pannus with **cartilage** destruction
D	Joint **deformity**	Endstage of arthritic destruction
E	**Erosions**	Pannus with bony destruction
S	Joint effusion (the first sign), soft-tissue **swelling**	Edema of synovium with fluid production

14. Can other radiographic studies be helpful in septic arthritis?
Other radiographic tests are especially helpful in visualizing joints that are deep or difficult to palpate (i.e., hip, sacroiliac, and sternoclavicular joints). They are also helpful early on in a septic process, when plain films do not yet demonstrate any abnormalities.

Specialized Radiographic Studies in Septic Arthritis

PROCEDURE	UTILITY
Technetium bone scan	Often positive in 24–48 hrs, but not specific for septic synovitis
Gallium scan	More specific than bone scan but less sensitive. Especially helpful in children when there is difficulty in establishing abnormalities in growth plate areas.
Indium scan	Less sensitive than bone scan but more specific because it relies on direct labeling of WBCs that migrate to area of infection. Especially helpful in evaluation of prosthetic joints.
CT	Visualizes bony changes, such as erosions, prior to plain films. Especially helpful in sacroiliac and sternoclavicular joints.
MRI	Provides early detection of soft-tissue changes, such as edema and effusions. Also demonstrates osteomyelitis.

15. How do you treat nongonococcal septic arthritis?
- Maintain a high index of suspicion in patients who are predisposed to septic arthritis.
- Choose effective antibiotic based on patient age, clinical situation, and Gram stain findings.
- Adequately drain the joint on a frequent basis (sometimes several times a day) by needle drainage unless open or arthroscopic drainage is required. Always send synovial fluid for cell count, Gram stain, and culture to make sure therapy is succeeding.
- Analgesics are useful as adjunctive therapy.
- Physical therapy is important.
    Immobilize the joint for first day or two.
    Passive range of motion after first 2 days.
    Active range of motion/weight-bearing as pain resolves.

16. Which antibiotic should you choose? How long do you treat nongonococcal septic arthritis?
Antibiotics should be started after cultures are obtained, with the choice of antibiotic determined by the organism and clinical situation. Parental therapy should be initiated for at least 2 weeks, followed by 2–6 weeks of oral therapy. The duration is variable and depends on the patient's clinical response.

Antibiotic Treatment of Nongonococcal Septic Arthritis

ORGANISM	ANTIBIOTIC OF CHOICE	ALTERNATIVES
Staphylococcus aureus	Nafcillin	Cefazolin Vancomycin Clindamycin
Methicillin-resistant *S. aureus*	Vancomycin	—
Streptococcus pyogenes or *S. pneumoniae*	Penicillin	Cefazolin Vancomycin Clindamycin
Enterococcus	Ampicillin plus gentamicin	Vancomycin plus aminoglycoside
Haemophilus influenzae	Ampicillin	Third-generation cephalosporin Cefuroxime Chloramphenicol
Enterobacteriaceae	Third-generation cephalosporin	Imipenem Aztreonam Ampicillin Aminoglycoside (not alone)
Pseudomonas	Aminoglycoside plus antipseudomonal penicillin	Aminoglycoside plus ceftazidime, imipenem, or aztreonam

17. When is surgical drainage absolutely indicated for a septic joint?
- Infected hip joints and probably shoulder joints
- Vertebral osteomyelitis with cord compression
- Anatomically difficult-to-drain joints (i.e., sternoclavicular joint)
- Inability to remove purulent fluid by needle drainage because fluid is too thick or loculated
- Joints failing to respond to needle drainage (i.e., persistent positive cultures of synovial fluid or failure of synovial WBC to decrease)
- Prosthetic joints
- Associated osteomyelitis requiring surgical drainage
- Arthritis associated with foreign body
- Delayed onset of therapy (>7 days)

18. What is the prognosis in patients with nongonococcal septic arthritis?
Despite better drainage and antibiotics, this remains a serious disease with a 5–15% mortality. Most of these patients (25–60%) have a chronic debilitating underlying disease that contributes

to the mortality. Of the surviving patients, up to 30% have a residual abnormality (pain or limited motion of the joint).

19. Do any factors suggest a poor outcome in nongonococcal septic arthritis?

Rheumatoid arthritis
Polyarticular sepsis
Positive blood cultures
Elderly age

Delayed diagnosis
Immunosuppressive therapy
Gram-negative organisms

20. How does septic arthritis differ in children?

- Age of patient is very helpful in determining likely organism.
- Arthritis is often secondary to adjacent osteomyelitis.
- Children have a higher incidence of hip involvement.

21. Discuss the important aspects in the association of rheumatoid arthritis (RA) and septic joints.

Previously damaged joints and the use of **immunosuppressive agents** are probably responsible for the increased risk of septic arthritis in patients with RA. The patients are usually those with long-standing seropositive disease, marked disability, and a history of corticosteroid use. Unfortunately, the steroids may blunt the typical symptoms of septic arthritis, causing it to be mistaken for a "flare" of RA. **Gram-positive organisms,** especially *Staphylococcus aureus,* account for 90% of infections. Rare organisms and polymicrobial infections have also been reported.

The most important feature is the poor **prognosis.** The mortality is 25%, with only half of those surviving attaining their preinfection level of functioning.

22. Are there any peculiarities about septic arthritis in intravenous drug abusers?

1. Higher incidence of gram-negative organisms, especially *Pseudomonas* and *Serratia*
2. More insidious course with longer duration of symptoms
3. Increased propensity to affect the axial skeleton (especially the lumbar vertebrae, sacroiliac joint, symphysis pubis, ischium, and sternocostal articulations)

23. What is the incidence of prosthetic joint infections? What are the risk factors?

The overall infection rate in total joint replacement is approximately 1%. Risk factors include impaired host defense, rheumatoid arthritis, revision arthroplasty, increased operative time, and superficial joint replacements (i.e., elbow shoulder, ankle).

24. What symptoms and signs suggest prosthetic joint infections?

Depending on the virulence of the organism, the presentation may be insidious or fulminant. Symptoms include pain (95%), fever (43%), swelling (38%), and drainage (32%). Pain, local inflammation, and radiographic signs of loosening should always suggest infection.

25. What is "pseudoseptic" arthritis?

Pseudoseptic arthritis is seen in the setting of poorly controlled rheumatoid arthritis in which the patient presents with one or more inflamed joints which very high synovial fluid WBC counts (> 100,000 cells/mm^3). The cultures are negative, and patients respond to increased corticosteroids rather than antibiotics. However, infection *always* needs to be ruled out first!

This presentation may also be seen in the crystal-induced arthritides and seronegative spondyloarthropathies.

26. Who is at risk for disseminated gonococcal infection (DGI)?

Unlike nongonococcal septic arthritis, the typical patient who develops gonococcal arthritis is a young, healthy person. Women are more commonly affected than men, and are more prone to develop DGI around menstruation and pregnancy.

27. How soon after infection do arthritic symptoms develop in DGI?
Arthritis complicates 1–3% of patients with gonorrhea. Typically, symptoms develop 1 day to several weeks after the sexual encounter.

28. What bacterial characteristics increase the potential for *Neisseria gonorrhoeae* to disseminate?
  1. Small, sharply bordered colonies with **surface pili** are more virulent than large colonies.
  2. The presence of **outer surface membrane 1A protein** increases its virulence and also its ability to disseminate.
  3. **Nutritional requirements**, in that organisms requiring arginine, hypoxanthine, and uracil (AHU) are more likely to disseminate.
  4. Some strains have **resistance to bactericidal effects** of human serum.
  5. **Antibiotic resistance** may be mediated by plasmids or chromosomal-mediated mutations.

29. What host factors enhance susceptibility?
  1. High-risk sexual practices (i.e., multiple partners and prostitutes)
  2. Local environment of the cervix (i.e., changes in pH that occur during menstruation)
  3. Congenital or acquired complement deficiencies, especially of C6–C8, predispose to recurrent neisserial infections. [**Pearl:** Always get a serum CH_{50} level in a patient with recurrent neisserial infections. If it is 0, work up the patient for complement deficiency.]
  4. Asplenia or reticuloendothelial dysfunction

30. What patterns of arthritis are associated with gonorrhea?

Migratory polyarthralgia	70%
Tenosynovitis	67%
Purulent arthritis	42%
Monoarthritis	32%
Polyarthritis	10%

An important diagnostic clue is **tenosynovitis.** It most commonly affects the hands, ankles, wrists, and knees, but the pain is often out of proportion to what is seen on physical examination.

31. Besides the articular complaints, what other symptoms are associated with DGI?
Only 25% of patients with DGI have **urogenital symptoms.** On the other hand, 67% or more present with **tenosynovitis, fevers,** and **dermatitis.** Classically, the dermatitis is maculopapular or vesicular. The lesions are often symptomatic and occur on the trunk and extremities. However pustules, hemorrhagic bullae, vasculitis, and erythema multiforme may be seen.

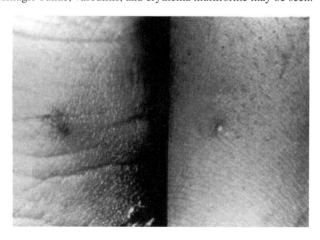

Vesicle and pustular rash of DGI. (From the Clinical Slide Collection on the Rheumatic Diseases. Atlanta, American College of Rheumatology, 1991, with permission.)

32. How useful are cultures and Gram stains in diagnosing gonococcal septic arthritis?
Unlike nongonoccal arthritis, in gonococcal arthritis the Gram stains of synovial fluid are positive in <25%. Cultures improve the diagnostic yield. Because urethritis is often asymptomatic, appropriate smears and urethral cultures should always be obtained.

Culture Positivity in DGI

SITE	ISOLATION RATE
Genitourinary	80%
Synovial fluid	25–30%
Rectum	20%
Pharynx	10%
Blood	5%
Skin	0%

Pearl: Specimens obtained from contaminated sites (genitourinary tract, pharynx, and rectum) should be cultured on Thayer-Martin media. Specimens from noncontaminated areas (synovial fluid and blood) should be cultured on chocolate agar. Always use culture plates that have been warmed to body temperature and plate specimens immediately, often at bedside.

33. Are other laboratory tests helpful in DGI?
Much like nongonococcal septic arthritis, in DGI leukocytosis and elevated sedimentation rates are common but nonspecific. Synovial fluid WBC counts range from 34,000–68,000 cells/mm^3 with a mean of 50,000/mm^3.

34. How is DGI treated?
In the past, a dramatic improvement on administration of penicillin was felt to be diagnostic of DGI. However, with the emergence of antibiotic-resistant strains, the initial drug of choice for gonorrhea has changed.

Local (cervicitis)   **Ceftriaxone,** 250 mg IM, followed by **doxycycline,** 100 mg orally twice daily for 7 days

DGI   **Ceftriaxone,** 1–2 gm IM or IV per day until signs and symptoms resolve, followed by daily outpatient therapy for 7 days with **cefuroxime,** 500 mg orally twice daily, or **amoxicillin calvulanate,** 500 mg orally three times daily

Alternate antibiotics include spectinomycin, ciprofloxacin, or norfloxacin. If the strain is not resistant to penicillin, parental penicillin or amoxicillin may be used. Repeated joint aspirations are necessary until the synovial fluid WBC count decreases to low level.

Patients and their partners should also receive empiric treatment for coexistent and/or silent *Chlamydia* infections (doxycycline, 100 mg orally twice daily for 7 days, or erythromycin if the patient is pregnant). Patients should also be tested for syphilis (VDRL) and human immunodeficiency virus (HIV).

BIBLIOGRAPHY

1. Baker DG, Schumaker HR Jr: Current concepts—Acute monarthritis. N Engl J Med 329:1013–1020, 1993.
2. Brancos MA, Peris P, Miro JM, et al: Septic arthritis in heroin addicts. Semin Arthritis Rheum 21:81–87, 1991.
3. Cassidy JT, Petty RE: Arthritis related to infection. In Cassidy JT, Petty RE (eds): Textbook of Pediatric Rheumatology, 2nd ed. New York, Churchill Livingstone, 1991, pp 489–521.
4. Cuckler JM, Star AM, Alavi A, Noto RB: Diagnosis and the management of the infected total joint arthroplasty. Orthop Clin North Am 22:523–530, 1991.
5. Epstein JH, Zimmerman B, Ho G Jr: Polyarticular septic arthritis. J Rheumatol 13:1105–1107, 1986.
6. Esterhai JL Jr, Gelb I: Adult septic arthritis. Orthop Clin North Am 22:503–514, 1991.
7. Goldenberg DL: Bacterial arthritis. Curr Opin Rheumatol 6:394–400, 1994.
8. Goldenberg DL: Bacterial arthritis. In Kelley WK, Harris ED, Ruddy S, Sledge CB (eds): Textbook of Rheumatology, 4th ed. Philadelphia, W.B. Saunders, 1993, pp 1449–1466.

9. Goldenberg DL: Gonococcal arthritis and other neisserial infections. In McCarty DJ, Koopman WJ (eds): Arthritis and Allied Conditions, 12th ed. Philadelphia, Lea & Febiger, 1993, pp 2025–2033.
10. Goldenberg DL, Reed JI: Bacterial arthritis. N Engl J Med 312:764–771, 1985.
11. Ho G Jr: Bacterial arthritis. Curr Opin Rheumatol 5:449–453, 1993.
12. Ho G Jr: Bacterial arthritis. In McCarty DJ, Koopman WJ (eds): Arthritis and Allied Conditions, 12th ed. Philadelphia, Lea & Febiger, 1993, pp 2003–2023.
13. Hughes RA, Rowe IF, Shanson D, et al: Septic bone, joint, and muscle lesions associated with human immunodeficiency virus infection. Br J Rheumatol 31:381–388, 1992.
14. Singleton JD, West SG, Nordstrom DM: Pseudoseptic arthritis complicating rheumatoid arthritis: A report of six cases. J Rheumatol 18:1319–1322, 1991.

43. LYME DISEASE

John Keith Jenkins, M.D.

1. How was Lyme disease recognized as a distinct clinical entity?

Lyme disease was first recognized as a distinct entity in Old Lyme, Connecticut in 1975. A neighborhood outbreak of juvenile rheumatoid (chronic) arthritis (JRA) was reported to the state public health department by the mothers of the affected children because they believed the neighborhood clustering of JRA to be more than coincidence. The outbreak in this rural community was consistent with an infectious etiology transmitted by an arthropod vector. To put things in perspective, Lyme disease is the most common vector-borne disease in the United States and the second most common in the world (malaria being the most common worldwide).

2. Name the infectious agent in Lyme disease.

Lyme disease is caused by an infection with the tick-borne spirochete *Borrelia burgdorferi,* which was discovered in 1982 by Dr. William Burgdorfer. As expected, the infection has many similarities to syphilis; it is a multisystem disease that occurs in stages that can imitate other diseases. *Borrelia* can only rarely be cultured from the blood or other infected tissues. The incubation period is 3–32 days.

3. What is the seasonal occurence of Lyme disease?

Lyme disease is most prevalent from April or May to November in the endemic areas. The peak incidence is in the late spring and early summer months of June and July.

4. What is the geographic distribution of Lyme disease in the United States? In what other countries has it been reported?

Lyme disease has been reported in virtually all 48 contiguous states, but most cases occur in the following areas:
- Northeast coast between Massachusetts and Maryland
- The midwest in Wisconsin and Minnesota
- Western coast of northern California and Oregon.

The disease also occurs in Europe, Scandinavia, China, Asia, Japan, and Australia.

5. Name the arthropod vector of *Borrelia burgdorferi.* Which animals are its hosts?

Ixodes dammini was the tick first described to carry the causative organism and is the vector in the northeast and midwest United States. The preferred host for the nymphal and larval stages of the tick is the white-footed mouse, whereas the preferred host for the adult tick is the white-tailed deer. *Ixodes pacificus* is the vector on the west coast, and its preferential host is the lizard, which is an incompetent reservoir for *Borrelia.* Other Ixodid species are the vector in other parts of the world: *I. ricinus* in Europe, where Lyme disease is common, and *I. persculatus* in the former Soviet Union and Asia. In general, small and large mammals are the preferred hosts.

6. How do Ixodid ticks transmit Lyme disease to humans?
The disease occurs through the bite of the Ixodid tick, an event remembered by only 50% of patients with Lyme disease—a key point to remember when taking a history. The tick is also very small (size of a freckle) and often simply overlooked. The intestinal tract of the tick is the reservoir for *Borrelia*. When attached, the tick has a slow, extended feeding cycle. Hours after feeding and upon regurgitation, *Borrelia* is transmitted to the host, either man or animal. Yes, "Spot" too can get Lyme arthritis through tick bites, and in endemic areas one of the most common reasons for a lame dog is Lyme disease.

7. What organ systems are involved in Lyme disease?
The disease is frequently thought of as a "rash-arthritis" complex, even though the arthritis may be a late manifestation and not all patients have either rash or arthritis. In addition to the *skin* and *joints*, the *nervous system* (both central and peripheral) and *cardiac system* are involved. A patient infected with *Borrelia* who develops the typical skin rash, erythema chronicum migrans (ECM), and who is not treated with antibiotics has a 10% chance of developing cardiac manifestations, 15% chance of developing neurologic manifestations, and a 60% chance of developing arthritis.

8. Describe the typical rash of Lyme disease.
In 80% of patients with Lyme borreliosis, the disease begins with ECM, which usually occurs at the site of the tick bite (most frequently the thigh, groin, or axilla). ECM begins as a red macule or papule that expands to form a *large annular lesion* up to 20 cm or more in diameter with *partial central clearing* and a bright red outer border (see figure). Atypical skin lesions can be seen and include diffuse erythema, urticaria, evanescent rashes, or a malar rash.

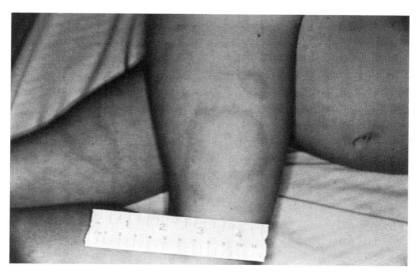

The lesions of eyrthema chronicum migrans. (From Steere AC, et al: Erythema chronicum migrans and Lyme arthritis: The enlarging spectrum. Ann Intern Med 86:685–698, 1977, with permission.)

9. What are the three stages of Lyme disease and their temporal relation? Which organ systems are predominantly involved in each stage?
Lyme disease has three stages:
- Localized ECM—skin

- Disseminated infection—nervous and cardiac systems, skin and musculoskeletal (and potentially any organ system) systems
- Persistent infection—musculoskeletal and nervous systems

After the incubation period, the first stage of Lyme disease or ECM occurs. Regional lymphadenopathy may occur, leading to confusion with tularemia. "Flu-like" symptoms such as headache, fatigue, and fever may occur, but ECM usually fades in several days to a few weeks. The second stage, or disseminated infection, may begin within days to several weeks after ECM occurs and is due to hematogenous spread. The third stage occurs a mean of 6 months after disease onset but may occur as soon as 2 weeks or as late as 2 years after disease onset.

10. What clinical manifestations occur in the second stage of Lyme disease?
Characteristically, the central nervous system is involved. Symptoms include those of meningitis, headache, cranial neuritis (especially Bell's palsy), motor or sensory radiculoneuritis, encephalitis, and mononeuritis multiplex. Cardiac manifestations occur during the second stage and include varying degrees of atrioventricular block (usually temporary) and myo- or pancarditis. Secondary skin lesions are common. Arthralgias, bursitis, and tendon involvement are common and transient. Frank arthritis is usually not prevalent until the third stage.

11. Describe the clinical manifestations of the third stage of Lyme disease.
The third stage of Lyme disease is persistent infection and usually involves *episodic attacks of an asymetric oligoarticular arthritis in the large joints,* especially the knee. With time the arthritis becomes more persistent and chronic, leading to attacks that last months rather than weeks. Fatigue frequently accompanies the arthritis episodes but in general fever and other systemic symptoms do not. Chronic nervous system involvement may occur in the third stage and is usually an encephalopathy (affecting memory, mood, and sleep) and/or a peripheral sensory neuropathy.

12. What is the natural history of ECM?
After the initial rash, secondary or satellite lesions may occur that resemble the initial rash (i.e., erythematous and annular). ECM may be seen during both the first and second stages of the disease but is much less common during the third stage. Less commonly in the United States than in Europe, a chronic skin rash occurs during the third stage called acrodermatitis chronica atrophicans. It is a blue-red area of the skin with swelling that may lead to skin atrophy. Thickened patches of skin called morphea may also occur in this stage.

13. How is ECM treated?
When treating ECM the physician needs to make sure that no other systemic manifestations suggesting disseminated infection are present (i.e., neurologic or cardiac). If none are present, then oral antibiotics are adequate when given for 10 days. In general, *Borrelia* species are less sensitive to penicillin by *in vitro* testing than to amoxicillin, doxycycline, and second- and third-generation cephalosporins. The drugs of choice are doxycycline (100 mg PO bid) or amoxicillin (500 mg PO qid). Azithromycin (500 mg) on the first day followed by 250 mg PO qd for 4 days is as effective as the other two oral regimens. Avoid doxycycline in children or pregnant women. In case of penicillin allergy, cefuroxime (500 mg PO bid), azithromycin, or erythromycin (250 mg PO qid) may be used. Erythromycin may be less effective clinically.

14. What diagnostic tests are available for Lyme disease?
Serologic testing by ELISA is the most commonly used. This test measures antibodies to *Borrelia* and is fraught with hazards. Clinical labs do not yet perform the test in a uniform manner, and the height of the titer does not imply the activity of the disease. As with much serologic testing, keep your brain or a salt shaker handy. The test is far from definitive, and the results are frequently misinterpreted.

Western blot analysis can be used to detect antibodies in a patient's serum to the various specific electrophoresed *Borrelia* proteins and may discriminate between antibodies crossreacting to some *Borrelia* proteins. Western blot analysis should not be used to screen for Lyme disease because of the cost and difficulty in interpreting the results. A new PCR-based test is being developed and may be useful in determining what type of treatment is needed in refractory or late disease.

15. Name the most common explanations for a false-negative Lyme test.
Specific antibodies to *Borrelia* may not be present early (such as during the first stage of the illness), leading to a false-negative result. These may be detectable by a Western blot analysis but not by the ELISA. It is helpful to draw acute and convalescent sera in this case. Additionally, antibiotics, either complete and adequate therapy or partial therapy with residual infection, may halt the immune response and subsequent development of measurable levels of specific antibody if given early in the first stage of Lyme disease.

16. Why might a false-positive serologic test for Lyme disease occur?
In endemic areas, a large percentage of the population may have had a subclinical infection and be seropositive without acute or chronic illness. Adequately treated patients may remain seropositive long after an infection with *Borrelia* is eradicated. Antibodies directed towards other spirochetes may crossreact to the *Borrelia* antigen(s) used in the ELISA. For example, patients with antibodies to syphilis (*Treponema pallidum*) or Rocky Mountain Spotted Fever or those who recently had a dental procedure that exposed them to spirochetes in the oral cavity (*Treponema denticola*) may have antibodies, usually IgM, that react positive in the Lyme ELISA. Not recognizing a false-positive result will lead to a patient being treated for borreliosis while his or her underlying disease goes untreated.

Interlaboratory variability and lack of standardization of the test may result in both false positives and false negatives. Serologic testing, though widely used, is of questionable value in diagnosing Lyme disease. In this author's opinion, the quality and nonspecificity of Lyme titers suggest that Lyme ELISAs should only be used in a confirmatory manner in patients suspected of having Lyme disease and should not be used in screening patients with multiple complaints of unclear etiology until better testing is available.

17. Describe laboratory abnormalities that may be seen in Lyme disease.
Antinuclear antibodies and rheumatoid factor are no more prevalent than in the general population. The neurologic manifestations of Lyme disease that occur during the second stage often involve symptoms of meningeal irritation. As one would expect, there may be a mild cellular pleocytosis and elevated protein in the CSF upon spinal tap. This may also occur in late stages of disease with chronic CNS symptoms that are not as suggestive of meningeal involvement. During episodes of arthritis, synovial fluid cell counts range from 1,000 to 100,000/mm^3 and are predominantly polymorphonuclear leukocytes.

18. How should the second stage of Lyme disease be treated and why?
There is not uniform agreement on how later stages of Lyme disease should be treated because the appropriate clinical trials have not been done. Before discovery of *Borrelia burgdorferi,* there were trials treating early disease with oral antibiotics and advanced disease with intravenous (IV) penicillin. In stage 2, intravenous antibiotics are indicated. For neurologic manifestations or a high degree of AV block, ceftriaxone (2 g IV qd for 2 to 4 weeks) or cefotaxime (2 g q 8hr for 2 to 4 weeks) is commonly used. Mild neurologic (Bell's palsy alone) or cardiac (first-degree AV block with a PR less than 0.3 seconds) disease may be treated with oral antibiotics as outlined in treatment for ECM above.

19. What is the treatment for stage 3 Lyme disease or chronic Lyme arthritis?
Again there are no definitive prospective trials extensively comparing different antibiotic regimens for the various manifestations of stage 3 Lyme disease. Oral antibiotics are used for 1 month if there is arthritis without neurologic manifestations: doxycycline (100 mg PO bid) or amoxi-

cillin with probenicid (500 mg of each, PO qid). Some physicians use the IV regimens outlined above in chronic Lyme arthritis.

Neurologic manifestations, which may occur after adequate treatment of arthritis with oral agents, are definitely thought to require IV antibiotics as outlined above for stage 2. Some consider ceftriaxone the drug of choice for any form of late Lyme disease, although doxycycline or amoxicillin plus probenicid for 1 month has been shown to work very well in arthritis. Intraarticular steroids and synovectomy can be used in refractory cases of arthritis.

20. Why does chronic Lyme arthritis not always respond well to antibiotic treatment?
The chronic arthritis may take a long time (up to 3 months) to respond to antibiotics, and the response may be incomplete. In some patients, the arthritis may not be due to persistent infection. A chronic immune process may have developed during the course of the infection that results in persistent arthritis. Supportive evidence for this hypothesis is that there appears to be a genetic predisposition to the development of chronic arthritis in patients with particular class II MHC genes (HLA-DR4 and DR2). A rational approach is to treat chronic arthritis with 1 month of oral antibiotics. If there is no response in 3 months, try one more antibiotic course of ceftriaxone (2 g/d IV for 2–4 weeks). If this is ineffective, consider synovectomy.

21. In view of the prevalence of Lyme disease, what prophylaxis should be used for tick bites?
At present there are no published recommendations, but the judicious physician should not use antimicrobial agents indiscriminately. Oral antibiotics are commonly used in endemic areas, but this may not be the correct approach. One study in an endemic area suggested that the chance of developing an adverse reaction to oral antibiotics for tick bites was as high as the likelihood of developing Lyme disease from the untreated bite. Excluding an epidemic in an area where most of the ticks are known to harbor *Borrelia,* the prudent thing to do is remove ticks promptly (it takes several hours to engorge and then regurgitate *Borrelia*), have an appropriate index of suspicion, and recognize and treat disease in its early stages.

BIBLIOGRAPHY

1. Bakken LL, Case KL, Callister SM, et al: Performance of 45 laboratories participating in a proficiency testing program for Lyme disease serology. JAMA 268:891–895, 1992.
2. Costello CM, Steere AC, Pinkerton RE, Feder HM Jr. Prospective study of tick bites in an endemic area for Lyme disease. J Infect Dis 159:136–139, 1989.
3. Kunkel MJ: Therapeutic considerations in the treatment of Lyme disease. Resident Staff Physician 38:71–76, 1992.
4. Lightfoot RW, Luft BJ, Rahn DW, et al: Empiric parental antibiotic treatment of patients with fibromyalgia and fatigue and a positive serologic result for Lyme disease: A cost effective analysis. Ann Intern Med 119:503–509, 1993.
5. Logigian EL, Kaplan RF, Steere AC: Chronic neurologic manifestations of Lyme disease. N Engl J Med 323:1438–1444, 1990.
6. Luft BJ, Gardner P, Lightfoot RW: The appropriateness of parenteral antibiotic treatment for patients with presumed Lyme disease—joint position paper of the American College of Rheumatology and the Council of the Infectious Diseases Society of America. Ann Intern Med 119:518, 1993.
7. Luger SW, Krauss E: Serologic tests for Lyme disease: Interlaboratory variability. Arch Intern Med 150:761–763, 1990.
8. Massarotti EM, Luger SW, Rahn DW, et al: Treatment of early Lyme disease. Am J Med 92:396–403, 1992.
9. Nocton JJ, Dressler F, Rutledge BJ, et al: Detection of *Borrelia burgforderi* DNA by polymerase chain reaction in synovial fluid from patients with Lyme arthritis. N Engl J Med 330:229–234, 1994.
10. Steere AC: Lyme disease. In Kelley WK, Harris ED, Ruddy S, Sledge CB (eds): Textbook of Rheumatology, 4th ed. Philadelphia, W.B. Saunders, 1993, pp 1484–1491.
11. Steere AC, et al: Erythema chronicum migrans & Lyme arthritis: The enlarging spectrum. Ann Intern Med 86:685–698, 1977.
12. Steere AC: Lyme disease. In Schumacher HR (ed): Primer on the Rheumatic Diseases, 10th ed. Atlanta, GA, Arthritis Foundation, 1993, pp 201–203.
13. Steere AC, Dwyer E, Winchester R: Association of chronic Lyme arthritis with HLA-DR4 and HLA-DR2 alleles. N Engl J Med 323:219–223, 1990.
14. Steere AC, Levin RE, Molloy PJ, et al: Treatment of Lyme arthritis. Arthritis Rheum 37:878–888, 1994.

44. MYCOBACTERIAL AND FUNGAL JOINT AND BONE DISEASES

William R. Gilliland, M.D.

1. What percentage of patients with tuberculosis have bone or joint involvement?

The number of cases of tuberculosis has risen because of its association with human immunodeficiency virus (HIV) infections. Extrapulmonary disease is now disproportionately represented (now seen in 16–18% as opposed to 7.8% in 1964). Approximately **1–3%** of current cases have osteoarticular involvement.

2. How does tuberculosis disseminate to the bone and joint?

Hematogenous spread
Lymphatic spread from distant focus
Contiguous spread from infected areas

Although joint involvement may be secondary to hematogenous spread, it usually is secondary to adjacent osteomyelitis. Therefore, tuberculous arthritis is usually a combination of bone and joint involvement.

3. Who is at risk for osteoarticular tuberculosis?

Alcoholics
HIV-positive patients
Immigrants from endemic countries
Drug abusers
Elderly nursing home patients
Immunosuppressed patients

4. Which bones and joints are commonly affected with osteoarticular tuberculosis?

Spine involvement (Pott's disease) accounts for 50% of cases. The thoracolumbar spine is more frequently involved than the cervical spine. It usually involves the anterior vertebral border and disc, ultimately progressing to disc narrowing, vertebral collapse, and kyphosis. Although tuberculosis may affect only the vertebral body, it usually will cross the disc and involve the adjacent vertebrae. Complications may include psoas abscess, sinus tract formation, and neurologic compromise. Sacroiliac joint involvement is unusual and usually unilateral when it occurs.

Peripheral joint involvement typically involves weight-bearing joints, usually the hip, knee, and ankle, and is monarticular. Subchondral bone involvement may precede cartilage destruction so that joint space narrowing is often a late finding. Adjacent osteomyelitis is common.

Osteomyelitis may only involve the appendicular skeleton. In adults, metaphyseal regions of the long bones are commonly affected. In children, metacarpals and phalanges are more likely to be affected.

5. What are the typical signs and symptoms of osteoarticular tuberculosis?

Spinal tuberculosis	Back pain, spasm, local tenderness, kyphosis, cord compression, mycotic aneurysm of aorta
Peripheral joints	Hip—pain in thigh, groin, or knee; limp (especially in children), muscle atrophy
	Knee—insidious pain, swelling, limp, stiffness
	Hand/wrist—carpal tunnel syndrome, swelling, pain
Osteomyelitis	Pain, lytic lesions on radiographs, dactylitis (especially in children)

Constitutional symptoms often are **not** present.

6. What is Poncet's disease?

In patient's with visceral or pulmonary tuberculosis, an acute polyarthritis (presumably reactive) may develop. Tuberculous organisms are not cultured from the involved joints.

7. How do you diagnose osteoarticular tuberculosis (TB)?

A definitive diagnosis is established by demonstrating *Mycobacterium tuberculosis* in tissue or synovial fluid. The yield for several common procedures is as follows:

Synovial fluid smear for TB	20%
Synovial fluid culture for TB	80%
Synovial biopsy and culture	>90%

Synovial fluid analysis reveals elevated protein in virtually all patients with arthritis, while low glucose is seen in 60%. Cell counts are highly variable and range from 1000–100,000 cells/mm^3, but most fall in the 10,000–20,000-cells/mm^3 range. Polymorphonuclear cells predominate. Synovial membrane biopsies typically show caseating granulomas. Osteomyelitis is diagnosed by needle biopsy, which usually reveals granulomata that may or may not be associated with caseating necrosis.

8. Does skin testing help in a patient with osteoarticular tuberculosis?

Purified protein derivative (PPD) skin testing is positive in virtually all patients with osteoarticular disease. However, skin testing may be difficult to interpret if anergy is present (as it may be in patients at risk for tuberculosis).

9. What are the characteristic radiographic features of osteoarticular tuberculosis?

No pathognomonic radiographic signs of tuberculosis exist. However, several signs may be helpful:
   Spine
   Narrowing of joint space with vertebral collapse
   Anterior vertebral scalloping
   Extensive vertebral destruction with relative preservation of disc space
   Peripheral joint
   Destructive lesions near joints with little periosteal reaction
   Soft-tissue swelling and osteopenia
   Subchondral erosions
   Joint destruction (late finding)

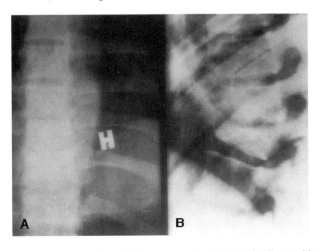

A, Abscess formation seen on anterior view of the thoracic spine. B, Vertebral collapse with angulation (Pott's disease) on lateral view. (From the Clinical Slide Collection on the Rheumatic Diseases. Atlanta, American College of Rheumatology, 1991, with permission.)

10. How do you treat osteoarticular tuberculosis?

Most information regarding treatment is derived from therapy for pulmonary disease. Although some authors still recommend long-term chemotherapy (1–2 years), many now recommend short-term (9 months) therapy as in pulmonary disease.

A typical long-term chemotherapy regimen includes **isoniazid** (5 mg/kg, up to 300 mg orally daily), **rifampin** (10 mg/kg, up to 600 mg orally daily), and **pyrazinamide** (15–30 mg/kg, up to 2 gm daily). Pyrazinamide is typically discontinued after 2 months. **Ethambutol** (15 mg/kg daily) should be added if there is a high likelihood of resistance or if the patient has previously been treated for tuberculosis.

For those with arthritis or minimal osteomyelitis, chemotherapy is often the only therapy needed. However, if bone involvement is extensive or there is neurologic compromise, surgery is often necessary to debride the abscess and hasten recovery.

11. What musculoskeletal problems can be caused by "atypical" mycobacteria?

Unlike *Mycobacterium tuberculosis,* the atypical mycobacteria have a propensity to involve the tendons and joints of the hands. In fact, 50% affect the hands, while only 20% affect the knees. Polyarticular disease is much less common.

Mycobacterium avium-intracellulare (MAI)

Most common systemic myobacterial infection in patients with HIV

Tenosynovitis, bursitis, and osteomyelitis are all well-described

Mycobacterium kansasii

Found primarily in the southwestern United States

May cause all of syndromes listed in MAI plus reactivation after total hip replacement

Mycobacterium marinum

An aquatic organism that is an occupational hazard of oyster shuckers, aquarium enthusiasts, and others

Tenosynovitis of the hands or wrist is the classic presentation, although synovitis and osteomyelitis have been reported.

12. What conditions predispose to infection with the atypical mycobacteria?

- Prior surgery or trauma
- Intra-articular steroid injections
- Open wounds in the hands or fingers

13. Are any musculoskeletal conditions associated with leprosy?

Erythema nodosum leprosum—It is seen in lepromatous leprosy and probably represents a "reactive" arthritis. Clinical manifestations include fever, subcutaneous nodules, arthralgias, or frank arthritis.

Symmetric polyarthritis—It is usually insidious and involves the wrist, small joints of the hands and feet, and knees. It is most often seen in tuberculoid or borderline leprosy.

Bony abnormalities secondary to neuropathy—These include resorption of the distal metatarsals, aseptic necrosis, "claw" hands, and Charcot joints.

Direct infection of the bone—This typically affects the distal phalanges.

14. How do fungal infections of the bones and joints present clinically?

Osteomyelitis is the most common fungal musculoskeletal syndrome. **Septic arthritis** may arise from direct extension from bone or, less frequently, from inoculation or hematogenous spread. Generally, the monarthritis is indolent with delays in diagnosis of months to years. Acute arthritis is unusual except in *Candida* and *Blastomyces* infections.

15. How helpful are synovial fluid analyses and cultures in a fungal septic arthritis?

As in tuberculosis, **cell counts** are highly variable. Typically, WBC counts range from 10,000– 60,000/mm^3 with either polymorphonuclear or mononuclear cells predominating.

Culture of synovial fluid is obviously important in establishing the diagnosis, but the colony counts are often low. Laboratory personnel must be alerted to the possibility of fungal disease so that they do not use inhibitory media.

16. What are the various fungi that can cause arthritis?

DEEP MYCOSES	OPPORTUNISTIC DEEP MYCOSES
Histoplasma capsulatum	Sporothrix schenckii
Cryptococcus neoformans	Candida species
Coccidioides immitis	Aspergillus fumigatus
Blastomyces dermatitidis	
Maduromycoses	

17. How and where are these fungi usually acquired?

Epidemiology of Fungi Causing Septic Arthritis

FUNGI	MODE OF INFECTION	GEOGRAPHIC AREA
Histoplasma capsulatum	Inhalation; aerosolized from soil rich in bird (esp. chicken) and bat feces	Worldwide, but highest in Ohio and Mississippi River valleys
Cryptococcus neoformans	Inhalation; aerosolized from pigeon droppings; also seen in immunosuppressed	Worldwide
Coccidioides immitis	Inhalation; especially in dry months; also seen in immunosuppressed and AIDS patients	Southwestern U.S., Central and South America (esp. in arid and semiarid regions)
Blastomyces dermatitidis	Usually inhalation, but rare case of dog-to-human, human-to-human, and inoculation reported; male to female ratio of 9:1	Mississippi and Ohio River basins, middle Atlantic states, Canada, Europe, Africa, and northern South America
Sporothrix schenckii	Cutaneous disease from scratch or thorn prick; systemic disease probably due to inhalation; also seen in immunosuppressed, alcohol abusers, and gardeners	Worldwide
Candida species	Endogenous; common in premature infants and other compromised hosts (malignancies, indwelling catheters, immunosuppression, wide-spectrum antibiotic use)	Worldwide
Aspergillus fumigatus	Inhalation of decaying matter or hospital air; also seen in surgical or trauma patients and immunocompromised	Worldwide
Madurella species	Implantation of aerobic bacteria or true fungi into uncovered feet	Worldwide, but typically in tropical climates where no shoes are worn (rare in U.S.)

18. How frequently is bone or articular involvement seen with these fungi? At what locations?

Histoplasma capsulatum—In the acute setting, polyarthritis with or without erythema nodosum can be seen. In the chronic setting, it is very rare.

Cryptococcus neoformans—Osteomyelitis occurs in 5–10% of infections. Arthritis is very rare and almost always involves the knee.

Coccidioides immitis—Bone and joint involvement is seen in 10–50% with extrathoracic disease. Osseous involvement may involve multiple sites. Monarthritis of the knee is the most common arthritis.

Blastomyces dermatitidis—Bone and joint involvement is seen in 20–60% of patients with disseminated disease. Osseous involvement typically affects vertebrae, ribs, tibia, skull, and feet. Synovitis is usually monarticular.

Sporothrix schenckii—Seen in 80% of systemic cases. Arthritis is mon- or pauciarticular.

Candida species—Rare, but the number is increasing with greater use of broad-spectrum antibiotics and indwelling catheters.

Aspergillus fumigatus—Osteomyelitis and arthritis are both rare.

Madurella species—Bone and joint involvement is common with spread of the soft-tissue infection to the bone, fascia, and joint.

19. How do you treat fungal septic arthritis?

Amphotericin B is the most effective therapy for most fungi. Its use is limited by its toxicity. Duration of therapy is dependent on the organism, extent of disease, clinical response, and toxicity, although it generally lasts 6–12 weeks or until 1–3 gm have been infused.

5-Flucytosine, ketoconazole, and fluconazole may also be useful. Because of the rapid occurrence of resistance to 5-flucytosine, it must be combined with amphotericin B. While the role for oral antifungal agents is expanding, their role in systemic mycoses is undefined. Surgical debridement is a useful adjuvant in resistant cases.

BIBLIOGRAPHY

1. Alarcon GS: Arthritis due to tuberculosis, fungal infections, and parasites. Curr Opin Rheumatol 4:516–519, 1992.
2. Almekinders LC, Greene WB: Vertebral Candida infections: A case report and review of the literature. Clin Orthop 267:174–178, 1991.
3. Bried JM, Galgiani JN: *Coccidioides immitis* infections in bones and joints. Clin Orthop 211:235–243, 1986.
4. Cuellar ML, Silveira LH, Espinoza LR: Fungal arthritis. Ann Rheum Dis 51:690–697, 1992.
5. Evanchick CC, Davis DE, Harrington TM: Tuberculosis of peripheral joints: An often missed diagnosis. J Rheumatol 13:187–189, 1986.
6. Garrido G, Gomez-Reino JJ, Fernandez-Dapica P, et al: A review of peripheral tuberculous arthritis. Semin Arthritis Rheumatol 18:142–149, 1988.
7. Marcus J, Grossman ME, Yunakov MJ, Rappaport F: Disseminated candidiasis, candida arthritis, and unilateral skin lesions. J Am Acad Dermatol 26:295–297, 1992.
8. Meier JL: Mycobacterial and fungal infections of bone and joints. Curr Opin Rheumatol 6:408–414, 1994.
9. Meier JL, Hoffman GS: Mycobacterial and fungal infections. In Kelley WK, Harris ED, Ruddy S, Sledge CB (eds): Textbook of Rheumatology, 4th ed. Philadelphia, W.B. Saunders, 1993, pp 1467–1483.
10. Messner RP: Arthritis due to mycobacteria, fungi, and parasites. In McCarty DJ, Koopman WJ (eds): Arthritis and Allied Conditions, 12th ed. Philadelphia, Lea & Febiger, 1993, pp 2035–2046.
11. Robert ME, Kauffman CA: Blastomycoses presenting as polyarticular septic arthritis. J Rheumatol 15:1438–1442, 1988.

45. VIRAL ARTHRITIDES

Cynthia Rubio, M.D.

1. List three general characteristics of viral arthritis.

• Viral arthritis often occurs during the viral prodrome, at the time of the characteristic skin rash.
• The most common viral arthritides in the United States generally present with symmetrical small joint involvement, although different patterns of joint and soft tissue involvement occur with each virus.
• In all instances, the arthritis associated with viral infections is nondestructive and does not lead to any currently recognized form of chronic joint disease.

HEPATITIS

2. Arthritis has been reported frequently with hepatitis B. Describe the general clinical course of hepatitis B virus (HBV) infection.

The recognition of the "Australia antigen" as a marker for HBV infection in the 1960s has aided studies that characterized this infectious disease. HBV is a double-stranded DNA virus consisting of a nucleocapsid core with two antigenically distinct constituents, hepatitis B core antigen (HBcAg) and hepatitis Be antigen (HBeAg). The core is surrounded by a nucleocapsid coat, or surface (HBsAg).

HBV is primarily transmitted parenterally. Most people exposed to it experience a clinically silent, self-limited infection resulting in an antibody response to HBsAg. Acute icteric infection occurs 40–180 days after exposure to the virus. In approximately 10% of cases, HBV infection proceeds to a chronic phase characterized serologically by HBeAg, anti-HBcAg, and HBsAg. Of these patients, 30% proceed to chronic active hepatitis.

3. What arthritic symptoms are associated with HBV infection?
Arthralgias and/or arthritis occur in 10–25% of patients with HBV infection. Joint symptoms typically are present during the prodromal phase of acute HBV infection and may precede to clinical jaundice by days to weeks. Articular symptoms usually have a rapid onset, occur in a symmetrical additive or migratory fashion, and primarily involve small joints of the hands and the knees. Early morning stiffness and pain are common, with symptoms persisting for 1–3 weeks. In patients with acute hepatitis, joint symptoms are self-limited and have not been associated with chronic joint disease or permanent damage. In patients with chronic active hepatitis, arthralgias and arthritis may be present or recur over long periods of time.

4. How does HBV infection produce these arthritic symptoms?
Arthritic manifestations are felt to be due to deposition of HBsAg–anti-HBs immune complexes in the synovial tissue, leading to a secondary nonspecific inflammatory response. This antibody response to HBsAg occurs earlier in the disease course in patients with arthritic symptoms compared to those without arthritic symptoms.

5. Name two other well-described rheumatic syndromes associated with HBV infection.
1. Polyarteritis nodosa
2. Mixed essential cryoglobulinemia

6. What serum antibodies and other laboratory findings are commonly seen with HBV infection and arthritic symptoms?
The diagnosis of HBV infection is made by confirming the presence of one or more HBV antigens or antibodies to these antigens in the sera of patients with HBV infection. Typically, during the period of joint involvement, free HBsAg is present in the serum. With the onset of jaundice and resolution of arthritic symptoms, the HBsAg titer falls and anti-HBsAg titer increases. Generally, liver function tests are abnormal; CH50, C3, and C4 may be normal or decreased; and synovial fluid appears inflammatory in nature with normal glucose levels, high protein, and high leukocyte counts. Patients may have a low-titer rheumatoid factor.

7. How do you treat a patient with HBV-associated articular symptoms?
Joint rest and anti-inflammatory therapy are the nonspecific therapies used to treat articular symptoms associated with acute HBV infection. One patient with chronic active hepatitis, persistent arthritis, and tenosynovitis was treated with interferon-alfa. After 14 weeks of therapy, the patient became HBsAg negative and anti-HBs positive, and resolution of his joint symptoms occurred several months later.

8. Which rheumatic symptoms have been associated with hepatitis B vaccination?
Although unusual, several rheumatic syndromes have occurred following recombinant hepatitis B vaccination: polyarthritis, erythema nodosum, and uveitis.

9. Is hepatitis A virus infection associated with any rheumatic manifestations?
Hepatitis A virus infections are not commonly associated with extrahepatic manifestations. Arthralgias and rash have been reported in 10–14% of patients and usually occur early during the acute phase of the disease.

10. Do rheumatic manifestations occur in hepatitis C virus infection?
Hepatitis C virus (HCV) accounts for 70–90% of non-A, non-B hepatitis. There is a clear association of HCV and essential mixed cryoglobulinemia. There have been a few case reports of non-A, non-B hepatitis–associated arthritis and, more recently, HCV-associated arthritis. Cases are limited, however, and the clinical syndrome is not clearly defined.

RUBELLA

11. Natural rubella infection or receipt of rubella vaccine is frequently associated with arthritic syndromes. When in the clinical course of natural rubella infection do the arthritic symptoms appear?
Rubella virus infection is symptomatic in 50–75% of individuals and is characterized by an acute mild to severe viral exanthem, consisting of a maculopapular rash, and significant lymphadenopathy. The incubation period is approximately 18 days. The rash appears first on the face as a light pink maculopapular eruption and then spreads centrifugally to involve the trunk and extremities, sparing the palms and soles. The onset of joint symptoms occurs rapidly and within several days either before or after the skin rash.

12. Who is usually affected by the arthritic manifestations?
Rubella infection associated with joint symptoms is seen most commonly in women who are 20–40 years old. Approximately 30% of female patients and 6% of male patients with rubella have joint symptoms.

13. What are the typical joint manifestations associated with natural rubella virus infection?
Joint involvement is usually symmetrical and affects the small joints of the hands, followed by the knees, wrists, ankles, and elbows. Periarthritis leading to tenosynovitis and carpal tunnel syndrome is a well-recognized complication of rubella infection. Joint symptoms are usually self-limited; however, there are case reports of chronic arthritis, without joint destruction, lasting several years.

14. Discuss the pathogenesis of the arthritic manifestations associated with rubella infection.
Wild-type rubella and some vaccine strains have been shown to replicate in synovial organ cultures. A number of case reports of rubella-associated arthritis have also demonstrated persistent rubella virus infection of synovial tissue. These data and others support the belief that active viral replication in synovial tissues may be responsible for the joint symptoms. Immune complexes, however, have also been isolated from involved joints. More recently, rubella virus has been isolated from lymphocytes of patients who had experienced rubella-associated arthritis years earlier. Virus in these lymphocytes would serve as a source for later direct viral seeding of the joint or for antigen release and subsequent immune complex formation.

15. Are any important laboratory abnormalities seen in rubella-associated arthritis?
Diagnosis of rubella infection may be confirmed by direct viral isolation from nasopharyngeal cultures or serologic methods employing hemagglutination inhibition (HI) or complement fixation (CF) assays. There are no other distinctive laboratory abnormalities in patients with rubella-associated arthritis. Synovial fluid has occasionally yielded rubella virus, with mildly elevated protein levels and leukocyte counts (predominately mononuclear cells).

16. How is it treated?
As with all virus-associated arthritides, no specific therapy is available. Restriction of activity and anti-inflammatory therapy are effective in most patients.

17. What are the arthritic symptoms associated with rubella vaccine?
Arthritic symptoms occur approximately 2 weeks after rubella vaccination, a time coincident with seroconversion and the ability to isolate rubella vaccine from the pharynx of inoculated people. Joint symptoms are similar to natural infection, however, and may involve the knees more frequently than the small joints of the hands. The rate of arthralgia or arthritis complicating vacci-

nation may be as high as 55% in adult women, with fewer women having prolonged joint symptoms (>8 months). In children, the frequency of joint manifestations is about 1–5%.

Joint symptoms are usually self-limited, lasting 1–5 days. Recurrences of joint symptoms are, however, not uncommon, being observed in approximately 1.3% of people with joint symptoms. Most studies have failed to demonstrate the development of any form of chronic arthritis.

18. What are the adverse side effects from pertussis and rubella vaccines?
In 1991 the National Academy of Sciences' Institute of Medicine found that available data were consistent with a causal relation between the RA 27/3 rubella vaccine strain (used in the United States since 1979) and chronic arthritis in adult women. They also noted that the evidence was limited in scope. In children, the risk for first occurrence of musculoskeletal symptoms was increased in girls but not in boys, with a relative risk of 3.5. Most of the episodes were mild and self-limiting.

OTHER VIRUS INFECTIONS

19. What diseases are associated with human parvovirus (HPV) B19 infection?
- **Transient aplastic crisis** in patients with hemolytic anemia is a well-described syndrome secondary to HPV infection.
- At the beginning of this century, pediatricians enumerated the rashes of childhood and numbered **erythema infectiosum** as "fifth disease." In children, the rash appears as bright red, "slapped cheeks." This is also now a well-recognized clinical disease associated with HPV infection.

20. What is the clinical course of HPV infection?
In a clinical experiment in human volunteers, HPV caused viremia 6 days after inoculation in those volunteers without anti-HPV IgG antibodies. Viremic volunteers developed anti-HPV IgM antibodies by the second week after inoculation. The experimental infection was biphasic, with some individuals developing a flu-like illness during the viremic stage and some remaining asymptomatic. Onset of anti-HPV IgM antibodies was associated with clearance of HPV and a clinical illness characterized by rash, arthralgia, and arthritis. In addition, there was an areticulocytosis and, in some individuals, neutropenia, lymphopenia, and thrombocytopenia.

21. Describe the arthritic symptoms in HPV infection.
The arthropathy associated with HPV infection is similar to that seen after natural rubella or vaccine-associated infection. There is rapid onset of symmetrical polyarthritis in peripheral small joints, primarily of the hands and wrists. Joint symptoms are more common in adults than children and in women than men. In general, the symptoms are self-limited, but they may persist for months or even years in certain individuals. As with other viral arthropathies, no long-term joint damage or significant functional disability has been reported after HPV infection.

The pathogenesis of joint symptoms appears to be secondary to immune-complex deposition and a nonspecific inflammatory response.

22. How is the serologic diagnosis of HPV B19 infection made?
Diagnosis of recent infection by HPV B19 may be confirmed by detecting the presence of anti-HPV IgM antibody. Elevated levels of virus-specific IgM antibody may persist for weeks or months, with IgG antibody developing several weeks after infection and then being maintained over a period of years. The presence of rheumatoid factor has not been noted in HPV infection.

23. Why is it important to make a diagnosis of HPV B19 infection?
The clinical presentation of HPV B19 infection may resemble adult or juvenile rheumatoid arthritis, especially in patients who do not present with the typical HPV exanthem and who have a clinical course of > 2 months' duration. Although there is no specific therapy, the diagnosis of HPV infection would avoid inappropriate treatment for other rheumatic conditions.

24. What five alphavirus infections have rheumatic complaints as a major feature?

ALPHAVIRUS	GEOGRAPHIC DISTRIBUTION
Chickungunya	East Africa, India, Southeast Asia, the Philippines
O'nyong-nyong	East Africa
Ross River	Australia, New Zealand, South Pacific islands
Mayaro	South America
Sindbis	Europe, Asia, Africa, Australia, the Philippines

25. Describe the clinical syndromes associated with alphavirus infection.
The illnesses arising from infection by the five alphaviruses share a number of clinical features, of which fever, arthritis, and rash are the most constant and characteristic. Arthritis may be severe. The joints most frequently affected are the small joints of the hands, wrists, elbows, knees, and ankles. The arthritis is generally symmetric and polyarticular. In the majority of alphavirus infections, joint symptoms resolve over 3–7 days. Joint symptoms persisting for >1 year have been reported, although there is no evidence of permanent joint damage.

26. Describe the clinical features and course of mumps virus infection.
Mumps virus is a member of the Paramyxoviridae family. It is a single-stranded RNA virus surrounded by a lipoprotein envelope. Subclinical infections with mumps virus are seen in 20–40% of patients. Some of the features of clinical infection include low-grade fever, anorexia, malaise, headache, myalgia, and parotitis. Epididymo-orchitis is the most common extrasalivary gland manifestation of mumps infections and is reported in 20–30% of postpubertal males. CNS involvement occurs in approximately 1 in 6,000 cases. Myocarditis is also not an uncommon finding.

27. When do the rheumatologic manifestations occur in patients with mumps viral infection?
Although rare, arthritis has been associated with mumps viral infection. Patients most commonly present 1–3 weeks after the clinical viral infection with a migratory polyarthritis that principally involves the large joints. The duration of symptoms is variable, usually resolving in approximately 2 weeks without residual joint damage.

28. Are any rheumatic symptoms associated with enterovirus infection?
Yes. Coxsackieviruses and echoviruses are among the enteroviruses causing a wide spectrum of clinical disease. Self-limited arthritis in both large and small joints has been reported in a limited number of patients with coxsackievirus or echovirus infections.

29. Is arthritis frequently associated with clinical infections by the herpetoviruses?
Arthritis is rarely reported as a complication of these infections. The Herpetoviridae family includes herpes simplex virus, varicella-zoster virus, Epstein-Barr virus, and cytomegalovirus.

BIBLIOGRAPHY

1. Biasi D, De Sandre G, Bambara LM, et al: A new case of reactive arthritis after hepatitis B vaccination. Clin Exp Rheumatol 11:215,1993.
2. Ford DK, Reid GD, Tingle AJ, et al: Sequential follow up observations of a patient with rubella associated persistent arthritis. Ann Rheum Dis 51:407, 1992.
3. Gran JT, Johnsen V, Myklebust G, Nordbo SA: The variable clinical picture of arthritis induced by human parvovirus B19. Scand J Rheumatol 24:174, 1995.
4. Howson CP, Katz M, Johnson RB Jr, Fineberg HV: Special report from the Institute of Medicine — Chronic arthritis after rubella vaccination. Clin Infect Dis 15:307, 1992.
5. Kelly WN, Harris ED Jr., Ruddy S, Sledge CB (eds): Textbook of Rheumatology, 3rd ed. Philadelphia, W.B. Saunders, 1989.
6. Miki NPH, Chantler JK: Differential ability of wild-type and vaccine strains of rubella virus to replicate and persist in human joint tissue. Clin Exp Rheumatol 10:3, 1992.
7. Naides SJ: Viral infection including HIV and AIDS. Curr Opin Rheumatol 5:468, 1993.

8. Nocton JJ, Miller LC, Tucker LB, Schaller JG: Human parvovirus B19-associated arthritis in children. J Pediatr 122:186, 1992.
9. Rotbart HA: Human parvovirus infections. Annu Rev Med 41:25, 1990.
10. Scully LJ, Karayiannis P, Thomas HC: Interferon therapy is effective in treatment of hepatitis B-induced polyarthritis. Dig Dis Sci 37:1757, 1992.
11. Siegel LB, Cohn L, Nashel D: Rheumatic manifestations of hepatitis C infection. Semin Arthritis Rheum 23:149, 1993.

46. AIDS-ASSOCIATED RHEUMATIC SYNDROMES

Daniel F. Battafarano, D.O.

1. What are the rheumatic manifestations associated with HIV?

Articular
  Arthralgias
  Reiter's syndrome
  Psoriatic arthritis
  Undifferentiated spondyloarthropathy
  AIDS-associated arthritis
  Painful articular syndrome

Muscular
  Myalgias
  Polymyositis/dermatomyositis
  Myopathy (i.e., HIV wasting, AZT-induced)

Sjögren's-like
Vasculitis
Infection
  Septic arthritis
  Osteomyelitis
  Pyomyositis

Miscellaneous
  Soft tissue rheumatism (i.e., tendinitis, bursitis)
  Fibromyalgia
  Avascular necrosis
  Hypertrophic osteoarthropathy

Adapted from Espinoza LR: Retrovirus-associated rheumatic syndromes. In McCarty DJ, Koopman WJ (eds): Arthritis and Allied Conditions, 12 ed. Philadelphia, Lea & Febiger, 1993, pp 2087–2100.

2. Does HIV infection have a direct role in the pathogenesis of rheumatic syndromes?
A direct role of the HIV infection in rheumatic syndromes has not been proved. Although the specific mechanism is unclear, the rheumatic syndromes typically occur in the presence of profound immunodeficiency. This suggests that the mechanism is CD4 cell independent and that CD8 cells may play a more central role in the pathogenesis. An acceptable hypothesis to explain Reiter's syndrome in AIDS is that the opportunistic infections can precipitate a reactive arthritis. Unfortunately, explanations for the other rheumatic syndromes are not easily simplified.

3. What role do autoantibodies have in AIDS-associated rheumatic syndromes?
Many autoantibodies have been identified in HIV-infected patients; however, no clinical correlation can be demonstrated with the rheumatic syndromes. The most common autoantibodies described are circulating immune complexes, antinuclear antibodies, rheumatoid factor, and anticardiolipin antibodies.

4. Name the rheumatic diseases that have a negative association with AIDS.
Systemic lupus erythematosus (SLE) and rheumatoid arthritis (RA). Both SLE and RA are mediated through a process involving the interaction of the MHC class II gene products and the CD4 lymphocytes. Therefore, SLE and RA do not develop or will become quiescent in an AIDS patient with low CD4 cell counts.

5. How does Reiter's syndrome typically present in an AIDS patient?
The incidence of Reiter's syndrome associated with HIV infection is 0.5–3%. The onset may precede the diagnosis of AIDS by up to 2 years, occur concomitantly, or most commonly present

with severe immunodeficiency. Oligoarthritis and urethritis are common, but conjunctivitis is rare. Enthesopathy, plantar fasciitis, dactylitis, and skin and nail changes are common. Stomatitis and balanitis may be seen. Axial skeletal involvement is unusual. The clinical course is typically one of mild arthritis with remissions and recurrences. Severe erosive arthritis does occur and can be very debilitating.

6. What is the frequency of HLA-B27 and Reiter's syndrome in the AIDS patient?

The frequency of HLA-B27 in HIV-infected Reiter's patients is the same as that found in other Reiter's patients of the same race.

7. What is conventional treatment for Reiter's syndrome in AIDS patients?

Nonsteroidal antiinflammatory agents (NSAIDs) are generally effective along with physical therapy modalities. Intra-articular and soft tissue cortisone injections are especially therapeutic for localized involvement. Low-dose corticosteroids and AZT have not been helpful for treating arthritis. Phenylbutazone (100–200 mg tid) or sulfasalazine may be the only effective agents for severe enthesopathy/arthritis. Methotrexate and other immunosuppressive agents should be used with caution because they may precipitate fulminant AIDS, Kaposi's sarcoma, or opportunistic infections.

8. What is the association of psoriasis and HIV infection?

Psoriasis is a poor prognostic sign in HIV patients because it often heralds recurrent and life-threatening infections. The full spectrum of psoriaform skin manifestations can be observed in the same patient.

9. What is the treatment for psoriatic arthritis?

Psoriatic arthritis is treated the same as the arthritis of Reiter's syndrome. Psoriatic skin disease in HIV-infected patients is often refractory to conventional therapy. Zidovudine (AZT) is very effective and considered the treatment of choice for psoriasis in these patients. Methotrexate and phototherapy are reserved only for severe psoriasis because they can precipitate worsening immunosuppression or the onset of Kaposi's sarcoma.

Pearl: Any patient with a severe unexplainable flare of psoriasis or the onset of psoriasis that is unresponsive to conventional therapy should be evaluated for HIV infection.

10. Why are many AIDS patients with arthritis categorized as having an undifferentiated spondyloarthropathy?

Many patients develop oligoarthritis, enthesitis, dactylitis, onycholysis, balanitis, uveitis, or spondylitis without sufficient criteria to be classified as Reiter's syndrome or psoriatic arthritis. These patients are given the diagnosis of an undifferentiated spondyloarthropathy.

11. What is AIDS-associated arthritis? How does it differ from the painful articular syndrome?

AIDS-associated arthritis is characterized by extreme disability and pain in the knees and ankles associated with noninflammatory synovial fluid. The symptoms tend to last 1 to 6 weeks and respond to rest, physical therapy and NSAIDs. The painful articular syndrome typically involves the knees, shoulders, and elbows and is short-lived, lasting only 2 to 24 hours. It is speculated that this may represent transient bone ischemia.

12. How is the Sjögren's-like syndrome associated with AIDS different than idiopathic Sjögren's syndrome?

The Sjögren's-like syndrome associated with AIDS is referred to as the diffuse infiltrative lymphocytic syndrome (DILS). It is characterized by xerophthalmia, xerostomia, parotid gland enlargement, persistent circulating CD8 lymphocytosis, and diffuse visceral lymphocytic infiltration in an HIV-infected patient. Pulmonary involvement as a result of lymphocytic interstitial pneumonitis is the most serious complication of DILS. Neurologic manifestations consist of cranial nerve palsies, aseptic meningitis, and symmetric, peripheral motor neuropathy. Hepatomegaly, elevated liver associated enzymes, and abdominal pain may be seen. Renal insufficiency, interstitial nephritis, hyperkalemia, and type IV renal tubular acidosis have been observed. Idiopathic Sjögren's syndrome is contrasted with DILS below.

	SJÖGREN'S	DILS
Extraglandular manifestations	Uncommon	Common
Infiltrative lymphocytic phenotype	CD4	CD8
Autoantibodies (RF, ANA, SSA, SSB)	Common	Rare
HLA association	B8, DR2, DR3	DR5 (Blacks)
	DR4 (RA)	DR6, DR7 (Caucasians)

13. What are the characteristic features of polymyositis associated with AIDS?
The clinical presentation and diagnosis are identical to those for idiopathic polymyositis: proximal muscle weakness, elevation of creatine phosphokinase (CPK), myopathic electromyography (EMG), and an inflammatory muscle biopsy. Most patients respond well to corticosteroid (30–60 mg/d) therapy for 8 to 12 weeks, and the dose is tapered and adjusted based on the clinical course. Corticosteroids and AZT may also be useful in combination. Methotrexate may benefit selected patients but should be used with caution.

14. What is AZT-induced myopathy?
Zidovudine (AZT)-induced myopathy occurs approximately 6 months after initiation of therapy. This syndrome is clinically indistinguishable from polymyositis. It is associated with an elevation of muscle enzymes, myopathic EMG, and abnormal muscle biopsy. The muscle biopsy reveals an AZT-induced toxic mitochondrial myopathy with the appearance of "ragged red fibers," which is indicative of abnormal mitochondrial and paracrystalline inclusions. Reduction of the dose or discontinuation of AZT will result in clinical improvement.

15. List the forms of vasculitis that have been described with AIDS.
• Polyarteritis
• Churg-Strauss
• Hypersensitivity vasculitis
• Henoch-Schönlein purpura
• Lymphomatoid granulomatosis
• Primary angiitis of the central nervous system

16. Is septic arthritis common in HIV-infected patients?
No. Case reports of septic arthritis and bursitis have been described, but this is an unusual infection in the AIDS patient. However, intravenous drug abusers and hemophiliacs are at increased risk for septic arthritis. Osteomyelitis is rare and may occur independently or coexistent with septic arthritis.

17. How does pyomyositis present clinically?
Pyomyositis presents with fever, local muscle pain, erythema, and swelling. This uncommon infection typically involves the quadriceps muscle, and a single abscess is present in 75% of cases. *Staphylococcus aureus* is identified in 90% of patients. Patients respond to conventional therapy.

18. What other miscellaneous rheumatic syndromes are associated with AIDS?
Arthralgias and myalgias are extremely common. Fibromyalgia has been reported in up to 30% of HIV-infected patients. Muscle atrophy and wasting associated with HIV can be prominent, especially in patients with an associated spondyloarthropathy. Tendonitis, bursitis, carpal tunnel syndrome, adhesive capsulitis, and Dupuytren's contracture may occur. Osteonecrosis has been reported in various joints.

BIBLIOGRAPHY

1. Berman A, Espinoza LR, Diaz JD, et al: Rheumatic manifestations of human immunodeficiency virus infection. Am J Med 85:59–64, 1988.

2. Calabrese LH: Vasculitis and infection with the human immunodeficiency virus. Rheum Dis Clin North Am 17:131–148, 1991.
3. Calabrese LH, Kelley DM, Myers A, et al: Rheumatic symptoms and the human immunodeficiency virus infection: The influence of clinical and laboratory variable in a longitudinal cohort study. Arthritis Rheum 34:257–263, 1991.
4. Espinoza LR: Retrovirus-associated rheumatic syndromes. In McCarty DJ, Koopman WJ (eds): Arthritis and Allied Conditions, 12th ed. Philadelphia, Lea & Febiger 1993, pp 2087–2100.
5. Espinoza LR, Aguilar JL, Berman A, et al: Rheumatic manifestations associated with the human immunodeficiency virus infection. Arthritis Rheum 32:1615–1622, 1989.
6. Espinoza LR, Aguilar JL, Espinoza CG, et al: Characteristics and pathogenesis of myositis in human immunodeficiency virus infection—distinction from azidothymidine-induced myopathy. Rheum Dis Clin North Am 17:117–129, 1991.
7. Fauci AS: The immunodeficiency virus: Infectivity and mechanisms of pathogenesis. Science 239:617–622, 1988.
8. Itescu S, Brancato LJ, Buxbaum J, et al: CD8 lymphocytosis syndrome in human immunodeficiency virus (HIV) infection: A host immunoresponse associated with HLA-DR5. Ann Intern Med 112:3–10, 1990.
9. Kaye BR: Rheumatologic manifestations of infection with human immunodeficiency virus (HIV). Ann Intern Med 111:158–167, 1989.
10. Solinger AM, Hess EV: Rheumatic diseases and AIDS—Is the association real? J Rheumatol 21:769–770, 1994.
11. Widrow CA, Kellie SM, Saltzman BR, et al: Pyomyositis in patients with immunodeficiency virus: An unusual form of disseminated bacterial infection. Am J Med 91:129–136, 1991.
12. Winchester R: AIDS and the rheumatic diseases. Bull Rheum Dis 39:1–10, 1990.
13. Winchester R, Bernstein DH, Fischer HD, et al: The co-occurrence of Reiter's syndrome and acquired immunodeficiency. Ann Intern Med 106:19–26, 1987.

47. WHIPPLE'S DISEASE

Cynthia Rubio, M.D.

1. When did Dr. Whipple first describe the disease and bacillus that now bears his name?

In 1907 Dr. George Hoyt Whipple reported a "hitherto undescribed disease" in a 36-year-old medical missionary with migratory arthritis, cough, diarrhea, malabsorption, weight loss, and mesenteric lymphadenopathy. In his original report, Whipple noted "great numbers of rod-shaped organism" in silver-stained sections of a lymph node and speculated that this organism might be the causative agent of the disease.

2. Describe the clinical presentation of patients with Whipple's disease.

Whipple's disease is a systemic illness affecting primarily middle-aged, white men who usually present with a history of intermittent arthralgia involving multiple joints over a period of years. Patients gradually develop diarrhea, steatorrhea, weight loss, and other organ involvement, including cardiac, central nervous system, and renal involvement. Hyperpigmentation of the skin is found in 50% of patients; low-grade fever and peripheral lymphadenopathy are common.

The multisystem manifestations of Whipple's disease can be remembered using the following mnemonic:

Wasting/Weight loss	**D**iarrhea
Hyperpigmentation (skin)	**I**nterstitial nephritis
Intestinal pain	**S**kin rashes
Pleurisy	**E**ye inflammation
Pneumonitis	**A**rthritis
Lymphadenopathy	**S**ubcutaneous nodules
Encephalopathy	**E**ndocarditis
Steatorrhea	

3. Describe the arthritis associated with Whipple's disease.

Seronegative migratory oligo- or polyarthritis is the presenting symptom in 60% of reported cases and is present in 90% of all patients. It does not correlate with intestinal symptoms and can precede other disease manifestations by a decade. Sacroiliitis is present in 7% and ankylosing spondylitis in 4% of cases. In addition, there is an increased association with HLA B27 (28% of Whipple's patients and 10% of healthy people); hence, Whipple's disease is often grouped among the spondyloarthropathies. Joint fluid examination may reveal PAS-positive material; however, joint fluid cultures are negative. Radiographs usually remain unremarkable.

4. Describe the synovial fluid and microscopic results from arthrocentesis and synovial biopsies of patients with Whipple's disease.

Arthrocentesis of patients with Whipple's disease and arthritis usually reveals an inflammatory fluid with white blood cell (WBC) counts between 2,000–30,000/mm^3 with greater than 50% polymorphonuclear cells. Repeat arthrocentesis after antibiotic therapy shows resolution of inflammation with WBC counts between 100 and 300/mm^3 and less than 50% polymorphonuclear cells. Synovial biopsy also demonstrates an inflammatory picture with focal synovial lining cell hyperplasia and moderate perivascular hymphocytosis. Importantly, there are also PAS-positive granules in macrophages within the synovial membrane consistent with bacilli infection.

5. What is the etiology of Whipple's disease?

Multiple tissues show periodic acid-Shiff (PAS) staining deposits. These deposits contain rod-shaped free bacilli that can be seen using electron microscopy. Recently, investigators have used the polymerase chain reaction to amplify a unique 16S rRNA sequence from tissue specimens of patients with Whipple's disease. According to phylogenetic analysis, the bacterium is a gram-positive actinomycetes that is not closely related to any known genus. The proposed name for the bacillus is *Tropheryma whippelii*. This microorganism has not been cultured *in vitro*, and the disease has not been reproduced in animals.

6. Describe the natural history of untreated Whipple's disease.

In 1955 a report of four cases of Whipple's disease and review of the 59 cases previously reported in the literature described the disease as being a "fatal condition." Prior to that time, patients had been followed conservatively or treated with "radiation" with little impact on the disease course. With the advent of corticosteroids, patients were treated with ACTH gel or adrenocorticosteroid therapy, again with limited success. In 1964 antibiotics were used successfully in the treatment of the disease.

7. How is the diagnosis of Whipple's disease most commonly made?

The diagnosis is established when microscopic examination of a biopsy of small intestinal mucosa shows infiltration of the lamina propria by large macrophages that contain diastase-resistant inclusions that are positive by PAS staining. Electron microscopy demonstrates that the PAS-positive material are rod-shaped bacilli. These bacilli can be found in multiple other tissues (lymph node, pericardium, myocardium, liver, spleen, kidney, synovium, and brain) and are located both intra- and extracellularly.

8. What is the currently recommended therapy for Whipple's disease?

Whipple's disease appears to be responsive to a variety of antibiotics. These include tetracycline, penicillin, erythromycin, and trimethoprim sulfamethoxazole (TMP/SMX). These antibiotics are continued for at least 1 year. Chlorambucil or TMP/SMX is used for central nervous system involvement.

9. How frequently do patients experience clinical relapses of disease following 1 year of treatment?

Follow-up data at least 1 year after completion of treatment or 2 years after diagnosis were obtained on 88 patients with documented Whipple's disease. Thirty-one patients relapsed. The mean time to relapse was 4.2 years. Sixteen patients had clinical relapses, 13 patients had central nervous system (CNS) relapses, five patients reported significant arthralgias, one patient had a gastrointestinal relapse, and two patients had cardiac relapses. All cardiac and CNS relapses occurred more than 2 years after diagnosis. In this review, tetracycline (TCN) therapy alone was followed by a 43% relapse rate. In comparison, the relapse rate for all other antibiotic regimens was 26%. Furthermore, of the 13 patients who developed a CNS relapse, 9 patients were initially treated with TCN alone. These findings lead the authors to conclude that TCN or oral penicillin alone is not adequate initial therapy for Whipple's disease. They recommended initial parenteral antibiotic therapy followed by 1 year of oral therapy, or oral TMP/SMX for 1 year.

10. How "rare" is Whipple's disease?
Whipple's disease was first described in 1907. By 1988 there were more than 300 case reports in the literature, and another 2,000 persons were estimated to have been afflicted during that same period. RARE! Probably the more relevant question is how many other rare diseases of unknown etiology will be found to have a definite infectious etiology susceptible to antibiotic therapy?

11. A 57-year old white man presents with a 6-year history of migratory polyarthritis, lymphadenopathy, abdominal pain, and an 18-kg weight loss over 3 years. A diagnosis of Whipple's disease is made, and the patient is treated with intravenous and then oral penicillin. During his initial treatment, the patient experiences a Jarisch-Herxheimer reaction. What does this mean?
The Jarisch-Herxheimer reaction was initially described as a systemic reaction that occurs 1 to 2 hours after the initial treatment of syphilis with effective antibiotics, especially penicillin. It consists of the abrupt onset of fever, chills, myalgias, headache, tachycardia, hyperventilation, vasodilation with flushing, and mild hypotension. It has been well correlated with the release from the spirochetes of heat-stable pyrogens. It is self-limited; however, it can be prevented by the administration of oral prednisone. It has been reported after initial treatment of a number of infectious diseases besides syphilis, including leptospirosis, Lyme disease, relapsing fever, and rat-bite fever.

BIBLIOGRAPHY

1. Chears WCJ, Ashworth CT: Electron microscopic study of the intestinal mucosa in Whipple's disease: Demonstration of encapsulated bacilliform bodies in the lesion. Gastroenterology 41:129, 1961.
2. Dobbin WO: Whipple's disease: An historical perspective. Q J Med 56:523, 1985.
3. Fleming JL, Wiesner RH, Shorter RG: Whipple's disease: Clinical, biochemical, and histopathologic features and assessment of treatment in 29 patients. Mayo Clin Proc 63:539, 1988.
4. Keinath RD, Merrell DE, Vlietstra R, Dobbins WO: Antibiotic treatment and relapse in Whipple's disease: Long-term follow up of 88 patients. Gastroenterology 88:1867, 1985.
5. Mandel G, Band J, Doli R (ed): Principles and Practice of Infectious Diseases. New York, Churchill Livingstone, 1995.
6. Relman DA, Schmidt TM, MacDermott RP, Falkow S: Identification of the uncultured bacillus of Whipple's disease. N Engl J Med 327:293–301, 1992.
7. Whipple GH: A hitherto undescribed disease characterized anatomically by deposits of fat and fatty acids in the intestinal and mesenteric tissues. Bull John Hopkins Hosp 18:382, 1907.
8. Wollheim FA: Enteropathic arthritis. In Kelley WN, Harris ED, Ruddy S, Sledge CB (eds): Textbook of Rheumatology, 4th ed. Philadelphia, W.B. Saunders, 1993, pp 985–997.
9. Young EJ, Weingarten NM, Baughn RE, et al: Studies on the pathogenesis of the Jarisch-Herxheimer reaction. J Infect Dis 146:606, 1982.

48. ACUTE RHEUMATIC FEVER

Cynthia Rubio, M.D.

1. When were the first published studies on acute rheumatic fever (ARF) written? When was the association with group A streptococci made?

The classic works in the field of ARF were published in 1836 by Jean-Bapite Bouillard and in 1889 by Walter B. Cheadle. They included extensive studies on "rheumatic arthritis" and carditis. The specific rheumatic lesion in the myocardium was described by Ludwig Aschoff in 1904. The introduction of Rebecca Lancefield's grouping system for beta-hemolytic streptococci in 1933 allowed clarification of the epidemiology of the disease by a number of investigators.

2. How is the diagnosis of ARF established?

The Jones criteria for guidance in the diagnosis of ARF were first published by T. Duckett Jones, M.D., in 1944 and have been revised over the years by the American Heart Association. The current guidelines are an update of these criteria and are designed to establish the initial attack of ARF.

Major Manifestations	Supporting Evidence of Antecedent Group A Streptococcal Infection	Minor Manifestations
Carditis	Positive throat culture or rapid	Clinical findings
Polyarthritis	streptococcal antigen test	Arthralgia
Chorea	Elevated or rising antibody titer	Fever
Erythema marginatum		Laboratory Findings
Subcutaneous nodules		Elevated acute phase reactants
		Erythrocyte sedimentation rate
		C-reactive protein
		Prolonged Pr interval

All patients should have evidence of a preceding group A streptococcal infection, with few exceptions, and the presence of two major manifestations or of one major and two minor manifestations. Fulfillment of these criteria indicates a high probability of ARF. "These guidelines represent recommendations to assist practitioners in the exercise of their clinical diagnosis and are not a substitute for clinical judgement."[4]

3. In which situations can the diagnosis of ARF be made without strict adherence to the Jones criteria?

There are three circumstances in which the diagnosis of rheumatic fever can be made without strictly adhering to the Jones criteria:

1. Chorea may occur as the only manifestation of ARF many months after the streptococcal pharyngitis and serologic evidence of an antecedent infection may be lacking.

2. Indolent carditis may also present as the only manifestation of ARF. Again, the prolonged latent period between clinical infection and the patient coming to medical attention may make documention of antecedent streptococcal infection difficult.

3. In patients with a history of ARF or rheumatic heart disease, a new episode of ARF may be difficult to diagnosis. Although most of the patients fulfill the Jones criteria, a different heart lesion would need to be present to distinguish between old and new cardiac pathology.

4. Describe the natural history of ARF and its relationship to the clinical and laboratory criteria necessary to establish a diagnosis.

There is usually a latent period of approximately 18 days between the onset of streptococcal pharyngitis and ARF. It is rarely less than 1 week or longer than 5 weeks. A positive throat culture for *Streptococcus* is found in only about 25% of patients with ARF and may be negative owing to the latent period. Several rapid group A streptococcal antigen detection tests are commercially available. These tests are generally very specific but may not be very sensitive. Neither throat culture nor antigen test for group A streptococci distinguishes between a carrier state and infection. As many as one third of patients with ARF do not remember having any illness in the month preceding the onset of rheumatic fever.

Streptococcal antibodies may be more useful because (1) they reach a peak titer at about the time of onset of rheumatic fever, (2) they indicate true infection rather than transient carriage, and (3) by performing several tests for different antibodies, any significant recent streptococcal infection can be detected.

5. What specific antibodies are used to help confirm a diagnosis of ARF?

The specific antibody tests that have been used are directed against extracellular products found in the supernatant broth of streptococcal cultures. They include antistreptolysin O, antideoxyribonuclease B, antistreptokinse, antihyaluronidase, and antiNADase. The normal ranges for all of these antibody titers depends on several factors, including the patient's age, geographical location, epidemiologic circumstances, and the time of the year. The most commonly used tests are antistreptolysin O, antideoxyribonuclease B, and antistreptokinase. If one looks for these three antibodies, there is an elevated titer for at least one in 95% of patients with ARF.

As a general reference, an antistreptolysin O titer is considered to be elevated at 240 Todd units in adults and 320 Todd units in children. Antideoxyribonuclease B titers of greater than 120 Todd units in adults and greater than 240 Todd units in children are also considered to be elevated. Samples should be drawn at 2- to 4-week intervals and all samples processed simultaneously.

6. What is the indirect evidence that the group A streptococcus causes ARF?

Group A streptococcus is clearly implicated as the causative agent in ARF. Group A streptococcus has not, however, been cultivated from lesions of patients with ARF, nor is there a satisfactory experimental model of the disease. Epidemiologic data supporting group A streptococcus as the etiologic agent in ARF include careful military studies over a period of 20 years showing a clear sequential relationship of outbreaks of streptococcal pharyngitis and rheumatic fever. Rheumatic fever does not occur without a streptococcal antibody response, and there is complete prevention of rheumatic recurrences by continuous chemoprophylaxis against streptococcal infection in rheumatic subjects and the prevention of initial attacks by prompt and effective penicillin therapy of streptococcal sore throat.

7. What is known about the biology of group A streptococcus and its relationship to ARF?

Streptococcus pyogenes (group A streptococcus) is a ubiquitous human pathogen that causes a wide array of infections. Streptococcal infections at other sites, such as skin, wound infections, puerperal sepsis, or pneumonia, have not been associated with rheumatic fever. The possibility that group A streptococci differ in their propensity to elicit acute rheumatic fever was investigated as early as 1935. It has become clear that changes in the biologic properties and clinical virulence of prevalent streptococcal strains influence the rheumatogenic potential of group A streptococci. The M protein is the chief virulence factor of group A streptococci, and antigenic differences are used to divide the group A streptococci into serotypes. Only streptococcal strains with certain M serotypes are known to be highly virulent and strongly associated with acute rheumatic fever. The degree of encapsulation varies greatly among strains of group A streptococci, and group A streptococcal strains that are both rich in M protein and heavily encapsulated are readily transmitted from person to person and tend to produce severe infections.

8. How does group A streptococcus cause ARF?

Many hypotheses have been advanced to explain the occurrence of ARF and exact genesis of rheumatic carditis and other clinical manifestations of disease. The most acceptable has been that the disease represents a damaging immune response on the part of the host to an antecedent group A streptococcal infection involving microbial antigens cross-reacting with target organs (molecular mimicry). The purification of the streptococcal M proteins and the identification of M protein peptides, which cross-react with cardiac myosin and are contained in some "rheumatogenic" M protein serotypes, may aid in confirming this hypothesis. Group A carbohydrate antibodies that cross-react the glycoprotein of the human heart were found to decrease in ARF patients post-valvectomy, but not after valvotomy. These so-called heart-reactive antibodies (HRA) are found in higher titers in patients with rheumatic heart disease compared to those without. Furthermore, immunoglobulin and complement have been found bound to the myocardium of children dying of rheumatic carditis, which suggests that circulating HRA may have pathogenetic significance. In addition, M protein and streptococcal pyrogenic exotoxin have been shown to function as "superantigens," capable of strongly activating a broad range of T lymphocytes. This suggests a potential mechanism mediating the unrestrained immunologic assault postulated to cause ARF.

9. Which host factors contribute to the pathogenesis of ARF?
ARF is most frequent among children in the 6- to 15-year-old group, and some observers have questioned whether repeated "primary" infections might be a prerequisite for the development of ARF. There is no clear-cut sex predilection, although there is a female preponderance in certain clinical manifestations (i.e., chorea). The attack rate of ARF after untreated streptococcal exudative tonsillitis ranges from 1–3%, and the disease may cluster in families. A statistically significant association has been reported between certain HLA Class II antigens (DR4 in whites and DR2 in blacks). Interestingly, a B lymphocyte alloantigen (designated 833) has been found in 75% of ARF patients and in only 16.5% of normals.

10. Describe the arthritis associated with ARF.
The arthritis of ARF usually involves the large joints, particularly the knees, ankles, elbows, and wrists and occurs in 75% of patients. The hips, spine, and smaller joints of the hands and feet are less commonly involved. In the classic attack, several joints are involved in quick succession and each for a brief period of time, resulting in the typical picture of a migratory polyarthritis accompanied by signs and symptoms of an acute febrile illness. Acute polyarthritis occurs early in the course of ARF, and is almost always associated with a rising or peak titer of streptococcal antibodies. Patients are usually symptomatic for 1 to 2 weeks, and only rarely exceed a 4-week course. ARF never causes permanent joint deformities, with the rare exception of Jaccoud type deformity which can occur in individuals who have had multiple attacks of ARF.

The pathologic changes of the joints in ARF include a serous effusion, with a thickened, erythematous synovial membrane covered by a fibrinous exudate. Microscopically, there is a diffuse cellular infiltrate of polymorphonuclear leukocytes (PMNs) and lymphocytes. Focal fibrinoid lesions and histiocytic granulomas may be late findings.

Subcutaneous nodules are similar to those found in rheumatoid arthritis and in systemic lupus erythematosus and are usually associated with a severe carditis and not arthritis.

11. Describe the treatment of ARF.
When the diagnosis of ARF is established, treatment with antibiotics adequate to eradicate the pharyngeal carriage of group A streptococci is indicated.

Current Recommendations for Treatment of ARF

ANTIBIOTIC	DOSE
Benzathine penicillin G	600,000 units for patients < 60 lb, IM, one dose
	1,200,000 units for patients > 60 lb, IM, one dose **or**
Penicillin V	250 mg 3 times daily by mouth for 10 days
For individuals allergic to penicillin:	
Erythromycin estolate	20–40 mg/kg/day in divided doses (maximum 1 g/day)
	given by mouth for 10 days **or**
Erythromycin ethylsuccinate	40 mg/kg/day in divided doses (maximum 1 gram/day)
	given by mouth for 10 days

Note: Massive antibiotic therapy will not alter the course of ARF or the frequency or severity of cardiac involvement.

The other objectives of therapy of ARF are to quiet inflammation, decrease fever and toxicity, and control cardiac failure. Analgesics without anti-inflammatory properties are recommended for patients with mild disease. This allows complete expression of the clinical manifestations to aid in diagnosis and also avoids post-therapeutic rebounds. Most patients, however, require salicylates. Salicylate levels of 20–30 mg/dl are required to control the inflammatory response. Controlled trials with other NSAIDs are not available. Corticosteroids may be indicated to control the joint and systemic symptoms in more severe cases, with special consideration to dose tapering to prevent rebound symptoms. Most patients with severe carditis or heart failure are treated with corticosteroids; however, it is not clear that this therapy alters the course of their disease.

12. What is the major sequela of ARF?
Most of the manifestations of ARF are transient without long-term sequelae, with cardiac involvement being the exception. Damage to heart valves may occur that may be chronic and progressive. Severe cardiac failure, total disability, and death may ensue years after the acute attack. In fact, the earliest structural change of rheumatic inflammation—fibrinoid degeneration—is found in the collagen of the connective tissues of the heart. The characteristic Aschoff nodule is now felt to be derived from connective tissue elements. Rheumatic carditis is characteristically a pancarditis involving the pericardium, myocardium, and free borders of valve cusps.

13. What is the recommended therapy for prevention of ARF?
Prevention of ARF in patients without a prior history of ARF involves antimicrobial therapy consisting of a single injection of 1.2 million units of benzathine penicillin G, or oral therapy with penicillin V, 250 mg three times a day, for 10 days. In penicillin-allergic patients, erythromycin estolate, 20–40 mg/kg/day (maximum 1 g/day), or erythromycin ethylsuccinate, 40 mg/kg/day (maximum 1 g/day), administered in two to four equally divided daily doses for 10 days.

Patients with a prior history of ARF are at increased risk of developing recurrent ARF and require continuous prophylaxis to prevent intercurrent streptococcal infections. The recommended regimens are as follows:

ARF Prophylaxis

ANTIBIOTIC	DOSE
Benzathine penicillin G	1,200,000 units, IM, every 4 w **or**
Penicillin V	250 mg twice daily **or**
Sulfadiazine	0.5 g once daily for patients < 60 lb.
	1.0 g once daily for patients > 60 lb
For individuals allergic to penicillin and sulfadiazine:	
Erythromycin stearate	250 mg twice daily

Note that sulfa medications can be used for prophylaxis but not for primary treatment of streptococcal infections. Patients with a history of ARF with cardiac involvement should receive lifelong antibiotic prophylaxis. Patients with a history of ARF without cardiac involvement should receive antibiotic prophylaxis for 5 years. If the ARF patient without cardiac involvement has frequent exposure to children (mother, day-care worker), then he or she should receive prophylaxis for as long as this exposure continues, even if longer than 5 years.

14. What is a reasonable differential diagnosis when confronted with a patient with migratory polyarthritis?
Gonococcal polyarthritis, subacute bacterial endocarditis, persistent viremias, rubella, Hepatitis B, and sarcoid arthritis.

It is important to bear in mind that ARF does not cause urticaria, angioneurotic edema, or clinically overt glomerulonephritis. In addition, serum complement levels are increased and antinuclear and other autoantibodies do not appear in the course of ARF, no matter how persistent the disease.

15. What is the world-wide impact of ARF?

The frequency and severity of ARF have been declining rapidly in North America, Europe, and Japan. These trends were beginning before the widespread use of antibiotics, and changes in social conditions have undoubtedly contributed to the decline. ARF is, however, rampant in the Middle East, the Indian subcontinent, and selected areas of Africa and South America. It has been estimated that there are 20 million new cases of ARF each year, and rheumatic heart disease accounts for 25–40% of all cardiovascular disease in many developing countries.

BIBLIOGRAPHY

1. Ayoub EM, Barrett DJ, Maclaren NK, Krischer JP: Association of class II human histocompatibility leukocyte antigens with rheumatic fever. J Clin Invest 77:2019, 1986.
2. Ayoub EM, Taranta A, Bartley TD: Effect of valvular surgery on antibody to the group A streptococcal carbohydrate. Circulation 50:144, 1974.
3. Bisno AL: Rheumatic fever. In Kelley WN, Harris ED, Ruddy S, Sledge CB (eds): Textbook of Rheumatology, 4th ed. Philadelphia, W.B. Saunders, 1993.
4. Coburn AF, Pali RH: Studies on the immune response of the rheumatic subject and it's relationship to activity of the rheumatic process. IV. Characteristics of strain of hemolytic streptococcus, effective and noneffective in initiating rheumatic activity. J Clin Invest 14:755, 1935.
5. Digenea AS, Ayoub EM, Barman F, et al: Guidelines for the diagnosis of rheumatic fever: Jones criteria, updates 1992. Circulation 87:302, 1993.
6. Dale J, Beached EH: Epitomes of streptococcal M proteins shared with cardiac myosin. J Esp Med 162:583, 1985.
7. Mandel G, Band J, Doli R (eds): Principles and Practice of Infectious Diseases. New York, Churchill Livingstone, 1995.
8. Markowitz M: Observations on the epidemiology and preventability of rheumatic fever in developing countries. Clin Ther 4:240, 1981.
9. Marrack P, Kappler J: The staphylococcal enterotoxins and their relatives. Science 248:705, 1990.
10. Stolerman GH: Rheumatogenic group A streptococci and the return of rheumatic fever. Adv Intern Med 35:1, 1990.
11. Tomai M, Kotb M, Majumdar G, et al: Superantigenicity of streptococcal M protein. J Esp Med 172:359, 1990.
12. Zabriskie JB: Rheumatic fever, the interplay between host genetics and microbe. Circulation 71:1077, 1985.
13. Zabriskie J, Lavenchy D, Williams RC, et al: Rheumatic fever–associated B cell alloantigens as identified by monoclonal antibodies. Arthritis Rheum 28:1947, 1985.

VIII. Rheumatic Disorders Associated with Metabolic, Endocrine, and Hematologic Diseases

Screw up the vise as tightly as possible—you have rheumatism; give it another turn, and that is gout.

Anonymous

49. GOUT
Robert W. Janson, M.D.

1. What is gout? How was the term derived?

Gout is a disease in which tissue deposition of monosodium urate (MSU) crystals occurs due to hyperuricemia (MSU supersaturation of extracellular fluids), resulting in one or more of the following manifestations:

- Gouty arthritis
- Tophi (aggregated deposits of MSU occurring in articular, osseous, cartilaginous, and soft tissue)
- Gouty nephropathy
- Uric acid nephrolithiasis

The term *gout* is derived from the Latin *gutta,* which means *a drop.* In the 13th century, it was thought that gout resulted from *a drop* of evil humour affecting a vulnerable joint.

2. Hyperuricemia is defined as a serum uric acid concentration above what levels in males and in females?

Serum uric acid concentrations are both age- and sex-dependent. Concentrations rise in association with the onset of puberty in males and menopause in females. Gout is rare in males under age 30 and in premenopausal females. The peak age of onset of gout in males is 40–50 years and in females is after 60 years. Hyperuricemia is defined as a serum uric acid concentration >7.0 mg/dl in males and >6.0 mg/dl in females.

3. How prevalent is gout? What is the ratio of males to females afflicted with gout?

Overall, the prevalence increases with age and increasing serum urate concentrations. The prevalence of gout is 5–28/1,000 for males and 1–6/1,000 for females. Thus, gout is the most common cause of inflammatory arthritis in men over 40 years of age. The male to female ratio is 2–7:1.

4. Uric acid is a product of the metabolism of which group of nucleotides?

Uric acid is the end product of the degradation of **purines.** Humans lack the enzyme uricase, which oxidizes uric acid to the highly soluble compound allantoin. The lack of this enzyme subjects humans to the potential risk of tissue deposition of uric acid crystals.

5. What pathogenic processes are responsible for the development of hyperuricemia?

- Overproduction of urate (endogenous or exogenous [dietary] purine precursors)
- Underexcretion of urate (abnormal renal handling of urate)
- A combination of both processes.

Most patients with hyperuricemia and primary gout (90%) are underexcreters of uric acid.

6. How do you determine if a patient with gout is an overproducer or underexcreter of uric acid?

A 24-hour urine collection is obtained for the determination of uric acid and creatinine excretion (to ensure an adequate 24-hour collection). On a regular purine diet, a urate value >800 mg/24 hrs suggests overproduction of uric acid. A 24-hour urate value <800 mg suggests underexcretion.

7. Name the two inherited enzyme abnormalities in the urate biosynthesis pathway that can cause urate overproduction.

- Superactivity of phosphoribosylpyrophosphate (PRPP) synthetase
- Partial deficiency of hypoxanthine-guanine phosphoribosyltransferase (HGPRT) (Kelley-Seegmiller syndrome)

These enzyme abnormalities, which cause uric acid overproduction, are inherited as X-linked traits. Patients with these abnormalities often present with early adult-onset gout (<30 years of age) and a high incidence of uric acid nephrolithiasis. Complete deficiency of HGPRT results in the **Lesch-Nyhan syndrome** (mental retardation, spasticity, choreoathetosis, and self-mutilation). In addition, patients with **glucose-6-phosphatase deficiency** (von Gierke's glycogen storage disease) also exhibit urate overproduction due to an accelerated breakdown of ATP during hypoglycemia-induced glycogen degradation. Inhibition of renal tubular urate secretion can also occur in this disease due to competitive anions from lactic acidosis.

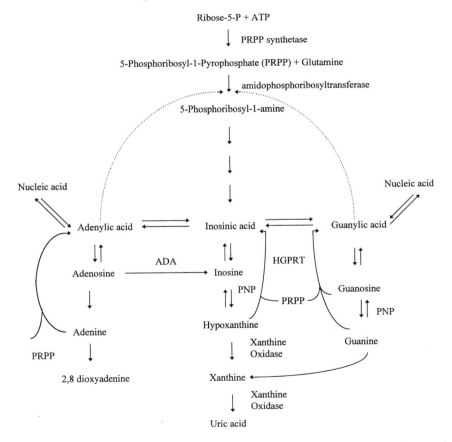

Urate biosynthesis. Broken arrows (- - - ->) represent feedback inhibition. HGPRT = hypoxanthine-guanine phosphoribosyltransferase; ADA = adenosine deaminase; PNP = purine nucleoside phosphorylase.

8. What are the acquired causes of hyperuricemia?
Urate overproduction: excess dietary purine consumption, accelerated ATP degradation in alcohol abuse, fructose ingestion in hereditary fructose intolerance, and increased nucleotide turnover in myeloproliferative and lymphoproliferative disorders.

Urate underexcretion: renal disease, lead nephropathy (saturnine gout), inhibition of tubular urate secretion (keto- and lactic acidosis), and miscellaneous causes such as hyperparathyroidism, hypothyroidism, and respiratory acidosis.

9. Name the drugs that cause hyperuricemia due to decreased renal excretion of urate.
The mnemonic **CAN'T LEAP** might be used to remember these drugs:

Cyclosporine	Lasix (furosemide) (and other loop diuretics)
Alcohol	Ethambutol
Nicotinic acid	Aspirin (low dose)
Thiazides	Pyrazinamide

Other drugs that can cause hyperuricemia by unknown mechanisms include levodopa, theophylline, and didanosine (ddI).

10. Why does excessive alcohol consumption often lead to hyperuricemia and gout?
Alcohol consumption is associated with the production of lactic acid, which reduces the renal excretion of urate. In addition, it increases the synthesis of urate by accelerating the degradation of ATP. Finally, beer contains a substantial amount of the purine guanosine.

11. What are the four stages of gouty arthritis?
- **Asymptomatic hyperuricemia.** Elevated serum uric acid level without gouty arthritis, tophi, or uric acid nephrolithiasis
- **Acute gouty arthritis**
- **Intercritical gout.** The intervals between acute attacks of gout
- **Chronic tophaceous gout.** Development of subcutaneous, synovial, or subchondral bone deposits of monosodium urate crystals

12. Describe the characteristics of an acute attack of gout.
Early episodes of acute gouty arthritis are typically **monoarticular** (85%) and begin abruptly, often during the **night** or **early morning.** The affected joint becomes exquisitely painful, warm, red, and swollen. A low-grade fever may be present. The **periarticular erythema and swelling** may progress to resemble a cellulitis termed gouty cellulitis. Acute gout may also occur in nonarticular sites, such as the olecranon bursa, prepatellar bursa, and Achilles tendon. Early attacks often spontaneously resolve over 3–10 days. Desquamation of the skin overlying the affected joint can occur with resolution of the inflammation. Subsequent attacks of gout can occur more frequently, become polyarticular, and persist longer.

13. Which joints are most commonly involved in gout?
The joints of the lower limbs are typically involved more often than those of the upper limbs. The **first metatarsophalangeal** (MTP) **joint of the great toe** is involved in >50% of initial attacks and over time is affected in >90% of patients. Acute gout of the first MTP is termed **podagra.** In order of frequency of involvement after the MTP joints are the insteps, ankles, heels, knees, wrists, fingers, and elbows. Attacks of gout at more axial sites (spine) are rare. Gout and tophi have a predilection for cooler, acral sites, where the solubility of monosodium urate crystals may be diminished due to the cooler temperature.

14. What events may trigger an acute attack of gout?

Alcohol ingestion	Hemorrhage
Dietary excess of purines	Acute medical illness including infections
Exercise	Drugs
Trauma	Radiation therapy
Surgery (typically during postoperative days 3–5)	

15. How is the diagnosis of gout established?

Fresh synovial fluid must be evaluated for the presence of monosodium urate crystals. The intra- or extracellular crystals are typically needle-shaped and negatively birefringent (yellow when parallel to the axis of the red compensator) on polarizing microscopy (see figure) (see Chapter 10). Extracellular crystals may be found in previously affected joints during the intercritical phases of gout.

The synovial fluid is inflammatory (typically 20,000–100,000 leukocytes/mm^3) with a predominance of neutrophils. Serum uric acid levels will be elevated at some time in almost all patients with gout, but the level can be normal at the time of an acute gouty attack. Since septic synovial fluids may contain urate crystals, synovial fluid cultures should be obtained if a clinical suspicion of a septic joint exists. Hematologic evaluation may show an elevated erythrocyte sedimentation rate, mild neutrophil leukocytosis, and possibly reactive thrombocytosis.

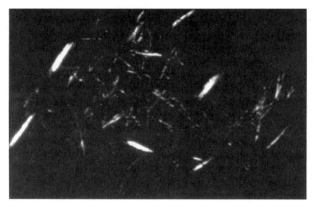

Polarized light microscopy showing needle-shaped uric acid crystals in synovial fluid.

16. What are the typical radiographic features of gout?

Soft tissue swelling around the affected joint can be seen in early acute attacks of gout. In chronic gout, **tophi** and **bony erosions** can be seen (see figure). Articular tophi produce irregular soft tis-

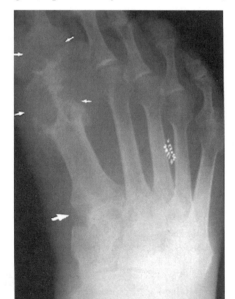

Radiograph of the foot showing erosive changes (*arrows*) of chronic tophaceous gout.

sue densities which occasionally are calcified. Bony erosions in gout appear "punched-out" with sclerotic margins and overhanging edges, sometimes termed **rat bite erosions.** The joint space is typically preserved until late in the disease, and juxta-articular osteopenia is absent.

17. After an initial attack of acute gout, what percentage of patients will experience a second attack within 1 year? At later points?
Only a small percentage of patients (7%) never experience a second attack of gout in 10 or more years.

<1 yr	62%
1–2 yrs	16%
2–5 yrs	11%
5–10 yrs	4%
≥10 yrs	7%

18. How long is it from the initial attack of gout until the appearance of tophi? Where do tophi commonly occur?
In untreated patients, tophi develop on average 10 years after the initial attack of gout. Tophi may occur at any site, with the common locations being the synovium, subchondral bone, digits of the hands and feet, olecranon bursa, extensor surface of the forearm, Achilles tendon, and, less commonly, the antihelix of the ear. Tophi can ulcerate through the skin and extrude a white, chalky material consisting of a dense concentration of monosodium urate crystals.

19. What medical conditions associated with hyperuricemia and gout must be excluded as part of your evaluation of a gouty patient?
The two most common medical conditions associated with hyperuricemia and gout:
- Obesity
- Alcohol abuse

Other medical conditions and causes of hyperuricemia:
- Drugs (see Question 9)
- Renal insufficiency
- Hypothyroidism
- Myeloproliferative disease, lymphoproliferative diseases, hemolytic anemias, polycythemia vera
- Hyperparathyroidism, diabetic ketoacidosis, diabetes insipidus, Bartter's syndrome
- Polycystic kidney, lead nephropathy
- Sarcoidosis, psoriasis
- Others (e.g., dehydration)

Other common medical conditions frequently seen in gouty patients:
- Hypertension
- Hyperlipidemia
- Atherosclerosis

Consequently, in addition to a good history and physical examination, appropriate laboratory evaluation of a patient with gouty arthritis should include a complete blood count, SMA18 (chemistries, creatinine and blood urea nitrogen, calcium, liver enzymes, serum uric acid), thyroid-stimulating hormone, lipid profile, urinalysis, and a 24-hour urine for creatinine and uric acid.

20. How do women with gout differ from male patients with regards to disease onset and clinical features?
Female patients develop gout at an older age (typically after menopause). Polyarticular acute gouty attacks are more common. Female patients frequently have osteoarthritis, hypertension, and mild chronic renal insufficiency or are being treated with diuretics. Tophi are particularly common in previously damaged joints, including Heberden's nodes, and in the finger pads.

21. Discuss the pathophysiology of acute gouty arthritis.
Acute gouty arthritis is triggered by the precipitation of monosodium urate crystals in the joint. The inflammatory nature of the crystals is thought to be determined by certain proteins which coat

the crystals; crystals coated with IgG react with Fc receptors on responding cells and promote an inflammatory response, whereas apolipoprotein-B coating of crystals inhibits phagocytosis and a cellular response. Urate crystals stimulate the production of chemotactic factors, cytokines (interleukins 1, 6, and 8 and tumor necrosis factor), prostaglandins, leukotrienes, and oxygen radicals by neutrophils, monocytes, and synovial cells in addition to activating complement and inducing lysosomal enzyme release.

22. Why are early attacks of acute gouty arthritis often self-limited?
The following mechanisms have been postulated:
- The cellular response may be modulated by different proteins coating the crystals.
- Phagocytosis and degradation of crystals by neutrophils decreases the crystal concentration.
- The heat associated with the inflammation results in increased urate crystal solubility.
- Enhanced ACTH secretion may suppress the inflammatory response.
- Proinflammatory cytokines (interleukin-1 and tumor necrosis factor) are balanced by the production of cytokine inhibitors and regulatory cytokines.

23. Name the types of renal disease associated with hyperuricemia.
- **Urate nephropathy.** Deposition of monosodium urate crystals in the renal interstitial tissue may cause mild and intermittent proteinuria and rarely causes renal dysfunction (associated hypertension is often the cause).
- **Uric acid nephropathy.** Precipitation of uric acid crystals in the collecting ducts and ureters results in acute renal failure, as in the acute tumor lysis syndrome.
- **Uric acid nephrolithiasis.** The frequency parallels the increase in serum and urinary concentrations of uric acid and in acidity of urine. Uric acid stones are radiolucent. The incidence of calcium stones is also increased in patients with gout, particularly those with hyperuricosuria. The uric acid serves as a nidus for calcium stone formation.
- **Other.** Polycystic kidney disease (one-third of patients have gout), lead intoxication, and familial urate nephropathy.

24. When should treatment of asymptomatic hyperuricemia be considered?
Asymptomatic hyperuricemia should only be treated in situations where there may be an acute overproduction uric acid, as in the acute tumor lysis syndrome, or where severe hyperuricemia exists (serum uric acid >12 mg/dl or 24-hr urinary uric acid >1100 mg). The prevalence of uric acid nephrolithiasis is 50% in this latter population.

25. Discuss the treatment options for acute gouty arthritis.
NSAIDs and **colchicine** are effective in the treatment of acute gout. In patients with contraindications to these medications or with acute gout refractory to these therapies, **corticosteroids** may be used to suppress the inflammatory response. Drugs that alter serum uric acid levels (allopurinol, probenecid) should never be started until after complete resolution of the acute gouty attack, nor should they be stopped if an acute gouty attack occurs while the patient is on these medications.

Medications Used in the Treatment of Acute Gouty Arthritis

TREATMENT OPTIONS	DOSAGE	COMMENTS
NSAIDs (Indomethacin)	50 mg po qid × 24–48 hr, then 50 mg po tid × 48 hr. Taper and discontinue after the attack subsides.	Indomethacin is the drug of choice. Other NSAIDs with short half-lives are probably as effective.
Colchicine*	0.6 mg po qh until symptoms ease, GI toxicity occurs, or a maximum dose of 10 tablets (6 mg) is reached	Most effective within the first 24 hr of an attack. Nausea, vomiting, diarrhea develop in 80% of patients. Contraindicated in the elderly and those with renal or liver insufficiency.
Intra-articular steroids (triamcinolone or methylprednisolone)	40 mg ia with lidocaine for large joints, 10–20 mg for small joints or bursae	Useful in the treatment of 1 or 2 involved joints or bursae. Effective within the first 12 hr of an attack in 90% of patients.

Medications Used in the Treatment of Acute Gouty Arthritis (Continued)

TREATMENT OPTIONS	DOSAGE	COMMENTS
Systemic corticosteroids	Prednisone, 30 mg/day with taper over 7–10 days or triamcinolone acetonide (Kenalog) 60 mg im, can repeat once	Rebound arthropathy may occur.
Adrenocorticotropic hormone (ACTH)	40–80 USP units im q12h as needed (1–3 doses typical)	More costly than alternative therapies

*Colchicine (see Chapter 88) can also be given intravenously. Dose is 1.0–2.0 mg in 20 ml of normal saline infused slowly over 5–10 min. Can be repeated once in 6–12 hrs if patient has normal kidney and liver function. Colchicine given iv is not associated with GI side effects, but can cause bone marrow depression, arrhythmias, and skin necrosis (if it extravasates from the vein). IV colchicine may soon no longer be manufactured due to its toxicities.

26. What are the indications for chronic treatment of symptomatic hyperuricemia?

Lifelong therapy with antihyperuricemic drugs (allopurinol or probenecid) is indicated in the following situations:

- >2 or 3 acute attacks of gout within 1–2 years
- Renal stones (urate or calcium)
- Tophaceous gout
- Chronic gouty arthritis with bony erosions
- Asymptomatic hyperuricemia with serum uric acid >12 mg/dl or 24 hr urinary excretion >1100 mg to decrease the risk of urate nephrolithiasis

The indications for allopurinol versus probenecid therapy, along with their dosing and side effects profiles, are discussed in Chapter 88.

27. Acute gouty attacks can be precipitated with the initiation of antihyperuricemic therapy. How can this risk be minimized?

The dose of the antihyperuricemic drug should be gradually increased, along with using either a low-dose NSAID twice daily or colchicine, 0.6 mg orally twice daily (decrease the dose in the setting of renal insufficiency) as prophylaxis for the first 6–12 months of therapy. In addition, these regimens are effective in reducing the overall frequency of acute attacks in patients with gout.

28. What is the treatment for tophaceous gout?

The goal of treatment is to lower the serum uric acid level substantially to permit urate resorption from the tophi. This result requires long-term treatment with allopurinol to keep the serum uric acid level ideally at least 1.0 mg/dl below the supersaturation threshold of 6.8 mg/dl. Prophylaxis with oral colchicine or NSAIDs is often helpful in these patients to reduce the frequency of acute gouty attacks.

29. Why is gout relatively common in organ transplant recipients?

Therapy with cyclosporine, which reduces urinary urate excretion, is probably the most significant factor. Treatment of acute attacks and normalization of the hyperuricemia is often problematic. NSAIDs are relatively contraindicated in the setting of cyclosporine therapy or renal insufficiency, and colchicine therapy with concomitant azathioprine may result in significant neutropenia. Intra-articular or systemic corticosteroids may be the safest treatment options for acute gouty attacks. Synovial fluid cultures should be performed routinely. Uricosurics are often ineffective in these patients due to a glomerular filtration rate <50 ml/min. Allopurinol, at a dose adjusted for renal function, can be used if the patient is not on azathioprine (see Chapter 88). Even if the dose of azathioprine is reduced by 50–75% while the patient is on allopurinol, it is a dangerous combination that may result in severe leukopenia or bone marrow failure.

30. Name some famous individuals who suffered with gout.

Isaac Newton, Michelangelo, Benjamin Franklin, William Pitt, and Charles Darwin, to name just a few!

BIBLIOGRAPHY

1. Alloway JA, Moriarty MJ, Hoogland YT, Nashel DJ: Comparison of triamcinolone acetonide with indomethacin in the treatment of acute gouty arthritis. J Rheumatol 20:111–113, 1993.
2. Baethge BA, Work J, Landreneau MD, McDonald JC: Tophaceous gout in patients with renal transplants treated with cyclosporine A. J Rheumatol 20:718–720, 1993.
3. Beutler A, Schumacher HR Jr: Gout and "pseudogout": When are arthritic symptoms caused by crystal deposition? Postgrad Med 95(2):103–116, 1994.
4. Cohen MG, Emmerson BT: Crystal arthropathies: Gout. In Klippel JH, Dieppe PA (eds): Rheumatology. London, Mosby, 1994, pp 7.12.1–7.12.16.
5. Groff GD, Franck WA, Raddatz DA: Systemic steroid therapy for acute gout: A clinical trial and review of the literature. Semin Arthritis Rheum 19:329–336, 1990.
6. Joseph J, McGrath H: Gout or "pseudogout": How to differentiate crystal-induced arthropathies. Geriatrics 50:33–39, 1995.
7. Kelley WN, Schumacher HR Jr: Gout. In Kelley WN, Harris ED Jr., Ruddy S, Sledge CB (eds): Textbook of Rheumatology, 4th ed. Philadelphia, W.B. Saunders, 1993, pp 1291–1336.
8. Kerolus G, Clayburne G, Schumacher HR Jr: Is it mandatory to examine synovial fluids promptly after arthrocentesis? Arthritis Rheum 32:271–278, 1989.
9. Pratt PW, Ball GV: Gout: Treatment. In Schumacher HR Jr (ed): Primer on the Rheumatic Diseases, 10th ed. Atlanta, Arthritis Foundation, 1993, pp 216–219.
10. Puig JG, Michan AD, Jimenez ML, et al: Female gout: Clinical spectrum and uric acid metabolism. Arch Intern Med 151:726–732, 1991.
11. Sells LL, German DC: An update on gout. Bull Rheum Dis 43:4–6, 1994.
12. Tate GA, Schumacher HR Jr: Gout: Clinical and laboratory features. In Schumacher HR Jr (ed): Primer on the Rheumatic Diseases, 10th ed. Atlanta, Arthritis Foundation, 1993, pp 213–216.
13. Terkeltaub RA: Gout and mechanisms of crystal-induced inflammation. Curr Opin Rheumatol. 5:510–516, 1993.
14. Terkeltaub RA: Gout: Epidemiology, pathology, and pathogenesis. In Schumacher HR Jr (ed): Primer on the Rheumatic Diseases, 10th ed. Atlanta, Arthritis Foundation, 1993, pp 209–213.
15. Wallace SL, Singer JZ, Duncan GJ, et al: Renal function predicts colchicine toxicity: Guidelines for the prophylactic use of colchicine in gout. J Rheumatol 18:264–269, 1991.

50. CALCIUM PYROPHOSPHATE DIHYDRATE DEPOSITION DISEASE

Matthew T. Carpenter, M.D.

1. What is calcium pyrophosphate dihydrate (CPPD)?

CPPD is a calcium salt ($Ca_2P_2O_7 \cdot 2H_2O$) that is deposited in cartilage, appearing as **chondrocalcinosis** on roentgenograms. CPPD can also be released as a crystal into a joint, causing an acute painful arthritis called **pseudogout.**

2. How common is chondrocalcinosis?

Up to 50% of the population has chondrocalcinosis on roentgenograms by the ninth decade of life. Asymptomatic chondrocalcinosis (or the "lanthanic" form of CPPD deposition disease) is the most common clinical presentation of CPPD deposition.

3. Is all chondrocalcinosis caused by CPPD deposition?

Calcium salts other than CPPD, such as calcium hydroxyapatite, can appear as chondrocalcinosis. For example, the calcification of the cartilage of intervertebral discs seen in ochronosis is largely calcium hydroxyapatite. Clinicians usually assume that certain radiographic patterns of chondrocalcinosis, such as the triangular fibrocartilage complex in the wrist or the hyaline cartilage and menisci in the knees, are due to CPPD deposition. Assuming isn't as precise a method as identifying the crystals in the laboratory.

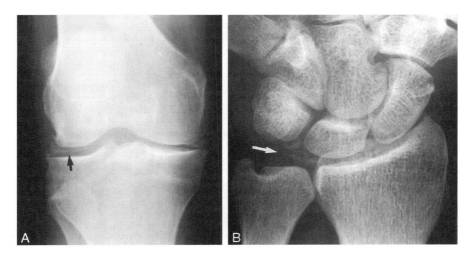

A, Chondrocalcinosis of the knee. *B*, Triangular fibrocartilage complex of the wrist.

4. Do all patients with CPPD deposition have chondrocalcinosis?
CPPD deposition can cause arthritis without showing up on roentgenograms as chondrocalcinosis. This is one reason that an acutely inflamed joint must be aspirated to identify the cause. An elderly patient who presents with an acutely inflamed knee could have gout or pseudogout as a cause of their arthritis, even if the roentgenogram is normal. The only way to tell is to aspirate the joint. The phrase "pyrophosphate arthropathy" has been used to describe structural damage to a joint associated with CPPD deposition, with or without chondrocalcinosis. Calcium pyrophosphate dihydrate deposition disease is the term for all problems associated with CPPD deposition, including chondrocalcinosis, pseudogout, and pyrophosphate arthropathy.

5. How can CPPD disease present clinically?
 Pseudogout
 Pseudo-rheumatoid arthritis
 Pseudo-osteoarthritis without superimposed acute attacks of pseudogout
 Pseudo-osteoarthritis with superimposed acute attacks of pseudogout
 Asymptomatic (lanthanic) radiographic disease
 Pseudo-Charcot or pseudo-neuropathic arthritis
These clinical presentations are frequently overlapping.

6. What is pseudogout? How does it present?
 Pseudogout is an acute arthritis caused by release of CPPD crystals into the joint space. Polymorphonuclear leukocytes engulf the CPPD crystals and release cytokines and other mediators, which cause intense inflammation of the joint. Symptoms of acute pseudogout are the same as any acute arthritis, with rapid onset of pain and swelling. Physical examination reveals warmth, swelling with effusion, tenderness, and limited motion of the involved joint(s). Overlying erythema may simulate cellulitis. Occasionally systemic symptoms such as malaise and fever will also raise suspicion for infection.
 The presentation of pseudogout can mimic gout, but the causative crystal is CPPD rather than monosodium urate. Attacks of pseudogout tend to be less painful and take longer to reach peak intensity than gout. Usually, only a single joint is affected, although oligoarticular and polyarticular pseudogout are described. Large joints are affected more commonly than small joints, with the knee being the most frequently involved joint. Untreated pseudogout is self-limited, resolving within a month. Patients are typically asymptomatic between attacks.

7. How is pseudogout diagnosed?

When a patient presents with an acute monarthritis or oligoarthritis, the critical and immediate diagnostic procedure is aspiration of the joint(s). The fluid obtained may appear yellow and cloudy or even opaque and chalky white from suspended crystals. Synovial fluid is sent to the laboratory for cell count and differential, as well as Gram stain and bacterial culture. Synovial fluid leukocytosis with a predominance of polymorphonuclear leukocytes (PMNs) is present. A specimen of synovial fluid is also promptly analyzed for crystals by **polarized light microscopy.** The presence of intracellular CPPD crystals confirms the diagnosis of pseudogout. Rarely, definitive diagnosis requires special methods of crystal identification such as x-ray diffraction.

8. How is polarized light microscopy done?

A drop of synovial fluid is placed on a clean microscope slide and covered with a cover slip. The slide is first examined under ordinary light microscopy. CPPD crystals tend to be rhomboid-shaped or rectangular. Compared to the monosodium urate crystals of gout, the ends of the CPPD crystals are blunt or squrae; monosodium urate crystals are needle-shaped or pointed.

Although a preliminary crystal identification may be made with light microscopy, definitive diagnosis requires polarized light microscopy with a first-order red compensator. CPPD crystals are referred to as **weakly positively birefringent.** This means that CPPD crystals appear blue when viewed under polarized light with the long axis of the crystal parallel to the *direction of slow vibration of light in the first-order red compensator.* (When rheumatologists talk about crystals, we just ask whether the crystal is aligned in the plane, rather than discussing the direction of slow vibration!) Usually, this axis is clearly indicated on the microscope to prevent confusion. Remember the mnemonic **ABC**—*A*ligned *B*lue *C*alcium—i.e., if the crystal is aligned with the red compensator and blue, then it is calcium pyrophosphate. CPPD crystals lying with their long axes at right angles to the direction of slow vibration will appear yellow rather than blue. If your microscope is equipped with a rotating stage, you can simply rotate the slide until the long axis of the crystal is properly aligned in order to see the expected color. (See Chapter 10.)

9. What are the pitfalls to be wary of when diagnosing acute pseudogout?

1. **Septic arthritis** can coexist with any acute crystalline arthritis, including CPPD. Enzymes that degrade cartilage can be released into the joint either from the infecting bacteria or the PMNs. These enzymes are able to "strip" crystals from the structures in and around the joint, causing an unwary clinician to miss a septic joint. This is why joint fluid is sent for Gram stain and culture on all arthrocenteses of acute arthritis.

2. It is possible for a patient to have simultaneous gout and pseudogout. Although rare, this condition is easily diagnosed with careful polarized light microscopy.

3. Acute pseudogout in the wrist of an elderly person may cause a carpal tunnel syndrome. Any patient with carpal tunnel syndrome requires a careful history and physical.

4. Acute pseudogout is frequently precipitated by an urgent medical illness, such as myocardial infarction, or by a surgical procedure. Fluid shifts with fluctuations in serum calcium levels are thought to play a role in such attacks. An elderly hospitalized patient who complains of new joint pain should be investigated for pseudogout. Note that most patients with idiopathic pseudogout are older than 55–60 years old.

10. How is pseudogout treated?

The principles of treating acute pseudogout are the same as those for treating acute gout, although the disease is not as well studied.

1. In some cases, **thorough aspiration** of the affected joint with removal of the offending

CPPD crystals is said to halt the attack. Most rheumatologists would offer other therapy in addition to thorough aspiration.

2. **NSAIDs** in full doses are the next mode of therapy. **Idomethacin** can be administered in doses of 50 mg po three or four times a day for 1–2 days and then tapered as symptoms subside. Indomethacin is the classic treatment for acute crystalline arthritis, although other NSAIDs in full doses are just as effective. However, the population who suffers from pseudogout is often elderly with multiple chronic illnesses, such as renal insufficiency or peptic ulcer disease, which complicate the use of NSAIDs. It is always prudent to check a creatinine before starting an NSAID.

3. In the patient at risk for a side effect from NSAIDs, an option is **joint injection** with a long-acting corticosteroid preparation, such as **triamcinolone hexacetonide.** Triamcinolone hexacetonide is widely available in a 20-mg/ml solution. 20–40mg is injected into large joints, such as the knee or shoulder. Smaller joints, such as the wrist, may be treated with 10–20 mg. Local injection is the best method to provide prompt, complete relief of the attack with little risk of systemic adverse effect. Because the patients are elderly and concomitant medical conditions often preclude other options, local injection is my favorite treatment.

4. If the patient is not already on chronic steroid therapy for another problem, such as asthma, an intramuscular or intravenous injection of 40 U of **ACTH** provides relief of symptoms within 5 days. As in gout, ACTH is less likely to be helpful if the attack is well established (i.e., symptoms present for more than a few days).

5. In acute gout one or two im injections of 60 mg **triamcinolone acetonide** have been shown to be as effective as indomethacin. Our preliminary data suggests that this same dose is equally effective in acute pseudogout. This approach has been useful in hospitalized patients with contraindications to NSAIDs who decline local injection.

6. Oral **prednisone** is used for acute gout by some clinicians. This has not been studied in pseudogout but could be considered if intra-articular or intramuscular injection is not desirable, as in a patient with a bleeding diathesis. The patient is started on 40 mg of prednisone po daily, which is tapered to discontinue in 10–14 days. Of course, the side effects of any steroid preparation must be kept in mind, including the potential for temporarily worsening diabetic glucose control or exacerbating an infection.

7. Both oral and intravenous **colchicine** are known to interrupt acute pseudogout attacks, with intravenous colchicine being more effective. Colchicine is not favored by rheumatologists for pseudogout because it has significant potential toxicity in the elderly population affected, and the other therapies noted are well-tolerated.

8. As in any acute arthritis, **resting the affected joint** is helpful, with gradual resumption of normal activities as the attack subsides.

9. Polyarticular attacks of pseudogout may be managed with NSAIDs, any of the systemic steroid regimens noted, or colchicine.

11. Can any therapy prevent attacks of pseudogout from occurring?

Fortunately, most patients only have a few attacks, which are widely separated in time, and thus require no prophylaxis against pseudogout. For patients with frequent attacks, colchicine, 0.6 mg twice a day, prevents recurrences. Some rheumatologists use daily low doses of an NSAID for the same purpose, although there are no reported studies of this approach.

12. Does any treatment retard or reverse the deposition of CPPD which is causing the arthritis?

Unfortunately, there is no therapy to prevent the deposition of CPPD or remove the CPPD deposits already present. Patients with chronic arthropathy from CPPD, in the pseudo-osteoarthritis or pseudo-rheumatoid pattern, are managed like those with osteoarthritis—with physical therapy, NSAIDs, or analgesics.

13. What conditions are associated with CPPD deposition and need to be ruled out in a patient with CPPD deposition disease?

Disease Associations of CPPD Deposition

ASSOCIATION STRONG	ASSOCIATION LIKELY	ASSOCIATION POSSIBLE
Hyperparathyroidism (primary and secondary)	Osteoarthritis	Hypothyroidism
Hemochromatosis	Amyloidosis	Ochronosis
Hypomagnesemia	Bartter's syndrome (secondary to resulting hypomagnesemia)	Paget's disease
Hypophosphatasia		Wilson's disease
Aging	Benign hypermobility	Acromegaly
Familial/hereditary forms	Hypocalciuric hypercalcemia	Diabetes mellitus
Post-traumatic, including surgery		Post-radiation therapy
		True neuropathic joints
		Gout
		X-linked hypophosphatemic rickets

* Adapted from Moskowtiz RW: Deposition of calcium pyrophosphate or hydroxyapatite. In Kelley WN, et al (eds): Textbook of Rheumatology, 4th ed. Philadelphia, W.B. Saunders, 1993.

14. Describe the appropriate laboratory workup in a patient with newly diagnosed CPPD deposition disease.

Most cases of CPPD deposition are sporadic or associated with normal aging. If the CPPD deposition is severe, affects many joints, or the patient is younger than 55 years, it is reasonable to search for a metabolic cause. Evaluations must be individualized for persons older than 55 years with hyperparathyroidism a primary consideration. Recommend laboratory studies include:

Calcium	Ferritin
Magnesium	Iron
Phosphorus	Total iron binding capacity
Alkaline phosphatase	Thyroid stimulating hormone (controversial)

15. Can CPPD deposition disease be confused with rheumatoid arthritis?

Differentiating CPPD disease and RA can be difficult. Up to 5% of patients with CPPD arthritis have involvement of multiple joints, particularly the knees, wrists, and elbows, with chronic low-grade inflammation persisting for weeks or months. This is called the **pseudo-rheumatoid pattern** of CPPD deposition disease. Joint involvement may be symmetric, and systemic symptoms such as fatigue or morning stiffness are present. Physical examination reveals synovial thickening, loss of joint motion, and flexion contractures. The ESR may be elevated.

Ten percent of patients with CPPD disease will test positive for rheumatoid factor (RF), as will healthy elderly patients. Usually RF is present in low titers in such individuals. Higher titers of RF, more widespread synovitis, involvement of the hands and feet, and characteristic erosions distinguish true RA from pseudo-RA.

Before making a diagnosis of seronegative RA, or RA with only a low positive RF, it is prudent to consider the possibility of CPPD deposition disease by reviewing roentgenograms and clincal features and by aspirating a joint to examine synovial fluid for crystals if necessary. This approach is particularly important in middle-aged men because about a third of patients with hemochromatosis present with arthralgias, which may be CPPD-associated. It is also important to remember that true seropositve RA with erosions and CPPD deposition has been reported to exist in the same patient.

16. How do you distinguish a CPPD pseudo-neuropathic joint (or pseudo-Charcot joint) from a truly neuropathic joint?

One feature suggestive of a true **neuropathic joint** is pain present in lesser degree than might be suggested by the severity of the clinical or roentgenographic findings. Patients with true neuropathic joints have abnormal neurologic examinations, with impaired sensation including vibration and proprioception. Patients with **pseudo-Charcot joints** from CPPD deposition have normal pain perception. The distinction is important because patients with true neuropathic joints are generally not offered total joint arthroplasties, while patients with pseudo-neuropathic joints are. Interestingly, patients with tabes dorsalis seem more likely to develop true neuropathic joints if they have underlying CPPD deposition.

17. Do any features suggest that a patient has pseudo-osteoarthritis from CPPD deposition rather than typical osteoarthritis?

Pseudo-osteoarthritis is seen in around half of patients diagnosed with CPPD deposition disease. The pattern of joint involvement is different from that seen in other types of osteoarthritis. CPPD pseudo-osteoarthritis results in severe degenerative changes in the metacarpophalangeal joints, wrists, elbows, and shoulders, as well as the knees. Of these joints, only the knees are typically involved in primary osteoarthritis.

In primary osteoarthritis the medial compartment of the knee is more commonly involved, resulting in varus changes or "bow legs." Pseudo-osteoarthritis is more likely to affect the lateral compartment, causing bilateral or unilateral valgus changes or "knock knees." Isolated patellofemoral osteoarthritis is also a common presentation. Flexion contractures in these joints are also said to be characteristic of CPPD pseudo-osteoarthritis. Psuedo-osteoarthritis is more likely to be symmetric than in primary osteoarthritis. Up to 50% of pseudo-osteoarthritis patients also suffer recurrent episodes of acute pseudogout. Radiographs typically show chondrocalcinosis and exuberant osteophyte formation.

BIBLIOGRAPHY

1. Alloway JA, Moriarty MJ, Hoogland YT, Nashel DJ: Comparison of triamcinolone acetonide with indomethacin in the treatment of acute gouty arthritis. J Rheumatol 20:111–113, 1993.
2. Doherty M, Dieppe P: Clinical aspects of calcium pyrophosphate dihydrate crystal deposition. Rheum Dis Clin North Am 14:395–414, 1988.
3. Fam AG: Calcium pyrophosphate crystal deposition disease and other crystal deposition diseases. Curr Opin Rheumatol 4:574–582, 1992.
4. Jacobelli SG, McCarty DJ, Silcox DC, et al: Calcium pyrophosphate dihydrate crystal deposition in neuropathic joints: Four cases of polyarticular involvement. Ann Intern Med 79:340–347, 1973.
5. Jones AC, Chuck AJ, Arie EA, et al: Disease associated with calcium pyrophosphate deposition disease. Semin Arthritis Rheum 22(3):188–202, 1992.
6. Meed SD, Spillberg I: Successful use of colchicine in acute polyarticular pseudogout. J Rheumatol 8:689–691, 1981.
7. Moskowitz RW: Deposition of calcium pyrophosphate or hydroxyapatite. In Kelley WN, Harris ED, Ruddy S, Sledge CB (eds): Textbook of Rheumatology, 4th ed. Philadelphia, W.B. Saunders, 1993.
8. Pritzker KPH: Calcium pyrophosphate dihydrate crystal deposition and other crystal deposition diseases. Curr Opin Rheumatol 6:442–447, 1994.
9. Reginato AJ: Calcium pyrophosphate dihydrate gout and other crystal deposition disease. Curr Opin Rheumatol 3:676–683, 1991.
10. Ritter J, Kerr LD, Valeriano-Marcet J, Spiera H: ACTH revisited: Effective treatment for acute crystal induced synovitis in patients with multiple medical problems. J Rheumatol 21:696–699, 1994.
11. Ryan LM: Calcium pyrophosphate dihydrate crystal deposition and other crystal deposition diseases. Curr Opin Rheumatol 5:517–521, 1993.
12. Ryan LM, McCarty DJ: Calcium pyrophosphate crystal deposition disease; pseudogout; articular chondrocalcinosis. In McCarty DJ, Koopman WJ (eds.): Arthritis and Allied Conditions, 12th ed. Philadelphia, Lea & Febiger, 1993.

51. HYDROXYAPATITE AND OTHER CRYSTALLINE DISEASES

Matthew T. Carpenter, M.D.

1. Are the crystals that cause gout and pseudogout the only crystals seen in synovial fluid?
While monosodium urate crystals, which cause gout, and calcium pyrophosphate dihydrate (CPPD) crystals, which cause pseudogout, are the most commonly identified crystals in synovial fluid, many other crystals or particles may be encountered during polarized light microscopy. Some of these crystals cause disease, and some are just interesting incidental findings.

Crystals and Particles Seen in Synovial Fluid

Monosodium urate crystals	Starch from examination gloves
Calcium pyrophosphate dihydrate (CPPD) crystals	Cholesterol crystals
Calcium hydroxyapatite crystals (and other	Lipid droplets
basic calcium phosphate crystals)	Foreign organic matter (e.g., plant thorns)
Calcium oxalate crystals	Metallic fragments from prosthetic joints
Injectable corticosteroid crystals	

2. What is calcium hydroxyapatite?
Calcium hydroxyapatite ($Ca_5(PO_4)_3 \cdot 2H_2O$) is a calcium-containing mineral found in bone. Hydroxyapatite and several other calcium-containing minerals may be found in soft tissue and tendon calcifications or in some forms of arthritis. Collectively, these calcium-containing minerals are referred to as **basic calcium phosphate** (BCP).

3. Do BCP crystals cause arthritis?
There are three groups of joint-related problems in which BCP may play a role:
Calcific tendinitis
Acute calcific periarthritis
BCP arthropathy (e.g., Milwaukee shoulder syndrome)
In acute calcific periarthritis, the BCP crystals are thought to cause the pain and swelling, much like monosodium urate crystals do in gout. In calcific tendinitis, it is not as clear whether the BCP crystals are the cause of the tendinitis or whether the BCP is deposited as a reaction to chronic strain in a poorly vascularized area. BCP deposition in the soft tissues also occurs in the calcinosis syndromes seen in systemic sclerosis and dermatomyositis.

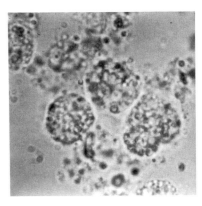

Aggregates of BCP crystals seen in neutrophils under light microscopy.

4. How are BCP crystals identified if they are suspected of causing a joint problem?

Identification of BCP crystals is difficult. If characteristic calcifications are observed on roentgenograms, BCP is often presumed to be the cause of symptoms. Aspiration of a calcific deposit may yield material that looks like toothpaste. Individual BCP crystals are so small that they cannot be seen. Ordinary light microscopy may reveal aggregated BCP crystals with an appearance described as "shiny coins."

BCP crystals are not birefringent and so are not seen on polarized light microscopy. Special stains, such as alizarin red, will confirm the presence of calcium in the aspirated material but are not widely available to clinicians and are not specific for BCP. Precise crystal identification requires techniques such as transmission electron microscopy, available only in large referral hospitals and not practical for the clinician.

5. Where is calcific tendinitis most often seen?

BCP deposition is common in the shoulder. Up to 5% of shoulder roentgenograms in adults will have periarticular calcium deposits, usually in the supraspinatus tendon. Tendons around other joints may also be affected.

6. Are such calcifications symptomatic?

Frequently, BCP deposits are noted as incidental findings. In the case of the supraspinatus tendon of the rotator cuff, the calcification is noted when a patient has a roentgenogram for symptoms of bursitis or impingement. The calcification may in fact be a *result* of chronic tendinitis rather than the cause.

7. How do you treat calcific tendinitis?

Of course, asymptomatic BCP deposits require no therapy. Patients with symptoms of bursitis or tendinitis are managed conservatively, with physical therapy and NSAIDs. Local injection with a short-acting corticosteroid such as betamethasone should be used sparingly, as steroids may promote calcification in the long-term. Occasionally, using a needle to disrupt the calcification causes more rapid dissolution of the deposit, by stimulating phagocytosis of the BCP. Surgical or arthroscopic debridement of very large or severely symptomatic calcific deposits may be necessary.

8. What is acute calcific periarthritis?

When BCP crystals are shed from a calcific deposit, there is an intense local inflammatory reaction to the crystals, similar to other crystalline arthritides. If this occurs around a joint, the clinical picture is an acute arthritis with pain, warmth, loss of motion, and swelling. Roentgenograms reveal the BCP deposit and thus identify the crystal causing the problem.

In young women, acute calcific periarthritis can occur in the first metatarsal phalangeal (MTP) joint, causing podagra identical to that seen in gout. It may be distinguished from gout by

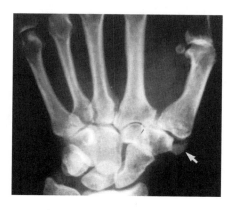

Amorphous homogeneous calcium deposits of BCP seen near the first CMC joint (*arrow*).

the premenopausal status of the patient, the absence of monosodium urate crystals in synovial fluid, and the characteristic calcifications around the joint on roentgenogram. This particular type of acute periarthritis is called **hydroxyapatite pseudopodagra.** Attacks of calcific periarthritis can occur in the setting of calcific tendinitis in the shoulder or other joints, either spontaneously or after trauma. Symptoms subside over several weeks, either spontaneously or with treatment. Interestingly, the calcific deposit may dissolve during the acute attack, leading to disappearance of calcification on followup roentgenograms.

9. Is any treatment for acute calcific periarthritis available?
Attacks of calcific periarthritis may be managed similarly to other crystalline arthritides. NSAIDs given in full doses are the mainstay of therapy. For acute crystalline arthritis, indomethacin 50 mg po four times daily for 1–2 days, followed by tapering doses, is the classic approach. Other NSAIDs are probably just as effective. The age of the patient, underlying renal disease (which may be occult in the elderly), and history of peptic ulcer disease are full factors that enter into the decision on whether to use NSAIDs. Colchicine, either oral or intravenous, is reported to be successful for acute calcific periarthritis. Aspiration of the joint with injection of a corticosteroid is often the most expedient way to provide relief. I favor triamcinolone hexacetonide for intra-articular injections and betamethasone for soft tissue injections.

10. How does Milwaukee shoulder syndrome (BCP-associated arthropathy) present?
Milwaukee shoulder syndrome is characterized by severe degenerative arthritis of the glenohumeral joint, with loss of the rotator cuff, associated with the presence of BCP crystals. Often, large joint effusions are present on physical examination. Patients with Milwaukee shoulder syndrome are usually women in their 70s. Bilateral shoulder involvement is common, with the dominant side more severely affected.

Symptoms vary from minimally symptomatic with shoulder motion to severe pain at rest. Physical examination reveals reduced active and passive range of motion with glenohumeral crepitus. Synovial fluid, which often has streaks of blood, is noninflammatory with few WBCs. Roentgenograms show severe osteoarthritis of the glenohumeral joint associated with upward migration of the head of the humerus, indicating a defect in the rotator cuff. Soft tissue calcifications may also be present.

BCP arthropathy can affect other joints as well, particularly the knees and hips. Lateral compartment joint-space loss in the knees distinguishes this from primary osteoarthritis, similar to CPPD-associated arthropathy.

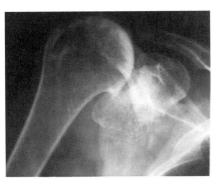

Milwaukee shoulder. Note upward migration of humeral head indicating rotator cuff tear.

11. How do you treat Milwaukee shoulder syndrome?
Treatment can be unsatisfactory. Some patients do well with a daily low-dose of NSAIDs. Local heat is frequently beneficial. If large effusions are present, repeated arthrocenteses sometimes re-

lieve symptoms. Joint usage needs to be reduced for severe symptoms. At the same time, physical therapy is vital to maintain range of motion and strengthen surrounding muscles. Surgical intervention may be considered for advanced degenerative changes.

12. Describe the appearance and clinical presentation of other crystals in synovial fluid.

- **Calcium oxalate crystals** are characteristically bipyramidal in appearance. They occur in effusions from patients with primary oxalosis or end-stage renal disease. Ascorbic acid is metabolized to oxalate, so dialysis patients taking ascorbate supplements are prone to this condition.
- **Cholesterol crystals** are found in synovial fluid from *chronic* joint effusions, usually rheumatoid arthritis. The crystals are square and plate-like with a single notched corner. Cholesterol crystals are beautifully birefringent, both positively and negatively. They do not cause inflammation. They are a sign of a chronic inflammatory effusion and form from the cholesterol in the neutrophils' cell membranes after they break down in the joint.
- **Steroid crystals** in synovial fluid may be confused with CPPD crystals because they are often small, irregularly shaped or rectangular, and weakly birefringent. Intracellular steroid crystals in synovial fluid are not uncommon. Careful polarized microscopy is necessary because steroid crystals may be positively or negatively birefringent (often both types are seen in the same field), whereas CPPD crystals are always weakly positively birefringent. The patient will also have an antecedent history of joint injection with a corticosteroid, possibly weeks earlier. Patients sometimes do not volunteer this information, so a specific question about previous joint injection must be asked.
- **Talc (or starch) particles** from examination gloves are a common artifact during preparation of synovial fluid slides. They resemble little beach balls when viewed with polarized light microscopy.

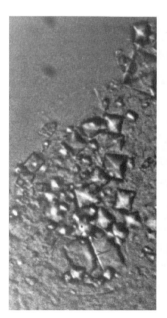 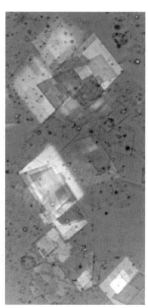 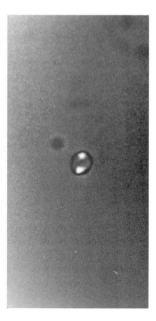

Other synovial fluid crystals. *Left,* Calcium oxalate crystals have a characteristic bipyramidal shape under ordinary light microscopy. (Courtesy of The Upjohn Company.) *Center,* Plane-shaped cholesterol crystals are strongly birefringent when viewed under polarized light microscopy. These crystals were obtained from aspiration of a knee effusion in a patient with rheumatoid arthritis. (Courtesy of Linda Sakai, M.D.) *Right,* Starch (talc) from examination gloves is a common artifact during slide preparation. (Courtesy of The Upjohn Company.)

• **Lipid droplets** have a "Maltese cross" appearance under polarized light microscopy. Lipid droplets in synovial fluid may represent a subchondral fracture or may be seen occasionally in medical conditions, including pancreatitis. Lipid droplets look like starch particles, although the size of starch particles is more variable.

There are many other types of particles or contaminants that can appear in synovial fluid, such as glass fragments from cover slips or specks of cartilage, so all synovial fluids must be examined carefully!

BIBLIOGRAPHY

 1. Dieppe P: Apatites and miscellaneous crystals. In Schumacher HR (ed): Primer on the Rheumatic Diseases, 10th ed. Atlanta, The Arthritis Foundation, 1993.
 2. Fam AG, Stein J: Hydroxyapatite pseudopodagra in young women. J Rheumatol 19:662–664, 1992.
 3. Fam AG: Calcium pyrophosphate crystal deposition and other crystal deposition disease. Curr Opin Rheumatol 4(4):574–582, 1992.
 4. Halverson PB, Carrera GF, McCarty DJ: Milwaukee shoulder syndrome: Fifteen additional cases and a description of contributing factors. Arch Intern Med 150:677–682, 1990.
 5. Halverson PB, McCarty DJ: Basic calcium phosphate (apatite, octacalcium phosphate, tricalcium phosphate) crystal deposition diseases. In McCarty DJ, Koopman WJ (eds): Arthritis and Allied Conditions, 12th ed. Philadelphia, Lea & Febiger, 1993.
 6. Halverson PB, McCarty DJ: Clinical aspects of basic calcium phosphate crystal deposition. Rheum Dis Clin North Am 14:427–439, 1988.
 7. Moskowitz RW: Diseases associated with deposition of calcium pyrophosphate or hydroxyapatite. In Kelley WN, Harris ED, Ruddy S, Sledge CB (eds): Textbook of Rheumatology, 4th ed. Philadelphia, W.B. Saunders, 1993.
 8. Pritzker KPH: Calcium pyrophosphate dihydrate crystal deposition and other crystal deposition diseases. Curr Opin Rheumatol 6:442–447, 1994.
 9. Reginato AJ: Calcium pyrophosphate dihydrate gout and other crystal deposition diseases. Curr Opin Rheumatol 3:676–683, 1991.
10. Ryan LM: Calcium pyrophosphate dihydrate crystal deposition and other crystal deposition diseases. Curr Opin Rheumatol 5(4):517–521, 1993.
11. Schumacher HR, Reginato AJ: Atlas of Synovial Fluid Analysis and Crystal Identification. Philadelphia, Lea & Febiger, 1991.

52. ENDOCRINE-ASSOCIATED ARTHROPATHIES

Edmund H. Hornstein, D.O.

1. What signs or symptoms should prompt a search for an occult endocrinopathy?
Entrapment neuropathy, particularly carpal tunnel syndrome
Calcium pyrophosphate dihydrate (CPPD) arthropathy
Diffuse myalgia with or without muscle weakness
Raynaud's phenomenon

2. Which endocrine diseases have well-described rheumatologic manifestations associated with them?

Diabetes mellitus   Hyperparathyroidism
Hypothyroidism   Acromegaly
Hyperthyroidism   Cushing's syndrome
Hypoparathyroidism

DIABETES MELLITUS

3. What rheumatologic syndromes are more common in patients with diabetes mellitus?
- Intrinsic complications of diabetes mellitus
  Diabetic hand syndrome of limited joint mobility (diabetic cheirarthropathy)
  Neuropathic arthropathy (Charcot joint) and diabetic osteolysis
  Diabetic amyotrophy
- Conditions with increased incidence in diabetes mellitus
  Periarthritis of the shoulder (frozen shoulder)
  Reflex sympathetic dystrophy (shoulder-hand syndrome)
  Flexor tenosynovitis
  Dupuytren's contractures
  Carpal tunnel syndrome
  Diffuse idiopathic skeletal hyperostosis (DISH)
  Septic joint/osteomyelitis

4. How does the diabetic hand syndrome of limited joint mobility (LJM) present?
This syndrome, also known as diabetic cheirarthropathy, presents with the insidious development of flexion contractures involving the small joints of the hands, starting with the distal (DIPs) and proximal interphalangeal joints (PIPs) and moving proximally over time. This condition occurs in both insulin-dependent (IDDM) and non-insulin-dependent (NIDDM) diabetics and correlates with disease duration, glucose control, and renal/retinal microvascular disease. It may be seen in as many as 30–50% of long-term diabetics.

The "prayer sign" observed on physical examination reflects the inability to fully extend the joints of the fingers (see figure). These finger contractures are attributed to excessive dermal collagen and collagen crosslinks, as well as to increased dermal hydration resulting in indurated and thickened skin around the joints. This condition can be confused with scleroderma. Laboratory serologies and hand radiographs are unremarkable. Treatment is physical therapy and control of the underlying diabetes. Contractures usually progress slowly but rarely limit function significantly.

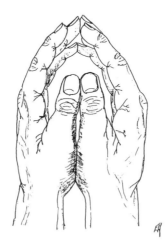

Prayer sign in a patient with LJM due to diabetes mellitus.

5. Discuss the relationship between Charcot joint and diabetes mellitus.
Charcot joint occurs in < 1% of all diabetics. It occurs in both males and females with equal frequency. Most patients (> 66%) are over age 40 and have had long-standing (> 10 yrs), poorly

controlled diabetes complicated by a diabetic peripheral neuropathy. Patients present with pain-less swelling and deformity usually of the foot (most commonly tarsometatarsal joints) and an-kle, although knee, hip, and spine can be involved. With progression of disease, the patient can develop "rocker bottom" feet due to midtarsal collapse. Skin over bony prominences can ulcer-ate and become infected without the patient's knowledge due to abnormal sensation resulting from their neuropathy.

Radiographs frequently show severe abnormalities characterized by the **5 Ds:** destruction, density (increased), debris, disorganization, and dislocation (see figure). The increased density and sharp margins of the bony debris help separate a Charcot joint from infection. Treatment in-cludes protected weight-bearing, soft casts, good shoes, and aggressive treatment and prevention of skin ulcerations. Charcot joints, however, usually progress. There is no role for surgery (fu-sion, arthroplasty) other than amputation for severe cases. Diabetes mellitus has replaced neu-rosyphilis as the most common cause of a Charcot joint today.

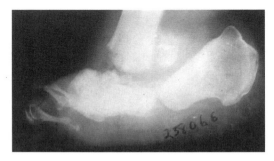

Charcot joints of foot and ankle.

6. What is diabetic osteolysis?
Diabetic osteolysis is a condition specifically occurring in diabetics. The osteolysis is character-ized by osteoporosis and variable degrees of resorption of distal metatarsal bones and proximal phalanges. Pain is variable. Radiographs have a characteristic "licked candy" appearance. The pathogenesis is unclear, as this syndrome can occur at any time during the course of diabetes. The major disease to rule out is infection. Treatment is conservative and includes protected weight-bearing. The process may terminate at any stage and in some cases may completely resolve.

7. How does diabetic amyotrophy present?
Diabetic amyotrophy present with severe pain and dysesthesias involving most commonly the proximal muscles of the pelvis and thigh. The condition may be bilateral in 50% of cases. Anorexia, weight loss, and unsteady gait due to muscle wasting and weakness may be seen. The typical patient is 50–60-year-old man with well-controlled, mild NIDDM of several years' dura-tion, although it can be the presenting sign of diabetes. Usually the patient has no evidence of di-abetic retinopathy or nephropathy but may have a distal symmetric sensory neuropathy.

Laboratory evaluation is usually unremarkable except for an elevated CSF protein. Elec-tromyography/nerve conduction velocity (EMG/NCV) testing demonstrates changes compatible with a neuropathy, and muscle biopsy shows muscle fiber atrophy without an inflammatory infil-trate. The etiology is unclear but may be due to an acute femoral mononeuritis. Treatment includes pain control and physical therapy. Over 50% recover within 3–18 months, although some patients progress or have recurrent episodes.

8. What is diabetic periarthritis of the shoulder?
Diabetic periarthritis of the shoulder is also known as **frozen shoulder** or **adhesive capsulitis.** It occurs in 10–33% of diabetics and is five times more common in diabetics than in nondiabetics.

The typical patient is female with NIDDM of long duration who presents with diffuse soreness and global loss of motion of the shoulder. Up to 50% of patients have bilateral involvement, although the nondominant shoulder is frequently more severely involved. Laboratory studies and radiographs are unremarkable. Treatment includes NSAIDs, rarely intra-articular steroids, and vigorous physical therapy to improve range of motion. For unclear reasons, this syndrome may spontaneously remit after weeks to months.

9. The shoulder-hand syndrome can be a complication of frozen shoulder. What is it?
When a frozen shoulder is accompanied by vasomotor changes of reflex sympathetic dystrophy, it is known as shoulder-hand syndrome. (See Chapter 69).

10. How commonly does flexor tenosynovitis or Dupuytren's contractures occur in patients with diabetes mellitus?
   Flexor tenosynovitis occurs in 5–33% of diabetic patients. Females with long-standing diabetes are more commonly affected than male. Patients complain of aching and stiffness in the palmar aspect of the hand. Symptoms are worse in the morning. A "trigger" finger may occur due to an inflammatory nodule getting caught in the proximal pulley at the base of the finger. The thumb of the dominant hand is most commonly involved (75%), although multiple fingers on both hands can be affected. Laboratory findings and radiographs are unremarkable. Treatment includes NSAIDs, local steroid injections, or surgery.
   Dupuytren's contractures occur in 33–60% of patients with IDDM. Patients present with nodular thickening of the palmar fascia, leading to flexion contractures usually of the fourth and fifth digits. Patients usually have long-standing diabetes, although there is no association with control of the diabetes. The pathogenesis is thought to be due to contractile myofibroblasts producing increased collagen secondary to microvascular ischemia. Treatment includes NSAIDs, physical therapy, vitamin E, local steroid injections, and rarely surgery.

11. What is the relationship between diabetes mellitus and carpal tunnel syndrome?
Carpal tunnel syndrome (CTS) commonly occurs in diabetic patients. Up to 15% of all patients with CTS will have diabetes. Patients present with numbness in the median nerve distribution. Nocturnal paresthesias, hand pain, and pain radiating to the elbow or shoulder (Valleix phenomenon) can also occur. Tinel's and Phalen's signs may be positive. Thenar atrophy is a late sign and indicates muscle denervation. The neuropathy may be from extrinsic compression or due to microvascular disease causing vasa nervorum ischemia. Treatment includes splints, NSAIDs, diuretics, local steroid injections into the carpal tunnel, and surgical decompression (See also Chapter 66).

12. What is DISH? How commonly does it occur in diabetes mellitus?
DISH is diffuse idiopathic skeletal hyperostosis, also known as Forestier's disease. It occurs in up to 20% of NIDDM patients who are typically obese and over age 50. Patients present with neck and back stiffness associated with loss of motion. Pain is not prominent. Radiographs are diagnostic and consist of at least four vertebrae fused together due to ossification of the anterior longitudinal ligament. Disc spaces, apophyseal joints, and sacroiliac joints are normal, helping to separate it from osteoarthritis and ankylosing spondylitis. Treatment is usually NSAIDs and physical therapy. (See Chapter 55).

13. What diabetes-associated rheumatologic syndromes have features in common with scleroderma?
   • The syndrome of limited joint mobility in which findings in the fingers are reminiscent of the sclerodactyly seen in the CREST syndrome
   • Scleroderma diabeticorum, also known as scleredema adultorum or Buschke scleredema, occurs as thickened, edematous areas of skin most commonly on the upper back and neck

THYROID DISEASE

14. Describe the arthropathy associated with severe hypothyroidism.

Myxedematous arthropathy usually affects large joints such as the knees. The patient presents with swelling and stiffness. Synovial thickening, ligamentous laxity, and effusions with a characteristic slow fluid wave (bulge sign) are common. The synovial fluid is noninflammatory with an increased viscosity giving a string sign of 1–2 ft instead of the normal 1–2 inches. Radiographs are typically normal.

Osteonecrosis can also occur (controversial). In adults, it typically involves the hip or tibial plateau. In children, abnormal epiphyseal ossification may occur, which can be confused with epiphyseal dysplasia or juvenile avascular necrosis (Legg-Calvé-Perthes disease) of the hip.

15. What other common rheumatologic syndromes are associated with hypothyroidism?
Think of **TRAP:**

     T—Tunnel (carpal) syndrome (7% of hypothyroid patients)
     R—Raynaud's phenomenon
     A—Aching muscles with findings indistinguishable from those of fibromyalgia
     P—Proximal muscle weakness and stiffness with an elevated creatine kinase

Although chondrocalcinosis has also been described, it probably does not occur more commonly than in age-matched controls.

16. What is the relationship between Hashimoto's thyroiditis and other collagen vascular diseases?
Hashimoto's thyroiditis occurs with increased frequency in several collagen vascular diseases. It has been described in SLE, Sjögren's, and rheumatoid arthritis, as well as mixed connective tissue disease, scleroderma, and polymyositis. The increased prevalence of HLA-B8, DR3 in patients with Hashimoto's thyroiditis accounts for its occurring with diseases that have similar HLA associations. Any patient with a collagen vascular disease should be followed closely for development of hypothyroid symptoms.

17. Which rheumatic problems occur in patients with hyperthyroidism?

     Thyroid acropachy
     Painless proximal muscle weakness (70% of hyperthyroid patients)
     Osteoporosis
     Adhesive capsulitis of the shoulders (controversial)

18. Describe thyroid acropachy.
Thyroid acropachy is a rare complication of Grave's disease consisting of soft tissue swelling of the hands, digital clubbing, and periostitis particularly involving the metacarpal and phalangeal

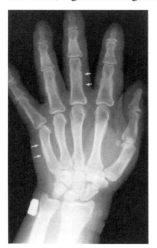

Thyroid acropachy. Note the periosteal reaction along shafts of the metacarpals and phalanges (*arrows*).

bones. Radiographs are characteristic (see figure). The symptoms usually occur after the patient becomes euthyroid. Pain is variable but usually mild. There is no effective therapy.

19. How do you differentiate hyperthyroid myopathy from the myopathies of hypothyroidism and idiopathic inflammatory myopathy (polymyositis)?

	TSH	T4	CK	PROXIMAL WEAKNESS	MUSCLE BIOPSY
Inflammatory myopathy	Normal	Normal	Increased	Mild-severe	Inflammation
Hypothyroidism	Increased	Decreased	Increased	Usually mild	Normal
Hyperthyroidism	Decreased	Increased	Normal	Usually mild	Normal

TSH, thyroid-stimulating hormone; T4, thyroxine; CK, creatine kinase.

PARATHYROID DISEASE

20. List the rheumatic syndromes associated with primary hyperparathyroidism.
- Painless proximal muscle weakness with normal muscle enzymes but a myopathic or neuropathic EMG
- Chondrocalcinosis with pseudogout attacks usually due to CPPD crystals
- Osteogenic synovitis due to subchondral bony collapse from thinning of bone (leading to osteoarthritis)
- Osteoporosis
- Ectopic soft-tissue calcifications

21. What are the skeletal ramifications of primary hyperparathyroidism?
Osteitis fibrosa cystica represents the classic sequela of prolonged hyperparathyroidism and is diagnosed by x-ray findings that are most prominent in the hands. Subperiosteal resorption with a blurring of the cortical margins is seen, accompanied by a decrease in bone diameter and resorption of the tufts of the distal phalanges (figure). **Diffuse osteopenia** is common and erosions may be seen in the joints of the hands and at the ends of the clavicles. Discrete lytic lesions due to focal aggregates of osteoclastic giant cells and fibrous tissue with decomposing blood may occur and are known as **brown tumors.** Spinal compression fractures are common.

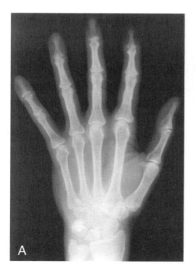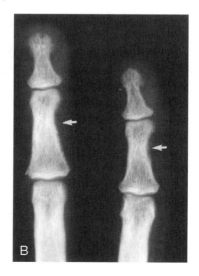

A, Radiograph of hand of a patient with hyperparathyroidism. *B*, Closeup of phalanges demonstrating subperiosteal resorption (arrows).

The full blown osteitis fibrosis cystica of primary hyperparathyroidism has become less common now that the diagnosis of this disorder is often made by the discovery of asymptomatic hypercalcemia on routine serum chemistry screen.

22. What is the relationship between chondrocalcinosis and primary hyperparathyroidism?
Up to 15% of patients with chondrocalcinosis will be found to have primary hyperparathyroidism. Conversely, over 50% of patients with long-standing primary hyperparathyroidism will have radiographic evidence of chondrocalcinosis.

23. What is the knuckle, knuckle, dimple, knuckle sign?
Patients with pseudo- and pseudo-pseudo-hypoparathyroidism may have a skeletal deformity with a short fourth metacarpal. When they clench their hand to form a fist, a dimple appears where the fourth knuckle should be, emphasizing the short fourth metacarpal bone. These patients also will have short stature and may have ectopic calcifications around weight-bearing joints.

ACROMEGALY

24. How often does arthropathy occur in acromegaly?
It is common and may be seen in up to 74% of affected patients. Degenerative disease is the most common manifestation, and crepitus on exam the most common finding. The knees, shoulders, hips, lumbosacral spine, and cervical spine are the most frequently symptomatic areas, but the hands reveal the most characteristic radiographic changes.

25. List the radiographic findings in the hands of patients with acromegaly.

Soft-tissue thickening	Deformation of epiphyses with squaring of
Enlarged terminal phalanx (spade-like)	phalanges
Increased joint space	Chondrocalcinosis (rare)
Periosteal apposition of tubular bones	

Acromegaly of the hand

26. What other rheumatologic syndromes may accompany acromegaly?
Carpal tunnel syndrome (up to 50% of patients)
Proximal muscle weakness with normal EMG and normal muscle enzymes
Raynaud's phenomenon (up to 33% of patients)
Chondrocalcinosis (rare)

CUSHING'S SYNDROME

27. List the rheumatic syndromes associated with excessive glucocorticoids.

Proximal muscle weakness	Osteoporosis
Osteonecrosis	Steroid withdrawal syndrome

28. Describe the myopathy seen with excessive glucocorticoids.
Proximal muscle weakness without muscle enzyme elevations can be seen in patients with Cushing's syndrome or in patients receiving > 10 mg of prednisone a day. EMG findings are usually normal or nonspecific. Muscle biopsy can show type 2b muscle fiber atrophy which is nonspecific and can be seen with disuse atrophy. Patients should be treated with physical therapy, as muscle-strengthening exercises may delay the onset or improve this myopathy.

29. What is the minimal dose of prednisone a person can take daily and not develop clinically significant osteoporosis?
This is controversial. Clearly, 10 mg of prednisone (or greater) a day will cause osteoporosis. Prednisone doses of 5 mg/day or less usually do not cause significant osteoporosis.

30. What is the steroid withdrawal syndrome?
This syndrome, sometimes called Slocumb's syndrome, is characterized by myalgias, arthralgias, and lethargy following too rapid a taper of corticosteroids. Sometimes patients can develop noninflammatory joint effusions, particularly in the knees. Low-grade fevers occasionally occur. This withdrawal syndrome can be confused with reactivation of the primary disease for which the corticosteroids were used. Increasing the corticosteroids, tapering the steroids more slowly, and using NSAIDs can all help the symptoms.

BIBLIOGRAPHY

1. Bland JH, Frymoyer JW, Newberg AH, et al: Rheumatic syndromes in endocrine disease. Semin Arthritis Rheum 9(1):23–65, 1979.
2. Brick JE, Brick JF, Elnicki DM: Musculoskeletal disorders: When are they caused by hormone imbalance? Postgrad Med 90(6):129–132, 1991.
3. De Ceulaer K: Bone and joint abnormalities in thyroid disorders. In Klippel JH, Dieppe PA (eds): Slide Atlas of Rheumatology. St. Louis, Mosby, 1994, sect 7, unit 2, pp 19.1–19.2.
4. Dixon RB, Christy NP: On the various forms of corticosteroid withdrawal syndrome. Am J Med 68:224–230, 1980.
5. Dorwart BB: Arthropathies associated with endocrine diseases. In Schumacher HR (ed): Primer on the Rheumatic Diseases, 10th ed. Atlanta, Arthritis Foundation, 1993, pp 242–243.
6. Forgacs SS: Acromegaly. In Klippel JH, Dieppe PA (eds): Slide Atlas of Rheumatology. St. Louis, Mosby, 1994, sect 7, unit 2, pp 17.1–17.6.
7. Forgacs SS: Diabetes mellitus. In Klippel JH, Dieppe PA (eds): Slide Atlas of Rheumatology. St. Louis, Mosby, 1994, sect 7, unit 2, pp 20.1–20.6.
8. Gray RG, Gottlieb NL: Rheumatic disorders associated with diabetes mellitus: Literature review. Semin Arthritis Rheum 6(1):19–34, 1976.
9. Hordon LD, Wright V: Endocrine disease. Curr Opin Rheumatol 5:85–89, 1993.
10. Lieberman SA, Bjorkengren AG, Hoffman AR: Rheumatologic and skeletal changes in acromegaly. Endocrinol Metab Clin North Am 21:615–631, 1992.
11. McGuire JL: The endocrine system and connective tissue disorders. Bull Rheum Dis 39(4):1–8, 1990.
12. McGuire JL, and Lambert RE: Arthropathies associated with endocrine disorders. In Kelley WK, Harris ED, Ruddy S, Sledge CB (eds): Textbook of Rheumatology, 4th ed. Philadelphia, W.B. Saunders, 1993, pp 1527–1540.
13. Pirisien M, Silverberg SJ, Shane E, et al: Bone disease in primary hyperparathyroidism. Endocrinol Metab Clin North Am 19:19–34, 1990.
14. Shagan BP, Friedman SA: Raynaud's phenomenon in hypothyroidism. Angiology 27:19–25, 1976.
15. Shagan BP, Friedman SA: Raynaud's phenomenon and thyroid deficiency. Arch Intern Med 140:832–833, 1980.
16. Turken SA, Cafferty M, Silverberg SJ, et al: Neuromuscular involvement in mild asymptomatic primary hyperparathyroidism. Am J Med 87:553–557, 1989.

53. ARTHROPATHIES ASSOCIATED WITH HEMATOLOGIC DISEASES

Matthew T. Carpenter, M.D.

1. What is a hemarthrosis?

Hemarthrosis is defined as extravasation of blood into a joint or its synovial cavity. The diagnosis may be readily apparent in the setting of hemophilia, but in other circumstances it is less clear. Streaks of blood, as opposed to the uniformly bloody fluid of a hemarthrosis, may be seen in the synovial fluid during routine arthrocentesis because of needle trauma to skin or other periarticular structures. Blood that appears in the synovial fluid at the end of an arthrocentesis is also because of trauma, particularly if the initial synovial fluid was not bloody. During an arthrocentesis, if frankly bloody fluid is seen initially on entering the joint, hemarthrosis must be suspected. The best option is to withdraw the needle and re-enter the joint at another site. If the original arthrocentesis was traumatic, synovial fluid obtained from the new site should become clear or be only blood-tinged. If diffusely bloody synovial fluid is seen again, hemarthrosis is likely. If you are still uncertain, check a hematocrit on the bloody synovial fluid. A hematocrit similar to peripheral blood is more likely from a traumatic arthrocentesis, whereas fluid from a hemarthrosis has a hematocrit less than peripheral blood.

2. What are causes of hemarthrosis?

Causes of Hemarthrosis

Trauma	**Miscellaneous**
Injury with or without fracture	Scurvy
Postsurgical	Sickle cell disease and other hemoglobinopathies
Post arthrocentesis	Myeloproliferative diseases with thrombocytosis
Bleeding disorders	Munchausen's syndrome
Hemophilia	Acute septic arthritis
Von Willebrand's disease	Lyme disease
Thrombocytopenia	Arteriovenous fistula
Excessive anticoagulation	Ruptured aneurysm
Thrombolytic therapy for myocardial infarction	Charcot arthropathy
Disorder of connective tissue	Gaucher's disease
Ehlers-Danlos syndrome	Amyloid arthropathy
Pseudoxanthoma elasticum	Acute crystalline arthritis
Tumors	Post dialysis
Pigmented villonodular synovitis	
Tumors metastatic to joints	
Secondary tumors of synovium	
Hemangiomas	

Adapted from Gatter RA, Schumacher HR: A Practical Handbook of Joint Fluid Analysis. Philadelphia, Lea & Febiger, 1991.

Any condition causing intense inflammation will cause synovial vessels to be congested and friable, predisposing patients to hemarthrosis after seemingly insiginificant trauma.

3. Is it safe to do arthrocentesis when a patient has a prolonged prothrombin time from warfarin therapy?

If a patient on warfarin develops an acute monarthritis, diagnostic aspiration is warranted, even if the prothombin time is excessively prolonged. Some authorities report that reversal of anticoagulation is not necessary if proper technique is carefully observed and an appropriately small gauge needle is used. However, bleeding into the joint may occur following such arthrocenteses. Caution should be observed, particularly in large joints where it is difficult to apply direct pressure, like the shoulder or knee. There are no specific published guidelines for reversal of anticoagulation before arthrocentesis. Small doses of vitamin K, 1–2 mg, given intravenously have been noted to reverse rapidly the effects of warfarin to allow surgical interventions where significant bleeding is not expected; however, this has not been studied for arthrocentesis.

4. What can be done for hemarthrosis in the setting of warfarin therapy?

Spontaneous hemarthrosis in the setting of warfarin therapy is uncommon, and almost always occurs with a prothombin time prolonged ≥2.5 times control. The knee is the most commonly affected joint. Typically, there is an underlying arthritis in the joint, such as osteoarthritis, which may be occult. The affected joint is rested. Ice may be applied and analgesia provided with acetaminophen or narcotics. Symptoms usually subside spontaneously if the prothrombin time is reduced from supratherapeutic to simply therapeutic. If the patient's underlying condition permits, complete reversal of anticoagulation will hasten recovery. Occasionally, an intra-articular injection of triamcinolone hexacetonide will be needed to control symptoms. Chronic destructive arthritis resulting from warfarin therapy has been reported.

5. Are there any rheumatologic manifestations of hemophilia?

- Acute hemarthrosis
- Subacute or chronic arthropathy
- End-stage arthropathy
- Intramuscular or soft-tissue hemorrhage (may cause pseudotumor or compartment syndrome)
- Septic arthritis

6. How does acute hemarthrosis present in a patient with hemophilia?

Prodromal symptoms of stiffness or warmth occur in the affected joint. As the joint capsule distends, severe pain follows with swelling from effusion and decreased range of motion. The swelling will eventually tamponade the bleeding, and the hemarthrosis will gradually resolve over a matter of days to weeks. Almost all patients with severe hemophilia (<5% of normal factor activity) will have recurrent hemarthroses spontaneously or following minor trauma. If factor levels are >5% of normal, hemarthroses tend to be less frequent or occur following more significant trauma. Hemarthroses first begin to occur in weight-bearing joints when a child is just learning to walk.

7. How do you treat an acute hemarthrosis in a patient with hemophilia?

Treatment consists of placing the joint at rest in as much extension as can be tolerated, with applications of ice packs and other local measures. Analgesics are given for pain. Glucocorticoids have been advocated by some authors. Arthrocentesis, after appropriate factor replacement, may help relieve symptoms.

The mainstay of therapy for acute hemarthrosis in hemophilia is rapid replacement of deficient factor to achieve a level of ≥30%. A useful rule of thumb is that each IU of factor VIII or IX infused per kilogram of body weight causes a rise in factor levels by 2% or 2 IU/dl. More specific information on factor replacement has recently been published. Therapy can be promptly instituted by the family at the first symptoms of hemarthrosis to decrease the risks of sequelae. Patient education and involvement are critical for the success of any treatment program.

8. When should a septic arthritis be suspected if a hemophiliac develops an acute monarthritis?

If the pain of a suspected hemarthrosis fails to improve after factor replacement, concomitant septic arthritis must be suspected and aspiration of the joint becomes mandatory.

Diagnostic Clues for Septic Arthritis Coexisting with Hemarthrosis

Failure of joint pain to resolve with factor replacement	Previous arthrocentesis in the same joint
Fever >38°C	Presence of arthroplasty
Peripheral leukocytosis	Underlying joint damage (chronic arthropathy)
HIV infection	Intravenous drug use

Adapted from Ellison RT, Reller LB: Differentiating pyogenic arthritis from spontaneous hemarthrosis in patients with hemophilia. West J Med 144:42–45, 1986.

Any synovial fluid obtained on routine aspiration of a hemarthrosis should be submitted for gram stain and culture.

9. Do recurrent hemarthroses have any long-term consequences?
As the patient approaches adulthood, acute hemarthroses become less frequent but chronic joint symptoms supervene. Recurrent hemarthroses lead to accumulation of hemosiderin in the joint lining tissues. Proliferative synovitis develops, and the joint cartilage is degraded. The end result is a chronically swollen joint, less painful than seen in acute hemarthroses, with decreased range of motion. Surrounding muscles become atrophic, and joint contracture is a frequent complication. Examination reveals bony enlargement, coarse crepitus, and deformity. Patients may be significantly disabled by chronic hemophilic arthropathy.

10. Are there any characteristic radiographic findings?
Radiographs in acute hemarthrosis will be remarkable only for soft-tissue swelling and effusion. Chronic arthropathy of hemophilia may have both inflammatory and degenerative features.

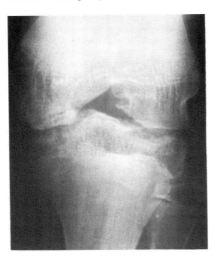

Knee of young patient with hemophilia. Note degenerative and erosive changes of both femoral condyles and the tibial plateau.

11. What is the treatment of chronic hemophilic arthropathy?

Treatment Principles for Chronic Hemophilic Arthropathy

Prophylactic infusions of factor VIII to prevent recurrences of hemarthrosis
Non–weight-bearing rest periods to allow synovitis to regress
Physical therapy to improve joint stability
Training in athletics to maintain muscle mass
Intra-articular glucocorticoids to reduce symptoms and recurrent hemarthroses
Nonacetylated salicylates for pain and swelling
Synovectomy for chronic synovitis unresponsive to conservative therapy
Total joint arthroplasty for end-stage joint disease

Adapted from Upchurch and Brettler.[14]

Treatment programs must be individualized for each patient. Although in small studies ibuprofen and choline magnesium salicylate have both been shown to decrease joint pain in hemophiliacs without decreasing platelet function or increasing bleeding time, exercise caution when using these agents. Difficult patients are frequently referred to specialized treatment centers.

12. Does sickle cell anemia have any rheumatologic manifestations?

- Hand–foot syndrome
- Bone infarction
- Avascular necrosis of bone
- Noninflammatory joint effusions adjacent to areas of bony crisis
- Chronic inflammation of joints
- Hyperuricemia and gout
- Hemarthrosis
- Septic arthritis
- Osteomyelitis
- Focal muscle necrosis
- Rhabdomyolysis

13. How does hand-foot syndrome present in a patient with sickle cell disease?

Hand-foot syndrome, or sickle cell dactylitis, is a problem in infants with sickle cell disease. Children present with acute pain and swelling diffusely in the fingers or toes, usually as a first manifestation of sickle cell disease. Fever and leukocytosis may accompany the dactylitis. The etiology is thought to be local bone marrow ischemia. Periostitis may be seen on radiographs of the metacarpal or metatarsal bones 2 weeks after the acute episode. Symptoms generally subside spontaneously in a few weeks.

14. Is avascular necrosis of bone a common problem in sickle cell disease?

Bony tenderness and fever are common indications of sickle cell crisis causing a bone infarction. If there is sufficient microvascular occlusion by sickled cells, or an end artery is occluded, avascular necrosis of bone is the result. Avascular necrosis of the femoral head is seen in up to 10% of patients with sickle cell disease. Initially, radiographs may be normal. Radioisotope bone scanning and magnetic resonance imaging are more sensitive methods to detect early avascular necrosis of bone.

The following, in decreasing order of frequency, are sites of avascular necrosis in sickle cell disease:

- Femoral head
- Humeral head
- Tibial plateau
- Fibula
- Radius
- Ulna

15. Can avascular necrosis be treated in the setting of sickle cell disease?

Treatment is very unsatisfactory. The affected area should be put on non–weight-bearing status in an attempt to allow revascularization and prevent collapse of the affected bone. An orthopedic surgeon should be consulted promptly. Core decompression of the femoral head may be attempted, although this procedure has not been systematically studied in avascular necrosis due to sickle cell disease. Prosthetic joint replacement is often the treatment used when joint damage is advanced, although results are suboptimal. In one series, 19% of total hip replacements for avascular necrosis of the femoral head in sickle cell disease required revision within 5 years.

16. Is gout seen frequently in sickle cell disease?

In children with sickle cell disease, hyperuricosuria without hyperuricemia occurs, probably as a result of increased red cell turnover associated with crises. Up to 40% of adult sickle cell patients will have hyperuricemia, caused by renal tubular damage with decreased uric acid excretion. However, gout is surprisingly uncommon. Occasionally, gout may be seen, so crystals should be looked for in joint effusions seen during sickle cell crisis.

17. What is the most common musculoskeletal infectious problem seen in sickle cell disease?

Osteomyelitis is seen more than 100 times more frequently in sickle cell disease than in normal persons. Because of functional asplenia, *Salmonella* infections account for 50% of osteomyelitis in sickle cell disease. Gram-negative organisms are also common. Fortunately, septic arthritis is infrequent. (See table next page.)

Factors Predisposing Sickle Cell Patients to Infection

Functional asplenia with decreased clearance of bacteria	Decreased opsonization
Tissue damaged by crisis	Decreased interferon-γ production
Decreased neutrophil function at lower oxygen tensions	Increased risk of nosocomial infection

18. What is the management of suspected osteomyelitis in sickle cell disease?

Management of Suspected Osteomyelitis in Sickle Cell Disease

1. Admit patient to hospital for thorough evaluation.
2. Immobilize affected bones to avoid pathologic fracture.
3. Check baseline CBC and ESR.*
4. Consult hematology and infectious disease services.
5. Obtain blood cultures.
6. Order febrile agglutinins and stool cultures for *Salmonella*.
7. Obtain plain radiographs of all involved bones; repeat these in 10–14 days if the originals are normal.
8. Obtain a radionuclide bone or gallium scan.†
9. Aspirate for culture any bones that are suspected for infection.
10. After a diagnosis is established, preoperative measures are instituted to decrease the risk of surgical complications (transfusions to achieve hemoglobin A level 60% of total hemoglobin, maintenance of adequate oxygenation and hydration).
11. All abscesses in bones should be promptly decompressed to restore blood supply.
12. Avoid tourniquets for intraoperative hemostasis.
13. Do not start antibiotics until adequate specimens of blood, bone, and pus are obtained for culture and Gram stain.
14. Initiate antibiotics based on gram stain results, considering the possibility of *Salmonella*.
15. Parenteral antibiotics are continued for 6–8 weeks.‡

Adapted from Epps CH Jr, Bryant DD, Coles MJM, Castro O: Osteomyelitis in patients who have sickle cell disease. Bone Joint Surg 73-A (9):1281–1294, 1991, with permission

*Erythrocyte sedimentation rate is more useful to follow response to treatment than for differentiating sickle crisis from osteomyelitis. Note that sickle cell disease is associated with an abnormally *low* ESR because the sickled cells cannot form good rouleaux.

†Radionuclide scans are not as useful for differentiating bony infarction and osteomyelitis but will identify affected areas in the spine or pelvis, or unsuspected multifocal involvement.

‡Prolonged therapy is necessary because both infection and sickle cell crisis impair blood flow to the affected bone.

19. How does osteomyelitis present in sickle cell disease?

Presentation of osteomyelitis may be subtle, mimicking sickle crisis or affecting multiple areas. Both sickle crisis and osteomyelitis may present with bone pain, fever, and leukocytosis, and radiographs may be identical. An absolute **band** neutrophil count >500/mm^3 is more suggestive of osteomyelitis than infarction; a band count >1000/mm^3 is even more specific for infection. The utility of radionuclide studies in distinguishing the two entities has not been firmly established. Combined technetium and gallium nuclear medicine scans performed over a period of 24 hours may identify all patients with osteomyelitis but is not specific. A recent study of 15 patients with osteomyelitis in sickle cell disease found that patients with osteomyelitis had a more striking clinical appearance than patients with simple bone infarction; they had more systemic signs and appeared more ill. In this study of osteomyelitis in sickle cell disease, findings included fever, malaise, and localized bone tenderness, with pain and swelling of the affected area.

20. Do the other hemoglobinopathies have any rheumatologic manifestations?

Hemoglobin SC disease and sickle β-thalassemia may develop similar manifestations to sickle cell disease, including hand-foot syndrome and gout. Avascular necrosis of bone has been reported in both conditions. Generally, rheumatologic manifestations are less common in these other hemoglobinopathies. There are case reports of avascular necrosis occurring in patients with sickle cell trait, but the incidence is the same as in age-matched controls with normal hemoglobin.

BIBLIOGRAPHY

1. Anand AJ, Glatt AE: Salmonella osteomyelitis and arthritis in sickle cell disease. Semin Arthritis Rheum 24(3):211–221, 1994.
2. Andersen P, Godal HC: Predictable reduction in anticoagulant activity of warfarin by small amounts of vitamin K. Acta Med Scand 198(4):269–270, 1975.
3. Andes WA, Edmunds JO: Hemarthroses and warfarin: Joint destruction with anticoagulation. Thromb Haemost 49(3):187–189, 1983.
4. Birnbaum Y, Stahl B, Rechavia E: Spontaneous hemarthrosis following thrombolytic therapy for acute myocardial infarction. Int J Cardiol 40(3):289–290.
5. Ellison RT, Reller LB: Differentiating pyogenic arthritis from spontaneous hemarthrosis in patients with hemophilia. West J Med 144(1):42–45, 1986.
6. Epps CH Jr, Bryant DD, Coles MJM, Castro O: Osteomyelitis in patients who have sickle-cell disease. J Bone Joint Sur 73-A(9):1281–1294, 1991.
7. Gatter RA, Schumacher HR: A Practical Handbook of Joint Fluid Analysis, Philadelphia, Lea & Febiger, 1991.
8. Kisker CT, Burke C: Double-blind studies on the use of steroids in the treatment of acute hemarthrosis in patients with hemophilia. N Eng J Med 282(12):639–642, 1970.
9. McCarty DJ: Synovial fluid. In McCarty DJ, Koopman WJ (eds): Arthritis and Allied Conditions, 12th ed, Philadelphia, Lea & Febiger, 1993.
10. Porter DR, Sturrock RD: Rheumatological complications of sickle cell disease. Baillière's Clin Rheumatol 5(2):221–230, 1991.
11. Shupak R, Teital J, Garvey MB, et al: Intra-articular methylprednisolone in hemophilic arthropathy. Am J Hematol 27(9):26–29, 1988.
12. Tozman ECS: Hematologic disorders in rheumatic diseases. Curr Opin Rheumatol 6(1):101–104, 1994.
13. Tozman ECS: Sickle-cell disease, hemophilia, and hematology. Curr Opin Rheumatol 5(1):95–98, 1993.
14. Upchurch KS, Brettler DB: Hemophilic arthropathy. In Kelley WN, Harris ED, Ruddy S, Sledge CB (eds): Textbook of Rheumatology, 4th ed, Philadelphia, W.B. Saunders, 1993.
15. Wild JH, Zvaifler NJ: Hemarthrosis associated with sodium warfarin therapy. Arthritis Rheum 19(1):98–102, 1976.
16. York JR: Musculoskeletal disorders in the haemophilias. Baillière's Clin Rheumatol 5(2):197–220, 1991.

54. MALIGNANCY-ASSOCIATED RHEUMATIC DISORDERS

Daniel F. Battafarano, D.O.

1. Is there a causal relationship between malignancies and rheumatic disorders?

It is uncommon for a rheumatic disease to mimic malignancy, but rheumatic syndromes have been associated with various malignancies, and patients with preexisting connective tissue disease (CTD) have developed malignancies. Approximately 15% of patients hospitalized with advanced malignancy will manifest a paraneoplastic syndrome. Endocrine syndromes secondary to ectopic hormone production account for one-third of all paraneoplastic syndromes followed by connective tissue, hematologic, and neuromuscular syndromes.

A causal relationship between some rheumatic syndromes and underlying malignancies has been established. For example, in patients with hypertrophic osteoarthropathy secondary to malignancy, the musculoskeletal symptoms resolve after resection of the underlying tumor. However, the majority of rheumatic syndromes associated with malignancies do not demonstrate dramatic clinical relationships and therefore have indirect relationships. In addition, the oncogenic risk associated with immunosuppressive drugs is variable.

2. What are the clinical relationships of polyarthritis and malignancy?

Polyarthritis can be the presenting manifestation of an occult malignancy. The association of polyarthritis and malignancy is suggested by:

1. A close temporal relationship (average, 10 months) between the onset of a seronegative arthritis and the diagnosis of malignancy
2. Improvement of the arthritis with treatment of the underlying cancer
3. Recurrence of the arthritis with tumor recurrence

Other clinical features suggesting an underlying malignancy are late age of onset of arthritis, asymmetric joint involvement, explosive onset, predominance of lower extremity involvement, and absence of rheumatoid factor or nodules.

3. What musculoskeletal paraneoplastic syndromes are associated with malignancy?

PARANEOPLASTIC SYNDROME	MALIGNANCY	CLINICAL ASSOCIATION
Myopathy		
Dermatomyositis-polymyositis	Adenocarcinoma	Cancer may precede, coincide, or follow diagnosis of myositis
Arthropathy		
Hypertrophic osteoarthropathy	Various types	Lung cancer is most common
Amyloidosis	Multiple myeloma	26% of primary (AL) amyloidosis is associated with multiple myeloma
Secondary gout	Myeloproliferative disorders	Tumor lysis syndrome
Carcinoma polyarthritis	Solid tumor or hematologic disorders	80% of women will have breast cancer
Jaccoud's-type arthropathy	Carcinoma of lung	Painless, nonerosive, deforming arthropathy with rapid onset
Miscellaneous presentations		
Lupus-like syndrome (polyarthritis, serositis, pleural effusion, positive ANA)	Various types, primary or recurrent	May have history of previously treated malignancy
Necrotizing vasculitis	Lymphoreticular disorders	Chronic unexplained necrotizing vasculitis
Cryoglobulinemia	Plasma cell dyscrasias	Refractory Raynaud's syndrome
Immune complex disease	Hodgkin's disease	Nephrotic syndrome
Reflex sympathetic dystrophy syndrome (RSDS) Shoulder-hand syndrome Palmar fasciitis and polyarthritis	Ovarian cancer	Rapid progressive RSDS
Scleroderma	Adenocarcinoma and carcinoid tumor	Women 3 times greater than men
Polyarteritis	Hairy-cell leukemia	Polyarteritis-like clinically and by arteriography
Polymyalgia rheumatica (PMR)	[Questionable relationship as malignancy and PMR share similar clinical features and both have an elevated ESR]	
Panniculitis	Pancreatic cancer	Subcutaneous nodules and arthritis, eosinophilia
Polychondritis	Hodgkin's disease	Rarely associated with malignancy
Pyogenic arthritis	Colon cancer	Intestinal flora cultured
	Multiple myeloma	Rare cause of primary septic arthritis
Digital necrosis	Various types	Severe Raynaud's syndrome of short duration
Erythromelalgia	Myeloproliferative disorders	Severe burning pain, erythema, and warmth primarily in feet

Modified from Caldwell DS: Musculoskeletal syndromes associated with malignancy. In Kelley WN, et al (eds): Textbook of Rheumatology. Philadelphia, W.B. Saunders, 1993, pp 1552–1566.

4. What are the accepted direct associations between musculoskeletal syndromes and malignancy?

Metastatic disease, leukemia, lymphoma, and primary synovial and bone tumors are directly associated with the pathologic mechanisms of the underlying tumor. **Bone metastases** typically involve the long bones or the axial skeleton and generally arise from primary breast and lung neoplasms. Monoarticular arthritis of the knee is the most common presentation of metastatic arthritis. Phalangeal metastasis can also occur.

Leukemia can present as a symmetric or migratory polyarthritis or as bone pain. The diagnosis is made by routine complete blood count and review of the peripheral smear. Articular manifestations in acute leukemia occur in approximately 14% of children and 4% of adults. Joint pain has been attributed to leukemic synovial infiltration and usually involves the ankle or knee. The joint pain is disproportionately more severe than the clinical findings. Synovial effusions are uncommon and are only mildly inflammatory with rare evidence of leukemic cells. Plain radiographs may be normal at the onset of the bone pain in at least 50%, but bone scintigraphy will detect osseous involvement early. At least 10% of patients with leukemia present with back pain. The joint or bone pain is optimally treated with systemic chemotherapy.

Nocturnal bone pain is the most common musculoskeletal complaint in patients with **lymphoma.** Arthritis occurs less commonly and usually exists as a consequence of adjacent bony invasion. Occasionally, patients with T-cell lymphoma may develop a chronic, nonerosive polyarthritis with erythroderma.

5. Discuss the occurrence of cancer in patients with dermatomyositis (DM) and polymyositis (PM).

Approximately 15% of adult patients with combined DM/PM demonstrate an underlying malignancy. Adults (age >40 years) with DM have an increased risk of having an underlying malignancy when compared to adults with PM. The onset of DM or PM may precede, coincide, or occur after the malignancy is diagnosed. Most patients have common malignancies, such as breast, ovarian, or lung cancer. The association of DM and malignancy in childhood is rare. Creatine kinase and muscle biopsy data are not useful for distinguishing DM and PM in patients with or without malignancy. It is recommended that all adult patients with new-onset PM or DM undergo a thorough history and physical examination, laboratory survey, chest x-ray, mammogram, gynecologic evaluation, and flexible sigmoidoscopy to screen for common malignancies.

6. What is the relationship of amyloidosis to multiple myeloma?

Amyloidosis is a disease characterized by the deposition of an insoluble proteinaceous material in the extracellular matrix of one or several organs. Multiple myeloma-associated amyloidosis closely resembles primary generalized amyloidosis in its age distribution (mean age, 55 years), sex predilection (M > F), and clinical presentation. The clinical features of both primary and multiple myeloma-associated amyloidosis are similar. Skin involvement is apparent in 50% of patients and manifests as waxy papules or plaques, nodules, or nonthrombocytopenic purpura. Renal failure and/or proteinuria is the next most common presentation, followed by restrictive cardiomyopathy. Neuropathic complications with sensorimotor symptoms occur in approximately 20% of patients and are frequently manifest by carpal tunnel syndrome. Hepatosplenomegaly, macroglossia, bronchioalveolar involvement, and an acquired factor X deficiency are also common. Most patients with myeloma-associated amyloidosis have both an intact paraprotein in the serum and Bence-Jones proteins in urine. Twenty-six percent of all primary amyloidosis cases are associated with myeloma and 6–15% of all multiple myeloma patients develop amyloidosis.

7. What is hypertrophic osteoarthropathy?

Hypertrophic osteoarthropathy (HOA) is a syndrome that includes (1) clubbing of fingers and toes, (2) periostitis of the long bones, and (3) arthritis. HOA is classified as primary or secondary. Primary HOA is hereditary and appears during childhood. The secondary form can be subdivided into generalized or localized. The secondary generalized form is most often associated with neoplasms or infectious diseases but can be seen with congenital heart disease, inflammatory bowel disease, cirrhosis, Grave's disease, or thalassemia. The secondary localized form of HOA has

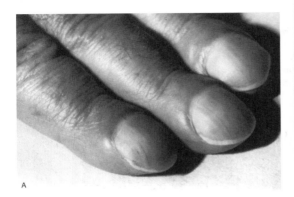
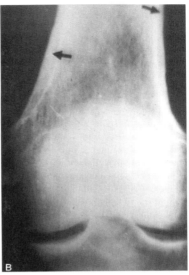

A, Clubbing of fingers. Soft tissue proliferation of the nailbed and distal tissues of the digits is seen. Usually the nail makes an angle of 20° or more with the projected line of the digit. When clubbing occurs, subungual proliferation causes diminution of the angle. *B,* Roentgenogram of the knee shows subperiosteal new bone formation of the lower femoral shafts (*arrows*). New bone is separated from the old cortex by a thin radiolucent line on the right; a later subperiosteal lesion is seen on the left. (From the Clinical Slide Collection on the Rheumatic Diseases. Atlanta, American College of Rheumatology, 1991; with permission.)

been associated with hemiplegia, aneurysms, infective arteritis, and patent ductus arteriosus. The etiology of HOA is still unclear but clubbing and HOA appear to result from peripheral impaction of megakaryocytes and platelet clumps in the fingers and toes.

8. Vasculitis occurs as a paraneoplastic syndrome with which malignancies?

Vasculitis is most often associated with leukemia and lymphomas but may occur with other solid tumors. Leukocytoclastic vasculitis is the most common clinical paraneoplastic presentation. Henoch-Schönlein purpura, systemic vasculitis involving medium-sized vessels, and granulomatous vasculitis have also been described. A polyarteritis nodosa-like vasculitis is the most common rheumatologic manifestation of hairy-cell leukemia. Vasculitis may precede, coincide, or follow the malignancy diagnosis. Proposed mechanisms for vasculitis as a paraneoplastic syndrome include immune complex formation, direct vascular injury by antibodies to endothelial cells, or a direct effect of leukemic cells (i.e., hairy cells) on the endothelium.

9. What is Sweet's syndrome?

This acute febrile neutrophilic dermatosis mimics vasculitis and is associated with malignancy in at least 15% of patients. It is most commonly seen with acute myelogenous leukemia but has been described with many malignancies. The cardinal features are:
- Abrupt onset of raised, often painful nodules or plaques on the extremities, face, neck, or trunk
- Fever
- Peripheral neutrophilic leukocytosis
- Dense dermal neutrophilic infiltrates without vasculitis on biopsy

10. Which rheumatic syndromes have been described with ovarian carcinoma?

Dermatomyositis-polymyositis   Carpal tunnel syndrome
Palmar fasciitis and arthritis   Adhesive capsulitis
Shoulder-hand syndrome   Fibromyalgia
Lupus-like syndrome   Positive antinuclear antibody
Acute febrile neutrophilic dermatosis (Sweet's syndrome)

11. Describe the features of palmar fasciitis and arthritis and the shoulder-hand syndrome.

Palmar fasciitis and arthritis and the shoulder-hand syndrome are considered to be clinical variants of reflex sympathetic dystrophy syndrome (RSDS).

Ovarian carcinoma is the classic malignant neoplasm associated with **palmar fasciitis and arthritis,** although this syndrome can be seen with other malignancies. The palmar fasciitis and arthritis syndrome has features of pain, swelling, limitation of motion, and vasomotor instability in the involved extremity similar to RSDS. The clinical characteristics of palmar fasciitis and arthritis that distinguish it from classic RSDS are (1) a severe symmetric inflammatory arthritis resembling rheumatoid arthritis, (2) bilateral extremity involvement (RSDS is bilateral in only 50%), and (3) its association with neoplasms. Plantar fasciitis can occur with lower extremity involvement. Histologic examination of the involved tissues reveals extensive fibrosis with increased fibroblast and mononuclear cell infiltration. There is no evidence of collagen deposition like that seen in scleroderma, and nailfold capillary examination is normal. Deposits of IgG in the palmar fascia and the presence of low-titer antinuclear antibodies in some patients suggest an immunopathologic mechanism. The response to NSAIDs, corticosteroids, ganglionic blockade, and/or physical therapy are variable. The presence of palmar fasciitis and arthritis portends a poor prognosis since it typically manifests after tumor metastasis. Successful removal of the underlying tumor may result in dramatic clinical improvement of the affected extremities.

The **shoulder-hand syndrome** is much milder than the palmar fasciitis and arthritis syndrome. This syndrome is most often described with ovarian carcinoma or with lung cancer localized to the superior sulcus (Pancoast tumor). Pain in the shoulder with loss of motion may result in adhesive capsulitis, and the hand of the involved side becomes puffy and stiff with vasomotor instability. Conventional treatment for RSDS provides variable relief.

12. Which malignancies are associated with preexisting connective tissue disease?

Preexisting Connective Tissue Disease Associated with Malignancy

CONNECTIVE TISSUE DISEASE	MALIGNANCY	CLINICAL ASSOCIATION
Systemic lupus erythematosus	Lymphoreticular disorders	Adenopathy, splenomegaly
Discoid lupus erythematosus	Squamous cell epithelioma	Found in plaques >20 years
Sjögren's syndrome	Lymphoreticular disorders (44 times normal risk)	May be primary or secondary Sjögren's
Rheumatoid arthritis (RA)	Lymphoreticular disorders (2–5 times normal risk even in the absence of immunosuppressive therapy)	Related more to the duration of RA than to severity
Scleroderma	Alveolar cell carcinoma	Pulmonary fibrosis
	Adenocarcinoma of esophagus	Barrett's metaplasia
	? Breast cancer	Case reports of breast cancer near onset of scleroderma
Osteomyelitis	Squamous cell carcinoma	Chronic osteomyelitis with cutaneous ulcer
Paget's disease	Osteogenic sarcoma	Occurs in <1% of preexisting Paget's lesions
Eosinophilic fasciitis	Lymphoid malignancy	Aplastic anemia, thrombocytopenia, Hodgkin's disease
Lymphomatoid granulomatosis	Lymphoma	At least 13% develop lymphoma

Modified from Caldwell DS: Musculoskeletal syndromes associated with malignancy. In Kelley WN, et al (eds): Textbook of Rheumatology. Philadelphia, W.B. Saunders, 1993, pp 1552–1566; with permission.

13. How do malignancy and the drugs used to treat connective tissue disease (CTD) relate?

The common immunosuppressive drugs used to treat CTDs include alkylating agents (i.e., cyclophosphamide and chlorambucil), a purine analogue (i.e., azathioprine), and a folic acid analogue (i.e., methotrexate). Prolonged daily treatment or a high cumulative dose of alkylating agents is clearly associated with an increased risk for hematologic malignancies years after the drug is discontinued. The prolonged use of oral **cyclophosphamide** also carries a significant increased risk for bladder carcinoma due to the acrolein metabolite excreted in the urine. Patients treated with parenteral pulse cyclophosphamide for systemic lupus nephritis or cerebritis are being monitored to determine the risk for the development of hematologic malignancies; current data suggest that parenteral pulse (monthly) cyclophosphamide has minimal risk when compared to oral daily cyclophosphamide.

High-dose **azathioprine** ($\geq$200 mg/day) increases the risk of lymphoproliferative malignancies in rheumatoid arthritis patients twofold over the risk due to rheumatoid arthritis alone. Low-dose oral weekly **methotrexate** has not been associated with an increase in oncogenic potential, although a few case reports have suggested that there may be an increased risk of developing non-Hodgkin's lymphoma, which may regress when the methotrexate is discontinued. Total lymphoid **irradiation** and total body irradiation have been reserved for refractory rheumatoid arthritis. The risk of myeloproliferative disorders is increased in this subset of patients, but rheumatoid arthritis alone and prior immunosuppressive therapy (either before or after irradiation) may also contribute to this risk.

Immunosuppressive Drugs/Agents Used in the Treatment of Connective Tissue Diseases and Their Potential Malignancies

TREATMENT	MALIGNANCIES
Cyclophosphamide	
Oral	Bladder carcinoma, hematologic malignancies
Parenteral	Hematologic malignancies
Alkylating agents	Acute myelogenous leukemia, non-Hodgkin's lymphoma
Azathioprine	Non-Hodgkin's lymphoma
Radiation therapy	Basal cell carcinoma
Total lymphoid/total body irradiation	Myeloproliferative disorders, osseous sarcoma
Methotrexate (low-dose)	Increased risk of non-Hodgkin's lymphoma?

BIBLIOGRAPHY

1. Abu-Shakra M, Guillemin F, Lee P: Cancer in systemic sclerosis. Arthritis Rheum 36:460–464, 1993.
2. Caldwell DS: Musculoskeletal syndromes associated with malignancy. In Kelley WN, Harris Jr ED, Ruddy S, Sledge CB (eds): Textbook of Rheumatology. Philadelphia, W.B. Saunders, 1993, pp 1552–1566.
3. Dickinson CJ: The etiology of clubbing and hypertrophic osteoarthropathy. Eur J Clin Invest 23:330–338, 1993.
4. Kyle RA, Gertz MA: Systemic amyloidosis. Crit Rev Oncol Hematol 10:49–87, 1990.
5. Moreland LW, Brick JE, Kovach RE, et al: Acute febrile neutrophilic dermatosis (Sweet syndrome): A review of the literature with emphasis on musculoskeletal manifestations. Semin Arthritis Rheum 17:143–155, 1988.
6. Naschitz JE, Rosner I, Rozenbaum M, et al: Cancer-associated rheumatic disorders: Clues to occult neoplasia. Senior Arhtritis Rheum 24:231–241, 1995.
7. Patel AM, Davila DG, Peters SG: Paraneoplastic syndromes associated with lung cancer. Mayo Clin Proc 63:278–287, 1993.
8. Pfinsgraff J, Buckingham RB, Killian PJ, et al: Palmar faciitis and arthritis with malignant neoplasms: A paraneoplastic syndrome. Semin Arthritis Rheum 16:118–125, 1986.
9. Rennie JAN, Auchterlone IA: Rheumatological manifestations of the leukaemias and graft vs host disease. Clin Rheumatol 52:231–251, 1991.
10. Sanchez-Guerrero J, Gutierrez-Urena S, V Daller A, et al: Vasculitis as a paraneoplastic syndrome: Report of 11 cases and review of the literature. J Rheumatol 17:1458–1462, 1990.
11. Schwarzer AC, Fryer J, Preston SJ, et al: Metastatic adenosquamous carcinoma presenting as an acute monoarthritis, with a review of the literature. J Orthop Rheum 3:175–185, 1990.
12. Sigurgeirsson B, Lindelof B, Edhag O, Alexander E: Risk of cancer in patients with dermatomyositis or polymyositis. N Engl J Med 326:363–367, 1992.
13. Silman AJ, Petrie J, Hazelman BL, Evans SJW: Lymphoproliferative cancer and malignancy in patients with rheumatoid arthritis treated with azathioprine: A 20 year follow-up study. Ann Rheum Dis 47:988–992, 1988.

IX. Bone and Cartilage Disorders

I cannot conceive why we who are composed of over 90 percent water should suffer from rheumatism with a slight rise in the humidity of the atmosphere.

John W. Strutt (Baron Rayleigh)
(1842–1919)
Bristish physicist, discoverer of argon

55. OSTEOARTHRITIS

Scott Vogelgesang, M.D.

1. What is osteoarthritis?
A slowly progressive musculoskeletal disorder that typically affects the joints of the hand (especially those involved with a pinch grip), spine, and weight-bearing joints (hips, knees) of the lower extremity. It is the most common articular disorder and accounts for more disability among the elderly than any other disease. It is characterized by joint pain, crepitus, stiffness after immobility, and limitation of motion. The clinical joint symptoms are associated with defects in the articular cartilage and underlying bone. There are no systemic symptoms, and joint inflammation, when present, is mild.

2. Give five other names for osteoarthritis.
Osteoarthrosis
Degenerative joint disease (DJD)
Hypertrophic arthritis
Degenerative disc disease (DDD, in the spine)
Generalized osteoarthritis (GOA) (Kellgren's syndrome)

3. Under what circumstances can osteoarthritis develop?
Osteoarthritis can develop when **excessive loads** (i.e., trauma) across the joint cause the articular cartilage or subchondral bone to fail. Alternatively, osteoarthritis may develop under **normal loads** if the cartilage, bone, synovium, or supporting ligaments and muscles are abnormal because of any one of a number of secondary causes.

4. What are the pathologic features of osteoarthritis?
Early
Swelling of articular cartilage
Loosening of collagen framework restraint
Chondrocytes increase proteoglycan synthesis but also release more degradative enzymes.
Increased cartilage water content
Later
Degradative enzymes break down proteoglycan faster than it can be produced by chondrocytes, resulting in diminished proteoglycan content in cartilage.
Articular cartilage thins and softens (joint-space narrowing on radiographs will be seen eventually.

Fissuring and cracking of cartilage. Repair is attempted but inadequate.

Underlying bone is exposed, allowing synovial fluid to be forced by the pressure of weight into the bone. This shows up as cysts or geodes on radiographs.

Remodeling and hypertrophy of the subchondral bone results in subchondral sclerosis and osteophyte (''spurs'') formation.

This pathology explains the joint-space narrowing, subchondral sclerosis, cysts/geodes, and osteophytes seen on radiographs in osteoarthritic patients.

5. List the clinical features of osteoarthritis.
1. Pain in involved joints
2. Pain worse with activity, better with rest
3. Morning stiffness (if present) <30 minutes
4. Stiffness after periods of immobility (gelling)
5. Joint enlargement
6. Joint instability
7. Limitation of joint mobility
8. Periarticular muscle atrophy
9. Crepitus

6. What is crepitus?
A creaking, cracking, or grinding noise made by joints having irregular cartilage that moves against a similar surface. Crepitus may be painless but most often is uncomfortable.

7. Name the joints typically involved in primary (idiopathic) osteoarthritis.
- Distal interphalangeal (DIP) joints of the hands
- Proximal interphalangeal (PIP) joints of the hands
- First carpometacarpal (CMC) joints of the hands
- Acromioclavicular joint of shoulder
- Hips
- Knees
- First metatarsophalangeal (MTP) joints of the feet
- Facet (apophyseal) joints of the cervical and lumbosacral spine

8. Name some joints *not* typically involved in primary (idiopathic) osteoarthritis.
- Metacarpophalangeal (MCP) joints of the hands
- Wrists
- Elbows
- Shoulders (glenohumeral joint)
- Ankles
- 2nd–5th MTP of the feet

Involvement of these atypical joints should prompt a search for secondary causes of osteoarthritis.

9. What laboratory features are seen in osteoarthritis?
Laboratory findings are nonspecific:
- Erythrocyte sedimentation rate (ESR) typically within normal limits
- Rheumatoid factor is negative
- Antinuclear antibodies (ANA) are not present
- Synovial fluid
  High viscosity with good string sign
  Color is clear and yellow
  White blood cell counts typically < 1000–2000/mm^3
  No crystals and negative cultures

10. What are the radiographic "ABCDES" of osteoarthritis?

A — No ankylosis
  Alignment may be abnormal

B — Bone mineralization is normal
  Bony subchondral sclerosis
  Bony spurs (osteophytes)

C — No calcifications in cartilage
  Cartilage space narrowing which is nonuniform (occurs in area of maximal stress in weight-bearing joints)

D — Deformities of Heberden's/Bouchard's nodes
  Distribution: involvement of typical joints vs. atypical joints (see Questions 7 and 8)

E — No erosions
  "Gull wing" sign in "erosive" osteoarthritis

S — Slow progression over years
  No specific nail or soft tissue abnormalities
  Vacuum sign in degenerative disc disease (a collection of nitrogen in a degenerated disc space)

Always obtain weight-bearing radiographs when evaluating for joint-space narrowing of lower extremity large joints (see figure).

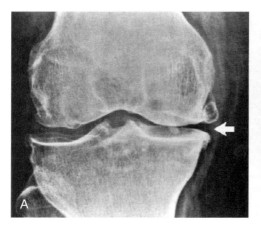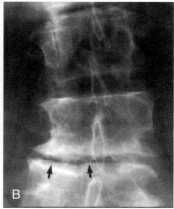

A, Radiograph of knee osteoarthritis, showing sclerosis, cysts, osteophytes, and medial joint space narrowing (*arrow*). *B,* Anterior radiograph of the lumbar spine with disc disease/osteoarthritis. Note disc space narrowing, osteophytes, and vacuum sign (*arrows*).

11. How is osteoarthritis classified?

• Primary, idiopathic osteoarthritis
  Localized
    Hands (Heberden's and Bouchard's nodes, first CMC)
    Hands (erosive, inflammatory)
    Feet (first MTP)
    Hip
    Knee
    Spine (including, diffuse idiopathic sclerosing hyperostitis [DISH]
  Generalized (Kellgren's syndrome)
• Secondary osteoarthritis

12. Are there any distinctive epidemiologic features of primary (idiopathic) osteoarthritis?
- Association with increased age
- More common in women than in men
- Radiographic evidence in > 50–80% of those > 65 years of age
- Estimated 2–3% of the adult population has symptomatic osteoarthritis.

13. Where do Heberden's and Bouchard's nodes occur?
Bony articular nodules (osteophytes or "spurs") located on the DIP joints are called **Heberden's** nodes. Such nodules on the PIP joints are **Bouchard's** nodes (see figure). Palmar and lateral deviation of the distal phalanx as a result of these nodules is not uncommon. Heberden's nodes are 10 times more frequent in women than in men. The tendency to develop Heberden's nodes may be familial with one estimate suggesting that a woman whose mother has Heberden's nodes is twice as likely to develop similar joint changes as a woman without such a family history. The clinical importance of Heberden's and Bouchard's nodes is that they usually signify that the patient has primary osteoarthritis and does not have a secondary etiology for the osteoarthritis.

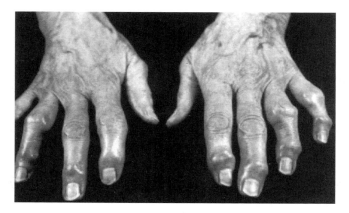

Herberden's (DIP joints) and Bouchard's (PIP joints) nodes in a woman with osteoarthritis. (From the Clinical Slide Collection on the Rheumatic Diseases. Atlanta, American College of Rheumatology, 1991; with permission.)

14. Who was Heberden?
William Heberden was an 18th-century physician who made substantial contributions to cardiology, preventive medicine, and rheumatology. He identified the interphalangeal nodular swellings seen in osteoarthritis that now bear his name. Heberden collected a set of clinical observations that became one of the first systems of differentiation of the arthritides.

15. List six risk factors for osteoarthritis.
Obesity
Heredity (especially osteoarthritis of DIP joints)
Age
Previous joint trauma
Abnormal joint mechanics (i.e., excessive knee varus or valgus)
Smoking (may contribute to degenerative disc disease)

16. Does obesity predispose to osteoarthritis? (*Controversy*)
Obesity is a clear risk factor for the development of osteoarthritis, especially of the knee but also, to a lesser degree, of the hand. Weight loss prior to the development of osteoarthritis is associated

with a decreased risk of osteoarthritis. One theory to explain this association is that obesity increases the force across the joint and speeds degeneration of the joint. This explanation, although intuitive, is not universally accepted and would seem to be at odds with the fact that obesity is not associated with osteoarthritis of the hip.

17. Does running or jogging predispose to osteoarthritis?
Previous joint injury and repetitive joint use predispose to the development of osteoarthritis, raising the question of whether runners are at increased risk for developing osteoarthritis in the knee and hip. Several studies attempting to address this question found no increase in the rate of knee and hip osteoarthritis or knee complaints in runners compared to controls. On the other hand, one uncontrolled study found that runners who developed osteoarthritis tended to have run more miles per week. Finally, one study found an increase of hip osteoarthritis in runners compared to controls. Although there is some disagreement in the literature, most of the present data suggest that in the absence of previous joint injury, runners do not develop osteoarthritis in the knee or hip at higher rates than others.

18. Are any factors protective against developing osteoarthritis?
Osteoporosis. It is postulated that the softened bone under the cartilage helps protect it from injury. Smoking may also be a negative risk factor, perhaps by contributing to osteoporosis.

19. What is erosive, inflammatory osteoarthritis?
A subset of primary osteoarthritis, sometimes called Crain's disease, which occurs primarily in women > 50 years of age. The involved joints include DIPs, PIPs, first CMCs, and first MTPs. There is a component of joint inflammation which is superimposed on the degenerative osteoarthritic symptoms. Painful inflammatory "flares" of the involved joints can occur.

These patients are frequently misdiagnosed as having rheumatoid arthritis. However, unlike rheumatoid arthritis, this disease is not accompanied by systemic symptoms; does not involve the MCPs, wrists, or second to fifth MTPs; and serologically has normal sedimentation rates and negative rheumatoid factors and ANAs. Additionally, radiographs are characteristic, showing osteophytes and central "erosions" with a hallmark "gull wing" or "inverted-T" appearance (see figure). Note that these are *not* true synovial-based erosions, which occur in the periarticular "bare areas" in patients with inflammatory arthritides like rheumatoid arthritis (see Chapters 11 and 19). Patients with erosive osteoarthritis also need to have superimposed gout and crystal arthritis/pseudogout ruled out when they have "flares."

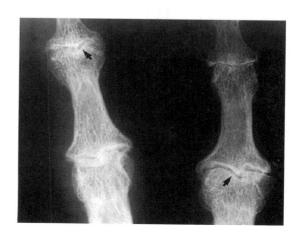

Radiograph of hands of a patient with "erosive" osteoarthritis of the DIP and PIP joints. Note "gull wing" sign (*arrows*) which is the hallmark of this disease.

20. Define generalized osteoarthritis.
A variant of osteoarthritis sometimes called Kellgren's syndrome in which individuals have several affected joints (≥ 4 joint groups) in the typical distribution for osteoarthritis. The disease frequently becomes manifest before age 40–50. Radiographic findings may be more severe than symptoms. Generalized osteoarthritis may simply be a more severe form of common osteoarthritis, although some researchers feel that a defect (such as an abnormal amino acid substitution) will be found in type II or IX collagens causing cartilage to degenerate more quickly.

21. What is DISH?
DISH stands for diffuse idiopathic skeletal hyperostosis, but this condition has also been called Forestier's disease and ankylosing hyperostosis. DISH can be confused with ankylosing spondylitis or osteoarthritis of the spine. It is, however, not an arthropathy in that there is no abnormality of articular cartilage, adjacent bone margins, or synovium. Instead, it is a bone-forming condition in which ossification occurs at skeletal sites subjected to stress. It occurs most frequently in the thoracic spine and can be associated clinically with pain or decreased motion. Involvement of the cervical spine can cause dysphagia. DISH occurs in approximately 12% of the elderly population and may coexist with other disorders, particularly type 2 diabetes mellitus.

22. Describe the radiographic findings in DISH.
Normal bone mineralization is seen in addition to "flowing" ossification of the anterior longitudinal ligament connecting at least four contiguous vertebral bodies. The calcification of the anterior longitudinal ligament is seen as a radiodense band separated from the anterior aspect of the vertebral bodies by a thin radiolucent line (see figure). Ossification of multiple tendinous or ligamentous sites in the appendicular skeleton may also be seen. Disc spaces, apophyseal joints, and sacroiliac joints are normal radiographically, helping to separate DISH from osteoarthritis and ankylosing spondylitis.

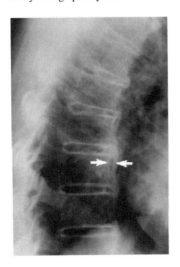

Lateral radiograph of thoracic spine showing calcification of the anterior longitudinal ligament connecting four vertebrae. Note the space between this calcified ligament and the anterior borders of vertebral bodies (*arrows*).

23. How does secondary osteoarthritis differ from primary osteoarthritis?
Secondary osteoarthritis has the same clinical features as idiopathic osteoarthritis except that it has an identifiable etiologic factor and may have a different joint distribution. Atypical joint involvement should prompt a search for an underlying disease process. A classic example is osteoarthritis seen in the MCP joints of the hands in association with hemochromatosis.

24. List some causes of secondary osteoarthritis.

Trauma

Congenital disorders
  Hip
    Legg-Calvé-Perthes
    Congenital hip dislocation
    Slipped capital femoral epiphysis
    Congenital shallow acetabulum
  Dysplasias
    Epiphyseal dysplasia
    Spondyloepiphyseal dysplasia
  Mechanical features
    Joint hypermobility
    Leg-length discrepancy
    Varus/valgus deformity
    Scoliosis

Metabolic diseases
  Hemochromatosis
  Ochronosis
  Gaucher's disease
  Hemoglobinopathy
Endocrine disorders
  Acromegaly
  Hypothyroidism
  Hyperparathyroidism
Neuropathic joints
  Diabetes mellitus
  Syphilis
Paget's disease
End result of any inflammatory
  arthropathy

25. Which medications are helpful in treating osteoarthritis?

No medication has been shown to stop or reverse the disease process underlying osteoarthritis. Medications are used, therefore, to alleviate symptoms and increase function. **NSAID**s are widely used. No single NSAID is more effective than another when evaluated in a large population, but efficacy in individuals may vary. Unfortunately, these medications may be associated with many side effects, some of which can be severe. Other therapeutic alternatives should be considered when possible. Nonacetylated **salicylates** can be useful and have much less gastrointestinal and renal toxicity. Analgesics such as **acetaminophen** may also be used effectively. A recent study has documented that acetaminophen was as efficacious as ibuprofen in the short-term treatment of osteoarthritis of the knee. There is no role for oral or parenteral corticosteroids.

26. How would you initiate medical treatment in a typical patient with osteoarthritis?

A reasonable approach to therapy in a patient with osteoarthritis is to start with acetaminophen, 650–1000 mg every 6 hours as needed. If this is unsuccessful, a trial of nonacetylated salicylates is warranted. Salsalate or choline magnesium trisalicylate can be used in typical doses of 1000 mg twice or three times a day. Salicylate levels can be followed to guide therapy. If unsuccessful, less-expensive, short-acting NSAIDs may be tried, such as ibuprofen or naproxen sodium. Using the smallest effective dose and/or intermittent dosing is prudent if possible.

27. Are there any surgical options for joints severely affected by osteoarthritis?

Surgery is most often employed in hip and knee osteoarthritis but is also helpful for osteoarthritis involving the first CMC joint, first MTP joint, and, less commonly, the DIP and PIP joints. Approximately 50% of all hip and knee replacements are done for osteoarthritis. Pain relief and satisfactory function result in approximately 90% of patients who undergo total joint replacement. Failure rates after total joint replacement, requiring revision of the prosthesis, are variable and occur in 10–30% at 10 years.

28. List the indications for total joint replacement for osteoarthritis of the hip or knee.

A person with hip or knee arthritis should be considered for total joint replacement if they meet one or more of the following:
- Severe pain unresponsive to medical therapy
- Loss of joint function
- Cannot walk more than one block due to pain
- Cannot stand in one place for > 20–30 minutes due to pain
- Consistently awakens from sleep due to pain

29. List other measures, beside medications or surgery, that may help someone afflicted with osteoarthritis.

Weight loss
Rest of affected joints
Exercise for muscle conditioning
Ambulatory aids (canes, crutches, walkers)
Splinting (CMC splints, knee sleeves, ankle sleeves)
Paraffin baths for hands (may be done at home)
Cervical collar
Cervical traction
Local corticosteroid injections
Diathermy
Topical irritants
Topical capsaicin (different than topical irritants in that it works by depleting nerve terminal of substance P, thereby decreasing pain)
Transcutaneous electrical nerve stimulator (TENS) (controversial but may help individual patients)
Superficial heat and cold
Patient education
Shock-absorbing insoles
Hydrotherapy

30. What is the role of exercise in osteoarthritis therapy?

A specific exercise program can play a significant role in improving joint range of motion, function, and pain. One recent study showed that a supervised program of fitness-walking resulted in improvement of pain and joint function. Other studies have shown participants also have improved psychological well-being. Caution is advised, however. Weight-bearing exercise may worsen the articular cartilage and subchondral bone.

The compromise should be an exercise that does not involve weight-bearing but does provide joint range of motion, muscle strengthening, and aerobic fitness. It is important that the individual select an exercise program that is enjoyable, easily done, and possible to accomplish. An ideal exercise for some is swimming. When done in a warm pool, the individual can move affected joints, strengthen periarticular muscles, and improve cardiovascular fitness, all without bearing weight on diseased joints. Other good options include bicycling, walking, and cross-country skiing.

31. Are serologic markers useful for diagnosing or following osteoarthritis?

Osteoarthritis is a degenerative disease of articular cartilage with subsequent changes in the subchondral bone. It has been suggested that serum or synovial levels of molecules involved with bone or cartilage matrix may facilitate diagnosis or help in following the progression of disease. Several candidates have been evaluated including proteoglycans, proteinases, cytokines, interleukins, and other matrix molecules. One of the best studied is keratan sulfate. Populations with osteoarthritis have higher levels of both synovial and serum keratan sulfate than controls. However, there is a large overlap between levels of both groups, and levels do not reliably change with disease activity. For these reasons, the value of these markers remains unclear, although they continue to be subjects of research interest.

32. What is the natural history of osteoarthritis?

Likely, the cartilage changes of osteoarthritis are asymptomatic for years. Despite this, osteoarthritis progresses with time in most individuals. The rate of progression, however, can be variable, and once symptomatic, the disease may seem to progress quickly. There may be rare individuals in whom the disease may remain stable or even improve somewhat. Nevertheless, osteoarthritis can lead to severe limitations in motion and eventual disability. Limitation in usual activities was noted by 60–80% of patients who reported having osteoarthritis according to the recent National Health Interview Survey.

BIBLIOGRAPHY

1. Altman RD: Criteria for classification of clinical osteoarthritis. J Rheumatol 18(suppl 27):10, 1991.
2. Belhorn LR, Hess EV: Erosive osteoarthritis. Semin Arthritis Rheum 22:298, 1993.
3. Bradley JD, Brandt KD, Katz BP, et al: Comparison of an anti-inflammatory dose of ibuprofen, and analgesic dose of ibuprofen and acetaminophen in the treatment of patients with osteoarthritis of the knee.
   N Engl J Med 325:87, 1991.
4. Buckwalter KA: Imaging of osteoarthritis and crystal deposition diseases. Curr Opin Rheumatol 5:503, 1993.
5. Bunning RD, Materson RS: A rational program of exercise for patients with osteoarthritis. Semin Arthritis Rheum 21:33, 1991.
6. Cushnaghan J, Dieppe P: Study of 500 patients with limb joint osteoarthritis: I. Analysis by age, sex and
   distribution of symptomatic joint sites. Ann Rheum Dis 50:8, 1991.
7. Dieppe P: Management of osteoarthritis of the hip and knee joints. Curr Opin Rheumatol 5:487, 1993.
8. Felson DT: Osteoarthritis. Rheum Dis Clin 16:499, 1990.
9. Felson DT, Zhang U, Anthony JM, et al: Weight loss reduces the risk for symptomatic knee osteoarthritis in women: The Framingham Study. Ann Intern Med 116:535, 1992.
10. Hamerman D: The biology of osteoarthritis. N Engl J Med 320:1322, 1989.
11. Harris WH, Sledge CB: Total hip and total knee replacement. N Engl J Med 323:725, 1990.
12. Lane NE, Bloch DA, Jones JJ, et al: Long-distance running, bone density and osteoarthritis. JAMA
    255:1147, 1986.
13. Malemud CJ: Markers of osteoarthritis and cartilage research in animal models. Curr Opin Rheumatol
    5:494, 1993.
14. Puett DW, Griffin MR: Published trials of nonmedicinal and noninvasive therapies for hip and knee os-
    teoarthritis. Ann Intern Med 121:133, 1994.
15. Resnick D, Shapiro RF, Wiesner KB, et al. Diffuse idiopathic skeletal hyptrophy (DISH). Semin Arthri-
    tis Rheum 7:153, 1978.

56. METABOLIC BONE DISEASE

Michael T. McDermott, M.D.

1. What are the major components of bone?

The main structural elements of bone are **osteoid,** which is a protein matrix, and **hydroxyapatite** (calcium phosphate) crystals, which are embedded in the osteoid. The major functional cells are **osteoclasts,** which resorb old bone, and **osteoblasts,** which form new bone.

2. What is osteoporosis?

Osteoporosis is a predisposition to skeletal fractures resulting primarily from a reduction in total or regional bone mass. Both hydroxyapatite and osteoid are reduced proportionately in osteo-porotic bone.

3. What fractures are most commonly associated with osteoporosis?

Fractures of the vertebrae, femoral neck, and distal radius (Colles' fractures) are characteristic, but any fracture may occur.

4. What are the major risk factors for osteoporosis?

Family history	Low calcium intake
Slender body build	Cigarette smoking
Fair skin	Excessive alcohol consumption (> 2 drinks/day)
Early menopause	Excessive caffeine consumption (> 2 cups/day)
Sedentary lifestyle	Medications (corticosteroids, L-thyroxine)

5. How is bone mass measured?

Standard roentgenography is inadequate for accurate bone mass assessment. Single photon absorptiometry, dual photon absorptiometry, and computed tomography (CT) are also available, but **dual-energy x-ray absorptiometry** (DEXA), the most recently developed technique, offers far greater accuracy and reproducibility than other methods.

6. How do you interpret a bone mass report?

The bone mass report includes three values at each skeletal site analyzed: absolute bone mass in gm/cm^2, T-score, and Z-score. The **T-score** is the number of standard deviations (SDs) that a patient's value lies above or below the mean peak value for young adults. Any T-score between -1 and -2.5 is termed **osteopenia** and any value below -2.5 is considered **osteoporosis**, which indicates a significantly increased risk of fracture at that site. The **Z-score** is the number of SDs that a patient's value lies above or below the mean value for age-matched adults. A value < -1 implies that bone loss exceeds what would be expected from age alone.

7. What types of bone are present at the three bone mass measurement sites?

The lumbar spine is predominantly trabecular (cancellous) bone, the mid-radius is mainly cortical (compact) bone, and the femoral neck is half trabecular and half cortical bone.

8. What are the accepted indications for bone mass measurement?
- Decision-making regarding the initiation or continuation of estrogen replacement therapy
- Evaluation of osteopenia or vertebral deformities discovered on routine x-rays
- Presence of modifiable conditions, such as steroid therapy and hyperparathyroidism, which may cause osteopenia

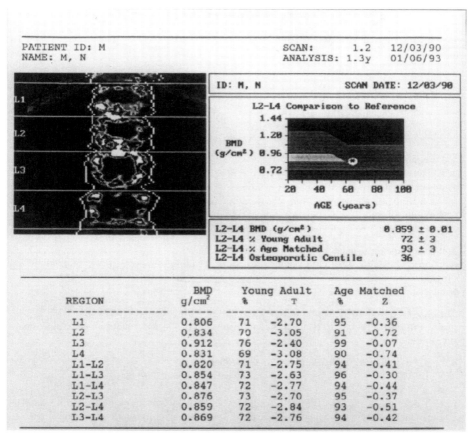

Bone density report for a DEXA study of the spine. The L2-L4 region, the most frequently evaluated, shows a bone mineral density (BMD) of 0.859 gm/cm^2, a T-score of -2.84, and a Z-score of -0.51. The very low T-score indicates osteoporosis with a significant fracture risk. The relatively normal Z-score indicates that age and menopause are likely the most important factors causing the low BMD.

9. Other than osteoporosis, what disorders must be considered as a cause of low bone mass?

Osteomalacia   Multiple myeloma
Osteogenesis imperfecta   Rheumatoid arthritis
Hyperparathyroidism   Renal failure
Hyperthyroidism   Idiopathic hypercalciuria
Cushing's syndrome

10. What are the most effective approaches currently available for the prevention and treatment of osteoporosis?

Treatment of Osteoporosis

BONE-RESORPTION–INHIBITING AGENTS	BONE-FORMATION–STIMULATING AGENTS
Calcium	Fluoride
Vitamin D	Calcitriol
Estrogen	Androgens
Calcitonin	Growth hormone
Bisphosphonates	Parathyroid hormone

The antiresorptive agents are in wide use because of their repeatedly demonstrated efficacy and safety. The formation-stimulating agents are still largely experimental. (See also Chapter 89.)

11. How can falls be prevented?
The major risk factors for falls include the use of sedatives, sensorium-altering drugs and antihypertensive medications, visual impairment, proprioceptive loss, and lower-extremity disability. Minimizing modifiable risk factors and removing obstacles to ambulation in the home are inexpensive and effective measures for reducing fractures due to falls. Simple measures such as carpeting slick surfaces and stairs, removing throw rugs and children's toys and installing railings and night lights can have a significant preventive effect.

12. How do corticosteroids cause osteoporosis?
Corticosteroids in supraphysiologic doses ($\geq$ 7 mg/day of prednisone) directly inhibit bone formation and indirectly increase PTH-mediated bone resorption through their antagonism of intestinal calcium absorption and promotion of renal calcium excretion. Because of these dual effects, significant osteoporosis may develop within 6 months of initiating corticosteroid therapy.

13. Can steroid-induced osteoporosis be prevented or treated?
Patients on corticosteroid therapy should receive calcium (1500 mg) and vitamin D (400 U) each day. If urinary calcium excretion exceeds 300 mg/day, a thiazide diuretic may be added. Calcitonin and bisphosphonate therapy have both been reported to reduce or prevent bone loss in these patients.

14. Describe vitamin D metabolism and action.
Vitamin D has two sources: 90% of the body's vitamin D comes from the skin in response to sunlight exposure, while 10% comes from dietary intake. Vitamin D from either source is converted by 25-hydroxylase in the liver to 25-hydroxyvitamin D and then by 1α-hydroxylase in the kidney to 1,25-dihydroxyvitamin D. The latter metabolite binds to peripheral vitamin D receptors to promote, among other things, intestinal absorption of calcium and phosphate.

15. What is osteomalacia?
The word *osteomalacia* means "soft bones." The condition results from impaired mineralization (deposition of hydroxyapatite) in mature bone.

16. What causes osteomalacia?
Osteomalacia results from an inadequate concentration of extracellular fluid phosphate and/or calcium or from a circulating inhibitor of mineralization.

Major Causes of Osteomalacia

Vitamin D deficiency	Hypophosphatemia
Low oral intake plus inadequate	Low oral phosphate intake
sunlight exposure	Phosphate-binding antacids
Intestinal malabsorption	Excess renal phosphate loss
Abnormal vitamin D metabolism	Inhibitors of mineralization
Liver disease	Aluminum
Renal disease	Bisphosphonates
Drugs (anticonvulsants, antituberculous	Fluoride
drugs, ketoconazole)	Hypophosphatasia

17. Describe the clinical manifestations of osteomalacia.

Osteomalacia causes pain and deformity, particularly in the long bones and pelvis. Laboratory abnormalities may include low serum calcium and/or phosphate, elevated serum alkaline phosphatase, reduced serum 25-hydroxyvitamin D levels, low urinary calcium excretion, and elevated urinary phosphate loss. Characteristic pseudofractures (milkman's fractures, Looser's zones) are seen radiographically at points where large arteries cross bones. Histologically, there is an increased amount of osteoid but significantly deficient hydroxyapatite deposition.

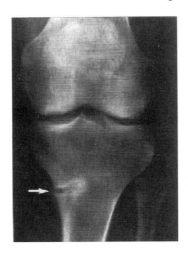

Pseudofractures (*arrow*) in osteomalacia involving the knee.

18. What causes rickets?

Rickets is a condition resulting from impaired mineralization of the skeleton during childhood. It may result from the same conditions that cause osteomalacia in adults as well as three congenital disorders:

1. Hypophosphatemic rickets is an inherited disorder, most commonly X-linked, in which excessive renal tubular phosphate losses result in serum phosphate levels too low to allow normal bone mineralization.

2. Congenital 1α-hydroxylase deficiency is caused by a genetic mutation in the 1α-hydroxylase gene. Deficiency of this renal enzyme results in inability to form 1,25-dihydroxyvitamin D, leading to inadequate intestinal calcium and phosphate absorption.

3. Congenital resistance to 1,25-dihydroxyvitamin D is caused by a genetic mutation in the vitamin D receptor gene. The defective or absent vitamin D receptor results in deficient 1,25-dihydroxyvitamin D–mediated intestinal absorption of calcium and phosphate.

19. What are the clinical manifestations of rickets?

The predominant clinical features are bone pain, deformities, and fractures, muscle weakness, and growth retardation. Deformities differ depending on the time of onset:

FIRST YEAR OF LIFE	AFTER FIRST YEAR OF LIFE
Widened cranial sutures	Flared ends of long bones
Frontal bossing	Bowing of long bones
Craniotabes	Sabre shins
Rachitic rosary	Coxa vara
Harrison's groove	Genu varum
Flared wrists	Genu valgum

Laboratory abnormalities may be similar to those seen in osteomalacia. Radiologic findings include delayed opacification of the epiphyses, widened growth plates, widened and irregular metaphyses, and thin cortices with sparse, coarse trabeculae in the diaphyses. Histologically, there is increased osteoid but deficient mineralization.

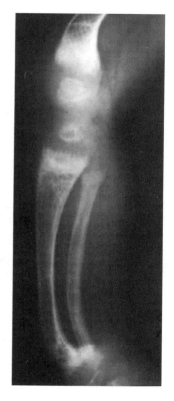

Radiologic findings in rickets. Lateral view of lower leg. Note flared end of bones, bowing of long bones, and osteoporosis.

20. How are osteomalacia and rickets treated?

Treatment of Bone Deposition Disorders

ETIOLOGY	TREATMENT
Simple nutritional vitamin D deficiency	Vitamin D, 5000 U/day until healing, then maintain 400 U/day
Malabsorption	Vitamin D, 50,000–100,000 U/day
Renal disease	Vitamin D, 50,000–100,000 U/day, or calcitriol, 0.25–1.0 μg/day
Hypophosphatemic rickets	Calcitriol, 0.25–1.0 μg/day, and oral phosphate
1α-hydroxylase deficiency	Calcitriol, 0.25–1.0 μg/day, and oral phosphate
Resistance to 1,25-dihydroxyvitamin D	Vitamin D, 100,000–200,000 U/day, or calcitriol, 5–60 μg/day, or IV calcium infusions

21. What is hypophosphatasia?

This rare congential disorder is caused by mutations in the gene that codes for the alkaline phosphatase isoform found in cartilage and bone. Affected patients present with rickets or osteomalacia and low serum alkaline phosphatase levels. The mineralization defect appears to be due to inability to break down inorganic pyrophosphate, a known inhibitor of mineralization. The disorder is frequently severe and often fatal. Patients with milder forms may be relatively asymptomatic until adulthood. There is no known effective treatment.

22. What is osteogenesis imperfecta?

Osteogenesis imperfecta results from mutations in one of the two genes that code for type I procollagen. Osteoblasts produce abnormal osteoid, resulting in osteopenic, fragile bones. Although four subtypes of varying severity have been described, there is actually a continuum ranging from a fatal infantile form to a mild adult form. Associated abnormalities often include blue sclerae, dentinogenesis imperfecta, and deafness. The diagnosis is made on clinical grounds. As there is no effective specific treatment, therapy involves mainly supportive, orthopedic, and rehabilitative measures.

23. Define osteopetrosis.

Osteopetrosis, or "marble bone disease," is caused by defective osteoclast function. An illustrative subset of patients have mutations in the gene for carbonic anhydrase II (CA II), resulting in CA II deficiency; osteoclasts in these patients are unable to generate the hydrogen ions (acidification) necessary for bone resorption. Failure of osteoclasts to resorb bone normally produces dense, chalky, fragile bones and bone marrow replacement with pancytopenia. Generalized osteosclerosis is seen on skeletal x-rays. There is a severe, usually fatal, infantile form and a more benign form that allows survival into adulthood. The most effective treatment for the infantile type is bone marrow transplantation, which provides normal osteoclasts. High-dose calcitriol may also be effective in some patients.

BIBLIOGRAPHY

1. Audan M: The physiology and pathophysiology of Vitamin D. Mayo Clin Proc 60:851, 1985.
2. Consensus Development Conference: Diagnosis, prophylaxis, and treatment of osteoporosis. Am J Med 94:646–650, 1993.
3. Favus MJ (ed): Primer on the Metabolic Bone Diseases and Disorders of Mineral Metabolism. New York, Raven Press, 1993.
4. Grisso JA, Kelsey JL, Strom BL, et al: Risk factors for falls as a cause of hip fracture in women. N Engl J Med 324:1326–1331, 1991.
5. Johnston CC Jr, Slemenda CW, Melton LJ: Clinical use of bone densitometry. N Engl J Med 324:1105–1108, 1991.
6. Lukert BP, Raisz LG: Glucocorticoid-induced osteoporosis: Pathogenesis and management. Ann Intern Med 112:352–364, 1990.
7. Manolagas SC, Jilka RL: Bone marrow, cytokines, and bone remodeling. N Engl J Med 332:305–311, 1995.
8. Prince RL, Smith M, Dick IM, et al: Prevention of postmenopausal osteoporosis: A comparative study of exercise, calcium supplementation, and hormone-replacement therapy. N Engl J Med 325:1189–1195, 1991.
9. Raisz LG: Local and systemic factors in the pathogenesis of osteoporosis. N Engl J Med 318:818–828, 1988.
10. Riggs BL, Melton LJ III: The prevention and treatment of osteoporosis. N Engl J Med 327:620–627, 1992.
11. Sambrook P, Birmingham J, Kelly P, et al: Prevention of corticosteroid osteoporosis: A comparison of calcium, calcitriol, and calcitonin. N Engl J Med 328:1747–1752, 1993.
12. Tinetti ME, Speechley M, Ginter SF: Risk factors for falls among elderly persons living in the community. N Engl J Med 319:1701–1707, 1988.

57. PAGET'S DISEASE OF BONE

David R. Finger, M.D.

1. What is Paget's disease?

Although evidence supports the existence of this disease in prehistoric times, it was not until the 19th century that Sir James Paget first described chronic inflammation of bone, using the term *osteitis deformans*. Paget's disease is a disorder of bone remodeling, with increased osteoclast-mediated bone resorption followed by increased bone formation. This process leads to a disorganized, mosaic pattern of woven and lamellar bone often associated with increased vascularity and marrow fibrosis.

2. Do we know what causes Paget's disease?

Many investigators suspect a viral infection, but this theory remains to be proved. Pagetic osteoclasts have been shown to contain intracellular particles resembling nucleocapsids of the paramyxovirus family of RNA viruses. Older studies have linked dog ownership to Paget's disease, although canine distemper virus antigen has been found in only half of patients and more recent studies have disproved this association.

3. Who gets Paget's disease?

Paget's is more common in whites of northern European ancestry. This disease is rare in the Far East, India, Africa, and Middle East. In the United States, it is more common in the north than in the south. Men have a slightly higher risk (3:2) than women.

4. How frequent is this disease?

The incidence doubles each decade from age 50, approaching 90% by age 90. The prevalence is 5% in England and 1–3% in the United States.

5. Is Paget's disease inherited?

Paget's disease is seven times more common in relatives of patients than in controls. This risk is further increased if the affected relative has severe disease or was diagnosed at an early age. There are no definite HLA associations.

6. Describe the clinical features of this disease.

Pain is the most common presenting manifestation (80%), though only one-third of patients are symptomatic. **Joint pain** is the second most common complaint (50%), usually involving the knee, hip, or spine. Affected areas often feel **warm** to palpation due to increased blood flow. **Bone deformities**, such as tibial bowing and skull thickening, may occur in advanced disease. Spontaneous **fractures**, most commonly in the femur, tibia, humerus, and forearm, may also occur.

7. Which part of the skeleton is most likely to be involved?

Paget's disease can be polyostotic (80%) or monostotic (20%) and has been noted to occur in every bone in the skeleton. The most common locations for monostotic disease include the tibia and iliac bones. Overall, the most common sites, in descending order, include the pelvis, lumbar spine, femur, thoracic spine, sacrum, skull, tibia, and humerus.

8. List some potential complications of Paget's disease.

Skeletal

Bone pain

Bone and joint deformities (bowing, frontal bossing)

Fractures

Neurologic
   Deafness (from ossification of the stapedius tendon or auditory nerve entrapment)
   Nerve entrapment (cranial nerves, spinal nerve roots)
   Spinal stenosis
   Basilar invagination
   Headaches
   Stroke (from blood vessel compression)
Vascular
   Hyperthermia
   Vascular steal syndrome (external carotid blood flow to the skull at the expense of the
      brain, resulting in apathy and somnolence)
Cardiac
   High cardiac output
   Congestive heart failure
   Hypertension
   Cardiomegaly
   Angina
Malignancy
   Osteogenic sarcomas (0.2–1.0%)
   Fibrosarcomas
   Benign giant cell tumors
Metabolic
   Hypercalcemia
   Hypercalciuria
   Nephrocalcinosis

9. How is Paget's disease usually diagnosed?

Asymptomatic patients are usually identified by an elevated alkaline phosphatase obtained on routine chemistry panels or by typical radiographic abnormalities noted on examination for some other complaint.

10. Which laboratory tests are abnormal in Paget's disease?

Paget's is characterized by accelerated bone turnover, which bone resorption and formation occurring simultaneously. Biochemical markers of each have been used in Paget's disease, but the most reproducible is **serum alkaline phosphatase**. These levels can be extremely elevated with skull involvement and high cardiac output, whereas other bony involvement (pelvis, sacrum, lumbar spine, femoral head) seems to be associated with lower levels. Alkaline phosphatase and **osteocalcin**, a less reliable index of disease activity, are markers of new bone formation. Levels correlate with the extent and activity of the disease process. Markers of bone resorption include urinary **hydroxyproline** and **pyridinoline cross-links**, which are usually elevated in Paget's disease. **Hypercalcemia** can occasionally be noted, usually in the presence of fracture or immobilization.

11. Identify the characteristic radiographic and scintigraphic findings seen in Paget's disease.

Paget's can be evaluated both by plain radiography and technetium bone scanning (^{99m}Tc-bisphosphonate); however, there is some discordance. Roughly 12% of lesions seen on bone scan will not be seen on radiographs, and 6% of radiographic abnormalities are absent on bone scan.

Plain radiographs reveal osteolytic, osteoblastic, or mixed lesions. Cortical thickening is usually present, along with adjacent trabecular thickening. The edge of lytic fronts in long bones gives a "blade of grass" appearance. Significant trabecular thickening of the iliopubic and ilioischial lines may be seen along the inner aspect of the pelvis in a "brim sign" or "pelvic ring" (see figure), while "osteoporosis circumscripta" refers to extensive lytic involvement in the skull (see figure). Lytic lesions can progress, but usually at a rate of less than 1 cm/year.

Paget's disease classically produces regions of focal increased uptake on **bone scan** (see figure). Scintigraphy is useful for evaluating the extent of disease and for detecting relapses following treatment. This disease does not spread to adjacent bones or "metastasize" to distant regions.

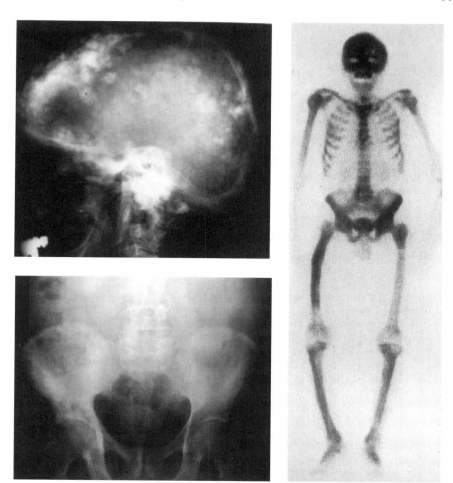

Skull radiograph showing a thickened cranium with regions of dense sclerosis and osteopenia resulting in a "cotton-wool" appearance. Pelvic radiograph showing right hemipelvic loss of normal trabeculation, sclerosis, and cortical thickening, along with sclerosis of the iliopectineal line. Full-body scintigraphy showing increased uptake in the skull, pelvis, lumbar spine, bilateral femurs with bowing of the right, tibias, scapula, and bilateral proximal humerus.

12. What is the differential diagnosis of Paget's disease?

Pagetic vertebrae may resemble lymphoma and metastatic cancers, especially prostate adenocarcinoma, but pagetic vertebrae are usually enlarged. In other affected bones, Paget's is often distinguished by the characteristic cortical thickening and adjacent thickened trabeculae. The progression of Paget's through different stages (lytic to sclerotic) also helps to differentiate it from osteoblastic metastatic lesions. Focal increased uptake on scintigraphy can be seen in many conditions besides Paget's disease, including osteomyelitis, arthritis, metastases, and fractures.

13. Describe the histopathologic findings seen in pagetic bone.

In the earliest stage of Paget's disease bone resorption occurs, mediated by numerous giant multinucleated osteoclasts. Vascular hypertrophy and medullary fibrosis are often associated with bone resorption. There is subsequently production of new lamellar and woven bone in a disorganized fashion, resulting in the characteristic mosaic appearance of bone seen in Paget's disease.

14. What are the indications to treat Paget's disease?
Involvement of the skull, vertebral bodies, long bones, and pelvis near the hip
Deafness
Neurologic compromise
High-output congestive heart failure
Disabling pain
Progressive skeletal deformity
Hypercalcemia, usually from immobilization
Planned surgery on pagetic bone

15. What treatments are available for Paget's disease?
NSAIDs, calcitonin, biphosphonates, mithramycin, and surgery have all been used successfully.
NSAIDs are used to treat pain often associated with osteoarthritis when Paget's occurs near joints.
Surgery is sometimes needed to relieve nerve compression and increase joint mobility. Specific
antipagetic therapy consists primarily of **calcitonin** and **biphosphonates**, as **mithramycin** has an
unacceptable toxicity profile. These agents directly suppress the activity of pagetic osteoclasts.
Etidronate is often the first drug used because it is an oral agent, less expensive, well tolerated,
and very effective. **Calcitonin** is often used when there is extensive lytic disease, disease in
weight-bearing bone, severe pain, or neurologic symptoms.

16. How are biphosphonates used in the treatment of Paget's disease?
Disodium etidronate, a first-generation biphosphonate, is currently the only agent in this category approved for use in the United States. It is available in 200- and 400-mg tablets and is given
in doses of 5–10 mg/kg/day. Over two-thirds of patients will experience a reduction in symptoms,
and there will be a 50% lowering of biochemical markers. Because this drug also inhibits bone
formation, it is generally given for 6 months followed by 6 months off therapy. Some patients experience a paradoxic increase in bone pain and develop generalized or focal regions of osteomalacia. **Pamidronate** (APD), a new parenteral second-generation biphosphonate that does not interfere with mineralization of newly formed bone, is also quite effective. In addition, these agents
can cause low-grade fever, transient leukopenia, flu-like symptoms, and gastrointestinal irritation.

17. How is calcitonin used in the treatment of Paget's disease?
Calcitonin was the first successful therapy for Paget's disease. It is available in human and salmon
parenteral preparations. A nasal spray has been developed but is not widely available. Calcitonin
is usually administered subcutaneously at 100 IU daily until clinical and biochemical improvement is seen, and then the dose is reduced to 50–100 IU every other day or three times a week.
Injections may be associated with flushing, nausea, and transient hypocalcemia in as many as
20%. Starting at lower doses (25–50 IU) and gradually increasing every 1–2 weeks will minimize
these side effects. Symptoms of Paget's disease usually diminish within a few weeks but return
when therapy is discontinued. A plateau phenomenon may occur due to neutralizing antibodies
to salmon calcitonin in up to 25% of patients. Human calcitonin will usually benefit those patients.

18. Can Paget's disease be cured?
There are many reports of long-term remissions following successful treatment of Paget's disease. Some investigators theorize that prolonged inactivation of multinucleated osteoclasts with
antiresorptive therapy could prevent recruitment of new cells. This cells mass of multinucleated
osteoclasts, which many believe to be infected with paramyxoviruses, would eventually die without replacements, leading to sustained remission or possible cures of Paget's disease.

BIBLIOGRAPHY

1. Bone HG, Kleerekoper M: Paget's disease of bone. J Clin Endocrinol Metab 75:1179–1182, 1992.
2. Burckhardt P: Biochemical and scintigraphic assessment of Paget's disease. Semin Arthritis Rheum
   23:237–239, 1994.

3. Franck WA, Bress NM, Singer FR, Krane SM: Rheumatic manifestations of Paget's disease of bone. Am J Med 56:592–603, 1974.
4. Gallacher SJ: Paget's disease of bone. Curr Opin Rheum 5:351–356, 1993.
5. Gordon MT, Mee AP, Sharpe PT: Paramyxoviruses in Paget's disease. Semin Arthritis Rheum 23:232–234, 1994.
6. Guyer PB, Chamberlain AT: Paget's disease of bone in two American cities. BMJ 280:985, 1980.
7. Hahn TJ: Metabolic bone disease. In Kelly WN, Harris ED, Ruddy S, Sledge CB (eds): Textbook of Rheumatology, 4th ed. Philadelphia, W.B. Saunders, 1993, pp 1619–1621.
8. Nagant de Deuxchaisnes C: Paget's disease of bone. In Klippel JH, Dieppe PA (eds): Rheumatology. St. Louis, Mosby, 1994, pp 7:39.1–39.6.
9. Nagant de Deuxchaisnes C, Krane SM: Paget's disease of bone: Clinical and metabolic observations. Medicine 43:233–266, 1964.
10. Siris ES: Epidemiological aspects of Paget's disease: Family history and relationship to other medical conditions. Semin Arthritis Rheum 23:222–225, 1994.
11. Siris ES: Paget's disease of bone. In Favus MJ (ed): Primer on the Metabolic Bone Diseases and Disorders of Mineral Metabolism, 2nd ed. New York, Raven Press, 1993, pp 375–384.

58. OSTEONECROSIS

Robert T. Spencer, M.D.

1. List some synonyms for osteonecrosis.

Avascular necrosis, aseptic necrosis, and ischemic necrosis.

2. How is osteonecrosis defined?

Osteonecrosis refers to death of the cellular component of bone (osteocytes) and contiguous bone marrow resulting from ischemia. Although inciting factors for such ischemia are varied, their end results are clinically indistinguishable.

3. What skeletal regions are predisposed to developing osteonecrosis?

Bones are most vulnerable in those areas having both limited vascular supply and restricted collateral circulation, which are areas that are also typically covered by articular cartilage. The area most frequently affected is the **femoral head**. At risk areas include:

Femoral head	Carpal bones (scaphoid, lunate)
Humeral head	Talus
Femoral condyles	Tarsal navicular
Proximal tibia	Metatarsals

4. What is the etiology of this disorder?

The etiology of osteonecrosis is most obvious and best understood in post-traumatic disruption of arterial blood supply. In those cases developing in the absence of trauma, various pathologic processes are capable of inducing hemostasis and, in turn, ischemia. Potential mechanisms include external vascular compression (due to marrow hypertrophy/infiltration, increased intraosseous pressure), thrombosis, embolization (fat/lipids, thrombi, sickle cells, nitrogen gas), osseous microfractures, and cytotoxic factors.

One etiologic factor theorized to be common to several associated conditions is that of fat/lipid embolization, which may occur in association with fatty liver (due to various causes), hyperlipidemia (particularly types II and IV), and disruption of fatty bone marrow (e.g., long-bone fracture). Conditions in which this is speculated to play a role include alcohol abuse, carbon tetrachloride poisoning, diabetes, hypercortisolism, hyperlipidemia, decompression illness, pregnancy, oral contraceptive use, hemoglobinopathies, and long-bone fractures.

5. What clinical conditions are associated with osteonecrosis?

Conditions Associated with Osteonecrosis

Nontraumatic	**Nontraumatic**
Juvenile	Sickle cell anemia
Slipped capital femoral epiphysis	Hemoglobinopathies
Legg-Calvé-Perthes	Caisson disease/decompression illness
Adult	Gaucher's disease
Corticosteroid administration	Radiotherapy
Cushing's disease	Carbon tetrachloride poisoning
Alcohol abuse	Tumor infiltration of marrow
Diabetes mellitus	Arteriosclerosis/vaso-occlusive disorders
Hyperlipidemia	**Traumatic**
Pancreatitis	Fracture of the femoral neck
Pregnancy	Dislocation or fracture-dislocation of the hip
Oral contraceptive use	Hip trauma without fracture or dislocation
SLE and other connective tissue disorders	Hip surgery
Renal transplantation	

6. Briefly describe the pathogenesis of osteonecrosis.

Etiologic factors initiate hemostasis directly or trigger a cascade resulting in hemostasis. Histologic findings indicate that the final common pathway for the various inciting factors involves local intravascular coagulation and resultant tissue ischemia. The end result is that of cancellous bone and bone marrow death. With subchondral cancellous bone death, collapse of the articular surface may or may not occur, depending on the extent of involvement.

Pain, the earliest symptom of osteonecrosis, may occur in the early stages of involvement, before any radiographic changes are noted. This pain is likely due to elevated intraosseous pressure, since such pain can be relieved by decompression. In some individuals, no symptoms develop until late stages of the disease process when collapse of the articular surface occurs and secondary degenerative changes develop. Others, in whom the area of infarction is small enough that collapse does not occur, may never develop symptoms. Radiographs in these patients reveal sclerotic areas often referred to as "bone islands" or "bone infarcts."

7. What clinical features would lead to suspicion of this disorder?

The signs and symptoms stemming from osteonecrosis are nonspecific. **Pain** is what leads affected individuals to seek medical evaluation. For the hip, the joint most commonly involved, pain is unilateral at onset and localizes to the groin, buttock, medial thigh, and medial aspect of the knee. Occasionally, knee pain is the only complaint in an individual with late-stage osteonecrosis. Typically, morning stiffness is absent or of short duration (< 1 hour), allowing differentiation from inflammatory monoarticular arthritides. Range of motion is not affected, except as limited by discomfort, until late degenerative changes develop. Although these findings are common to other potential etiologies, their occurrence in the setting of a patient with a predisposing risk (e.g., recent trauma, high-dose steroid use) should suggest underlying osteonecrosis.

8. What are the epidemiologic features of osteonecrosis?

- An estimated 15,000 new cases develop each year in the United States.
- Of cases of nontraumatic osteonecrosis, steroid use and alcohol abuse may be responsible for > 50% of cases; in up to 40%, there is no identifiable risk factor (idiopathic).
- Males are affected more frequently than females at a ratio of approximately 8:1, possibly reflecting a higher incidence of trauma in males.
- Most cases develop in the < 50-year-old age group. One exception to this observation is seen in osteonecrosis of the knee (femoral condyles, proximal tibia), to which women over age 50 are predisposed (F:M ratio of about 3:1).

9. What is the role of plain radiographs in the diagnosis of osteonecrosis?

Initially plain films are normal. Later, a region of generalized osteopenia may develop (a nonspecific finding). Eventually, after bone repair mechanisms have had time to work, a mottled appearance develops in the affected area due to the presence of "cysts" (regions of dead bone resorption) and contiguous sclerosis (regions of bone repair).

Early collapse of the cancellous bone beneath the subchondral plate is apparent as a pathognomonic radiolucent line frequently referred to as the **crescent sign**. (See figure). Once in this stage, further collapse is almost inevitable, and it thus represents the earliest irreversible lesion of osteonecrosis. Once the articular surface has collapsed and flattened, secondary degenerative changes develop, resulting in joint-space narrowing and secondary involvement of other bones within the articulation (e.g., acetabulum).

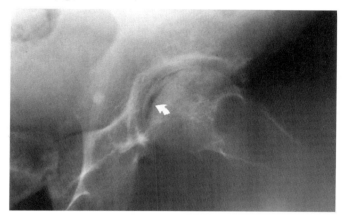

Plain radiograph of hip showing crescent sign (*arrow*) of osteonecrosis.

10. How is radionuclide bone scanning used in the diagnosis?

This technique is much more sensitive than plain radiography and is thus capable of detecting osteonecrosis at earlier and potentially treatable stages. However, the "hot spot" seen in osteonecrosis is nonspecific. On occasion a "cold" area (representing necrotic tissue) is seen within the area of enhanced uptake (a "cold-hot" lesion), and this finding is highly specific for osteonecrosis. Overall, the bone scan is being used less frequently in evaluation of this disorder due to the enhanced specificity and sensitivity of MRI.

11. How good is magnetic resonance imaging in the diagnosis of osteonecrosis?

Compared to other diagnostic studies, MRI has been found to have the highest sensitivity and best diagnostic accuracy, thus nearly obviating invasive diagnostic procedures such as biopsy and bone marrow pressure determinations. Sensitivity and diagnostic accuracy appear to be > 95%.

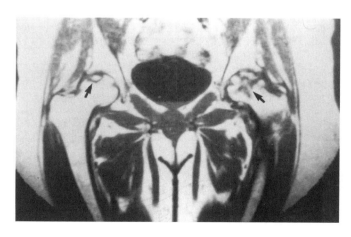

MRI of bilateral hips showing necrotic bone (*arrows*) in both femoral heads consistent with osteonecrosis.

The characteristic MRI finding is an area or **line of decreased signal** on both T1 and T2 images (see figure on previous page). This area appears to correspond with the demarcation between live regenerating bone and necrotic tissue.

12. How often does osteonecrosis occur in a bilateral fashion?
In the hips, bilateral involvement occurs in 50–90% of cases by MRI determination. Similar frequencies would be expected in osteonecrosis of the humeral head and knee.

13. Describe the staging scheme for osteonecrosis of the femoral head.

Staging of Osteonecrosis of the Femoral Head

STAGE	PLAIN RADIOGRAPHIC FINDINGS	MRI/BONE SCAN
0	Normal	Normal
I	Normal	Abnormal
II	Osteopenia, bony sclerosis, cystic changes	Abnormal
III	Subchondral collapse ("crescent sign") without articular surface flattening	Abnormal
IV	Flattening of the articular surface without joint-space narrowing	Abnormal
V	Flattening of the articular surface with joint-space narrowing and/or acetabular involvement	Abnormal
VI	Advanced degenerative changes	Abnormal

14. Can osteonecrosis be prevented?
Yes. Some of the predisposing risk factors can be manipulated—e.g., steroid dose, alcohol intake, speed of decompression, and control of diabetes and hyperlipidemia. As an example, the vast majority of cases of corticosteroid-related osteonecrosis occur in patients who have received the equivalent of ≥ 20 mg of prednisone/day. In rheumatoid arthritis, where prednisone doses rarely exceed 10–15 mg/day, osteonecrosis is rarely seen. In contrast, in SLE in which higher doses of steroids are frequently used, up to 50% of patients may expect to develop some degree of osteonecrosis.

15. Describe the medical management of osteonecrosis.
The goal in treating osteonecrosis is to prevent bony collapse and subsequent deformity. Thus, effective treatment is contingent upon diagnosis while osteonecrosis is still in its early stages (stage II and less). Recommended medical management is unfortunately limited to having the patient **discontinue weight-bearing** on the affected side for 4–8 weeks and administering **analgesics** for relief of associated pain. There have been reports of promising results obtained utilizing pulsing electromagnetic field therapy, but this technique is still under investigation.

16. Describe surgical management for this disorder.
In **early, reversible stages** of osteonecrosis, several surgical procedures have been developed with the hope of preventing progression. Of these, **core decompression** of the femoral head has been most commonly performed and investigated. The rationale for this operation is that if increased intraosseous pressure can be relieved, vascular perfusion can then be enhanced and help prevent progression of the lesion. Several studies comparing core decompression to nonoperative management have shown favorable results, with success rates in the range of 33–100%. Because no other surgical procedures have been as well studied, core decompression should be the procedure of choice when surgery is recommended.

In the **nonreversible stages** of osteonecrosis (particularly stages IV–VI), the goal of surgical intervention is to restore joint function and relieve associated pain. The effectiveness and reliability of **total hip arthroplasty** (replacement) have made earlier procedures attempting to achieve these goals obsolete.

BIBLIOGRAPHY

1. Chang CC, Greenspan A, Gershwin ME: Osteonecrosis: current perspectives on pathogenesis and treatment. Semin Arthritis Rheum 23:47, 1993.
2. Jones JP: Osteonecrosis. In McCarty DJ, Koopman WJ (eds): Arthritis and Allied Conditions, 12th ed. Philadelphia, Lea & Febiger, 1993.
3. Mazières B: Regional bone diseases: Osteonecrosis. In Klippel JH, Dieppe PA (eds): Rheumatology. London, Mosby, 1994.
4. Resnick D, Niwayama G, Sweet DE, Madewell JE: Osteonecrosis. In Resnick D (ed): Bone and Joint Imaging. Philadelphia, W.B. Saunders, 1989.
5. Steinberg ME, Steinberg DR: Osteonecrosis. In Kelley WN, Harris ED, Ruddy S, Sledge CB (eds): Textbook of Rheumatology, 4th ed. Philadelphia, W.B. Saunders, 1993.

X. Hereditary, Congenital, and Inborn Errors of Metabolism Associated with Rheumatic Syndromes

The law of heredity is that all undesirable traits come from the other parent.
Anonymous

59. HERITABLE COLLAGEN DISEASES

John Keith Jenkins, M.D.

1. What are the most prevalent types of collagen in the body? Where are they located?
Type I collagen accounts for 60–90% of the dry weight of skin, ligaments, and demineralized bone. Type II collagen accounts for >50% of the dry weight of articular cartilage and also occurs in substantial amounts in the vitreous, nucleus pulposus, and nasal and auricular cartilages. Type III is found in blood vessels and in tissues that have type I collagen (except for bone). Type IV occurs in most basement membranes. Type VII collagen is also a basement membrane collagen found in the skin.

2. Describe the important features of collagen synthesis.
Collagen synthesis is complex and requires normal expression of the different collagen genes in the right proportion. The molecules must also be functional. Nucleated growth of the nascent collagen fibrils requires the correct primary structure as well as post-translational modifications of the procollagen molecules. For example, type I collagen is formed from two procollagen type I α_1 chains and one procollagen type I α_2 chain. The three chains combine at one end and will only zip together to form the triple helix (nucleated growth) after adequate post-translational modification of the proline residues. Fibrils are arranged in a quarter stagger array to form a large fiber.

3. How do abnormalities in collagen synthesis cause clinical disease?
   1. With mutations in collagen genes, the location of the collagen type that is abnormal determines which organs will be involved.
   2. Mutations that simply diminish production of a particular collagen type may give a milder phenotype than does a high level of expression of a structurally abnormal protein.
   3. The principle of nucleated growth explains why structurally abnormal molecules lead to devastating and potentially lethal clinical results.
   4. Different amino acid substitutions in the same collagen gene may affect different functions of the molecule and lead to different clinical manifestations, but there may be significant overlap in the syndromes.

4. What is osteogenesis imperfecta? Which organs are involved and why?
Osteogenesis imperfecta (OI), known as "brittle bone" disease, is actually a group of diseases defined by similar clinical manifestations (brittle bones and blue sclerae) in differing degrees, a suspected similar etiology, and variable inheritance patterns. A surprising result of recent research is that >90% of all OI patients studied thus far have a mutation in one of the two genes encoding type I collagen. Type I collagen is prevalent in bone and is necessary for its structure and physical properties. The collagen abnormality results in osteopenia and brittleness, leading to frequent fractures. Diminished collagen in the sclerae leads to its translucency and apparent blueness.

5. Because type I collagen mutations cause brittle bones, is there a molecular defect in collagen in osteoporosis?

Molecular defects in type I collagen recently have been shown to cause some forms of familial osteoporosis in Europe and the United States. Some investigators suspect that women at risk for osteoporosis may have an as-yet-undefined abnormality of collagen that predisposes them to "premature" osteoporosis.

6. How can a defect in type I collagen lead to brittle bone disease in one patient and familial osteoporosis in another?

Collagen is a complex molecule containing multiple domains with different functions. The clinical manifestations of its abnormalities vary depending on the function or structure interrupted. In recent years, investigators have found overlap between milder OI and osteoporosis syndromes and between OI and Ehlers-Danlos syndromes. Defining the molecular defect in a specific collagen does not necessarily allow one to determine the precise clinical diagnosis. These diseases demonstrate the Orwellian principle that some collagens are created more equal than others. The first corollary of this principle is that one still has to learn clinical syndromes for board examinations.

7. What is the Sillence classification of OI?

The Sillence classification groups OI into four clinical categories of severity. Multiple mutations may be responsible for each Sillence type.

Type I OI (mild): Patients have bone fragility with a moderate number of fractures (leading to wormian bones), blue sclerae, and short stature.

Type II OI (usually lethal): Patients have multiple in utero fractures and blue or gray sclerae. In utero or neonatal death is common.

Type III OI (severe deforming): Patients have major skeletal deformities, such as bone fragility, scoliosis, and joint laxity with a high number of fractures. They may have gray or blue sclerae and osteopenia and are not usually ambulatory.

Type IV OI (moderate severity): Patients have a moderate number of fractures and wormian bones, normal (white) or gray sclerae, osteopenia, and bone deformity but are ambulatory.

Type III OI is autosomal recessive, and types I, II, and IV are autosomal dominant. Dental abnormalities (dentinogenesis imperfecta) may accompany types I, III, and IV, and hearing loss may accompany forms I and IV.

8. Describe the clinical manifestations of the Ehlers-Danlos syndromes.

The Ehlers-Danlos syndromes (EDS) comprise a group of uncommon disorders primarily involving the joints and skin and characterized by **increased joint mobility** and **increased skin fragility and hyperextensibility.** There is a wide variability in the joint, skin, and internal organ

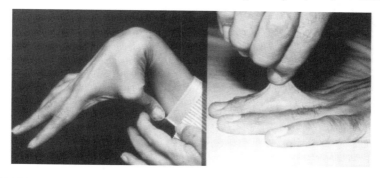

Patient with Ehlers-Danlos syndrome demonstrating hyperextensibility of joints and skin. (From the Clinical Slide Collection on the Rheumatic Diseases. Atlanta, American College of Rheumatology, 1991; with permission.)

involvement depending on the type of EDS. EDS types I (gravis) and II (mitis) have the typical skin and joint disease.

9. What is the significance of increased joint mobility and skin hyperextensibility?

Increased joint mobility is frequently associated with a lack of stability leading to dislocation. This laxity results in congenital hip dislocation and habitual dislocation later in life. Hemarthritic disability may occur as a result of recurrent dislocation with hemorrhage. Regarding the skin, these patients may have gaping wounds from minor trauma and do not retain sutures well (fragility).

10. How is EDS inherited?

The genetic defect is known for only a few types of EDS. In most cases, the defect is inherited in an autosomal dominant manner and results in diminished or defective collagen in some way. One exception is EDS type VI (oculo-scoliotic) which involves a recessive defect in lysyl hydroxylase, the vitamin C-requiring enzyme necessary for forming the hydroxylysine needed in cross-linking collagen. In addition to joint and skin hyperextensibility, scoliosis and rupture of the ocular globe occur in this form. The defect, though, still affects collagen.

11. What is the arterial form of EDS?

EDS type IV (arterial form) involves a defect in production of type III collagen, which is found in blood vessels. Skin and joint disease is less than with types I and II, but arterial or bowel rupture may be dramatic and lethal. Defects in type III collagen have been shown to be a rather common cause of premature aneurysms in the cardiovascular (abdominal aortic) and cerebrovascular (proximal to the circle of Willis) systems. Rare diseases such as EDS and OI may simply represent the most severe phenotypes of mutations in structural proteins that otherwise manifest late in life as premature bone, joint, or vascular disease.

12. How is abnormal joint laxity determined in EDS and other syndromes?

There are six simple tests for joint laxity, i.e., hyperextensibility, done during the physical examination:

1. Genu recurvatum or extension of the knee beyond $10°$
2. Extension of the elbow $>10°$ past normal
3. Extension of the thumb to touch the anterior surface of the forearm (see Question 8)
4. Extension of fingers backward so that they are parallel with the posterior forearm
5. Trunk flexion so that the palms of the hands can be placed flat on the ground
6. Dorsiflexion of the foot beyond the normal $20°$ past a right angle

Hyperextensibility in EDS patients may be greater in the small joints than large joints and may diminish with age. Signs of laxity/hyperextensibility in other organs include Gorlin's sign (ability to touch the nose with the tip of the tongue) and skin laxity (loss of ability of stretched skin to return and papyraceous-appearing skin over the knees).

13. What is the benign hypermobility syndrome?

Formerly EDS type III. This syndrome is characterized by varying degrees of joint laxity without instability or disability. It is an important cause of periarticular complaints. Arthralgias (hands, knees, and hips) occur with unusual physical activity, there is a familial tendency, and frequent ankle or wrist sprains may occur. Young girls are the most common patients with this disorder, and joint effusions do occur. A patient needs at least three of the six physical examination signs of hyperextensibility to have the hypermobility syndrome diagnosed.

14. What are the primary organ systems involved in the Marfan syndrome? Why?

Marfan syndrome commonly involves primarily the ocular, skeletal, and vascular systems, but the skin and pulmonary systems are also involved. A defect has been found in the gene for fibrillin in all patients studied. The inheritance pattern is autosomal dominant, and the prevalence is probably $>6/100,000$.

Marfan syndrome was long suspected to be a defect in elastin, a specialized connective tissue providing elasticity and prominent in ligaments, but no abnormality in elastin has ever been found in this syndrome. Fibrillin, found in soft connective tissues, is a constituent of extracellular microfibrils which form the substructure for elastin. Organs involved in the Marfan syndrome are those in which elastic fibers (and therefore fibrillin) are important and include the elastic wall of arteries (especially the aorta), zonula fibers of the eye, ligaments, skin and lung parenchyma.

15. Describe the phenotype and skeletal manifestations of the Marfan syndrome.

Patient's with the Marfan syndrome have a characteristic phenotype that can be recognized easily: tall stature, long thin extremities, arachnodactyly, and diminished subcutaneous fat. Skeletal manifestations include arachnodactyly (spider digits), pectus excavatum or carinatum, excessively tall stature, dolichostenomelia (abnormally low ratio of upper to lower body segments, < 0.85), loss of thoracic kyphosis, and scoliosis. Other manifestations include a gothic (high, arched) palate and dolichocephaly (long, narrow face).

Several prominent athletes as well as Abraham Lincoln are said to have had the Marfan syndrome. The Olympic sports in which persons with the Marfan syndrome are said to excel are volleyball and basketball. In fact, a U.S. Olympic volleyball star, Flo Hyman, died in 1986 of vascular complications of the Marfan syndrome.

16. How is arachnodactyly recognized?

Look at the hands. However, there are three simple, and probably more definitive, methods by which to determine its presence.

- The **thumb sign,** or Steinberg's sign, is a protrusion of the thumb past the hypothenar border when the hand is clenched in a fist.
- The **wrist sign,** or Walker-Murdoch sign, is overlap of the fifth finger and thumb when they encircle the wrist of the opposite hand.
- The **metacarpal index** is a radiographic measure of arachnodactyly. It is the average of the lengths divided by the midpoint widths of the second through fourth metacarpals (5.4–7.9 is normal, >8.4 occurs in Marfans).

All these signs indicate long, thin (spider-like) digits.

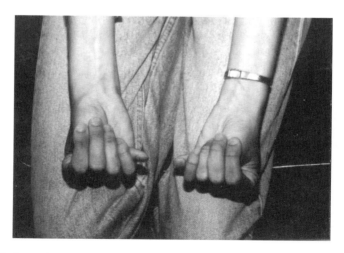

Patient with Marfan syndrome demonstrating Steinberg's thumb sign. (From the Clinical Slide Collection on the Rheumatic Diseases. Atlanta, American College of Rheumatology, 1991; with permission.)

17. How good a measure of the Marfan syndrome is arachnodactyly? What is its differential diagnosis?
Arachnodactyly is present in about 90% of cases of Marfan syndrome, is not diagnostic, and may be seen in other diseases. Nonasthenic Marfan syndrome may be a *forme fruste* of the disease; patients have a more normal-appearing phenotype with arachnodactyly and may have the same mutation as that in other more severely affected family members. Marfanoid hypermobility syndrome has skeletal features of the Marfan phenotype, such as arachnodactyly, but also has hyperelastic skin and hyperextensible joints as in Ehlers-Danlos syndrome. Congenital contractural arachnodactyly is another autosomal dominant disease with tall stature, arachnodactyly, joint contractures and unknown etiology. Homocystinurics may also demonstrate tallness, arachnodactyly, and spinal abnormalities.

18. What are the nonmusculoskeletal manifestations of the Marfan syndrome? Which cause significant morbidity and mortality?
Ectopia lentis occurs in over half of patients. Cardiovascular complications are multiple and common. Aneurysmal dilatation of the ascending aortic with dissection is the most common cause of death in patients, with the average lifespan being 32 years in these patients. Mitral valve prolapse with regurgitation or aortic insufficiency is detectable in 60% of patients by auscultation and in >80% by echocardiography. Pulmonary manifestations include cystic disease and spontaneous pneumothorax. The primary cause of morbidity is skeletal disease of the spine. Scoliosis is a major management problem and may be rapidly progressive during adolescence, requiring surgery.

19. How is Marfan syndrome treated?
Genetic counseling is in order, and preventative measures are taken to monitor cardiovascular problems. Because the disease is autosomal dominant, 50% of offspring will be affected. Echocardiography is needed to determine the presence of mitral and aortic valvular disease. Infective endocarditis occurs in patients with mitral or tricuspid disease, and they should receive prophylaxis. Echocardiography is performed yearly to follow aortic dilatation; when the size exceeds 50% of normal, echocardiography is recommended at 6-month intervals. Propranolol may retard progression of aortic dilatation. Vigorous exercise is contraindicated. Pregnancy is generally safe unless aortic dilatation is present.

20. What are the clinical features of pseudoxanthoma elasticum?
Pseudoxanthoma elasticum is a rare autosomal recessive disease that involves degeneration and calcification of elastic fibers. The molecular defect is undefined but is somewhere in the structure of elastic fibers. There is moderate heterogeneity in the clinical findings. Occasionally autosomal dominant forms manifest clinical features late in life.

Xanthomatoid papules occur in flexural skinfolds and is the classic finding. **Angioid streaks** occur in the fundus. Visual loss may occur from a maculopathy and retinal lesions. **Calcific deposits** in the lungs and cardiac involvement mimicking cardiomyopathy may occur. **Arterial rupture** occurs in the gastrointestinal tract. Abnormal elastic fibers usually do not impair wound healing until late in life.

21. What is cutis laxa?
Cutis laxa refers to a group of disorders with a common finding of lax, redundant skin. The skin may appear wrinkled, aged, or sagging in loose folds. A similar skin appearance may occur after penicillamine use or subsequent to inflammatory skin diseases. The skin appears to have lost elasticity and does not recoil when stretched, unlike EDS skin which does recoil. Cardiopulmonary manifestations may occur, including bronchiectasis and emphysema. There is no abnormality of skin fragility with bleeding, so surgery is safely performed (again, unlike Ehlers-Danlos syndrome).

22. What is the Stickler syndrome?
The Stickler syndrome, or hereditary arthro-ophthalmopathy, is an hereditary disease of unknown etiology in which patients have skeletal and ocular abnormalities. It is thought to be relatively

common, and the inheritance pattern is autosomal dominant. Half of families in one study were shown to have an abnormality in type II collagen, the most common collagen in cartilage. The syndrome includes myopia, retinal detachment and other eye problems, cleft palate, mandibular hypoplasia, hyper- and hypomobile joints, epiphyseal dysplasia, and disability from joint problems. The diagnosis should be suspected in any young adult with degenerative hip arthritis or any infant with congenitally swollen joints. Other clinical syndromes involving widespread cartilage disease that may be associated with abnormal type II collagen include primary generalized osteoarthritis, chondrodysplasia, and spondyloepiphyseal dysplasia.

23. Where is the molecular defect in Alport's syndrome?

Alport's syndrome includes hereditary glomerulonephritis and deafness. The defect is in a nonfibrillar basement membrane collagen, type IV collagen. Type VII is another basement membrane collagen important in anchoring the dermis of the skin, and it may be abnormal in some blistering skin diseases.

BIBLIOGRAPHY

1. Barker DF, Hostikka SL, Zhou J, et al: Identification of mutations in the COL4A5 gene in Alport syndrome. Science 248:1224–1227, 1990.
2. Beighton P: The dominant and recessive forms of cutis laxa. J Med Genet 9:216–221, 1972.
3. Hermann J, France TD, Spranger JW, et al: The Stickler syndrome (hereditary arthroophthalmopathy). Birth Defects 11:76–103, 1975.
5. Kornberg M, Aulicino P: Hand and wrist joint problems in patients with Ehlers-Danlos syndrome. J Hand Surg 10:193–196, 1985.
6. Kuivaniemi H, Tromp G, Prockop DJ: Mutations in collagens: Causes of rare and some common disorders in humans. FASEB J 5:2052–2060, 1991.
7. Leier CV, Call TD, Fulkerson PK, Woolery CF: The spectrum of cardiac defects in the Ehlers-Danlos syndrome, types I and III. Ann Intern Med 92:171–178, 1980.
8. Marchase P, Holbrook R, Pinnell SR: A familial cutis laxa syndrome with ultra-structural abnormalities of collagen and elastin. J Invest Dermatol 75:399–403, 1980.
9. Pope FM, Narcisi P, Nicholls AC, et al: Clinical presentations of Ehlers-Danlos syndrome type IV. Arch Dis Child 63:1016–1025, 1989.
10. Powell JT, Adamson J, MacSweeney STR, et al: Genetic variants of collagen III and abdominal aortic aneurysm. Eur J Vasc Surg 5:145–148, 1991.
11. Prockop DJ: Osteogenesis imperfecta: Model for genetic causes of osteoporosis and perhaps several other common diseases of connective tissue. Arthritis Rheum 31:1–8, 1988.
12. Pyeritz RE: Heritable disorders of connective tissue. In Schumacher HR (ed): Primer on the Rheumatic Diseases, 10th ed. Atlanta, Arthritis Foundation, 1993; pp 249–255.
13. Pyeritz RE: Maternal and fetal complications of pregnancy in the Marfan syndrome. Am J Med 71:784–790, 1981.
14. Pyeritz RE, McKusick VA: The Marfan syndrome: Diagnosis and management. N Engl J Med 300:772, 1978.
15. Rowe DW, Shapiro JR: Disorders of bone and structural proteins. In Kelley WK, Harris ED, Ruddy S, Sledge CB (eds): Textbook of Rheumatology, 4th ed. Philadelphia, W.B. Saunders, 1993, pp 1567–1592.

60. INBORN ERRORS OF METABOLISM AFFECTING CONNECTIVE TISSUE

John Keith Jenkins, M.D.

1. What are the homocystinurias?

There are three clinically (and biochemically) distinct disorders of amino acid metabolism resulting in elevated serum and urine levels of homocystine. The most common form of homocystinuria is due to an autosomal recessive defect in methionine metabolism because of absence of activity of the enzyme cystathionine β-synthase. This enzyme is involved in the transsulfuration pathway from methionine to cysteine. Two other less common forms are due to defective remethylation of homocystine to methionine.

2. How common is homocystinuria?

Cystathionine β-synthase deficiency probably occurs in about 1 in 200,000 (or less) livebirths in this country, prompting some states to require newborn homocystine screening. In comparison, newborn screening for phenylketonuria, which most states require, detects 1 case in 10,000 livebirths. Heterozygotes for cystathionine β-synthase deficiency (1 in 70 in the general population) have been thought to be unaffected but may be at risk for premature peripheral and cerebral vascular disease.

3. How is homocystinuria diagnosed?

Homocystine is increased in the blood and urine in all three known defects. The cyanide-nitroprusside test detects sulfhydryl-containing amino-acids in the urine, so it is not specific for the particular enzymatic defect. The pathway is from homocystine to methionine to cysteine. Plasma methionine levels are high in cystathionine β-synthase deficiency but normal or low in the premethionine defects causing homocytinuria. The other known defects are in synthesis of the cofactors (methyl vitamin B12 and methyltetrahydrofolate) needed for methionine synthesis. A combination of homocystine and methionine levels in urine and blood must be measured. Precise tissue (e.g., cultured skin fibroblasts) enzyme assays can then be performed.

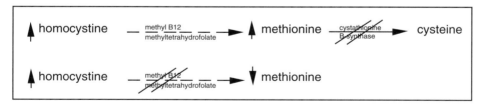

Biochemical pathways leading to homocystinuria. *Top,* Cystathionine β-synthase deficiency leads to increased homocystine and methionine levels. *Bottom,* Deficiency of other cofactors leads to decreased methionine and increased homocystine.

4. List the major clinical manifestations of homocystinuria.

Ectopia lentis (dislocated lens)—hallmark finding
Thromboembolism
Mental retardation
Connective tissue disorder

5. What are the musculoskeletal manifestations of homocystinuria?

The appearance is similar to that of Marfan syndrome—tall, arachnodactyly (dolichstenomelia), ectopia lentis, and chest wall and spinal deformity. Osteoporosis (generalized) and tight joints occur. Spinal osteoporosis occurs in 36–64% by age 15. Spinal disease is prominent and is usually a combination of osteoporotic fractures, degenerative disc/joint disease, and scoliosis. Joint fluid is normal.

6. How does homocystinuria affect connective tissue?

Cysteines are necessary for proper cross-linking (to cystine) of structural proteins such as collagen and fibrillin in connective tissue and bone, the suprasensory ligament of the eye, and the extracellular milieu of endothelial cells. On this basis, altered collagen may be responsible for the lens dislocation and osteoporosis, while altered proteins in the elastomeric complex or its substructure (fibrillin) may be responsible for the phenotypic similarity to the Marfan syndrome. Altered endothelial ground substance is responsible for the thrombosis and subsequent mental retardation.

7. How is homocystinuria treated? Which symptoms can be expected to respond?

Effective treatment requires early diagnosis to prevent mental retardation, which is the basis of newborn screening for inborn errors of metabolism. B6, B12, and folate are cofactors for the different enzymes involved in methionine metabolism. One-half of patients are B6-responders. Large doses of vitamin B6 (15–500mg of pyridoxine per day) lowers blood methionine, raises blood cysteine, and improves symptoms in patients with cystathionine β-synthase deficiency, presumably by augmenting a small amount of residual enzyme activity.

8. Do symptoms regress with therapy?

Development of ectopia lentis, osteoporosis, and retardation may be mitigated with therapy, but they will not remit if already present.

9. What causes alkaptonuria? What is the inheritance pattern?

Alkaptonuria (also known as ochronosis) is a rare defect in tyrosine catabolism due to a deficiency in homogentisic acid oxidase. This enzyme catabolizes homogentisic acid to molecules that can be used in the TCA cycle. Deposition of homogentisic acid produces a gray to blue-black pigment in tissues, hence the name *ochronosis*. Alkaptonuria is a favorite board question because it was the first human disease shown to be autosomal recessive. Heterozygotes are unaffected even when challenged with high doses of the precursor amino acids.

10. How is the diagnosis of alkaptonuria made?

The clinical diagnosis is suggested by the typical triad of findings:
- Degenerative arthritis (premature)
- Abnormal pigmentation
- Urine that turns blue-black on standing (alkalinization or ferric chloride addition).

Homogentisic acid binds collagen and is therefore deposited in connective tissues. If you see blue-black (skin, ears, sclerae, cartilage), think ochronosis. A specific enzyme assay for homogentisic acid oxidase, as well as thin layer chromatography for homogentisic acid, can be performed.

11. Describe the musculoskeletal manifestations of alkaptonuria.

Degenerative joint disease occurs in the third decade with typical symptoms of pain, stiffness, and limited range of motion of large joints and spine. The most common site involved is the spine, followed by the knees, hips, and shoulders. Abnormal calcification and ossification occur. Tendinitis has been reported. Dense calcification of the intervertebral discs is said to be pathognomic. The vacuum sign is prominent in discs also. Synovial fluid does not darken on alkalinization as urine does, but it may have a characteristic ground-pepper appearance. Calcium pyrophosphate deposition disease has been noted to coexist with ochronotic arthritis.

12. How is ochronotic arthritis treated?
Symptomatic treatment of the arthritis as for osteoarthritis is the standard therapy: patient education, physical therapy and/or local therapy, analgesia, etc. Dietary restriction of phenylalanine and tyrosine are indicated. Surgical procedures (including arthroplasty) and arthroscopy have been of benefit for removal of osteochondral loose bodies in the knee. Large doses of vitamin C have been used, but there are no studies of its efficacy.

13. What is Menkes' kinky hair syndrome? What is its inheritance pattern?
Menkes' is an X-linked recessive disorder of copper metabolism in which the clinical abnormalities are primarily neurologic: seizures, abnormal reflexes, spasticity, mental retardation, and pili torti (beaded, brittle, and sparse hair).

14. What is the cause of the rheumatic or musculoskeltal manifestations in Menkes'?
Abnormal copper metabolism affects copper-requiring metalloenzymes involved in collagen and elastin synthesis. It therefore affects connective tissues. The rheumatic manifestations may be either cutis laxa-like or Ehlers-Danlos-like with highly extensible skin and joints.

BIBLIOGRAPHY

1. Albers SE, Brozena SJ, Glass R, Fenske NA: Alkaptonuria and ochronosis: Case report and review. J Am Acad Dermatol 27:609–614, 1992.
2. Gordan DA: Storage and deposition diseases. In Schumacher HR (ed): Primer on the Rheumatic Diseases, 10th ed. Atlanta, Arthritis Foundation, 1993, pp 227–228.
3. Hunter T, Gordon D, Ogryzlo MA: The ground pepper sign of synovial fluid: A new diagnositic feature of ochronosis. J Rheumatol 1:45–53, 1974.
4. Mudd SH, Skovby F, Levy HL, et al: The natural history of homocystinuria due to cystathionine beta-synthase deficiency. Am J Hum Genet 37:1–31, 1985.
5. Pyeritz RE: Heritable disorders of connective tissue. In Schumacher HR (ed): Primer on the Rheumatic Diseases, 10th ed. Atlanta, Arthritis Foundation, 1993, pp 249–255.
6. Rowe DW, Shapiro JR: Disorders of bone and structural proteins. In Kelley WK, Harris ED, Ruddy S, Sledge CB (eds): Textbook of Rheumatology, 4th ed. Philadelphia, W.B. Saunders, 1993, pp 1567–1592.
7. Sakkas L, Thomas B, Smyrnis P, Vlahos E: Low back pain and ochronosis. Int Orthop 11:19–21, 1987.

61. STORAGE AND DEPOSITION DISEASES

Mark Jarek, M.D., FACR

1. What is the pattern of inheritance for primary hemochromatosis? Wilson's disease? Alkaptonuria (ochronosis)?
All are inherited as autosomal recessive traits with heterozygotes being asymptomatic carriers. Wilson's disease occurs in about 1 in 30,000, and alkaptonuria in about 1 in 200,000 individuals. Alkaptonuria was the first human disease shown to be inherited as an autosomal recessive trait.

2. Which human leukocyte antigens (HLA) are associated with hemochromatosis?
The genetic basis for hemochromatosis was introduced by Simon and coworkers in 1976. The hemochromatosis gene is located on the short arm of chromosome 6, near the HLA-A locus. The HLA-A3 alloantigen is present in about 70% of patients with hemochromatosis and approximately 20% of whites (relative risk = 23). The basis for this association probably relates to a mutation in ancient northern Europe which initially provided a nutritional advantage in an iron-poor environment. Other HLA haplotypes linked to hemochromatosis are HLA-A2, A29, B7, and B14.

3. How common is hemochromatosis?

Recent screening studies suggest that the hemochromatosis gene occurs in 5% of whites, giving a carrier (heterozygote) frequency of approximately 10% and a disease (homozygote) frequency of 1–3/1000. Studies in Scandinavian families have identified the frequency of homozygosity to be as high as 1%, making this one of the most commonly inherited metabolic diseases. Expression of the disease is modified by several factors, most notably blood loss in women associated with menstruation and pregnancy. This blood loss accounts for the five times more frequent clinical expression of disease in males than in females. Given the frequency of hemochromatosis in the general population, many physicians recommend screening iron studies in all men by age 40.

4. How does the typical patient with hemochromatosis present?

Clinical manifestations usually appear between ages 40–60 years, but the disease severity is quite variable. A few patients may develop full clinical expression as early as age 20, while some homozygotes never develop clinical symptoms.

Hemochromatosis typically presents with **asymptomatic abnormal liver function tests** or **hepatomegaly.** Liver disease often progresses to hepatic cirrhosis in untreated cases. A characteristic **arthropathy** occurs in 20–50% of patients and may be the initial manifestation, although more often it occurs later in the disease and may even develop after treatment has been initiated. Other manifestations include a slate-gray or brown **skin pigmentation** due to melanin deposition, **diabetes mellitus,** and **hypogonadism** manifested by decreased libido, impotence, amenorrhea, or sparse body hair. **Constitutional symptoms** such as weakness or lethargy are also common. Cardiac involvement, manifested most commonly by **congestive heart failure,** is present in about 30% of patients and is the principal cause of death in untreated patients.

5. What are some clinical features of the arthropathy of hemochromatosis?

Most joints can be affected, but pain and stiffness affecting the second and third metacarpophalangeal joints (MCP) are the most characteristic complaints. Other joints affected are the proximal interphalangeal joints, wrists, knees, hips, ankles, shoulders, and occasionally metatarsophalangeal joints. Joint examination usually reveals firm swelling with mild tenderness, but warmth and erythema are absent, helping to distinguish it from rheumatoid arthritis.

6. Describe the typical radiographic abnormalities seen in the arthropathy of hemochromatosis.

Radiographs show osteoarthritis-like changes with sclerotic margins, joint-space narrowing, and osteophyte formation which is characteristically hook-like, particularly when found at the MCP joints. Chondrocalcinosis is present in 30–60% of patients and can occur without the degenerative arthropathy.

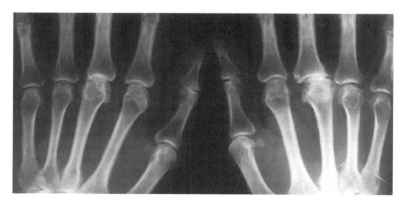

Hand radiographs of a patient with hemochromatosis. Note degenerative arthritis of the MCP joints with hook-like osteophytes.

7. Generalized osteopenia is common in hemochromatosis. What are its possible causes?
- Increased synovial iron (comparable to serum levels) directly inhibits bone formation.
- Pituitary iron infiltration decreases gonadotropin levels, leading to hypogonadism.
- Hepatic cirrhosis leads to testicular atrophy and hypogonadism.

8. Now that you have made the diagnosis of hemochromatosis, outline a treatment plan.
Phlebotomy is performed once or twice weekly until the transferrin saturation and ferritin levels become normal (2–3 years) and then is performed as required to maintain these levels within the normal range. Life expectancy of symptomatic patients is extended considerably by removal of excessive iron stores (90% 5-year survival vs. 33% survival without therapy). With therapy, hepatosplenomegaly improves, liver function studies return to normal, pigmentation decreases, and cardiac failure improves or stabilizes. Diabetes mellitus improves in about 50%. Phlebotomy has little effect on hypogonadism or arthropathy. Hepatic fibrosis may improve, but cirrhosis is irreversible. Hepatocellular carcinoma, a late sequela in one-third of those who develop hepatic cirrhosis, is not diminished by phlebotomy. Because the life expectancy of homozygotes diagnosed and treated before the development of cirrhosis is the same as that of the normal population, the importance of family screening and early therapy cannot be overemphasized. Chelation therapy and the use of antioxidants such as α-tocopherol may also be of some benefit in patients with cardiac involvement.

9. Once a proband case of hemochromatosis is identified, who should be screened and by what method?
All first-degree relatives (>10 years old) of the proband should be screened every 2–5 years by measuring a transferrin saturation (iron/total iron-binding capacity [TIBC]). If the transferrin saturation rises to >50%, then a serum ferritin is obtained. If the ferritin level is elevated, a liver biopsy with iron quantification should be performed. Because of the strong genetic association, HLA typing may be a more cost-effective method for screening first-degree relatives. Affected siblings usually have both HLA haplotypes identical with those of the proband. Siblings sharing only one HLA haplotype probably will not develop clinically evident iron overload. When children of a proband are affected, a homozygous-heterozygous mating probably occurred.

10. Liver disease is the first clinical manifestation in approximately 50% of patients with Wilson's disease (hepatolenticular degeneration). What are the clinical presentations of liver involvement?
Transient hepatitis, fulminant hepatitis, chronic active hepatitis, and cirrhosis.

11. Are there other common clinical features in Wilson's disease?
In addition to hepatic manifestations, Wilson's disease, which usually presents between ages 20 and 40, can also have neurologic manifestations, arthropathy, and hemolytic anemia. The most common neurologic manifestations are movement disorders arising from ganglion degeneration, but many other neurologic and psychiatric disorders have been described. Gynecologic manifestations include amenorrhea and infertility.

12. Describe Kayser-Fleischer rings. What is their significance?
Kayser-Fleischer rings are green or brown deposits of copper in Descemet's membrane of the cornea which do not interfere with vision. Their presence is such a reliable predictor of neurologic involvement in Wilson's disease that if they are absent on slitlamp examination in a patient with a neurologic or psychiatric disorder, the diagnosis of Wilson's disease is unlikely. Kayser-Fleischer rings can occasionally be seen in other causes of hepatic cirrhosis and therefore are not specific for Wilson's disease.

13. What is the biochemical defect in Wilson's disease? How is a diagnosis confirmed?
Wilson's disease results from excessive copper accumulation in association with a ceruloplasmin deficiency. The capacity of hepatocytes to store copper is exceeded, and excessive copper is deposited in the liver and at extrahepatic sites such as the brain, kidneys, urine, and serum. De-

creased serum ceruloplasmin (<20 mg/dl) and copper levels (<80 μg/dl) with elevated urinary copper excretion (>100 μg/24 hrs) is suggestive of Wilson's disease. An elevated hepatic copper concentration (>250 μg Cu/gm) is the most reliable test early in the course of the illness.

14. A young person complaining of arthritis has been referred to you by an ophthalmologist who identified Kayser-Fleischer rings. What might you find on the musculoskeletal examination?
Pain and swelling of the MCPs, wrists, elbows, shoulders, knees and hips resembling hemochromatosis may occur, although asymptomatic radiographic changes are equally as common.

15. Suspecting the diagnosis of Wilson's disease, you order radiographs of the involved joints. What do the radiographs reveal?
Subchondral and cortical fragmentation, as well as marginal, subchondral, and central bony sclerosis of the wrist, hand, elbow, shoulder, and knee help to distinguish this arthropathy from primary osteoarthritis. Unlike hemochromatosis, involvement of the hip and MCP joints is uncommon. Less common radiographic findings include osteochondritis dissecans, chondrocalcinosis, chondramalacia patellae, vertebral wedging, and generalized osteoporosis or osteomalacia.

16. Osteopenia and/or osteomalacia are present in 25–50% of patients with Wilson's disease. What is a possible mechanism for this?
Osteopenia and osteomalacia are probably a result of renal tubular acidosis or Fanconi syndrome, both of which are common renal diseases seen in Wilson's disease.

17. How would you treat your patient with Wilson's disease?
Life-long penicillamine chelation therapy can prevent virtually every manifestation of the disease. If irreversible intolerance to penicillamine develops, trientine or hepatic transplantation can be considered.

18. What is the biochemical defect underlying alkaptonuria?
Alkaptonuria is a disorder of tyrosine catabolism caused by a deficiency of homogentisic acid oxidase, leading to excretion of large amounts of homogentisic acid in urine and accumulation of oxidized homogentisic acid pigment in connective tissues (ochronosis). The tendency of the patient's urine to darken upon standing due to excessive homogentisic acid is characteristic.

19. List five locations where ochronotic pigment may deposit.
Foci of gray-brown ochronotic pigment can be found in the skin, sclera, arterial walls, prostate, and ear (concha, antihelix, and cerumen). These deposits can lead to aortic stenosis, conduction hearing loss, and prostatic calculi. Deposition in articular cartilage and intervertebral discs eventually leads to ochronotic arthropathy.

20. Discuss the clinical features of ochronotic arthropathy.
Ochronosis typically presents between ages 20–30 as a chronic progressive spondylosis with decreased range of motion of the lumbosacral spine. The posture of such a patient can be quite similar to that of a patient with ankylosis spondylitis (AS)—forward stoop, loss of lumbar lordosis, loss of height, flexed hips and knees, and wide-based stance—but patients lack the typical radiographic features of AS such as annular ossification or sacroiliac joint fusion. Ochronotic pigment deposition in the nucleus pulposus predisposes to herniation of the intervertebral disc, which can present as acute-onset low-back pain clinically indistinguishable from typical cases of herniated disc disease without alkaptonuria. A degenerative arthritis of the peripheral joints occurs less frequently than the spinal disease. Peripheral joints most commonly affected are the knees, shoulders, and hips. Pain, stiffness, and limited range of motion are the most common features, similar to hemochromatotic arthropathy. However, ochronosis spares the small joints of the hands, wrists, and feet.

21. What are the characteristic findings on spinal radiographs in ochronosis?

Lumbosacral radiographs show premature degenerative changes, dense calcifications of the intervertebral discs, and narrowing of the intervertebral spaces. Prominent intervertebral disc calcification can also be seen in hemochromatosis, hyperparathyroidism, calcium pyrophosphate deposition disease, paralytic poliomyelitis, and amyloidosis. The radiographic appearance of the large peripheral joints in ochronotic arthritis is virtually indistinguishable from that of primary osteoarthritis.

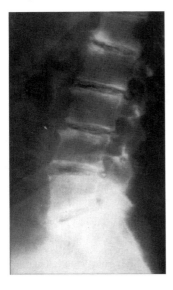

Lateral radiograph of the spine in a patient with ochronosis. Note the vertebral disc space calcification at multiple levels.

22. Is there a beneficial treatment for patients with ochronosis?

Numerous therapies, such as ascorbic acid, and diets low in protein, phenylalanine, and tyrosine have been studied, but to date no therapy has been proved to be beneficial.

BIBLIOGRAPHY

1. Bothwell TH, Charlton RW, Cook JD, Finch CA: Iron Metabolism in Man. Oxford, Blackwell, 1979.
2. Bothwell TH, Charlton RW, Motulsky AG: Hemochromatosis. In Scriver CH, Beaudet AL, Sly WS, et al (eds): The Metabolic Basis of Inherited Disease, 6th ed. New York, McGraw-Hill, 1989, pp 1433–1462.
3. Edwards CQ, Kushner JP: Screening for hemochromatosis. N Engl J Med 328:1616–1620, 1993.
4. Edwards CQ, Skolnich MH, Kushner JP: Hereditary hemochromatosis: Contributions of genetic analysis. Prog Hematol 12:43–71, 1981.
5. Gordon DA: Storage and deposition diseases. In Schumacher HR (ed): Primer on the Rheumatic Diseases, 10th ed. Atlanta, Arthritis Foundation, 1993, pp 225–230.
6. Lalouel JM, Jorde LB: Idiopathic hemochromatosis: Significance and implications of linkage and association to HLA. Ann NY Acad Sci 526:34–46, 1988.
7. Lambert RE, McGuire JL: Iron storage disease. In Kelly WN, Harris ED, Ruddy S, Sledge CB (eds): Textbook of Rheumatology, 4th ed. Philadelphia, W.B. Saunders, 1993, pp 1435–1443.
8. Niederau C, Fischer R, Sonnenberg A, Stremmel W et al: Survival and causes of death in cirrhotic and noncirrhotic patients with primary hemochromatosis. N Engl J Med 313:1256–1262, 1985.
9. Olsson KS: Hemochromatosis. In Klippel JH, Dieppe PA (eds): Rheumatology. London, Mosby, 1994, pp 7:18.1–7:18.4.
10. Powell LW, Isselbacher KJ: Hemochromatosis. In Wilson JD, et al. (eds): Harrison's Principles of Internal Medicine, 12th ed. New York, McGraw-Hill, 1991, pp 1825–1829.
11. Resnick D, Berthiaume MJ, Sartoris D: Diagnostic tests and procedures in rheumatic diseases. In Kelly WN, Harris ED, Ruddy S, Sledge CB, (eds): Textbook of Rheumatology, 4th ed. Philadelphia, W.B. Saunders, 1993, pp 627–628.
12. Rosenberg LE: Storage diseases of amino acid metabolism. In Wilson JD, et al. (eds): Harrison's Principles of Internal Medicine, 12th ed. New York, McGraw-Hill, 1991, pp 1875–1876.
13. Scheinberg IH: Wilson's disease. In Wilson JD, et al (eds): Harrison's Principles of Internal Medicine, 12th ed. New York, McGraw-Hill, 1991, pp 1843–1845.

14. Schumacher HR: Ochronosis, hemochromatosis, and Wilson's disease. In McCarty DJ, Koopman WJ (eds): Arthritis and Allied Conditions, 12th ed. Philadelphia, Lea & Febiger, 1993, pp 1913–1925.
15. Baer DM, Simons JL, Staples RL, et al: Hemochromatosis screening in asymptomatic ambulatory men 30 years of age and older. Am J Med 98:464–468, 1995.

62. RHEUMATOLOGIC MANIFESTATIONS OF THE PRIMARY IMMUNODEFICIENCY SYNDROMES

Mark Malyak, M.D.

1. Why are primary immunodeficiency syndromes of concern in rheumatology?

Primary immunodeficiency syndromes may be associated with a variety of problems in addition to an increased risk of infection, including autoimmune manifestations, allergy, and increased risk of lymphoid and epithelial neoplasms. Autoimmunity may manifest as a recognized autoimmune disease, such as systemic lupus erythematosus in congenital deficiency of C4. Alternatively, various autoantibodies may be present in the absence of clinically expressed autoimmune disease, such as rheumatoid factor (anti-IgG antibodies) or anti-nuclear antibodies (ANA) in selective IgA deficiency.

2. Which components of the immune system are involved in the primary immunodeficiency syndromes?

- B cells (humoral immunodeficiency)
- T cells (cell-mediated immunodeficiency)
- Natural killer (NK) cells
- Phagocytes
- Complement proteins

The individual primary immunodeficiency syndromes may be due to dysfunction of a single component of the immune system, such as C4 deficiency, or dysfunction of multiple components, such as impairment of B-cell, T-cell, and phagocyte function in certain severe combined immunodeficiencies.

3. The types of recurrent infection in a particular patient offer a clue to the underlying primary immunodeficiency syndrome. Which microorganisms are responsible for recurrent infection in B-cell immunodeficiency syndromes?

B-cell immunodeficiency, such as X-linked (Bruton's) agammaglobulinemia, results in inadequate immunoglobulin production, leading to recurrent infection with extracellular, encapsulated, pyogenic bacteria, particularly *Streptococcus pneumoniae* and *Haemophilus influenzae*. These organisms typically cause acute and chronic infections of the upper and lower respiratory tracts, meningitis, and bacteremia.

4. Which organisms are responsible for infections in primary T-cell immunodeficiency, such as thymic hypoplasia (DiGeorge syndrome)?

- Viruses (e.g., herpesviruses)
- Intracellular bacteria (e.g., mycobacteria)
- Fungi (e.g., *Candida* species, *Pneumocystis carinii*)

Primary T-cell immunodeficiency results in inadequate cell-mediated immunity, leading to infections similar to those encountered in patients with HIV infection, the prototypic acquired T-cell immunodeficiency state.

5. What laboratory tests are performed to evaluate the integrity of the humoral immune system (B-cell function)?

Laboratory Evaluation of B-cell Function

CATEGORY	SPECIFIC TESTS	COMMENTS
In vivo functional tests (routine screening tests)	Isohemagglutinin titers (anti-blood group A and B)	Naturally occurring; predominantly IgM
	Diphtheria and tetanus booster immunization	Serum antibodies assayed prior to and 2 weeks later; assesses capacity to synthesize IgG antibodies against protein antigens
	Pneumococcal immunization	Serum antibodies assayed prior to and 3 weeks later; assesses capacity to synthesize antibodies against poly-saccharide antigens
Immunoglobulin quantitation	IgM, IgG, IgA levels	Various immunoassays may be used; readily available
	IgG subclass, IgE levels	ELISA and RIA available (expensive)
In vitro tests (expensive)	Peripheral blood B-cell quantitation	Anti-Ig antibodies and specific mono-clonal antibody may be used
	Bone marrow pre-B-cell quantitation	Measures surface Ig-negative, cyto-plasmic μ-chain-positive cells
	In vitro immunoglobulin synthesis	Peripheral blood mononuclear cells stimulated in vitro with pokeweed mitogen

ELISA = enzyme-linked immunosorbent assay; RIA = radioimmunoassay.

A reasonable screening evaluation of B-cell function is to determine the serum IgA level and perform the inexpensive in vivo functional tests. If all these tests are normal, clinically significant B-cell dysfunction may be excluded. If any of these tests is abnormal, quantitation of IgG and IgM levels, and possibly in vitro testing, will be necessary to determine the cause of the underlying primary immunodeficiency syndrome.

6. What laboratory tests can be used to evaluate the integrity of the cellular immune system (T-cell function)?

Laboratory Evaluation of T-Cell Function

CATEGORY	SPECIFIC TESTS	COMMENTS
In vivo functional tests (skin testing for delayed-type hypersensitivity) (routine screening tests)	*Candida* skin test	Examine degree of induration 48–72 hr later
	PPD, *Trichophyton,* mumps, tetanus/diphtheria toxoid, keyhole-limpet hemocyanin	If *Candida* skin test is negative, testing with at least 4 of these antigens must be performed to determine if cell-mediated immunity is inadequate
Absolute lymphocyte count (routine screening test)	Determine from total WBC count and % lymphocytes	Severe cell-mediated immunity disorder unlikely in setting of normal lymphocyte count
In vitro tests (expensive)	Quantitation of: Total T cells CD4+ cells CD8+ cells NK cells	Specific monoclonal antibody may be used
	Lymphocyte blastic transformation	Assessment of radiolabeled thymidine uptake following stimulation with lectins (such as PHA), specific antigen (such as *Candida*), or one-way mixed lymphocyte reaction
	Quantitate ability of T cells to synthesize IL-2 and IL-2 receptors	These and lymphocyte blastic transformation assay are indicators of successful T-cell activation.

PPD = purified protein derivative (for tuberculosis); WBC = white blood cell; PHA = phytohemagglutinin; IL = interleukin.

A reasonable screening evaluation of T-cell function is to determine the absolute lymphocyte count and perform a *Candida* skin test. If these are both normal, clinically significant T-cell dysfunction may be excluded. If the *Candida* skin test is negative, negative delayed-type skin testing with at least four other antigens is necessary to demonstrate that T-cell function is inadequate. If these screening tests are abnormal, more sophisticated in vitro tests may be necessary to define the underlying primary immunodeficiency disorder. HIV testing should be performed as part of the screening evaluation to exclude this acquired T-cell disorder.

7. Which organisms are responsible for septic arthritis in patients with hypogammaglobulinemia due to primary B-cell immunodeficiency?

Selective IgA deficiency, X-linked (Bruton's) agammaglobulinemia, common variable immunodeficiency, and immunoglobulin deficiency with increased IgM (hyper-IgM) account for >99% of the primary hypogammaglobulinemic states (B-cell immunodeficiency). These patients are susceptible to septic arthritis due to the usual organisms encountered in B-cell immunodeficiency states: *Streptococcus pneumoniae, Haemophilus influenzae,* and *Staphylococcus aureus.* In addition to these typical infectious agents, patients are also susceptible to joint infections with *Ureaplasma urealyticum* and other *Mycoplasma* organisms. The incidence of septic arthritis in these B-cell disorders is unknown but is less than that for the more frequently encountered infections of the upper and lower respiratory tract and gastrointestinal tract.

8. Which primary immunodeficiency syndromes are most commonly associated with autoimmune phenomena?

Selective IgA deficiency, common variable immunodeficiency, X-linked agammaglobulinemia, and hyper-IgM syndrome are the B-cell immunodeficiency syndromes commonly associated with autoimmune phenomena. Complete absence of certain complement components (C2, C4) is also associated with autoimmune phenomena, particularly systemic lupus erythematosus (SLE). Finally, chronic granulomatous disease, a primary disorder of neutrophils, is associated with the presence of ANA, and, less commonly, SLE. For the most part, patients with predominantly T-cell immunodeficiency do not manifest autoimmune phenomena, due at least in part to the fact that many of these patients do not survive infancy.

9. What are the rheumatologic manifestations of X-linked agammaglobulinemia?

Rheumatologic Manifestations of X-linked Agammaglobulinemia

Septic arthritis	Occurs in 20% of cases
Extracellular, encapsulated bacteria (*S. pneumoniae,* *H. influenzae, S. aureus*)	
Mycoplasma, particularly *Ureaplasma urealyticum*	
Enteroviruses, particularly echovirus and coxsackievirus	
Aseptic, possibly autoimmune, arthritis	Usually mono- or oligoarticular; involves large joints; rarely destructive; RF and ANA absent
Dermatomyositis-like syndrome associated with progressive enterovirus CNS infection	Presents with rash and muscle weakness

X-linked (Bruton's) agammaglobulinemia is a rare disorder characterized by absent or near-absent levels of serum IgG, IgM, and IgA and by abnormal *in vivo* B-cell functional tests. Cell-mediated immunity is intact. The cellular abnormality appears to be failure of maturation of the B-cell line, and therefore peripheral B cells are absent. Arthritis occurs in approximately 20% of patients, with half of these cases due to infection with the typical pyogenic bacteria. In addition, patients appear vulnerable to infections with enterovirus and *Mycoplasma.*

There are cases of arthritis in X-linked agammaglobulinemia in which an infectious agent cannot be detected despite rigorous evaluation. These cases may represent infection due to a fastidious organism that cannot be identified or may represent a true autoimmune disorder, such as juvenile rheumatoid arthritis. Overall, autoimmune phenomena occur much less frequently in X-linked agammaglobulinemia than in selective IgA deficiency or common variable immunodeficiency.

10. What are the rheumatologic manifestations of selective IgA deficiency?
- Autoantibodies, particularly RF and ANA, in the absence of clinically expressed autoimmune disease
- Systemic autoimmune disorders (SLE, aseptic, possibly autoimmune arthritis, etc.)
- Organ-specific autoimmune disorders (diabetes mellitus type I, myasthenia gravis, etc.)

IgA deficiency is the most common primary immunodeficiency syndrome, with a prevalence as high as 1/330 in the general population. It is characterized by absent or near-absent levels of serum and secretory IgA, accompanied by normal levels of serum IgG and IgM. Cell-mediated immunity is intact. Patients may be asymptomatic, have recurrent respiratory and gastrointestinal tract infections, or manifest autoimmune phenomena. In most cases, IgA deficiency is likely a genetic disorder that is present at birth and remains persistent. Some cases may be acquired later in life, often associated with drug therapy or viral infection, and are often transient.

11. List the autoantibodies seen in patients with selective IgA deficiency without clinically expressed autoimmune disease.
The presence of autoantibodies in the absence of clinically expressed autoimmune disease commonly occurs in IgA deficiency. RF and ANA are most consistently observed. Other autoantibodies that may be present include antibodies against double-stranded and single-stranded DNA, cardiolipin, thyroglobulin, thyroid microsomes, smooth muscle, gastric parietal cell, striated muscle, acetylcholine receptor, and bile canaliculi. Autoantibodies against IgA occur in up to 44% of patients.

12. What systemic and organ-specific autoimmune diseases are associated with selective IgA deficiency?

SYSTEMIC	ORGAN-SPECIFIC
Systemic lupus erythematosus*	Diabetes mellitus type I*
Juvenile rheumatoid arthritis*	Myasthenia gravis*
Rheumatoid arthritis*	Inflammatory bowel disease
Sjögren's syndrome	Autoimmune hepatitis
Scleroderma	Pernicious anemia
Dermatomyositis	Primary adrenal insufficiency
Vasculitic syndromes	

*Most likely associations. Other conditions have been noted in case reports, but their true association with IgA deficiency remains to be proved.

13. Describe the rheumatologic manifestations of common variable immunodeficiency (CVID).

Rheumatologic Manifestations of Common Variable Immunodeficiency

Septic arthritis
Extracellular, encapsulated bacteria (*S. pneumoniae, H. influenzae, S. aureus*)
Mycoplasma, particularly *Ureaplasma urealyticum*
Aseptic, possibly autoimmune, arthritis
Organ-specific autoimmune disorders (pernicious anemia, autoimmune hemolytic anemia, idiopathic thrombocytopenic purpura)

CVID is an heterogeneous group of disorders characterized by IgG, IgM, and IgA hypogammaglobulinemia, often resulting in the very low levels seen in X-linked agammaglobulinemia. Features distinguishing CVID from X-linked agammaglobulinemia include equal sex distribution, onset of symptoms later in life, and presence of circulating B cells. Although the underlying immunologic defect is heterogeneous, most patients manifest a primary B-cell defect resulting in failure to mature into Ig-secreting plasma cells. Like selective IgA deficiency, CVID is likely a genetic disorder in most cases, although some cases may be truly acquired and secondary to a viral infection or an adverse drug effect.

Septic arthritis due to *Staphylococcus aureus,* the usual extracellular encapsulated bacteria, and *Mycoplasma* species occurs with increased frequency in CVID. Because cell-mediated immunodeficiency sometimes occurs in CVID, fungi and mycobacteria must also be considered as potential pathogens.

The presence of autoantibodies in the absence of clinically expressed autoimmune disease appears less often than in selective IgA deficiency. Regardless, autoimmune disorders are not unusual in CVID. Polyarthritis in which an infectious agent cannot be detected despite rigorous evaluation has been described. Characteristics include involvement of the large and medium-sized joints with sparing of the small joints of the hands and feet. Rheumatoid nodules, erosions, and significant articular cartilage destruction are not features of this syndrome. This form of arthropathy often responds to treatment with intravenous gammaglobulin.

14. What mechanisms may explain the presence of aseptic arthritis and other autoimmune phenomena in the primary immunodeficiency syndromes?

The mechanisms responsible for autoimmune phenomena in the primary immunodeficiency syndromes remain unknown. The following possibilities exist:

1. Aseptic arthritis in the primary B-cell immunodeficiency states may be due to infection with a fastidious organism that cannot be identified by available methods.

2. Absence of secretory IgA in the primary B-cell immunodeficiency syndromes may lead to:
   - Excessive absorption of antigen from the gut, leading to the formation of immune complexes (in disorders other than X-linked agammaglobulinemia) and subsequent immune complex disease. Additionally, immune complexes may lead to the formation of rheumatoid factor.
   - Excessive absorption of superantigen from the gut, which may lead to activation of T cells containing particular V_β families on their T-cell receptors. If one of these clones also reacts against self-antigen, an autoimmune state may result.
   - Excessive absorption of a particular antigen from the gut, leading to autoimmunity as a result of molecular mimicry.

3. Coexistence of primary immunodeficiency and autoimmunity may be coincidental rather than causal. Common HLA extended haplotypes often present in selective IgA deficiency and common variable immunodeficiency are also commonly present in autoimmune disorders such as SLE, diabetes mellitus type I, and myasthenia gravis.

15. Discuss the therapy for X-linked agammaglobulinemia, common variable immunodeficiency (CVID), and selective IgA deficiency.

X-linked agammaglobulinemia: Intravenous immunoglobulin (IVIG) and aggressive treatment of bacterial infections with appropriate antibiotics are the recommended therapy. IVIG is usually administered in a dose of 200–600 mg/kg every month.

CVID: IVIG is also recommended for patients with CVID who have low IgG levels and recurrent infections. Occasionally, patients with CVID have complete absence of IgA, along with anti-IgA antibodies, placing them at risk for anaphylaxis with IVIG therapy.

Selecive IgA deficiency: The mainstay of therapy is rigorous treatment of active bacterial infections with antibiotics. IVIG should *not* be administered, since many patients have autoantibodies against IgA, including IgE anti-IgA, which may result in severe, occasionally fatal anaphylaxis. Patients should ideally receive blood products obtained from other patients with IgA deficiency.

16. How do you screen for homozygous complement deficiency associated with a rheumatologic disorder?

Homozygous deficiency of certain complement components is associated with a number of rheumatologic disorders. The **total hemolytic complement assay** (CH_{50}) assesses the integrity of the classic pathway of complement activation. Patient's sera is added to a standardized suspension of sheep red blood cells (RBC) coated with rabbit antibody. These "immune complexes" allow activation of the classic pathway, resulting in lysis of the sheep RBC. The CH_{50} is the reciprocal of the serum dilution that lyses 50% of the sheep RBC. Because specific deficiencies that lead to rheumatologic manifestations are usually in the classic, rather that the alternative, pathway, CH_{50} is the ideal, inexpensive screening test. Homozygous deficiency of a complement component in the classic pathway results in a CH_{50} of 0; individual complement levels may then be determined by immunoassay.

17. What are the rheumatologic manifestations of homozygous complement deficient states?

Deficiencies of the early components of the classic pathway (C1, C4, C2) are associated with immune complex disease, particularly SLE. This may be due to inability to maintain circulating immune complexes in a soluble state and inability to remove circulating immune complexes. C2 deficiency is the most common deficiency.

Deficiencies of components of the membrane attack complex (C5–9) are associated with recurrent *Neisseria* infections, both *N. meningitidis* and *N. gonorrhoeae*. Patients with recurrent bouts of neisserial infection, particularly when systemic, should be evaluated for the presence of a complement deficiency.

BIBLIOGRAPHY

1. Buckley RH: Specific immunodeficiency diseases, excluding AIDS. In Kelley WN, Harris ED Jr, Ruddy S, Sledge CB (eds): Textbook of Rheumatology, 4th ed. Philadelphia, W.B. Saunders, 1993, pp 1264–1282.
2. Lee AH, Levinson AI, Schumacher HR Jr: Hypogammaglobulinemia and rheumatic disease. Semin Arthritis Rheum 22:252, 1993.
3. Liblau RS, Bach J-F: Selective IgA deficiency and autoimmunity. Int Arch Allergy Immunol 99:16, 1992.
4. Ruddy S: Complement deficiencies and rheumatic diseases. In Kelley WN, Harris ED Jr, Ruddy S, Sledge CB (eds): Textbook of Rheumatology, 4th ed. Philadelphia, W.B. Saunders, 1993, pp 1283–1289.
5. Waldmann TA, Nelson DL: Inherited immunodeficiencies. In Frank MM, Austen KF, Claman HN, Unanue ER (eds): Samter's Immunologic Diseases, 5th ed. Boston, Little, Brown & Company, 1995, pp 387–429.

63. BONE AND JOINT DYSPLASIAS

Edmund H. Hornstein, D.O.

1. What exactly is a bone or joint dysplasia?

Dysplasia is a term literally meaning abnormal growth. Applied to the skeletal system, the term encompasses a group of conditions in which abnormalities of growth can affect the epiphysis, metaphysis, physis, or diaphysis of developing bone. These abnormalities may be devastatingly symptomatic or fatal, but they can also exist as mere radiologic curiosities. Broadly, these syndromes are grouped under the heading of **osteochondrodysplasias.** The vast majority of these syndromes are exceedingly rare and are not of practical importance in most clinical situations.

2. Why should bone and joint dysplasias even be covered in a rheumatology text?

- Dysplastic syndromes may present with musculoskeletal pain or dysfunction that mimic other rheumatologic disorders.

- Early recognition of some dysplasias may allow the initiation of therapy which can prevent or reduce later pain and disability.
- Many osteochondrodysplasias are inherited, and an accurate diagnosis may allow appropriate genetic counseling to be offered.

3. How are the osteochondrodysplasias classified?

A variety of complicated classification schemes exist for these syndromes. It is useful and practical, however, to group these disorders by where the most prominent abnormalities in growth occur. The mnemonic **EMPD** (empty) can help to broadly group these syndromes.

E —Epiphyseal dysplasias: The epiphysis is at the end of tubular bone and is formed as a secondary site of ossification. Normal development of the epiphysis is required if the joint surface is to be normal.

M—Metaphyseal dysplasias: The metaphysis is the wider part of a tubular bone between the diaphysis and physis.

P —Physeal dysplasias: The physis, or epiphyseal cartilage plate, separates the metaphysis from the epiphysis during growth. It is the primary site responsible for elongation of tubular bones.

D —Diaphyseal dysplasia: The diaphysis is the shaft of a long or tubular bone. It is composed of the spongiosa and cortex and is covered with periosteum.

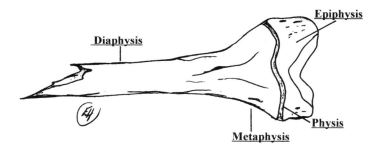

4. What are the distinguishing features of the epiphyseal dysplasias?

Epiphyseal dysplasia is characterized by abnormal ossification of the developing epiphysis. The resulting morphologic abnormalities of the ossification centers are used to differentiate the various subtypes within this category. The most important epiphyseal dysplasias from a rheumatologic standpoint are multiple epiphyseal dysplasia and spondyloepiphyseal dysplasia.

5. How does a patient with multiple epiphyseal dysplasia present clinically?

Usually, the patient complains of symmetric joint pain in the hips, knees, wrists, and ankles. These complaints are commonly accompanied by back pain. Limitation in range of motion of affected joints is frequent. Radiographs reveal irregular, flattened, small epiphyseal ossification centers during childhood and a deformed articular surface after physeal closure. The long bones of the legs and arms are most prominently affected. Vertebrae are often flattened (platyspondyly) with irregular appearing endplates. Adult stature is generally diminished and is proportionate to the severity of involvement. Disabling early degenerative arthritis is a common end result. Symptoms usually occur before adolescence but may not become apparent until early adulthood, depending on the severity of epiphyseal deformity.

6. What other conditions can be confused with multiple epiphyseal dysplasia?

Inflammatory arthritis: The pain and symmetry of involvement are sometimes mistaken for inflammatory arthritis. On closer evaluation, the absence of signs and symptoms of inflammation usually suffice to rule out this condition.

Hypothyroidism: Occult hypothyroidism can lead to developmental skeletal abnormalities which may closely resemble some of the hereditary epiphyseal dysplasias. Thyroid function should always be checked when a diagnosis of epiphyseal dysplasia is being considered.

Juvenile osteochondrosis: These disorders, including Legg-Calvé-Perthes disease, may have a radiographic appearance similar to epiphyseal dysplasia but is usually limited to a single joint.

7. Describe the radiographic abnormalities typical for spondyloepiphyseal dysplasia.
The spondyloepiphyseal dysplasias are a diverse group of disorders linked by the radiographic findings of marked **platyspondyly** (short flat vertebrae) in association with abnormalities of **epiphyseal ossification.** Spinal abnormalities are prominent, and impaired spinal growth often leads to the diagnosis.

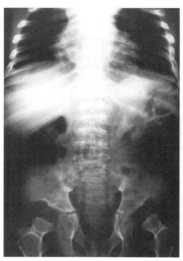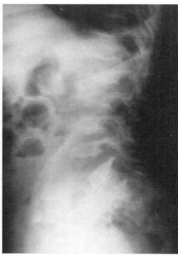

8. Spondyloepiphyseal dysplasia tarda and spondyloepiphyseal dysplasia tarda with progressive arthropathy can sometimes be confused with juvenile rheumatoid arthritis. Why?
Both of these X-linked recessive disorders are accompanied by enlargement of the ends of the tubular bones in the hands, which may be mistaken for JRA on visual inspection.

9. What abnormality characterizes the metaphyseal dysplasias?
These dysplasias are characterized by a failure either to form or absorb the spongiosa of developing bone. Important disorders from a rheumatologic standpoint within this category of dysplasias include the hypophosphatasias and craniometaphyseal dysplasias.

10. What is the primary differential diagnosis in the hypophosphatasias?
The hypophosphatasias may look like **rickets** in children and **osteomalacia** in adults. Subtle radiographic findings may allow the distinction to be made, but the diagnosis of hypophosphatasia is ultimately based on the findings of an exceptionally low serum alkaline phosphatase in conjunction with high urine and serum phosphorylethanolamine levels. Consideration of hypophosphatasia is warranted in any case of suspected rickets or osteomalacia.

11. List the clinical findings that link the various forms of craniometaphyseal dysplasias.
Joint pain, muscle weakness, scoliosis, pathologic fractures, genu valga, and Erlenmeyer-flask deformity of long bones. Cranical abnormalities include supraorbital bossing, a broad flat nose, hypertelorism, dental malocclusion, and a sclerotic thickened skull.

12. One of the most common of the osteochondrodysplasias is considered a physeal dysplasia and leads to dwarfism. Name this syndrome.
Achondroplasia. This physeal dysplasia is transmitted as an autosomal dominant trait, though spontaneous mutation is probably responsible for most cases. It is considered a disproportionate

dwarfism with rhizomelic (shorter proximal compared to distal) short limbs, macrocephaly with prominent frontal bossing, and some midface hypoplasia. An exaggerated lumbar lordosis is usually seen as well as flexion contractures at the elbows and hips. Intelligence is normal. Mean adult height is approximately 52 inches in men and 49 inches in women. Rheumatologic complaints may stem from a narrowed spinal canal and symptoms of spinal stenosis or from ligamentous laxity of the knees, leading to complaints of pain and premature degenerative disease.

13. Where is the abnormality of bone formation found in the diaphyseal dysplasias?
Diaphyseal dysplasias result from abnormal formation of endosteal or periosteal bone. These dysplasias can be subclassified as hyperplasias or hypoplasias. Osteogenesis imperfecta is considered a hypoplastic diaphyseal dysplasia (see Chapter 59).

14. A 21-year-old man complains of lower leg pain and swelling that has been gradually increasing. An x-ray is obtained and appears below. What is this disorder?

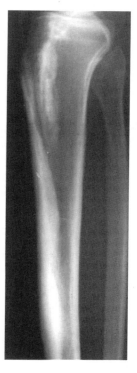

Melorheostosis, a nonhereditary idiopathic diaphyseal hyperplasia. Clinically, the patient complains of joint pain with onset usually in late childhood or early adulthood. Decreased range of motion, joint contracture or ankylosis, growth disturbances, foot deformities, and dystrophic skin, muscle, and soft tissue changes overlying affected bone are other features of this unusual disorder. The x-ray is characteristic and reveals dense, wavy, periosteal bony excrescences which have been described as resembling wax flowing down the side of a candle.

15. Another diaphyseal hyperplasia has radiographic and clinical features in common with hypertrophic pulmonary osteoarthropathy, including clubbing of the digits, painful swollen joints, and periosteal bony apposition, but it is also associated with thickened, wrinkled elephant-like skin. Name this disorder.
Pachydermoperiostosis. A literal translation of the term describes the major clinical manifestations of the disorder.

16. A 15-year-old boy is seen complaining of thoracic back pain with no clear history of trauma. The pain is worse with activity, improves with rest, and is not associated with significant morning stiffness. Physical exam is remarkable only for a hint of increased thoracic kyphosis with some lower thoracic tenderness to palpation in the midline and mild paravertebral muscle spasm. Workup reveals a normal ESR, serum chemistries, and CBC. An x-ray report lists that the findings are most consistent with Scheuermann's disease. What the heck is that?

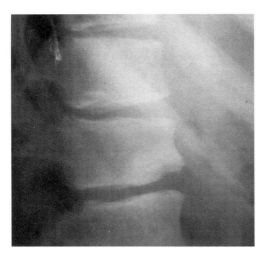

Radiograph of the spine showing irregular vertebral endplates in a patient with Scheuermann's disease.

Vertebral osteochondritis, or Scheuermann's disease, is a developmental abnormality of ossification of the endplates of vertebrae seen most often in the thoracic spine but also seen in the thoracolumbar and lumbar regions. It occurs during adolescence and is symptomatic in up to 60% of those affected, though it may also be found by chance on plain spine or chest x-rays requested for other reasons. The x-ray shows anterior wedging of multiple vertebrae with Schmorl's nodes and irregular vertebral endplates. Though the pathogenesis is uncertain, a hereditary weakening of the vertebral endplates present in affected patients is believed to allow disc material to encroach into the vertebral bodies. This then leads to abnormal growth and the x-ray changes described. Therapy is usually symptomatic and aimed at minimizing the tendency toward kyphosis. Occasionally, surgical intervention is required.

17. A newborn girl has a reproducible "click" as you flex and abduct her right hip (Ortolani's sign). You suspect that the child may have congenital dislocation of the hip. How can you verify this suspicion? What do you tell the parents?
Congenital hip dislocation or dysplasia is screened for shortly after birth using physical exam maneuvers such as Ortolani's sign and by inducing dislocation and reduction of an unstable hip (Barlow's sign). Plain films may not be easily interpretable in the first weeks of life, and modalities

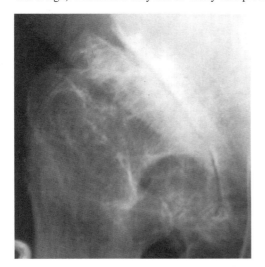

Hip radiograph from an adult with congenital hip dysplasia which was not treated during childhood. Note severe degenerative changes, shallow acetabulum, and malformed femoral head.

such as ultrasound, CT, or MRI generally offer better sensitivity. Congenital hip dysplasia has an excellent prognosis if recognized soon after birth. Treatment usually involves splinting the legs in abduction, thus allowing the shallow acetabulum to fully contain the femoral head. If the diagnosis is missed, however, later therapy is often much more involved and may require extensive orthopedic surgery. Untreated, this condition leads to premature osteoarthritis and may require early total hip replacement.

BIBLIOGRAPHY

 1. Altman RD, Tenenbaum J: Hypertrophic osteoarthropathy. In Kelley WK, Harris ED, Ruddy S, Sledge CB (eds): Textbook of Rheumatology, 4th ed. Philadelphia, W.B. Saunders, 1993, pp 1545–1563.
 2. Borenstein DG, Wiesel SW: Vertebral osteochondritis. In Borenstein DG, Wiesel SW, Boden SD (eds): Low Back Pain: Medical Diagnosis and Comprehensive Management. Philadelphia, W.B. Saunders, 1989, pp 227–229.
 3. Clark RN: Congenital dysplasias and dwarfism. Pediatr Rev 12(5):149–159, 1990.
 4. Horton WA, Hall JG, Scott CI, et al: Growth curves for height for diastrophic dysplasia, spondyloepiphyseal dysplasia congenita and pseudoachondroplasia. Am J Dis Child 136:316–319, 1982.
 5. Kozlowski K: Metaphyseal and spondylometaphyseal chondrodysplasias. Clin Orthop 114:83–93, 1976.
 6. Lateur LM: Bone and joint dysplasias. In Klippel JH, Dieppe PA (eds): Slide Atlas of Rheumatology. St. Louis, Mosby, 1994, sect 7, unit 3, pp 45.3–45.10.
 7. Lowe TG: Scheuermann disease. J Bone Joint Surg 72A:940–945, 1990.
 8. Pyeritz RE: Heritable disorders of connective tissue. In Schumacher HR (ed): Primer on the Rheumatic Diseases, 10 ed. Atlanta, Arthritis Foundation, 1993, pp 249–255.
 9. Scott CI: Achondroplastic and hypochondroplastic dwarfism. Clin Orthop 114:18–30, 1976.
10. Spranger J: The epiphyseal dysplasias. Clin Orthop 114:47–59, 1976.
11. Steinberg ME, Steinberg DR: Osteonecrosis. In Kelley WK, Harris ED, Ruddy S, Sledge CB (eds): Textbook of Rheumatology, 4th ed. Philadelphia, W.B. Saunders, 1993, pp 1628–1650.
12. Townsend DJ, Tolo VT: Congenital dislocation of the hip. Curr Opin Rheumatol 6:183–186, 1994.
13. Wenger DR: Legg-Perthes disease. In Klippel JH, Dieppe PA (eds): Slide Atlas of Rheumatology. St. Louis, Mosby, 1994, sect 7, unit 3, pp 42.1–42.4.

XI. Nonarticular and Regional Musculoskeletal Disorders

It would be a great thing to understand pain in all its meanings.

Peter Mere Latham
(1789–1875)

The lower back is at the crossroads where the psyche meets the soma.

Voltaire
(1694–1778)

64. APPROACH TO THE PATIENT WITH NECK AND LOW BACK PAIN

Danny C. Williams, M.D.

1. Which rheumatic disorders commonly involve the neck?

DISORDER	FEATURE
Rheumatoid arthritis	C1–C2 (atlantoaxial) subluxation
Juvenile chronic arthritis	C2–C3 fusion, C1–C2 subluxation
Ankylosing spondylitis	Ankylosis, C5–C6 fracture
Diffuse idiopathic skeletal hyperostosis	Anterior longitudinal ligament ossification
Osteoarthritis	C5–C7 spondylosis
Polymyositis	Flexor muscle weakness
Polymyalgia rheumatica	Pain and stiffness
Fibromyalgia	C2, C5–C7 tenderpoints

2. When assessing range of motion of the cervical spine, what does "partial" versus "global" loss signify?

Global loss of range is suggestive of *total* joint involvement, which is a feature of *inflammatory* rheumatic diseases (e.g., rheumatoid arthritis). In contrast, *mechanical* or *degenerative* disorders (e.g., osteoarthritis) will *partially* limit range to a few planes of movement. The same principle applies to the thoracic and lumbar spine.

3. When evaluating a patient with neck pain, how can you differentiate between a "bony" or "muscular" disorder?

Comparison of *active* and *passive* range of motion is useful for differentiating articular from soft-tissue disorders. *Passive* neck range of motion is best performed by supporting (cradling) the head while the patient is supine. Full range of the cervical spine may then be tested: flexion, extension, lateral rotation, and lateral bending. During lateral rotation and bending, *ipsilateral* discomfort elicited in the direction of movement is suggestive of *bony* pain. Pain and/or tightness produced on the *contralateral* side implicates a muscular disorder. Finally, palpable tenderness of the spinous processes and/or facet joints is usually indicative of *bony* pathology.

Passive range of motion should *not* be performed if instability of the cervical spine is suspected!

4. What is Spurling's maneuver?

Nerve root compression, within the foramina of the cervical vertebrae, may be physically demonstrated by Spurling's maneuver. With the patient seated, downward pressure is uniformly applied to the patient's cranium while the head is gently rotated or flexed toward the side of the suspected lesion. The immediate development of pain and paresthesias with radiation to the upper limb (see below) is indicative of cervical radiculopathy.

Spurling's maneuver should *not* be performed if cervical spine instability or fracture is suspected.

5. What physical findings enable you to identify the *approximate* level of common, cervical nerve root lesions?

NERVE	SENSORY LOSS	MOTOR WEAKNESS	REFLEX
C5 (5%)	Lateral arm	Deltoid, biceps	Biceps
C6 (35%)	Lateral forearm, thumb, index finger	Wrist extensors, biceps	Radial*
C7 (35%)	Middle finger	Wrist flexors, finger extensors, triceps	Triceps
C8 (25%)	Medial forearm, ring finger, little finger	Finger flexors, thumb extensor	None
T1 (rare)	Medial arm	Finger abductors	None

*Radial = brachioradialis.

6. What is Lhermitte's sign?

Lhermitte's sign is the reported sensation of an "electric-like shock" propagating down the spine as a result of brisk neck flexion. This maneuver may also induce limb paresthesias and weakness. Lhermitte's sign is observed is some patients with spinal cord compression.

7. Compare and contrast cervical myelopathy with cervical radiculopathy.

FEATURE	MYELOPATHY	RADICULOPATHY
Etiology	Spinal cord compression	Nerve root compression
Neck pain	Variable	Variable
Cranial nerve involvement	Occasional	Never
Sensory loss	Stocking–glove paresthesias/numbness (all limbs)	Light touch/pinprick (upper limb dermatome)
Weakness (early)	All limbs (diffuse)	Upper limb myotome
Weakness (late)	Spastic paraparesis, quadriparesis	Upper limb myotme
Deep tendon reflexes	Upper limbs (decreased), lower limbs (increased)	Upper limb (decreased)
Pathologic reflexes	*Babinski's* sign, *Hoffmann's* sign	None
Lhermitte's sign	Occasional	Never
Bladder disturbance	Urine retention, urine incontinence	None
Spinal automaticity	"Jumping legs"	None

8. What are the major categories of low back pain?

- Inflammatory
- Degenerative
- Traumatic
- Metabolic
- Infectious
- Neoplastic
- Congenital
- Psychogenic

9. List the important questions that should be asked when obtaining a history from a patient with low back pain.

One can use the helpful mnemonic **P-Q-R-S-T** (the components of an electrocardiogram tracing) when approaching any patient with pain:

P Provocative and palliative factors
   Is pain worse with flexion or extension?
   Is pain better or worse with lying down? with sitting? with standing?
   What makes pain more intense? Less intense?
   Do symptoms get worse with coughing, sneezing, or Valsalva maneuvers?

Q Quality of pain
Is pain dull, sharp, burning, or associated with tingling or numbness?
R Radiation of pain
Does pain radiate into legs?
Is there any bowel or bladder dysfunction?
S Severity of pain and associated systemic symptoms
Does pain cause patient to lie quietly supine or is patient writhing in pain?
Is there associated fever or weight loss?
T Timing of pain
When did pain begin?
Is there pain at night?
Has the patient injured his or her back before?

10. How may back pain be categorized on the basis of historical symptoms?

FEATURE	MECHANICAL	INFLAMMATORY	SOFT TISSUE	INFILTRATIVE
Location	Diffuse	Diffuse	Diffuse	Focal
Symmetry	Unilateral	Bilateral	Generalized	Mid-line
Onset	Variable	Subacute	Subacute	Insidious
Likely precipitant	Trauma, spondylosis	HLA-B27?	Poor sleep, stress	Infection, cancer
Morning stiffness	< 30 min	> 1 h	Variable	None
Activity response	Worsens symptoms	Improves symptoms	Variable	Persistent symptoms
Rest response	Improves symptoms	Worsens symptoms	Variable	Persistent symptoms
Nocturnal pain	Mild	Moderate	Moderate	Severe
Systemic disease	No	Yes	No	Possible

Mechanical (osteoarthritis); Inflammatory (ankylosing spondylitis); Soft Tissue (fibromyalgia); Infiltrative (infection or malignancy).

11. What are the symptoms and signs that indicate that a patient's low back pain may be from a serious cause?

Most low back pain is mechanical in nature and should resolve in a few days to 1–2 months. The following are symptoms/signs that suggest more serious causes of low back pain:

- Unrelenting pain not changed by position, improved by rest, or relieved by the supine position with hips flexed (infection, cancer, osseous lesions)
- Fever, chills, weight loss (infection, cancer)
- Patient writhing on exam table and unable to lie still due to pain (aortic dissection, kidney stone, ruptured viscous)
- Pain worse with walking, radiating into legs, exacerbated by spinal extension, and eased with sitting in forward flexion (spinal stenosis)
- Pain and stiffness (>30 minutes) worse in the morning in a patient less than age 40 (spondyloarthropathy)
- Bilateral radiation of pain (cancer, central disk herniation, spondyloarthropathy)
- Abnormal neurologic exam: sensory/motor deficit, bowel/bladder dysfunction, saddle anesthesia, Babinski sign, ankle clonus (nerve root compression, cancer, central disk herniation)
- Pain lasting more than 2 months

12. What is sciatica?

The simplest definition for *sciatica* is back pain that *radiates* down one leg below the knee. The character of the pain is usually sharp, lancinating, or burning. Occasionally, dermatomal numbness and paresthesias of the lower limb are also reported. *Valsalva* maneuvers or flexion and extension of the lumbosacral spine may exacerbate these symptoms. Sciatic pain is suggestive of nerve root irritation and usually occurs as a consequence of lumbar spondylosis.

13. What physical findings enable you to identify the *approximate* level of common, lumbar nerve root lesions?

NERVE	SENSORY LOSS	MOTOR WEAKNESS	REFLEX
L4	Anterior leg, medial foot	Tibialis anterior (ankle dorsiflexion)	Patellar
L5	Lateral leg, web of great toe	Extensor hallucis longus (great toe extension)	None
S1	Posterior leg, lateral foot	Peroneus muscles (foot eversion)	Achilles

14. What is the difference between *straight-leg raising* and the *femoral stretch test?*
Both maneuvers are used to elicit signs of nerve root irritation in the lumbosacral spine. The *femoral stretch test* is performed to evaluate the upper lumbar roots (L2–L4). With the patient prone, the examiner maximally flexes the knee while gently extending the hip. Anterior thigh (L2, L3) or medial leg (L4) pain is suggestive of a lumbar root lesion. In contrast, *straight-leg raising* evaluates the sciatic nerve roots (L4-S1) and is performed with the patient supine. The examiner passively raises the extended leg, by the foot, until it is elevated 70°. Dermatome pain occurring between 30° and 70° of elevation indicates sciatic nerve irritation.

15. What is spinal stenosis?
Lumbar spinal stenosis is a neural compression disorder that may clinically present as radiculopathy, pseudoclaudication, or cauda equina syndrome. Spinal stenosis results from luminal narrowing of the spinal canal generally attributed to lumbar osteophytosis and spondylosis. The typical patient has symptoms of lower limb claudication (neurogenic) in absence of peripheral vascular disease. Symptoms are exacerbated by back extension and relieved with flexion, thus creating the classic "simian" posture.

16. What is Schober's test?
Schober's test measures mobility of the thoracolumbar spine in the direction of extension and flexion. Two midline marks are drawn (10 cm apart), originating from and proximal to the "dimples of Venus" (posterior, superior iliac spines), on an upright patient. The marks are again measured with the patient's back at maximal flexion. A difference of less than 5 cm between extension and flexion is suggestive of spondylitis. Limitation of lateral flexion and rotation also supports the diagnosis. See figure in chapter 38.

17. How can you clinically demonstrate sacroiliitis?
Sacroiliitis may be physically demonstrated by pelvic compression, **Patrick's test,** and **Gaenslen's sign.** Bilateral compression of the anterior iliac crests toward the midline, on a supine patient, may produce pathologic sacroiliac joint pain. Patrick's test is performed by having the patient **F**lex, **AB**duct, and **E**xternally **R**otate (**FABER**) the hip such that the ipsilateral heel rests on the contralateral knee. Pressure is then exerted on the ipsilateral knee and the contralateral iliac crest. Pain arising from the contralateral pelvis is suggestive of sacroiliitis. Gaenslen's maneuver is performed with the patient supine and both hips and knees in flexion. The patient then moves one buttock off the examining table edge while extending the leg over the side. Sacroiliitis is suspected if the maneuver provokes sacroiliac discomfort. See figures in chapter 38.

18. What is cauda equina syndrome?
Cauda equina syndrome is the clinical complex of low back pain, lower limb motor weakness and saddle anesthesia with bowel and bladder incontinence. The syndrome most commonly results from central intervertebral disc herniation into the sacral nerve roots. Rarely, advanced ankylosing spondylitis and malignancy may cause cauda equina syndrome. The diagnosis of this syndrome in a patient with mechanical back pain constitutes a surgical emergency.

19. What are the indications for obtaining a lumbosacral spine radiograph in a patient with low back pain?
- Unimproved or increasing symptoms, especially if lasting more than 1 month and not improved with therapy

- Acute onset of pain without prior trauma in patient less than 15 or greater than 50 years old
- Back pain after significant trauma
- Severe pain
- History and physical examination consistent with sacroiliitis
- Pain not significantly improved with bed rest
- Patients with known malignancies that have a propensity for going to bone (prostate, breast, kidney, lung, thyroid)
- Constitutional symptoms of fever or weight loss
- Spinal deformity
- Previous vertebral fracture or spinal surgery

20. Define spondylosis, spondylitis, spondylolysis, and spondylolisthesis.

Spondylosis refers to degenerative disease (e.g., osteoarthritis) of the intervertebral disc and/or the apophyseal (facet) joints. The natural, lordotic curves of the spinal column, about C5 and L3–L5, seem predisposed to these degenerative changes. Spondylosis of the cervical spine is the most common cause of neck pain.

Spondylitis literally means inflammation of the vertebral column, a classic feature of the spondyloarthropathies (e.g., ankylosing spondylitis). The inflammatory lesion of spondylitis occurs at the vertebral enthesis.

Spondylolysis is characterized by a defective (separated) pars interarticularis, the bony bridge joining the superior and inferior articular processes of the vertebrae. The pars defect usually results from congenital dysplasia, degenerative disease, and/or trauma.

Spondylolisthesis occurs when the pars defect (spondylolysis) allows forward displacement (subluxation) of the proximal vertebra. Spondylolysis, with or without spondylolisthesis, is the most common *structural* cause of low back pain.

21. When should an electromyogram (EMG) be ordered for a patient with low back pain?
An EMG is obtained in a patient with low back pain who has signs and symptoms of a radiculopathy. The EMG is usually done at least 3 weeks after onset of symptoms when the diagnosis is in question, the severity of the nerve injury needs to be assessed, or the anatomic location of the disc compressing a nerve root needs to be documented before surgery. The results of an EMG are helpful only when combined with the clinical presentation, physical examination, and radiographic tests. Surgical removal of a disc has the most likelihood of improving symptoms if the physical examination, EMG, and radiographic studies all agree on the anatomic location of the disc compressing the nerve root.

22. When should a CT-myelogram or MRI of the spine be ordered for a patient with low back pain?
Certainly most patients with low back pain do *not* need an expensive imaging procedure of their lumbar spine. Diagnostic imaging should only be done when the diagnosis is unclear or if the diagnosis is known but the results are important for the management of the patient's low back pain. For example, a patient with a history and physical examination consistent with lumbar radiculopathy who is getting better with conservative therapy does not need an imaging procedure of his or her back. However, a patient with lumbar radiculopathy who is not improving with current treatment may need an imaging study to better define the etiology (disc, tumor, osteophyte) and site of the radiculopathy before possible surgery. All imaging procedures must be interpreted in conjunction with the clinical history, physical examination, laboratory results, and electrophysiologic studies.

23. What is the sensitivity and specificity of the various diagnostic tests used to document a herniated lumbar disc? How often are they abnormal in individuals without low back pain?
The diagnostic tests used to evaluate low back pain have the following sensitivity and specificity in patients with surgically documented herniated lumbar discs causing a compressive radiculopathy:

	Sensitivity	Specificity
Electomyography	92%	38%
CT scan	92%	88%
Myelography	90%	87%
MRI scan	93%	92%

It is important to note that a significant number of asymptomatic individuals *without* low back pain will have an abnormal CT scan or myelogram (30–40%). MRI studies have shown that 25–50% of individuals *without* low back pain will have a disc bulge or protrusion at one or more lumbar disc levels. Consequently, disc bulges/protrusions on MRI in patients with low back pain are *usually* coincidental, whereas disc extrusion, especially with compression of the lumbar nerve, is usually a significant cause of back pain.

24. What exercises are good for patients with mechanical low back pain?

Exercise is important in any rehabilitation program for mechanical low back pain. People who are more fit have fewer episodes of low back pain and recover from an episode of back pain more quickly. Exercise is important in maintaining the strength of the spinal segments.

Flexion exercises (Williams' exercises) are prescribed to decrease the load on the posterior facet joints and to open the intervertebral foramina. Extension exercises (MacKenzie's exercises) decrease compression load on the intervertebral disc and are consequently useful for patients with radiculopathies due to a herniated or degenerative disc. Exercises to improve lower limb flexibility and strength are important for normal lumbopelvic motion when squatting, bending, and lifting.

25. What is the prognosis of patients with mechanical low back pain?

It is estimated that up to 80% of all individuals will develop back pain during their life. Despite the potential number of people affected, the overall prognosis is good. Within 1 week of an acute episode, 50% of patients have symptomatic improvement; 75% will improve after 1 month; and 87% improve at three months. By 6 months, 93% are better. The remaining 7% have persistent symptoms and will develop chronic back pain.

BIBLIOGRAPHY

1. Borenstein DG, Wiesel SW: Low Back Pain. Philadelphia, W. B. Saunders, 1989.
2. Chang DJ, Paget SA: Neurologic complications of rheumatoid arthritis. Rheum Dis Clin North Am 19:955, 1993.
3. Deyo RA, Loeser JD, Bigos, SJ: Herniated lumbar intervertebral disc. Ann Intern Med 112:598, 1990.
4. Doherty M, Doherty J: Clinical Examination in Rheumatology. London, Wolfe Publishing Ltd. 1992.
5. Doherty M, Hazelman BL, Hutton CW, et al: Rheumatology Examination and Injection Techniques. London, W. B. Saunders, 1992.
6. Frymoyer JW: Back pain and sciatica. N Engl J Med 318:291, 1988.
7. Hoppenfeld S: Physical Examination of the Spine and Extremities. Norwalk, Appleton-Century-Crofts, 1976.
8. Kelly WN, Harris ED, Ruddy S, Sledge CB (eds): Textbook of Rheumatology, 4th ed. Philadelphia, W. B. Saunders, 1993.
9. Klippel JH, Dieppe PA (eds): Rheumatology. London, Mosby-Year Book Europe Limited, 1994.
10. McCarty DJ (ed): Arthritis and Allied Conditions, 11th ed. Philadelphia, Lea & Febiger, 1989.
11. Jensen MC, Brandt-Zawadzki MN, Obuchowski N, et al: Magnetic resonance imaging of the lumbar spine in people without back pain. N Engl J Med 331:69–73, 1994.

65. FIBROMYALGIA

Mark Malyak, M.D.

1. Define soft tissue rheumatism.

Soft tissue rheumatism refers to a group of musculoskeletal pain syndromes that results from pathology of extra-articular and extraosseous periarticular structures. These "soft tissue" structures include bursae, tendons and their synovial sheaths, entheses, muscles, and fasciae. A major point conceptually is that pain from soft tissue rheumatism is not due to pathology of structures within the true joint (i.e., arthritis). Soft tissue rheumatism may manifest as well-defined pathology of a single periarticular site, regional myofascial pain syndrome, or fibromyalgia.

Examples of involvement of **single periarticular sites** include bursitis, tendinitis, tenosynovitis, and enthesitis or enthesopathy (e.g., plantar fasciitis). Although diffuse connective tissue disorders, such as rheumatoid arthritis and seronegative spondyloarthropathy, may involve these soft tissue structures, involvement of a single or few periarticular sites in the absence of articular disease suggests the syndrome is due to chronic low-grade repetitive trauma or acute overexertion (e.g., the weekend warrior).

Regional myofascial pain syndrome is a localized soft tissue pain syndrome characterized by the presence of a trigger point within a muscle that, on palpation, results in severe local tenderness and radiation of pain into characteristic regions. Though the discomfort of the myofascial pain syndrome remains regional, it is usually more widespread than bursitis or tendinitis. Regional myofascial pain syndrome most commonly involves the lower back, neck, shoulder, or hip region. This syndrome is sometimes referred to as **localized fibromyalgia.**

2. Define fibromyalgia.

Criteria for Diagnosis of Fibromyalgia

Always present	Often present
History	History
Chronic, diffuse pain	Morning stiffness
Physical examination	Fatigue
Characteristic tender points	Sleep disturbance
Otherwise unremarkable	Depression
Laboratory tests	Anxiety
All normal	Headache
	Paresthesias
	Raynaud's phenomenon

Fibromyalgia is a chronic (> 3 months) noninflammatory and non-autoimmune diffuse pain syndrome of unknown etiology with characteristic **tender points** present on physical examination. In addition to diffuse chronic musculoskeletal pain, patients subjectively often have morning stiffness, severe fatigue, nonrestorative sleep, paresthesias, and Raynaud's phenomenon. Physical examination and pathologic investigation reveal no evidence of articular, osseous, or soft tissue inflammation or degeneration. Fibromyalgia may occur alone, or may be associated with a number of other disorders. Fibromyalgia is sometimes referred to as generalized fibromyalgia or fibrositis.

3. What are tender points? Where are they located in fibromyalgia patients?

The classification criteria for fibromyalgia require detection of 11 out of 18 tender points. Tender points should exist both above and below the waist and be present for at least 3 months.

Tender points are specific regions on the surface anatomy that are exceedingly tender when point pressure (4 kg/cm^2, or enough pressure to blanch your thumbnail) is applied by the examiner. Tender points in patients with fibromyalgia are more sensitive to pressure than in control patients and when compared to other, nontender point sites (**control points**) in the same patient. Palpation of tender points usually does not result in radiation of pain and thus can be distinguished from the trigger points characteristic of myofascial pain syndrome.

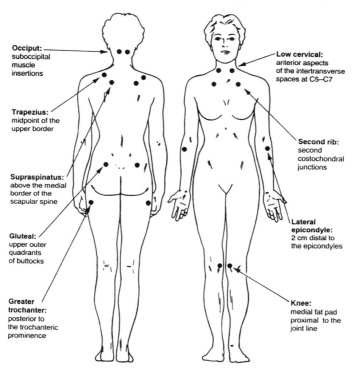

Occiput: suboccipital muscle insertions

Trapezius: midpoint of the upper border

Supraspinatus: above the medial border of the scapular spine

Gluteal: upper outer quadrants of buttocks

Greater trochanter: posterior to the trochanteric prominence

Low cervical: anterior aspects of the intertransverse spaces at C5–C7

Second rib: second costochondral junctions

Lateral epicondyle: 2 cm distal to the epicondyles

Knee: medial fat pad proximal to the joint line

Location of the 18 (9 pairs) specific tender points in fibromyalgia patients. (Freundlich B, Leventhal L: The fibromyalgia syndrome. In Schumacher HR Jr, Klippel JH, Kooopman WJ (eds): Primer on the Rheumatic Diseases, 10th ed. Atlanta, Arthritis Foundation, 1993, pp 247–249; with permission.)

4. What are control points?

Control points are areas that are not normally painful when pressure is applied. They are located on the: mid-forehead; thumbnail; volar surface, mid-forearm; and anterior mid-thigh. Control points are not tender in fibromyalgia patients but are frequently painful in patients with somatization disorders.

5. Who generally develops fibromyalgia? At what age?

Though there is lack of good population-based studies, the prevalence of fibromyalgia in the general adult population is probably 0.5–5%. **Females** account for 70–90% of patients. The observation that **whites** represent >90% of patients with fibromyalgia may represent selection bias. The average **age of onset** is approximately 35–40 years, but the range is great, with onset occurring most commonly between 10–55 years (i.e., menarche to menopause). Fibromyalgia symptoms occurring for the first time in a patient older than 55–60 years is usually due to a disease other than fibromyalgia (e.g., infection, neoplasia, arthritis).

6. How can the pain of fibromyalgia be distinguished from the pain of widespread arthritis?

Patients with fibromyalgia generally have diffuse pain that may be perceived to originate within joints, muscles, or both, and thus it may be confused with a diffuse arthritis syndrome, such as rheumatoid arthritis or ankylosing spondylitis. Pain involving the **axial skeleton** is universally present in fibromyalgia, with patients experiencing lower back, cervical spine, and/or thoracic spine pain. Patients with fibromyalgia also commonly experience **bilateral pain** in the upper and lower extremities. True arthritis may often be excluded by the physical examination, and therefore the joint exam in fibromyalgia should reveal **absence of effusion,** synovial proliferation, deformity, and warmth. The multiple widespread **tender points** present in fibromyalgia are also helpful in distinguishing fibromyalgia from a diffuse arthritis syndrome. Finally, laboratory and radiographic findings are normal in fibromyalgia.

Fibromyalgia may occur alone or may coexist with numerous other medical syndromes, including arthritis. Therefore, the presence of an arthritis syndrome does not exclude the presence of coexistent fibromyalgia, and vice-versa. In these cases, the diagnosis of superimposed fibromyalgia may be considered if subjective pain and constitutional symptoms exceed that expected for the degree of objective arthritis as determined by physical examination, radiographs, and laboratory tests. The presence of diffuse tender points also suggests the diagnosis of coexistent fibromyalgia.

7. Discuss the sleep disorder associated with fibromyalgia.

Non-REM sleep progresses through four stages that can be identified by electroencephalography. Quiet wakefulness with closed eyes is characterized by alpha-waves (8–13 Hz), whereas alert wakefulness with eyes open and bright lights is characterized by beta-waves (14–25 Hz). Non-REM stage I sleep is a transition from wakefulness and is associated with predominantly theta-wave activity (4–7 Hz). As deeper sleep is reached, the frequency of brain waves slows further, so that by non-REM stage IV sleep, delta-waves (<4 Hz) account for >50% of brain wave activity. It is delta-wave or non-REM stage IV sleep that is responsible for restful and restorative sleep.

The sleep disturbance associated with fibromyalgia, termed **alpha-delta sleep,** is characterized by disruption of delta-wave sleep by frequent alpha-wave intrusion, such that non-REM stage IV sleep is significantly reduced. This sleep pattern is not specific for fibromyalgia and may be present during periods of emotional stress, in chronic painful conditions such as rheumatoid arthritis and osteoarthritis, in sleep apnea syndrome, and in some otherwise normal individuals. Alpha-delta sleep is clinically associated with nonrestorative sleep.

8. Though fibromyalgia is a noninflammatory disorder, patients often have morning stiffness and other subjective findings suggestive of an inflammatory disorder, which may lead to difficulty in arriving at the correct diagnosis. Discuss other subjective findings in fibromyalgia that are often considered to represent inflammatory rather than noninflammatory disorders.

Most patients with fibromyalgia have severe, often debilitating, **fatigue.** Fatigue is often most severe upon arising in the morning and is exacerbated by minor physical exertion. Confusion may arise because fatigue is a common constitutional symptom in systemic inflammatory disorders, such as rheumatoid arthritis, and is usually absent in noninflammatory disorders, such as osteoarthritis. Fatigue in chronic inflammatory disorders is likely due to circulating proinflammatory cytokines. Fatigue in fibromyalgia is probably not due to circulating cytokines but is rather associated with alpha-delta sleep disturbance.

Approximately 50% of patients perceive **subjective soft tissue swelling** of joints, suggesting a true arthritis. Physical examination reveals no swelling or other evidence of arthritis.

Paresthesias, which may suggest impingement of neural structures or a neuropathy secondary to an inflammatory condition, are present in approximately 50% of patients with fibromyalgia. Paresthesias may be localized or diffuse and may or may not occur in dermatomal distributions. Subjective muscle weakness is also common. Neurologic examination is unremarkable in these patients, as is nerve conduction velocity/electromyographic examination.

Raynaud's phenomenon occurs in approximately 10% of patients. Though this symptom may occur in otherwise normal individuals, it is a characteristic finding in systemic sclerosis and may be present in other diffuse connective tissue diseases including rheumatoid arthritis and systemic lupus erythematosus.

Dry eyes and **dry mouth** occur in 15% of patients. Confusion may arise because these sicca complaints are common manifestations of primary and secondary Sjögren's syndrome. Other common subjective findings in fibromyalgia include tension headache, migraine headache, symptoms of irritable bowel syndrome, primary dysmenorrhea, depression, and anxiety.

9. Fibromyalgia often occurs independently, but there are well-described associations with other disorders. What are these associated medical disorders?
Fibromyalgia may occur in the setting of numerous **painful syndromes,** including rheumatoid arthritis and osteoarthritis. The chronic pain from the associated syndrome may result in disruption of normal sleep patterns, which may be related to the pathophysiology of fibromyalgia. In these cases, fibromyalgia may be truly secondary. In a similar fashion, fibromyalgia may be associated with **obstructive sleep apnea.**

Fibromyalgia is also associated with **irritable bowel syndrome, tension headaches, migraine headaches, depression,** and primary **dysmenorrhea.** These conditions share a number of features, including female predominance, muscle pain, and lack of abnormal laboratory tests or pathologic features. Thus, these conditions may form a collection of disorders, labeled the **affective spectrum disorders,** that share common pathophysiologic mechanisms.

Fibromyalgia also appears associated with the **chronic fatigue syndrome,** and in fact, these two syndromes may represent the same disorder. Finally, **hypothyroidism** and **Lyme disease** have been associated with fibromyalgia.

10. What is the chronic fatigue syndrome (CFS)? How is it related to fibromyalgia?
CFS is a disorder of unknown etiology and pathophysiology characterized by severe, chronic, debilitating fatigue leading to an inability to perform usual activities. Numerous additional symptoms are commonly present, including joint and muscle pain, headache, and sleep disturbance. Like fibromyalgia, it is not associated with any consistent abnormality on pathologic examination, and specifically, there is no evidence of chronic inflammation accounting for the symptoms. Numerous reports in the past have attempted to associate CFS with chronic active viral infection, most recently Epstein-Barr virus (EBV), but to date there is no evidence to suggest that viral infection is responsible for symptoms in the vast majority of patients. Various studies have reported numerous but subtle immunologic abnormalities, including elevation of certain antibodies against EBV, abnormal T-cell subset ratios, reduced natural killer cell function and number, decreased immunoglobulin subset quantities, and reduced delayed-type hypersensitivity. Although not studied in detail, some of these abnormalities have also been detected in patients with fibromyalgia. Abnormalities of the hypothalamic-pituitary-adrenal axis have also been described.

Numerous hypotheses may explain the symptoms and observed immunologic findings in CFS. Chronic active viral infection remains a possible but unlikely explanation for most patients. Neuro-psycho-immuno-endocrine interrelations are now well-recognized, and dysfunction of any one aspect of this system may lead to abnormalities within the other three. Thus, a primary psychiatric disorder conceivably could lead to the symptoms and abnormal immunologic and endocrinologic findings in CFS. Finally, CFS and fibromyalgia may represent the same disorder or be manifestations of the affective spectrum disorders.

11. Why is it important to determine if fibromyalgia is coexistent in a patient with an underlying inflammatory disorder such as rheumatoid arthritis?
The possibility of fibromyalgia should be ascertained to prevent overtreatment of the rheumatoid arthritis. If articular pain and subjective joint swelling, morning stiffness, and fatigue are manifestations of active rheumatoid arthritis, antirheumatic treatment is inadequate, and more aggressive therapy should be considered to control these inflammatory symptoms and prevent articular destruction. If these same symptoms are due to coexistent fibromyalgia, treatment of this disorder should be instituted, thereby avoiding more aggressive and more toxic antirheumatic therapy.

12. What laboratory tests should be obtained in patients with suspected fibromyalgia?
Laboratory tests in fibromyalgia unassociated with another disorder are normal. Thus, laboratory tests are performed to exclude disorders that may mimic fibromyalgia and to investigate for possible associated conditions.

- Complete blood count, erythrocyte sedimentation rate (ESR), creatinine, liver function tests, thyroid-stimulating hormone, creatine kinase, and urinalysis in all patients
- Rheumatoid factor and antinuclear antibody (ANA) (obtain only if there are supporting data for rheumatoid arthritis, SLE, or other diffuse connective tissue disease)
- Plain radiography (to check for underlying or coincidental arthritis or other pathology)
- Nerve conduction velocity (NCV), electromyography (EMG), MRI, CT, and muscle biopsy usually not necessary
- Formal sleep studies (to evaluate for obstructive sleep apnea in patients with compatible symptoms or signs)

13. Discuss the differential diagnosis of fibromyalgia.

Differential Diagnosis of Fibromyalgia

DISEASE	HISTORY	PHYSICAL EXAMINATION	LABORATORY TESTS
Diffuse connective tissue disease			
Rheumatoid arthritis	Morning stiffness Peripheral joint pain, swelling Fatigue	Synovitis Joint deformities Rheumatoid nodules	Rheumatoid factor Inflammation indicators[†] Plain radiographs
Systemic lupus erythematosus	Fatigue Peripheral joint pain, swelling Raynaud's phenomenon Headache Rash, serositis, etc.*	Rash Synovitis Neuropathy	ANA dsDNA, Sm, Ro antibodies C3, C4 Urinalysis Inflammation indicators
Systemic sclerosis	Raynaud's phenomenon Fatigue Peripheral joint pain, swelling Esophageal, pulmonary symptoms*	Scleroderma Edematous hands Abnormal nailfold on microscopy	ANA Centromere, Scl-70 antibodies Esophageal motility studies PFTs Inflammation indicators
Sjögren's syndrome	Peripheral joint pain, swelling Fatigue Dry eyes, dry mouth Raynaud's phenomenon	Enlarged salivary glands KCS Synovitis	ANA Ro, La antibodies Schirmer's and Rose bengal tests Salivary gland biopsy Inflammation indicators
Polymyositis	Muscle weakness Muscle pain Fatigue	Muscle weakness	CK, aldolase ANA EMG/NCV Muscle biopsy Inflammation indicators
Polymyalgia rheumatica/giant cell arteritis (GCA)	Morning stiffness Shoulder, hip girdle, and neck pain Headache	Tender temporal artery with GCA	ESR Inflammation indicators Temporal artery biopsy for suspected GCA
Seronegative spondyloarthropahty			
Ankylosing spondylitis	Morning stiffness Lower back pain Cevical spine pain Peripheral joint pain/swelling	Limitation of motion of lumbar/cervical spine Peripheral synovitis Iritis	Sacroiliac joint radiograph Spine, peripheral joint radiographs Inflammation indicators

Differential Diagnosis of Fibromyalgia (Continued)

DISEASE	HISTORY	PHYSICAL EXAMINATION	LABORATORY TESTS
Colitic arthritis	Abdominal pain, diarrhea Axial musculoskeletal pain Peripheral joint pain/swelling	Peripheral synovitis Limitation of motion of lumbar, cervical spine Gross/occult blood in stool	Colonoscopy/radio- contrast studies Spine, peripheral joint radiographs Inflammation indicators
Other			
Obstructive sleep apnea	Fatigue Nonrestorative sleep	Unrevealing	Sleep studies
Hypothyroidism	Fatigue Peripheral joint pain/swelling	Thyromegaly	TFTs

*Symptoms not present in fibromyalgia, whereas all other features under history are commonly present in fibromyalgia; not all listed subjective and objective findings are necessarily present in an individual patient with these disorders

†Inflammation indicators include anemia of chronic inflammation, elevated ESR, leukocytosis, thrombocytosis, hypoalbuminemia, and elevated serum globulins.

Abbreviations: KCS, keratoconjunctivitis sicca; PFTs, pulmonary function tests; CK, creatine kinase; TFTs, thyroid function tests.

The fatigue and generalized pain of fibromyalgia are nonspecific symptoms common to many medical conditions. Though the symptoms of these other disorders may mimic fibromyalgia, objective data obtained from physical examination and laboratory evaluation will lead to the correct diagnosis. Except for the mandatory laboratory tests (see Question 12), other tests should be obtained only if the disorder being evaluated is clinically suspected through information obtained from the history, physical examination, and general laboratory tests.

14. Which psychological disorders are sometimes confused with fibromyalgia? Why?

Functional psychiatric disorders, such as the somatoform disorders, often result in symptoms identical to those of fibromyalgia. The term *functional* suggests the syndrome has no organic basis and is due to purely psychologic factors or conflicts. It is conceivable that in some patients fibromyalgia originates as a functional disorder, but then the objective clinical, sleep, and neuro-trans-mitter abnormalities become manifest due to neuro-psycho-immuno-endocrine interrelationships. Thus, although a "functional" psychiatric disorder may precipitate fibromyalgia, "organic" pathophysiologic mechanisms are likely responsible for the symptoms of fibromyalgia. The alternative possibility is that the chronic pain and fatigue of a somatoform disorder are purely functional in certain patients. It is unclear if these patients would have tender points on physical examination, alpha-delta sleep disturbance, or neurotransmitter abnormalities.

Organic psychiatric disorders, such as major depression, have also been associated with fibromyalgia, with up to 50% of patients either having or having had major depression. Alternatively, many patients diagnosed with major depression experience sleep disturbance, fatigue, and diffuse musculoskeletal pain. Three potential explanations may account for this association. (1) Depression and fibromyalgia may both be clinical manifestations of the affective spectrum disorders, and their presence in an individual patient is coincidental rather than causal. (2) Major depression may lead to alterations of the neuro-psycho-immuno-endocrine system such that it leads to the development of fibromyalgia. In a similar fashion, fibromyalgia may lead to the development of major depression. (3) Fibromyalgia and major depression may represent a single syndrome, with the diagnosis in a particular patient dependent on the major clinical manifestations present.

Finally, the **anxiety** and **mild depression** often present in fibromyalgia may be a psychologic response to concerns regarding financial and personal independence in the setting of chronic pain and disability. This association may be present in any chronic pain or debilitating syndrome.

15. Is the etiology of fibromyalgia known?

No. Although patients often report no precipitating event prior to the onset of fibromyalgia, fibromyalgia is occasionally preceded by an acute viral syndrome, physical or emotional trauma, a localized pain syndrome such as myofascial pain syndrome, or withdrawal from certain medications (particularly glucocorticoids). Although it is possible that these disorders may precipitate fibromyalgia, it is less likely that they play a primary role in the maintenance or pathophysiology of the syndrome.

16. What abnormalities in the central nervous system have been implicated in fibromyalgia?
- Descending analgesia system
- Alpha-delta sleep disturbance
- Endorphin/enkephalin system
- Affective spectrum disorder
- Somatoform disorder

17. Discuss the descending analgesia pathway and its potential role in the pathophysiology of fibromyalgia.
The descending analgesia system is a physiologic mechanism by which the transmission of pain is inhibited at the dorsal horn and other locations within the CNS (see figure). Projections from the origin of this pathway within the hypothalamus, utilizing enkephalin as a neurotransmitter, reach the raphe magnus nucleus within the pons and medulla. The raphe nucleus sends projections into the dorsal horn, utilizing serotonin as a neurotransmitter, where they stimulate interneurons whose neurotransmitter is again enkephalin. These axons innervate the presynap-

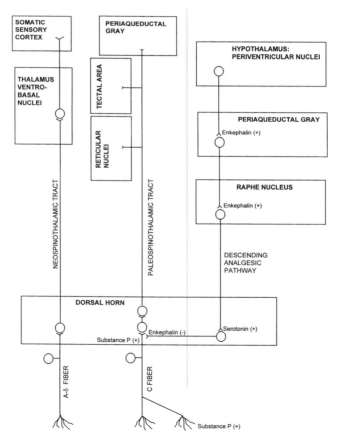

Pain pathways.

tic region of incoming pain fibers, leading to the presynaptic inhibition of transmission of painful sensation to second-order pain fibers, most likely through the inhibition of calcium channels.

The implication of the descending analgesia system in the pathophysiology of fibromyalgia has been suggested by studies that have demonstrated decreased serotonin or serotonin availability within the CNS. It remains unclear if the observed serotonin abnormality is a primary dysfunction or secondary to another process within the neuro-psycho-immuno-endocrine system. It further remains unclear if the serotonin abnormality is in fact associated with dysfunction of the descending analgesia system.

18. What mechanisms originating in the peripheral musculoskeletal system may be important in the etiology and pathophysiology of fibromyalgia?
- Muscle microtrauma
- Muscle deconditioning
- Substance P
- Alpha$_2$-adrenergic receptors

To date, there is no evidence that patients with fibromyalgia have an inflammatory or metabolic disorder of skeletal muscle. There is evidence that patients with fibromyalgia are deconditioned, which is likely due to disuse as a result of chronic pain. It is postulated that deconditioned muscle is more susceptible to microtrauma as a result of minor activity. This microtrauma may then result in greater pain which would further reduce activity, resulting in a vicious cycle of muscle inactivity, deconditioning, microtrauma, and pain.

Substance P is the neurotransmitter of type C pain fibers in the dorsal horn. In addition to transmitting "slow" pain, stimulation of type C fibers may also lead to the secretion of substance P from peripheral nerve fibers in an antidromic fashion, where it may lead to a localized inflammatory response. Excessive substance P, either as a primary or secondary disorder, conceivably could lead to a chronic pain syndrome. Interestingly, elevated substance P levels have been found in the cerebrospinal fluid of some fibromyalgia patients.

In patients with fibromyalgia, there appears to be a correlation between Raynaud's phenomenon and increased alpha$_2$-adrenergic receptors on platelets. This observation suggests that elevated concentrations of these adrenergic receptors within muscle, lacrimal glands, salivary glands, and peripheral digital vessels may lead to excessive adrenergic activity even in the presence of normal catecholamine levels, resulting in muscle pain due to relative ischemia, dry eyes, dry mouth, and Raynaud's phenomenon, respectively.

19. List the six components of nonmedicinal therapy for fibromyalgia.
- Patient education
- Aerobic exercise
- Correction of sleep disturbance
- Analgesia
- Physical therapy
- Treatment of associated disorders

Although the etiology and pathophysiology of fibromyalgia remain unknown and many of the therapeutic interventions have been inadequately studied, a logical multidisciplinary approach to the treatment of this disorder is possible and necessary if meaningful results are expected.

20. What three major points regarding the disease process should be emphasized in patient education programs?
1. Fibromyalgia is a "real" and objective disease. This fact provides relief to the many patients whose chronic symptoms were labeled as purely psychologic or imagined.
2. A serious underlying disorder such as malignancy or destructive arthritis is not responsible for the symptoms of fibromyalgia (unless fibromyalgia is secondary to one of these conditions).
3. Although fibromyalgia is a real disease, the patient has substantial control over many components that may modulate the resultant symptoms. Discussion of an hypothesis of fibromyalgia in lay terms is appropriate, emphasizing those components that may be modified by the patient, e.g., the roles of the sleep disturbance and muscle deconditioning in the positive feedback loop resulting in amplified pain (see figure next page). Provision of lay literature may also be helpful.

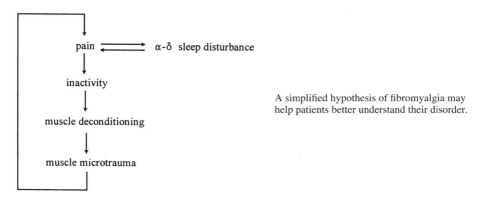

pain $\rightleftharpoons$ α-δ sleep disturbance

inactivity

muscle deconditioning

muscle microtrauma

A simplified hypothesis of fibromyalgia may
help patients better understand their disorder.

21. What is the goal of exercise programs in fibromyalgia patients?

Aerobic exercise improves muscle conditioning, which may lead to less muscle microtrauma and thus may interrupt the positive feedback loop. Aerobic exercise may furthermore improve restorative sleep and increase endogenous endorphins within the CNS. Because patients with fibromyalgia often experience severe postexercise pain, the intensity of exercise must be initially low and only gradually increased as tolerated. Exercise should be aerobic and nonimpact, such as swimming, water aerobics, walking with proper footwear, or bicycling. Patients often find group exercise programs to be beneficial. Physical therapy consultation may be helpful in designing the optimal exercise program for a particular patient.

22. Which physical therapy modalities should be considered in treating a patient with fibromyalgia?

It is reasonable to try safe, relatively inexpensive interventions such as massage and the application of local heat in patients with fibromyalgia. The more expensive interventions, such as transcutaneous electrical nerve stimulation, hypnotherapy, EMG biofeedback, and acupuncture, have been inadequately tested and cannot be recommended for routine use but may be considered in patients whose symptoms are resistant to more conventional therapy. In the unusual patient with fibromyalgia who is experiencing regional pain associated with a local very painful tender point (or trigger point) out of proportion to generalized pain, it is reasonable to treat as one would with a myofascial pain syndrome, including trigger point injection with a local anesthetic and possibly a glucocorticoid preparation followed by stretching of the muscle.

23. Discuss the medicinal approach to therapy for fibromyalgia.

1. **Tricyclic antidepressants (TCA).** Low-dose TCAs administered before bedtime have been objectively demonstrated to improve the sleep disturbance, pain, and tender points in a proportion of patients with fibromyalgia. An example of such a regimen is the administration of amitriptyline at a dosage of 10–25 mg 1–3 hours prior to bedtime. This dose may be increased by 10–25-mg increments at 2-week intervals; the usual effective dose is 25–100 mg daily. Adverse effects are common and are due to the TCA's anticholinergic and antihistamine activities. They include morning drowsiness, dry mouth, and constipation. If amitriptyline fails to provide an adequate response, another TCA such as cyclobenzaprine may be tried.

Although the mechanism of action of the TCAs in the treatment of fibromyalgia remains unclear, the small dosages used and the rapid onset of action suggest it is not due to treatment of underlying depression. Since TCAs inhibit the reuptake of serotonin (and norepinephrine) at synaptic junctions, it is hypothesized that the greater availability of serotonin may be responsible for improved stage IV sleep in addition to providing a central analgesic effect through potentiation of the descending analgesic pathways. TCAs may also have an effect on CNS endorphins as well as on peripheral pain receptors.

2. **Analgesia.** It is reasonable to recommend **acetaminophen** to patients who do not respond

to nonmedicinal interventions and TCAs. If acetaminophen provides no benefit and pain persists, low-dose **NSAID** therapy may be considered, keeping in mind that NSAIDs have common potentially life-threatening adverse effects and have not objectively been demonstrated to be of benefit in fibromyalgia. If low-dose NSAID therapy fails, there probably is no benefit, but potential harm, in using anti-inflammatory doses of NSAIDs. Narcotic analgesics should be avoided in the treatment of fibromyalgia.

24. What is the prognosis for fibromyalgia?

Outcome studies suggest that the majority of patients continue to experience symptoms despite specific treatment. The poor outcome reported in these studies may reflect more severe disease since they originate from tertiary care centers. The only community-based study reported that 25% of patients were asymptomatic and an additional 25% were substantially improved after conventional therapy. Despite these discouraging data, a sympathetic patient-physician interaction and an organized approach to therapeutic intervention will lead to substantial improvement in many patients with fibromyalgia.

BIBLIOGRAPHY

1. Bennett RM: Fibromyalgia and the facts: Sense or nonsense. Rheum Dis Clin North Am 19:45–59, 1993.
2. Bennett RM: The fibromyalgia syndrome: Myofascial pain and the chronic fatigue syndrome. In Kelley WN, Harris ED Jr, Ruddy S, Sledge CB (eds): Textbook of Rheumatology, 4th ed. Philadelphia, W. B. Saunders, 1993, pp 471–483.
3. Carette S: Fibromyalgia 20 years later: What have we really accomplished? J Rheumatol 22:590–594, 1995.
4. Carette S, Bell MJ, Reynolds WJ, et al: Comparison of amitriptyline, cyclobenzaprine, and placebo in the treatment of fibromyalgia: A randomized, double-blind clinical trial. Arthritis Rheum 37:32–40, 1994.
5. Freundlich B, Leventhal L: The fibromyalgia syndrome. In Schumacher HR Jr, Klippel JH, Kooopman WJ (eds): Primer on the Rheumatic Diseases, 10th ed. Atlanta, Arthritis Foundation, 1993, pp 247–249.
6. Goldenberg DL: Fibromyalgia. In Klippel JH, Dieppe PA (eds): Rheumatology. St. Louis, Mosby, 1994, pp 5:16.1–12.
7. Goldenberg DL: Fibromyalgia, chronic fatigue syndrome, and myofascial pain syndrome. Curr Opin Rheumatol 7:127–135, 1995.
8. Goldenberg DL: Fibromyalgia: Why such controversy? Ann Rheum Dis 54:3–5, 1995.
9. Granges G, Zilko P, Littlejohn GO: Fibromyalgia syndrome: Assessment of the severity of the condition 2 years after diagnosis. J Rheumatol 21:523–529, 1994.
10. Hudson JI, Pope HG Jr: Fibromyalgia and psychopathology: Is fibromyalgia a form of "affective spectrum disorder?" J Rheumatol 16 (suppl 19):15–22, 1989.
11. Reichlin S:Neuroendocrine-immune interactions. N Engl J Med 329:1246–1253, 1993.
12. Wilke WS: Treatment of "resistant" fibromyalgia. Rheum Dis Clin North Am 21:247–260, 1995.
13. Wolfe F: When to diagnose fibromyalgia. Rheum Dis Clin North Am 20:485–501, 1994.
14. Yunus MB, Masi AT: Fibromyalgia, restless leg syndrome, periodic limb movement disorder, and psychogenic pain. In McCarty DJ, Koopman WJ (eds): Arthritis and Allied Conditions, 12th ed. Philadelphia, Lea & Febiger, 1993, pp 1383–1405.

66. REGIONAL MUSCULOSKELETAL DISORDERS

Scott Vogelgesang, M.D.

1. What is bursitis?

- A bursa is a sac with a potential space that makes it easier for one tissue to glide over another. There are 78 bursa on each side of the body.
- Occasionally, a bursa may communicate with a nearby joint.

- Most bursae differentiate during development, but new ones may form in response to stress, inflammation, or trauma.
- Bursitis is the condition when a bursa becomes inflamed or infected.

2. What is tendinitis?

Many tendons pass through a sheath with lining tissue that is vascular and resembles synovium (joint lining). Tendinitis occurs when at least one of the following occurs:

Synovial tendon sheaths become inflamed

Trauma induces ischemia and subsequent inflammation

Crystal deposition into the tendon (especially basic calcium pyrophosphate crystals) cause inflammation called calcific tendinitis

Most of these conditions can be classified as "overuse" syndromes. Aging can decrease the integrity of the tendon, making it more prone to injury.

3. What is a nerve entrapment syndrome?

A syndrome of pain, paresthesias, and possibly weakness that occurs because a nerve becomes compressed by an anatomic structure (e.g., a band of tissue, a bony prominence, or swollen surrounding tissue). (See Chapter 68).

4. Name four nonarticular causes of shoulder pain.

- Rotator cuff tendinitis/supraspinatus tendinitis
- Impingement syndrome
- Subacromial bursitis
- Bicipital tendinitis

5. Describe the shoulder impingement syndrome. How does it occur?

The shoulder impingement syndrome is a chronic pain condition of the shoulder that results from a real or relative encroachment of the tendons of the rotator cuff (most commonly the supraspinatus) occurring with glenohumeral motion. Impingement of the tendons occurs most commonly with shoulder abduction. Abduction elevates the greater tuberosity of the humerus and rotator cuff tendon insertions toward the coracoacromial arch. The coracoacromial arch is made up of the acromion, the coracoid process of the scapula, and the stout coracoacromial ligament which connects the two. Etiologies include sporting activities, occupational overuse, and idiopathic, approximately 33% for each. It also can result from a single traumatic episode with post-traumatic tendon inflammation.

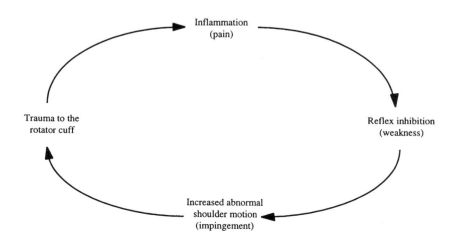

Vicious cycle in impingement syndrome.

In the normal functioning shoulder, the rotator cuff serves as a dynamic stabilizer of the joint. Its principal function lies in humeral head depression. It also assists with early abduction to 0–30° and with internal and external rotation. The biceps tendon long head also crosses the shoulder joint and serves as an additional humeral head depressor. When the rotator cuff is inflamed secondary to chronic repetitive microtrauma or acute post-traumatic tendon strain, it becomes relatively ineffective at shoulder depression, a characteristic called reflex inhibition. This results in increased superior translation of the humeral head with contraction of the deltoid muscle (the prime mover of the shoulder joint), thus setting up the vicious cycle of impingement. With continued motion and increased superior humeral head translation, there is impingement of the tendons on the coracoacromial arch, which leads to tendon inflammation and increased reflex inhibition. Eventually, this can lead to rotator cuff tears or voluntary decreased motion to avoid pain with resultant adhesive capsulitis (frozen shoulder).

6. What are the stages of shoulder impingement syndrome?

Impingement syndrome is divided into 3 stages that correspond to patient age and duration of symptoms:
- Stage I occurs usually under 25 years of age and is characterized by tendon inflammation and edema.
- Stage II occurs at 25–40 years and is characterized by some tendon degeneration.
- Stage III develops at over 40 years of age and is characterized by full-thickness rotator cuff tears.

Stages I and II are reversible with appropriate treatment.

7. How is impingement syndrome treated?

The mainstays of management are physical therapy and anti-inflammatory medications. Regaining full shoulder motion and rotator cuff strength are the therapy goals. The inflammatory changes in the tendons are addressed with oral NSAIDs or local injection of corticosteroid into the subdeltoid bursa. Nonoperative management should be pursued for 9–12 months before consideration of surgical decompression, unless a full-thickness rotator cuff tear is present.

8. Name the muscles of the rotator cuff.

Remember the mnemonic **SITS:**
> S—Supraspinatus
> I—Infraspinatus
> T—Teres minor
> S—Subscapularis

9. How does the impingement syndrome present clinically?

- Pain with active shoulder movement (patient moves arm), especially flexion (between 60°–120°) and internal rotation
- Much less or no pain with passive movement (examiner moves arm)
- Absence of swelling, redness, or warmth at shoulder joint
- Radiographically, the space between the humeral head and inferior surface of the acromion may be < 8 mm

10. What is the impingement sign?

This maneuver produces pain in patients with the impingement syndrome. The examiner stands behind the patient. With one hand, the examiner prevents scapular movement and, with the other, flexes the shoulder. If there is pain with this maneuver that is relieved with injection of local anesthetic, the diagnosis of impingement is supported.

11. Describe with the clinical aspects of subacromial bursitis.

1. Pain with active shoulder movement, especially abduction
   > 90° (motions such as combing hair or reaching with arms over head)
2. Much less or no pain with passive movement

3. Absence of swelling, redness, or warmth at shoulder joint
4. Focal tenderness when area of bursa is palpated (see figure)
5. Pain is worsened with resisted abduction

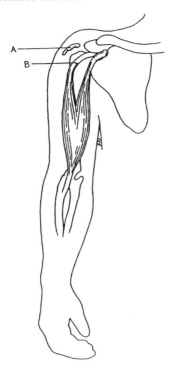

Shoulder anatomy. *A,* Subacromial bursa; B, Biceps tendon, long head.

12. Describe the clinical aspects of bicipital tendinitis.
1. Anterior shoulder pain
2. Pain worsened with active shoulder movement
3. Positive Yergason's manuever and Speed's test
4. Less pain with passive movement
5. Absence of swelling, redness, or warmth at shoulder joint
6. Focal tenderness when area overlying long head of biceps tendon is palpated (see figure)

13. What are Yergason's maneuver and Speed's test?
Both of these clinical signs support the diagnosis of bicipital tendinitis:
Yergason's maneuver—Pain in the area of the long head of the biceps tendon is elicited by resisted supination of the forearm when the elbow is held at the side and flexed to 90°.
Speed's test—Pain in the area of biceps tendon occurs when downward pressure is put on the arm when it is raised anteriorly to 90° with the palm held up.

14. What is a "frozen shoulder?"
Also called adhesive capsulitis or pericapsulititis, frozen shoulder is any cause of shoulder pain that leads to the affected individual restricting shoulder movement because of pain. With little movement, the shoulder joint capsule and surrounding structures contract, making range of motion physically restricted in addition to being painful. Arthrography shows decreased volume of the joint capsule. It is rarely seen before age 40 and, if not treated, can be permanent.

15. Give three causes of nonarticular elbow pain.

> Lateral epicondylitis (tennis elbow)
> Medial epicondylitis (golfer's elbow)
> Olecranon bursitis

16. List the clinical features of lateral epicondylitis.

- Lateral elbow pain, especially with motions such as turning a screwdriver, shaking hands, etc.
- Pain is worsened with extension of the wrist, especially against resistance
- Pain is elicited by palpation at the origin of the wrist extensors (see figure)
- There may be swelling, redness, and warmth at the point of maximum tenderness
- Pain is caused by tendinitis of the wrist extensors

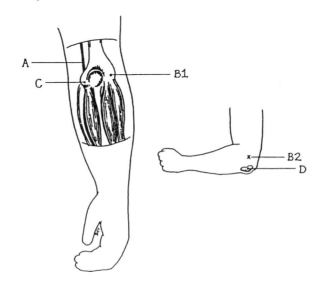

Anatomy of elbow. A, Ulnar nerve; B1 and B2, Lateral epicondyle; C, Medial epicondyle; D, Olecranon bursa.

17. List the clinical characteristics of medial epicondylitis.

- Medial elbow pain
- Pain is worsened with flexion of the wrist, especially against resistance
- Pain is elicited by palpation at the origin of the wrist flexors (see figure)
- There may be swelling, redness, and warmth at the point of maximum tenderness
- Pain is caused by a tendinitis of the wrist flexors

18. Describe the clinical features of olecranon bursitis.

- Pain, swelling, warmth at the location of the olecranon bursa on the extensor surface of the elbow (see figure)
- May be fluctuant and full
- Unless the bursa is extremely tense with fluid, the elbow has normal range of motion.
- Can be secondary to: trauma, rheumatoid arthritis, crystalline arthropathies (gout, CPPD), dialysis, or infection, especially if break in surrounding skin.

19. What is deQuervain's tenosynovitis?

- Tendinitis involving the abductor pollicis longus (APL) and extensor pollicis brevis (EPB) tendons
- Most frequently described as pain at the base of the thumb
- APL/EPB tendons form the palmar side of the anatomic snuffbox

20. What is the Finkelstein maneuver?

The Finkelstein maneuver suggests the diagnosis of deQuervain's tenosynovitis when it reproduces the pain at the base of the thumb. To perform it, the patient touches the thumb to the base of the fifth finger, then wraps the other fingers around the thumb and abducts of the wrist (the fist moves toward the ulnar side).

21. How does trochanteric bursitis present clinically?

Patients complain of "hip pain." When asked to localize the pain, they point to the lateral aspect of the pelvis, with the area of greatest pain typically overlying the greater trochanter on the femur. Pain is exacerbated by lying on the affected side, walking, climbing stairs, and external rotation of the hip.

22. What is "weaver's bottom"?

- Also called ischial bursitis
- Bursa lies superficial to the ischial tuberosity
- Secondary to prolonged sitting on hard surfaces, especially in thin individuals

23. Give the common name for prepatellar bursitis.

Housemaid's knee.

24. What is prepatellar bursitis?

- Pain, swelling, and warmth in the prepatellar bursa
- Located superficial to the patella (see figure)
- Caused by repetitive trauma or overuse such as kneeling
- Can be infected, especially after breaks in the skin

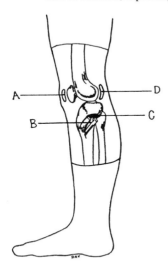

Anatomy of the knee. *A,* Prepatellar bursa; *B,* Conjoined tendons; *C,* Anserine bursa; *D,* Posterior fossa (where Baker's cyst will be felt).

25. Where do you find the pes anserinus?

Literally meaning "goose's foot," it is the anatomic location of the conjoined tendons of the sartorius, gracilis, and semitendinosus muscles in the knee (see figure). The anserine bursa (see figure) lies between these tendons and the medial collateral ligament and can become inflamed.

26. What is anserine bursitis?

Inflammation of the anserine bursa located at the medial aspect of the knee approximately 2 inches below the joint line (see figure). It is frequently described as knee pain, but it is typically noticed when lying on one's side in bed when the knees are opposed. It is more common in obese individuals. Pain is elicited by palpating the bursa and may have associated redness and warmth.

27. What is a Baker's cyst?
Also called a popliteal cyst, this is swelling or fullness in popliteal fossa with minimal tenderness (see figure). Its proposed etiology, in some individuals, involves a communication between the semimembranosus/gastrocnemius bursa and the knee joint. Some have postulated a one-way valve effect in which synovial fluid moves from the knee to the bursa. Baker's cyst can occur secondary to any process that produces synovial fluid (most commonly rheumatoid arthritis, osteoarthritis, or trauma). A ruptured cyst can occasionally dissect down the calf. It may be confused with deep venous thrombosis and is diagnosed with ultrasound or arthrography.

28. Name five causes of heel pain.
(1) Achilles tendinitis, (2) Achilles enthesitis, (3) Achilles or retrocalcaneal bursitis, (4) heel spur, and (5) plantar fasciitis.

29. What is enthesitis?
An **enthesis** is the place where a tendon or ligament inserts into bone. These areas can become inflamed in the spondyloarthropathies such as Reiter's syndrome or ankylosing spondylitis. Achilles enthesitis is another cause of heel pain and is characterized by swelling, erythema, warmth, and pain where the Achilles tendon inserts into the calcaneus (see figure).

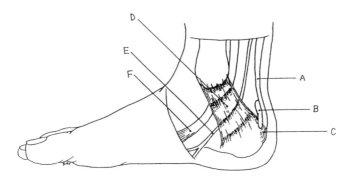

Anatomy of medial ankle and foot. *A*, Achilles tendon; *B*, Achilles bursa; *C*, Achilles enthesis; *D*, Flexor retinaculum; *E*, Posterior tibial nerve; *F*, Posterior tibial tendon.

30. Describe the clinical features of Achilles tendinitis.
- Heel pain, sometimes described as posterior leg pain
- Dorsiflexion and plantarflexion increase the pain
- Area of most tenderness is 2–3 cm proximal to the insertion into the calcaneus (see figure)
- Tendon may be swollen with thickening, especially 2–3 cm proximal to the insertion
- May rupture spontaneously
  Sudden onset of pain during dorsiflexion
  Audible pop or snap
  Positive "Thompson test"

31. How is the Thompson test done?
The patient kneels on a chair with the feet extending back over the edge. As the examiner squeezes and pushes the calf toward the knee, normally you should see plantarflexion of the foot, but in rupture of the Achilles tendon, there will be no movement.

32. How does Achilles or retrocalcaneal bursitis present clinically?

- Heel pain
- Fullness or swelling just proximal to the insertion of the Achilles tendon into the calcaneus (see figure)
- Pain on palpation of the bursa

33. What is posterior tibial tendinitis?

Inflammation of the posterior tibial tendon and its synovial sheath. Pain is located more prominently on the medial side of the ankle. The pain and swelling are localized to the path of the posterior tibial tendon (see figure), with increased pain on resisted foot inversion.

34. What are some clinical features of dysfunction or rupture of the posterior tibial tendon?

Acquired pes planus—Also called a flat foot, in which the normal contour of the longitudinal arch becomes flattened.

"Too many toes" sign—Caused from hind-foot valgus and forefoot abduction. When the foot is viewed from behind the heel, you can see more toes over the lateral side of the affected foot than on the unaffected side.

"Heel-rise" sign—the inability to rise to the ball of the affected foot while lifting the unaffected foot.

35. Describe the clinical features of plantar fasciitis.

Some may describe heel pain, but most affected individuals complain of pain along the plantar surface of the foot. The pain is worsened by pressure on the bottom of the foot (i.e., walking, running, palpation). It is also worse with the first steps taken after getting out of bed in the morning.

36. What is the significance of a heel spur?

Many people complain of heel pain. In many, it appears to be secondary to irritation of the subcutaneous tissue underneath the thick skin of the heel. It is worsened by pressure on the bottom of the foot (i.e., walking, running, palpation). Radiographically, an osteophyte (spur) can be seen to protrude from the calcaneus, and the pain is frequently attributed to the osteophyte irritating the surrounding tissue. Unfortunately, many people without heel spurs have similar pain, and some individuals with a heel spur seen radiographically are asymptomatic.

37. What causes a "bunion"?

Lateral deviation of the first toe (called hallux valgus). It may cause swelling, redness, and pain of the bursa on the medial aspect of the metatarsophalangeal (MTP) joint. A bunion is commonly associated with osteoarthritis of the first MTP joint. Obesity and wearing high-heeled shoes with pointed toes may predispose individuals.

38. How can the regional musculoskeletal syndromes be treated?

1. Avoid the precipitating movements or actions: Bursitis and tendinitis can frequently be caused by repetitive motions or movements (e.g., biceps tendinitis caused by carrying a heavy briefcase daily).
2. Rest the affected area: However, intermittent range of motion needs to be maintained, or the joint may contract or "freeze."
3. Anti-inflammatory or analgesic medications: NSAIDs probably have a more important role than just analgesia.
4. Splinting of the affected area (e.g., an elastic forearm band in epicondylitis)
5. Local corticosteroid injections
6. Superficial heat and cold
7. Deep heat (ultrasound)
8. Range of motion/flexibility exercises
9. Strengthening exercises
10. Ambulatory aids (cane, crutches, or walker)
11. Surgery (bursectomy, tenosynovectomy, reattachment of ruptured tendons)

ACKNOWLEDGMENT

Illustrations by Debra Vogelgesang.

BIBLIOGRAPHY

1. Bland JH, Merritt JA, Boushey DR: The painful shoulder. Semin Arthritis Rheum 7:21–47, 1977.
2. Ege Rasmussen KJ, Fano N: Trochanteric bursitis: Treatment by coritcosteroid injection. Scand J Rhe-
   matol 14:417–420, 1985.
3. Furey JGF: Plantar fasciitis. J Bone Joint Surg 57A:672–673, 1975.
4. Hulstyn MJ, Weiss APC: Adhesive capsulitis of the shoulder. Orthop Rev (Apr):425–433, 1993.
5. Hunter SC, Poole RM: The chronically inflamed tendon. Clin Sports Med 6:371–388, 1987.
6. McAfee JH, Smith DL: Olecranon and prepatellar bursitis: Diagnosis and treatment. West J Med
   149:607–610, 1988.
7. Neer CS II: Impingement lesions. Clin Orthop 173:70–77, 1983.
8. Nirschl RP: Elbow tendinosis/tennis elbow. Clin Sports Med 11:851–870, 1992.
9. Reilly JP, Nicholas JA: The chronically inflamed bursa. Clin Sports Med 6:345–370, 1987.
10. Smith DL, Campbell SM: Painful shoulder syndromes: Diagnosis and management. J Gen Intern Med
    7:328–339, 1992.
11. Supple KM, Hanft JR, Murphy BJ, et al: Posterior tibial tendon dysfunction. Semin Arthritis Rheum
    22:106–113, 1992.

67. SPORTS MEDICINE AND OCCUPATIONAL INJURIES

John A. Reister, M.D.

1. What is the difference between a sprain and a strain?

A **sprain** is an acute traumatic injury to a **ligament.** There are three grades of sprains:

First-degree—mild pain due to tearing a few ligamentous fibers

Second-degree—moderate pain, swelling, and disability

Third-degree—severe pain from a complete rupture of the ligament causing joint instability

A **strain** is an acute traumatic injury to the **muscle-tendon junction.** It is commonly called a "pull." Strains are also classified according to three grades:

First-degree—mild

Second-degree—moderate injury associated with a weak and painful contraction of the involved muscle

Third-degree—complete tear of the muscle–tendon junction resulting in severe pain and
an inability to contract the involved muscle

2. How do overuse injuries and a sprain or strain differ?

Strains and sprains are acute and traumatic in cause. Overuse injuries are nonacute injuries to the soft tissue structures due to chronic, repetitive microtrauma. Overuse injuries can involve the ligaments or the muscle–tendon junction. Microscopically, local tissue breakdown occurs with tissue lysis, lymphocytic infiltration, and blood extravasation.

Overuse injuries are reported to exist in 30–50% of the athletic population and are classified by four grades of injury:

Grade I—pain after activity only

Grade II—pain during and after activity but which does not interfere with performance

Grade III—pain during and after activity with interference with performance

Grade IV—constant pain that interferes with activities of daily living

3. **List some common overuse injuries of ligaments and tendons occurring in athletes.**

Ligaments	Tendons
Little leaguer's elbow	Achilles tendinitis
Swimmer's knee	Suprapatellar tendinitis
Iliotibial band syndrome	Posterior tibialis tendinitis
Jumper's knee	de Quervain's tenosynovitis
Plantar fasciitis	Lateral epicondylitis (tennis elbow)
	Supraspinatus (rotator cuff) tendinitis
	Bicipital tendinitis

4. **Is there any difference between tendinitis, tendinosis, and tenosynovitis?**

Tendinitis is usually due to tendon trauma with associated vascular disruption and acute, subacute, or chronic inflammation.

Tendinosis is noninflammatory, intratendinous atrophy and degeneration which is often associated with chronic tendinitis. Tendinosis can lead to partial or complete tendon rupture.

Tenosynovitis is inflammation of the paratendon, which is the outermost sheath that is lined in some tendons by a synovial membrane (e.g., extensor tendons of thumb in de Quervain's tenosynovitis).

5. **What is tennis elbow?**

Tennis elbow, better termed **lateral epicondylitis,** is an overuse syndrome that presents with lateral elbow pain. Etiologically, few patients who present with this disorder have acquired it through playing tennis. The differential diagnosis of lateral elbow pain includes local conditions, elbow arthritis, loose body in the elbow, nerve compression of the radial nerve or posterior interosseous nerve, and cervical spondylosis with radiculitis.

Presently, lateral epicondylitis is believed to be an inflammatory process and/or microtearing involving the origin of the extensor carpi radialis brevis muscle. Provocative testing of forced middle-finger extension against resistance should reproduce pain, as the muscle in question inserts on the base of the middle-finger metacarpal. Treatment is conservative, with a tennis elbow band (Chopat strap) which anchors the muscle in the proximal forearm and unloads the true origin during activities; this is worn for 9–12 months. Oral NSAIDs are also used, as is local corticosteroid injection and physical therapy.

6. **Golfer's elbow and little leaguer's elbow sound similar mechanically to tennis elbow. Are they?**

Golfer's elbow, better termed a **medial epicondylitis,** results from an overuse injury to the tendinous origin of the flexor pronator muscle mass. This area is placed under valgus stress at the top of a backswing in golfing and proceeds through the downswing until impact with the golf ball. Pain is elicited over the elbow's medial epicondyle and is increased with resisted wrist flexion and forearm pronation. Management includes rest, ice, NSAIDSs, and splints. Steroid injections and surgery are rarely required.

Little leaguer's elbow is a **medial apophysitis** seen mostly in young pitchers between ages 9–12 years. It occurs due to valgus stress, often from throwing curve balls. The person experiences microtearing of the flexor pronator muscle group and, in severe cases, fragmentation of the medial epicondylar apophysis. Treatment is 2–3 weeks of rest, no throwing for 6–12 weeks, and rarely surgery if the medial apophysis is displaced.

7. **What clinical test is used to diagnose a rotator cuff tear?**

The diagnosis is made by combining the history, physical examination, and imaging results. On the history, rotator cuff tear (RCT) can present as a single post-traumatic finding (shoulder dislocation in a patient over age 40) or as the end result of the impingement syndrome. If the tear is large, then the rotator cuff will have lost its mechanical function and a positive **drop arm test** will result. A drop arm test is performed by allowing the patient to bring the arm down from a position of full abduction. When 90 ° of abduction is reached, the arm drops involuntarily toward the patient's side. Pain is not a part of this test.

If the cuff tear is small, as in early stage III impingement, it will retain enough of its mechanical function so that the drop arm sign will not be positive; but patients may exhibit a similar response secondary to pain. Weakness can usually be demonstrated if the pain is removed. Therefore, to aid in diagnosis, a subacromial bursal injection of lidocaine is used to anesthetize the rotator cuff. Once done, strength of resisted abduction at 90° is tested. A small RCT will usually exhibit weakness compared to the opposite side.

8. How is radiographic imaging used to diagnose rotator cuff tears?

Imaging modalities are quite useful for the diagnosis of RCT. **Plain films** will often show superior migration of the humeral head toward the acromion, with an acromiohumeral distance of < 7 mm being suggestive of RCT. This is due to loss of the rotator cuff humeral head depression function. **Ultrasound** can be used to diagnose a RCT, but is operator-dependent. **MRI** is gaining popularity and can show full-thickness tears, tendinitis, and sometimes partial-thickness tears. However, the gold standard test is the **arthrogram,** in which dye is injected into the joint. In a patient with RCT, dye will be visualized traversing the rotator cuff into the subacromial/subdeltoid bursae. The diagnosis of a complete RCT is obvious on physical examination and does not require supporting imaging modalities to make the diagnosis.

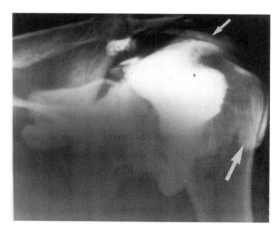

Rotator cuff tear with contrast extending into the subacromial (*short arrow*) and subdeltoid (*long arrow*) bursae.

9. What is a stinger (burner) injury?

The stinger is well known in football, resulting from forced lateral deviation of the neck and inferior force on the ipsilateral shoulder. This occurs with tackling, blocking, or ground contact. A traction injury to the brachial plexus results, predominately affecting the upper extremity. Players complain of significant shoulder and arm pain involving the lateral aspect of the entire upper extremity. Occasionally, shoulder pain is the only complaint. Motor weakness of the involved C5 and C6 root innervated muscles is commonly associated. A stinger should be managed by rest and avoidance of sports participation until normal strength has returned.

10. What is a hip pointer?

A hip pointer refers to a contusion of the iliac crest which usually results from a direct blow to the iliac crest during a contact sport (i.e., football). The athlete experiences severe localized pain, and an audible pop or snap commonly occurs at the time of injury. Frequently, the athlete cannot walk. Physical examination reveals tenderness, swelling, and often ecchymosis which can migrate down the leg. Treatment is ice, analgesics, and a supervised stretching program.

11. Is a snapping hip the same as iliotibial band friction syndrome?

A **snapping hip** occurs when the patient reports sounds or sensations of internal hip clicking with flexion and extension as the iliotibial band moves over the greater trochanter. The patient usually does not have pain unless there is an associated trochanteric bursitis. This usually occurs due to a tight iliotibial band or muscle imbalance.

The **iliotibial band (ITB) friction syndrome** causes lateral knee pain and is related to irritation and inflammation at the distal portion of the iliotibial band as it courses over the lateral femoral condyle. There is increased pain on palpation of this band distally and as the knee goes from flexion to extension. The patient usually has a positive **Ober test.** The Ober test is done by placing the patient on his or her side with the affected leg upward. The injured leg is flexed to 90° at the knee and fully abducted. The leg is released and allowed to adduct. Pain or tightness on adduction is considered a positive test.

The ITB syndrome is usually caused by running excessively or running uphill or on slanted surfaces. Treatment consists of stretching the iliotibial band, ice, modalities, NSAIDs, better training techniques, and rarely corticosteroid injections.

12. How do swimmer's knee, jumper's knee, and runner's knee differ from each other?

Swimmer's knee (breaststroker's knee) is knee pain due to the valgus stress placed on the knee by the whip kick used in swimming the breaststroke. This usually results in medial collateral ligament stress/strain causing pain.

Jumper's knee is an accepted term for **patellar tendinitis.** It is common in high jumpers and volleyball or basketball players. This injury is characterized by pain at the inferior pole of the patella at its attachment to the patellar tendon. It is due to repetitive stress whose frequency of occurrence exceeds the body's rate of natural repair or healing.

Runner's knee is more correctly called **patellofemoral syndrome.** This is the most common injury in runners and accounts for up to 30% of running injuries. Pain is due to compression of nerve fibers in the subchondral bone of the patella or from a synovitis. It is not due to chondromalacia patellae.

13. How is a diagnosis of chondromalacia patellae made?

By visually inspecting the cartilage surface of the patella at the time of surgery. The term chondromalacia patellae refers to a degenerative condition of the articular surface of the patella that progresses from softening, through fibrillar changes and full-thickness cracks, to exposed subchondral bone. It is graded from I to IV, according to the Outerbridge classification system, using the above descriptors, as well as the size of the lesion.

14. List the differential diagnosis for anterior knee pain.

For many years chondromalacia patella was used as a catch-all term for patients with anterior knee pain. Patellofemoral syndromes (PFS) was the next generalized title that evolved for this group of patients. The current accepted diagnosis is anterior knee pain. The differential diagnosis is extensive:

Chondromalacia patellae	Symptomatic plica of the knee
Patellar malalignment	Fat pad syndrome (Hoffa's disease)
Patellar tracking abnormality	Bursitis, infrapatella/prepatellar
Tendinitis quadriceps/patellae	Pes anserine bursitis
Tight iliotibial band	Retinacular neuroma
Meniscal pathology	Tight lateral retinaculum
Painful bipartite patella	Post-surgical neuroma
Blunt trauma, occult fracture	Referred pain from hip
Osteochondritis dissecans (patella)	Radicular pain from lumbosacral spine
Sindig-Larsen-Johansen syndrome	

15. What is the most common condition giving rise to anterior knee pain?

Patellar maltracking due to a relative weakness of the vastus medialis portion of the quadriceps. This maltracking leads to increased pressure on the lateral facet of the patella and pain. With time, it can lead to chondromalacia. It is common in young adults and responds to directed rehabilitation of the quadriceps and stretching of the hamstrings. Adjunctive modalities of oral NSAIDs and patellar centralizing bracing or taping can also be effective.

Other common conditions that affect the patella and give rise to anterior knee pain are true patellar malalignment and tendinitis.

16. What physical exam tests are most sensitive and specific for the diagnosis of an anterior cruciate ligament (ACL) injury?

The best-known test for ACL deficiency is the **anterior drawer sign** which measures anterior translation subjectively.

The most sensitive test is the **Lachman test.** The relaxed knee is placed in 20° of flexion, the distal femur is stabilized by one of the examiner's hands, and the proximal tibia is then translated anteriorly by the other hand. ACL-deficient knees exhibit increased translation and a soft or mushy endpoint, as compared to the opposite, uninjured knee.

The most specific test is the **pivot shift test.** It is performed by applying a valgus and internal rotation force on the tibia with the knee in full extension and hip abducted 10–20°. The knee is then gently flexed. A clunk of tibial rotation is appreciated as the knee passes 20–30° of flexion. This must be compared to the opposite side. The appreciable clunk occurs when the tibia which is abnormally subluxated (anterior and internally rotated secondary to ACL absence) is pulled back into its normal position by the secondary restraints. This test is highly dependent on patient relaxation and is not recommended in the acutely injured, unanesthetized knee.

17. What is the "terrible triad" of knee injury?

An ACL tear, complete medial collateral ligament tear, and a tear of the medial meniscus. This combination is almost always a result of sporting activities, particularly football. The knee in these injuries exhibits a markedly positive anterior drawer test, a positive Lachman's and pivot shift test, and marked valgus angulation with applied stress in full extension. The knee will be stable to varus stress testing because the lateral collateral ligament and posterior cruciate ligament remain intact. Effusion from hemarthrosis may be mild secondary to medial capsular tearing, which allows the traumatic bleeding to exit the knee joint. Suspicion of an injury of this magnitude should lead to the prompt referral to an orthopedic surgeon.

18. Name two lower extremity tendon injuries commonly occurring in runners.

Achilles tendinitis
Posterior tibialis tendinitis

19. What is the best treatment for acute rupture of the Achilles tendon?

Acute Achilles tendon rupture usually results from a forced contraction of the gastrocnemius muscle against resistance, which occurs either during sports participation or from a fall. It is not rare, and these are not subtle injuries. The patient usually presents with pain most notable in walking and with weakness in the pushoff phase of gait.

The best treatment remains controversial. Options include closed treatment with placement in a long or short leg cast with the foot in equinus (plantar-flexed by gravity). A percutaneous suture repair has been reported with good results but may risk some injury to the sural nerve. The third option is open direct primary surgical repair.

Many long-term studies have compared surgical versus nonsurgical treatment. The healing rate is excellent with all techniques. The closed technique requires longer cast immobilization and results in more ankle stiffness in the short-term. The biggest question revolves around the rate of rerupture. Rerupture rates are reported to be 1–5% with surgical treatment and 8–16% with closed-cast treatment. Therefore, selection of the best treatment option is individualized, with age, activity level, patient and surgeon interests, and experience as guiding parameters. The best treatment for rerupture is not controversial and universally accepted to be open surgical repair.

20. What is the relationship of plantar fasciitis to the plantar heel spur seen on the lateral foot x-ray?

This is an area of uncertainty. For years, the heel spur was believed to be a significant cause of heel pain, and surgical excision was common treatment. Now, with more information from anatomic dissection and clinical studies, the relationship, if any, becomes less clear.

Anatomically, the spur is located in the origin of the flexor digitorum brevis, located inferiorly on the anteromedial aspect of the calcaneal tuberosity just deep to the origin of the plantar fascia. Overuse of either of these two structures is thought to produce reactive inflammatory bone production or spur formation secondary to traction, but it is not clear which (if not both) mechanisms are responsible. In either case, the spur is secondary to an overuse phenomenon and treatment should be directed at the cause and not the result.

21. How do a "shin splint" and a stress fracture differ?

Shin splint is an overuse injury caused by chronic traction and inflammation of the tibial periosteum. It may involve either tibialis muscles or the soleus muscle and is characterized by anteromedial or posteromedial leg pain of gradual onset. Pain occurs at the start of running, then decreases, and returns after the athlete stops running. Tenderness is found on palpation of the posterior medial border of the tibia, usually at the junction of the middle and distal thirds. Pain is increased with resisted dorsiflexion. Radiographs are normal, but a bone scan shows fusiform uptake of tracer. Shin splint is sometimes called **medial tibial stress syndrome.**

A **stress fracture** is an overuse injury that occurs when periosteal resorption exceeds bone formation. The tibia is the most common site for stress fractures (30%) in runners, but other areas can be affected depending on the activity or sport. A tibial stress fracture causes pain in runners the entire time they are running as well as afterward. There is often a focal area of tenderness along the anterior tibia. The pain is increased if a vibrating tuning fork is put over the site. Radiographs are usually negative at onset but become abnormal after 5 or more weeks. A bone scan shows uptake, and CT scan/MRI scans are abnormal. Avoidance of activity is necessary to permit repair and to prevent progression to complete fracture.

22. What are some hand injuries that can occur in athletes?

1. **Mallet finger.** Extensor tendon avulsion with or without fracture involving the distal interphalangeal (DIP) joint. The athlete cannot extend the DIP joint.

2. **Jersey finger.** Avulsion of the flexor digitorum profundus tendon causing inability to flex the DIP joint. Usually occurs from grabbing a jersey when tackling in football.

3. **Gamekeeper's thumb.** Rupture of the ulnar collateral ligament of the first metacarpophalangeal (MCP) joint.

4. **Boxer's knuckle.** Longitudinal tear of the extensor digitorum communis tendon overlying the metacarpal head (usually the third MCP), resulting in extensor weakness of that finger.

23. How common are occupational overuse injuries?

Repetitive movements for prolonged periods can lead to overuse injuries in several professions. Approximately 10–20% of musicians, typists, keypunch/calculator/cash register operators, and assembly-line workers will experience a repetitive strain syndrome. The most common problems are bicipital tendinitis, carpal tunnel syndrome, and deQuervain's tendinitis. Patients presenting with tendinitis need to have a complete occupational history obtained to determine if their work is causing their problems.

24. What occupations are associated with osteoarthritis?

Several occupations can cause stress and trauma to joints, leading to early osteoarthritis. This occurs most likely in joints that have been previously injured, have an abnormal joint alignment, or are unstable due to ligamentous injury. Examples include ballet dancers (ankle, feet); farmers (hips); miners, riveters, or metal workers (elbows); pneumatic tool operators (hands or wrists); and coal miners (knees).

25. Discuss the principles of treatment of tendinitis and overuse injuries.

The general principles of management can be remembered with the mnemonic **PRICES:**

Primary Therapies	Secondary Therapies
P = Protection	**P**hysical modalities
R = Rest	**R**ehabilitation
I = Ice	**I**njections
C = Compression	**C**ross-training
E = Elevation	**E**valuation and re-evaluation
S = Support	**S**alicylates

Treatment of soft-tissue injuries with early control of pain and inflammation is critical. Sustained inflammation decreases soft-tissue healing and leads to gradual deconditioning and functional disability. With acute problems, relative rest is important. Ice is an effective anti-inflammatory in the first hours after an injury. Heat is often preferred after the acute injury. Orthotics, splinting, braces, or taping may be used to facilitate protected motion.

26. When are medications useful?

NSAIDs are often used, and all NSAIDs are equally effective. After acute injuries, there is little evidence to support using them for longer than 72 hours. More prolonged use is recommended for chronic overuse conditions.

Corticosteroid injections for chronic conditions are not definitive treatment but should be used to facilitate rehabilitation. Injections should be done by clinicians experienced in performing these procedures and who are familiar with the side effects. Corticosteroids can increase the rate of collagen degradation, decrease new collagen formation, lower tendon tensile strength, and lead to tendon rupture if the procedure is performed incorrectly or too often. The patient should be advised to restrict activity of the affected area for 2–3 weeks after an injection.

BIBLIOGRAPHY

1. Crenshaw AH (ed): Campbell's Operative Orthopaedics, 8th ed. Philadelphia, Mosby, 1992.
2. Fulkerson JP: Patellofemoral pain disorders: Evaluation and management. JOAAOS 2:124–132, 1994.
3. Graham CE: Painful heel syndrome. Foot Ankle 3:261, 1983.
4. Hadler N: Industrial rheumatology. Arthritis Rheum 20:1019–1025, 1977.
5. Jobe FW, Ciccotti MG: Lateral and medial epicondylitis of the elbow. JOAAOS 12:1–8, 1994.
6. McDermott F: Repetition strain injury: A review of current understanding. Med J Aust 14:196–200, 1986.
7. O'Connor FG, Sobel JR, Nirschl RP: Five-step treatment for overuse injuries. Phys Sports Med 20(10):128–142, 1992.
8. Pullman S, Mooar P: Sports and occupational injuries. In Schumacher HR (ed): Primer on the Rheumatic Diseases, 10th ed. Atlanta, Arthritis Foundation, 1993, pp 295–298.
9. Renstom P, Johnson RJ: Overuse injuries in sports: A review. Sports Med 2:316–333, 1985.
10. Swain RA, Kaplan BK: Practice and pitfalls of corticosteroid injections. Phys Sports Med 23(3):27–40, 1995.
11. Torg JS, Glasgow SG: Criteria for return to contact activities following cervical spine injury. Clin J Sports Med 1:12–26, 1991.

68. ENTRAPMENT NEUROPATHIES

David R. Finger, M.D.

1. What are entrapment neuropathies and how do they occur?

Entrapment neuropathies occur when a peripheral nerve is compressed within an enclosed anatomic space. Entrapment can occur from increased pressure, stretch, angulation, ischemia, or friction; previously damaged nerves, such as from alcoholism or diabetes, are more vulnerable. The nerve damage is characterized by physiologic slowing, demyelination, and remyelination; exposure of the involved nerve often reveals swelling proximal to the site of entrapment.

2. Do entrapment neuropathies occur in rheumatoid arthritis (RA)?
Inflammation and swelling of synovium, bursae, ligaments, or tendon sheaths cause pressure on adjacent nerves. Entrapment neuropathies have been reported to occur in nearly half of chronic RA patients at some point in their lifetime. Interestingly, there does not appear to be any correlation with duration of disease, positive rheumatoid factor, level of acute phase reactants (sedimentation rate), functional class, or extra-articular disease. Carpal tunnel syndrome (CTS) occurs with a frequency of 23–69% in RA.

3. List the differential diagnoses of entrapment neuropathies.
- Polyneuropathies
- Brachial plexopathy
- Radiculopathy
- Raynaud's phenomenon
- Reflex sympathetic dystrophy
- Vasculitis
- Overuse syndromes (tendinitis)

4. How are entrapment neuropathies usually diagnosed?
The presence of characteristic symptoms along with provocative maneuvers (Tinel's sign) are usually adequate to support the diagnosis. Electrodiagnostic studies (nerve conduction velocities and electromyography) are often used to confirm and localize the site of entrapment.

5. When are electrodiagnostic studies indicated?
- When the diagnosis is uncertain
- To exclude radiculopathy or polyneuropathy
- To follow the course of patients being treated conservatively
- Prior to surgery

6. Describe characteristic clinical features of entrapment neuropathies.
- Dysesthesias, usually localized to the sensory distribution of the involved nerve
- Symptoms described as burning, tingling, pain, or "pins and needles"
- Symptoms not use-related
- Tenderness of the involved area not a feature
- Symptoms usually worse at night and while at rest
- Muscle weakness and atrophy are late findings
- Often unilateral, with the exception of idiopathic CTS
- Swelling or vasomotor abnormalities absent

7. Describe physical exam signs indicative of an entrapment neuropathy.
A positive **Tinel's sign** occurs when tapping the nerve at the site of entrapment produces pain and dysesthesias radiating into the sensory distribution of the nerve distally. In CTS, this test has a sensitivity of 60% and a specificity of 67%. **Phalen's test** is performed to elicit CTS, and a positive test occurs when maximal passive wrist flexion for 1 minute produces or worsens paresthesias in the median nerve distribution. It has a 75% sensitivity and 47% specificity for CTS. A recently described sign, the **volar hot dog** (swelling at the wrist on the ulnar side of the palmaris longus tendon), was noted in 61 of 63 patients with CTS.

8. What is the carpal tunnel syndrome (CTS)?
Carpel tunnel syndrome (CTS) is easily the most common entrapment neuropathy, with a prevalence of 0.2–1%. CTS occurs when the median nerve is compressed by the flexor retinaculum at the wrist, producing characteristic nocturnal dysesthesias but occasionally progressing to sensory loss and weakness of thumb abduction (see figure below). This condition is bilateral in half of patients and occurs with increased frequency in occupations associated with high levels of repetition and force (meatpackers, shellfish packing, musicians).

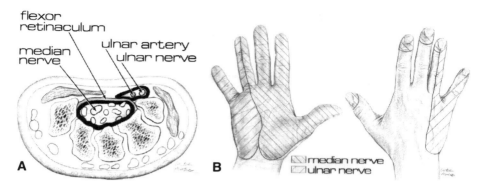

A, Wrist anatomy showing the median nerve through the carpal tunnel in close proximity to Guyon's canal, where the ulnar nerve passes. *B*, Median and ulnar nerve sensory distributions.

9. List some diseases associated with CTS.
Use the mnemonic **PRAGMATIC.**
Pregnancy (20%)
Rheumatoid arthritis (any inflammatory arthritis)
Acromegaly
Glucose (diabetes)
Mechanical (overuse, occupational)
Amyloid
Thyroid (myxedema)
Infection (TB, fungal)
Crystals (gout, pseudogout)

10. What are the treatment options for CTS?
Nonsurgical therapy consists of avoidance of repetitive wrist motion, cock-up wrist splints for night (and work), along with anti-inflammatory medications. Local corticosteroid injections result in excellent short-term relief (80%). Indications for **surgical therapy** (sectioning of the transverse carpal ligament) include failure of conservative therapy, lifestyle limiting symptoms, and muscle weakness or atrophy. Surgical results are favorable in 90% of patients.

11. Where else can median nerve entrapment occur?
The **anterior interosseous nerve syndrome** occurs when this nerve, a purely motor branch of the median nerve, is compressed 6 cm distal to the lateral epicondyle. The resulting loss of distal thumb and index finger flexion produces a characteristic **flattened pinch sign** (inability to form an "O"). The **pronator teres syndrome** occurs when the median nerve is compressed by the pronator teres muscle at the forearm, resulting in proximal forearm, that is worsened by grasping and pronation.

12. Describe the various ulnar nerve entrapment syndromes.
Ulnar nerve compression at the elbow, the second most common entrapment neuropathy of the upper extremity, can occur from external pressure at the medial epicondylar groove (synovitis, osteophytes, anesthetized patients with prolonged resting of the elbow on a flat surface), flexion dislocation, and compression at the aponeurosis of the flexor carpi ulnaris, the so-called cubital tunnel (see figure). **Cubital tunnel syndrome** results in paresthesias in an ulnar nerve distribution, weakness in pinching and grasping, and hypothenar atrophy. Ulnar nerve entrapment is often exacerbated by elbow flexion. Therapy consists of avoidance of prolonged elbow flexion, local steroid injections (in RA), and surgical release in severe cases. **Ulnar tunnel syndrome** occurs when the ulnar nerve is compressed in Guyon's canal at the wrist (see preceding figure), resulting in symptoms similar to those seen in the cubital tunnel syndrome. When ulnar nerve entrapment occurs insidiously, with few dysesthesias or sensory changes, this is referred to as **tardy ulnar palsy.**

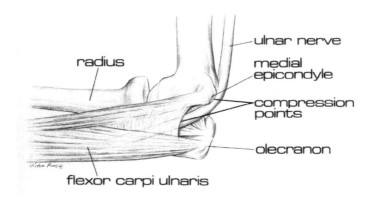

radius

ulnar nerve

medial epicondyle

compression points

olecranon

flexor carpi ulnaris

Anatomy of the ulnar nerve at the elbow, showing sites of common entrapment at the medial epicondyle and the cubital tunnel.

13. What is the thoracic outlet syndrome?

This rare syndrome can occur in the vasculopathic and/or neurogenic form. Occlusion of the subclavian artery results in ischemic symptoms, whereas venous occlusion results in edema, engorged superficial veins, and thrombosis. Brachial plexus impingement can occur from a cervial rib (35%), fibrous tissue bands, scalene muscles, or an elongated transverse process of C7. This results in weakness of the intrinsic muscles of the hand along with sensory loss in the ulnar distribution over the hand and forearm. The **Adson maneuver** is performed by palpating the radial pulse while the patient inhales deeply and extends the neck, turning the head to the side being examined. A positive Adson maneuver occurs when there is diminution of the radial pulse and reproduction of symptoms. The **hyperabduction maneuver,** another provocation test for thoracic outlet syndrome, is performed with the arm abducted to 180 degrees in external rotation. This syndrome is difficult to diagnose because electrodiagnostic studies are usually normal, and many normal people have false-positive physical exam provocation tests. Treatment consists of range of motion and strengthening exercises to improve posture, avoidance of hyperabduction, and surgery for rare patients with severe, refractory symptoms (cervical rib or fibrous band resection).

14. How does radial nerve entrapment occur?

Improper positioning during anesthesia or sleeping on the arm can result in prolonged compression of the nerve along the radial groove on the humerus. This results in wrist drop, referred to as **Saturday night palsy** because it often occurs while the patient is intoxicated. The **posterior interosseous nerve,** a motor branch of the radial nerve, can be impinged at the elbow with resulting weakness in finger extension.

15. What is meralgia paresthetica?

Meralgia (Greek for "pain in the thigh") paresthetica results when the lateral cutaneous nerve of the thigh, a sensory nerve, is compressed at the inguinal ligament just medial to the anterior superior iliac spine. This syndrome results in burning pain and dysesthesia over the anteriolateral thigh (see figure). Common causes include obesity, pregnancy, trauma, surgical injury (appendectomy or inguinal herniorrhapy), tight-fitting clothing (belts), and diabetes mellitus. This syndrome usually is self-limiting, and treatment is conservative, involving weight loss, avoidance of tight clothing, and occasional local steroid injections at the site of compression.

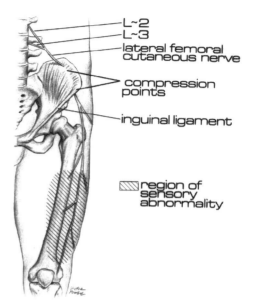

L~2
L~3
lateral femoral cutaneous nerve
compression points
inguinal ligament

▨ region of sensory abnormality

Anatomy of the lateral femoral cutaneous nerve. The inguinal ligament and the anterior superior iliac spine are most likely points of entrapment.

16. Describe the piriformis syndrome.

This controversial syndrome refers to sciatica that arises from entrapment of the sciatic nerve by the piriformis muscle. Symptoms include pain over the buttocks radiating down the back of the leg. It occurs more commonly in women and is usually precipitated by trauma. Physical examination reveals pain and sciatica on resisted hip external rotation (sometimes on internal rotation) along with tenderness of the piriformis muscle on rectal or vaginal examination. Local steroid injections can be beneficial.

17. A 50-year-old woman presents with pain and burning between her third and fourth toe. Symptoms are worsened by walking on hard surfaces and wearing high heels. The region between her third and fourth metatarsal heads is tender to palpation. What is the most likely diagnosis?

A **Morton's neuroma,** caused by entrapment of the interdigital plantar nerve most commonly by the transverse metatarsal ligament, usually located between the third and fourth metatarsal heads. This occurs more commonly in women who wear tight-fitting shoes. Treatment consists of wearing more supportive shoes, padding the metatarsal heads, and local steroid injections.

18. Which nerve is most likely to be compressed in a patient presenting with a painless foot drop?

The common peroneal nerve. **Peroneal nerve palsy** usually occurs following compression over the head of the fibula from prolonged leg crossing, squatting, leg casts and braces. The distal lateral leg often has decreased sensation, and foot eversion (superficial peroneal nerve) and dorsiflexion (deep peroneal nerve) are affected because the lesion occurs proximally in the common peroneal nerve.

19. One of your patients with rheumatoid arthritis presents with burning dysesthesias of toes and sole extending proximally to the medial malleolus; it is worse at night but somewhat relieved by walking. What syndrome does this patient most likely have?

The **tarsal tunnel syndrome.** This syndrome occurs when the posterior tibial nerve is compressed at the flexor retinaculum, located posterior and inferior to the medial malleolus (see following figure). A positive **Tinel's sign** (obtained by percussing posterior to the medial malleolus) and a positive **tourniquet test** (applying pressure over the flexor retinaculum) can be noted to reproduce the symptoms. This occurs more often in women, and is associated with trauma, fracture, valgus deformity, hypermobility, inflammatory arthritis (seen in up to 25% of RA patients), diabetes, and occupational factors. Treatment consists of anti-inflammatory medications, local steroid injection, and orthotics. Surgical release is indicated when conservative measures fail.

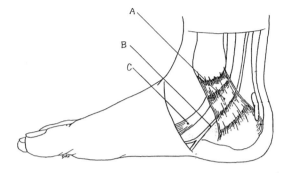

Diagram showing the posterior tibial nerve (B) and posterior tibialis tendon (C) as they descend inferior to the medial malleolus and underneath the flexor retinaculum (A). (Illustration by Debra Vogelgesang.)

BIBLIOGRAPHY

 1. Chang DJ, Paget SA: Neurologic complications of rheumatoid arthritis. Rheum Dis Clin North Am 19:955–973, 1993.
 2. Dawson DM: Entrapment neuropathies of the upper extremities. N Engl J Med 329:2013–2018, 1993.
 3. Grabois M, Puentes J, Lidsky M: Tarsal tunnel syndrome in rheumatoid arthritis. Arch Phys Med Rehabil 62:401–403, 1981.
 4. Hadler NM: Nerve entrapment syndromes. In McCarty DJ, Koopman WJ (eds): Arthritis and Allied Conditions, 12th ed. Philadelphia, Lea & Febiger, 1993, pp 1619–1624.
 5. Herbison GJ, Teng C, Martin JH, et al: Carpal tunnel syndrome in rheumatoid arthritis. Am J Phys Med 52:68–74, 1973.
 6. Katz JN, Larson MG, Sabra A, et al: The carpal tunnel syndrome: Diagnostic utility of the history and physical examination findings. Ann Intern Med 112:321–327, 1990.
 7. Nakano KK: Entrapment neuropathies and related disorders. In Kelly WN, Harris ED, Ruddy S, Sledge CB (eds): Textbook of Rheumatology, 4th ed. Philadelphia, W.B. Saunders, 1993, pp 1712–1727.
 8. Nakano KK: The entrapment neuropathies of rheumatoid arthritis. Orthop Clin North Am 6:837–860, 1975.
 9. Nashel DJ: Entrapment neuropathies. In Klippel JH, Dieppe PA (eds): Rheumatology, 1st ed. St. Louis, Mosby, 5:19.1–19.12, 1994.
10. Shuman S, Osterman L, Bora FW: Compression neuropathies. Semin Neurol 7:76–87,1987.

69. REFLEX SYMPATHETIC DYSTROPHY SYNDROME

David H. Collier, M.D.

1. How is reflex sympathetic dystrophy (RSD) defined?
  There is no uniformly accepted definition. Most definitions include four general criteria:
   Diffuse pain, usually in a nonanatomic pattern and often unrelenting
   Swelling in the involved extremity
   Loss of function in the area due to pain and/or skin and bone changes
   Autonomic dysfunction with vasomotor signs, including a cool or occasional warm skin
    temperature and moist/sweaty or dry/scaly skin
  Some definitions include relief of pain by a sympathetic block. Others describe RSD in terms of signs and symptoms.

2. What are the classic signs and symptoms of RSD?

- Pain and swelling in an extremity
- Trophic skin changes in the same extremity
  Skin atrophy or pigmentary changes
  Hypertrichosis
  Hyperhidrosis
  Nail changes
- Signs and symptoms of vasomotor instability
- Pain and/or limited motion of the ipsilateral shoulder
- A precipitating event, e.g., trauma, surgery, myocardial infarction, spinal disc disease

The pain is often described as burning and severe. It generally involves an entire area such as a hand or foot, although any site on the body can be involved. **Allodynia,** pain from an usually nonnoxious stimulation such as light touch or even a breeze, is commonly present. **Hyperpathia,** prolonged pain on stimulation, is also usually present. The vasomotor instability is manifested by a blue and cool area (but occasionally can be warm and erythematous) along with unusual sweating in the area (but occasionally can be dry and scaly). Dystrophic skin changes, such as atrophy of subcutaneous tissue with overlying tight, shiny, hairless skin, may develop later during evolution of RSD. Contractures of the flexor surface of the hand may occur in the late stage of this disease, leaving a claw-like, nonfunctional hand.

3. What are some synonyms for RSD?

Causalgia, major or minor
Acute atrophy of bone
Sudeck's atrophy
Sudeck's osteodystrophy
Peripheral acute toponeurosis
Traumatic angiospasm
Traumatic vasospasm
Post-traumatic osteoporosis
Postinfarctional sclerodactyly

Shoulder-hand syndrome
Reflex dystrophy
Reflex neurovascular dystrophy
Reflex sympathetic dystrophy
Sympathalgia
Algodystrophy
Algoneurodystrophy
Hyperpathic pain
Sympathetic maintained pain
Complex regional pain syndrome

4. Who was Silas Weir Mitchell?

Silas Weir Mitchell was a neurologist and an assistant surgeon in the U.S. Army during the Civil War. He was in charge of Turner's Lane Hospital, in Philadelphia, to which war wounded with neurologic injuries were brought. In October 1864, during the beginning of Sherman's march from Atlanta to the sea and while Grant was besieging Petersburg, Dr. Mitchell and two colleagues, George Morehouse and William Keen, published one of the classics in medical literature, *Gunshot Wounds and Other Injuries of Nerves*. In this book are clear detailed descriptions of RSD. He emphasized the association with trauma, yet the lack of direct injury to the nerve, and the articular nature of this syndrome. In 1867, Dr. Mitchell coined the word *causalgia* (from the Greek words for heat and pain) for this illness in an article in the *United States Sanitary Commission Memoirs*. He is the father of RSD in this country.

5. Who gets RSD?

There is an equal incidence of RSD in men and women. When individual inciting factors are examined that are more common in one sex than another (e.g., myocardial infarction in men), the statistics become skewed toward that sex. Adults get RSD much more often than children. The highest incidence is in the 40–60-year age group with a mean age of 50 years. The incidence in children is thought to be under-reported because it often goes unrecognized, sometimes being diagnosed as a psychiatric condition. It is, in general, a more benign disease in children. About 75% of the time, there is a clear precipitating factor that causes the development of RSD.

6. What are some precipitating factors for the development of RSD?
Inciting factors

Trauma

 Fractures

 Lacerations

 Crush injuries

Contusions

 Sprains

Immobilization in a cast

Myocardial infarctions

Strokes and other CNS injury

Pleuropulmonary diseases

Surgery (esp. for carpal
   tunnel and Morton's neuroma)

Chemical burns

Electrical burns

Postherpetic neuralgia

Cervical spine pathology

Subcutaneous injections

Drugs (barbiturates)

Malignancies

Pregnancy

Peripheral nerve diseases

Emotional stress

Predisposing factors

Diabetes mellitus

Hyperparathyroidism

Hyperthyroidism

Multiple sclerosis

Neurovegetative dystonia

Hypertriglyceridemia

Alcohol abuse

Tobacco use

7. How soon after a precipitating event, such as trauma, will a patient develop RSD?
RSD usually begins days to weeks after the inciting event. In about 80% of cases, it occurs within 3 months of a traumatic episode, but in many cases, RSD begins over 6 months later

8. What is the shoulder-hand syndrome?
This term was coined by Dr. Otto Steinbrocker in 1947 to describe the concomitant shoulder involvement seen with hand RSD. The ipsilateral shoulder will commonly become diffusely painful, develop limited range of motion in all directions, and may progress to adhesive capsulitis.

9. What are the stages of RSD?
   Dr. Steinbrocker was the first to divide RSD into three stages. Some recent authors may add a fourth stage:
   Stage 1 (acute stage): typically lasts 3–6 months after the development of RSD;
         characterized by:
      Pain in the extremity or shoulder
      Swelling in the extremity
      Color change of the extremity
      Pain on movement
      Early osteoporosis on x-rays
   Stage 2 (dystrophic phase): persists an additional 3–12 months; characterized by:
      Pain usually continues
      Swelling changes to brawny hard edema
      Beginning of atrophy of subcutaneous tissue and intrinsic muscles
      Progression of osteoporosis
   Stage 3 (atrophic stage): classically described beginning 9–18 months after the RSD starts;
         characterized by:
      Pain remains constant or diminishes
      Extremity becomes stiff
      Swelling changes to periarticular thickening
      Skin becomes smooth, glossy, and drawn
      Brittle nails
      Progression of osteoporosis with pathologic fractures
   Stage 4 (psychological): untreated or passively treated patients may develop severe depression,
      suicidal ideation, and/or undergo unnecessary surgery with further aggravation of pain.

Although these stages can be useful, it is often difficult to place an individual patient into one of them. Most often, stages 1 and 2 are merged or fluctuate back and forth. A patient may stay in one stage for months or years, and another patient may progress rapidly through the stages. The earlier stages are much easier to treat than the later stages.

10. What factors may maintain the pain syndrome through the stages?

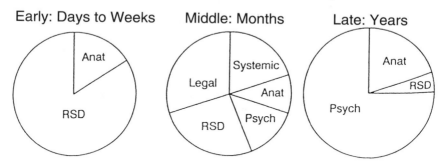

Anat = anatomic factors, such as the injury with which the RSD is associated; Psych = psychological factors; Systemic = systemic factors and associated diseases, such as diabetes mellitus, stroke or myocardial infarction; Legal = litigation involving personal injury suits, worker's compensation, and other forms of secondary gain. (From Amadio PC, Mackinnon SE, Merritt WH, et al: Reflex sympathetic dystrophy syndrome: Consensus report of an ad hoc committee of the American Association for Hand Surgery on the definition of reflex sympathetic dystrophy syndrome. Plast Reconstr Surg 87:371–375, 1991, with permission.)

11. Discuss the bilateral involvement of RSD.
Bilateral involvement in patients with RSD has been described in 18–100% of patients, depending on the type of measurements and criteria used. Using an algometer on involved joints may demonstrate abnormalities bilaterally in almost all patients, whereas using bone scans may show bilateral involvement in 22% of cases of RSD. The side secondarily involved tends to have less signs and symptoms than the originally involved side. Bilateral involvement is usually symmetric, with the same area of involvement on each side, but the side secondarily involved can occasionally have a patchy pattern of involvement.

12. Are there notable plain radiographic findings in RSD?
The characteristic radiologic appearance is soft tissue swelling and regional patchy or mottled osteopenia. This appearance is especially evident when comparing the involved side to the contralateral side. This x-ray pattern was first described by Sudeck in 1900 and is often referred to as **Sudeck's atrophy.** This patchy osteopenia is helpful in making the diagnosis but is actually seen in less than half the patients in most series.
Fine-detailed radiography has actually revealed five patterns of bone resorption:
1. A thinning of the trabecular or cancellous bone of the metaphyseal regions, producing bandlike, patchy, or periarticular osteoporosis.
2. Subperiosteal cortical bone resorption resulting in a corrugated appearance of the outer margins of the diaphyses.
3. Endosteal bone resorption resulting in irregularity of the endosteal surface and variation in the thickness of the cortices.
4. Intracortical bone resorption resulting in excessive striation or tunneling within the cortex paralleling the longitudinal axis.
5. Subchondral and juxta-articular erosions visible as small periarticular erosions and intraarticular gaps in the subchondral bone.

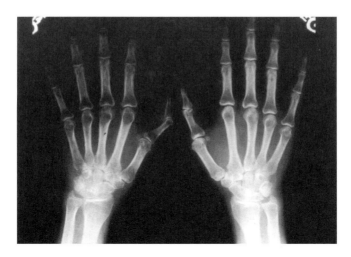

Radiograph of the hands showing RSD of left hand. Note marked periarticular osteoporosis compared to the right hand.

13. What are the scintigraphic findings in RSD?

The results of a three-phase bone scan using technetium-99m pertechnetate can vary greatly depending on how early in the course of the disease the study is performed. In **stage 1,** there is an increase in blood velocity and blood pooling with early and delayed hyperfixation. The bone scan is abnormal about 80% of the time in this stage. In **stage 2,** there is normalization of blood velocity and blood pooling but a persistence of early and delayed hyperfixation. The bone scan is abnormal about half the time in this stage. In **stage 3,** there is reduced blood velocity and blood pooling, and a minority of patients have early and delayed hyperfixation. Thus, a bone scan performed early in the disease is usually abnormal, but as the disease progresses, scans can be normal. A normal bone scan does not exclude the diagnosis of RSD.

14. Discuss the use of a thermogram in RSD.

Some authors believe that infrared thermography is the most sensitive test in the diagnosis of RSD (90% accuracy). It documents the temperature differences and subtle temperature gradients in different parts of the skin. If the sympathetic nervous system is behaving abnormally due to RSD, the thermogram picks up these cold or hot areas, usually in a regional pattern. Most patients will have a decrease of subcutaneous temperature associated with the RSD, but some patients have an increase.

Other authors emphasize the nonspecificity of the thermogram. Vascular problems unrelated to sympathetic abnormalities can give regional coolness. Secondly, sympathetic hyperfunction is not a prerequisite for the diagnosis of RSD, and patients may have normal or even subnormal levels of sympathetic function.

15. Does synovial biopsy yield any typical findings in RSD?

RSD is an arthritic problem. The involved joints tend to be more tender than the periarticular areas. The synovium has been shown to be clearly abnormal. Findings include synovial edema, proliferation and disarray of synovial lining cells, proliferation of capillaries, fibrosis in the deep synovial layers, and occasional infiltration with chronic inflammatory cells (chiefly lymphocytes).

16. What is the pathophysiology of RSD? (*Controversial*)

Over the years, various theories have explained specific findings in RSD (e.g., allodynia, bilateral involvement), and both central and peripheral nervous system mechanisms have been evoked to explain sympathetically mediated pain. However, there is no one accepted theory to explain RSD. A synthesis of various hypotheses to explain the traditional therapeutic approach to RSD is as follows:

The afferent nerves consist of A fibers (α, β, δ) and C fiber (polymodal nociceptors). The A fibers are mainly involved in nonpainful sensation (except for some A-δ fibers). The C fibers relay pain. The A fibers are myelinated, and current flows much faster in them than in the unmyelinated pain fibers.

Wall and Melzach have proposed a **gate control theory** in which dorsal horn cells of the spinal cord can modulate the transmission of sensory information. The pattern of impulses allowed to go through this "gate" determines the rate of firing of the "action system" or spinal transmission neurons. In certain laminae (3 and 4) of the dorsal horn are wide dynamic range fibers that can transmit painful or nonpainful information to the brain depending on information coming from the peripheral and central nervous systems. The stimulated A fibers are thought to inhibit information from C type polymodal nociceptors until a specific number C fibers firing at a rapid frequency can break through the gate and impart painful information. This system is designed so that normal touch is not perceived as pain. When polymodal nociceptors are stimulated, the neuropeptide substance P is released around the receptor where the painful stimulus began. Substance P is pro-inflammatory and causes histamine release, neutrophil migration, vasodilation and vasopermeability, and the release of bradykinin which can stimulate prostaglandin production. Thus, the stimulation of pain fibers can promote inflammation.

When afferent nerves are damaged, two responses can happen. Myelinated A fibers will not send information to the dorsal horns, thus not acting as inhibitory neurons. Unmyelinated C fibers behave oppositely. They will spontaneously fire and become sensitive to certain chemicals, such as norepinephrine, from sympathetic fibers. Thus, painful messages are sent to the dorsal horn. The wide dynamic range fibers then send messages of pain to the brain. The sympathetics become stimulated, releasing chemicals that stimulate the polymodal nociceptors, and thus we have RSD.

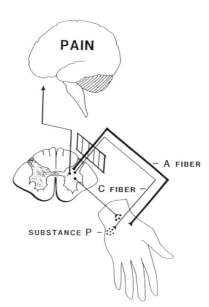

17. Describe a rational approach to the treatment of RSD.

Stimulation of inhibitory neurons
  Physical therapy
  Massage, counterirritants
  Ultrasound
  Transcutaneous nerve stimulators
  Spinal cord stimulator

Anti-inflammatory agents
  NSAIDs
  Ketorolac in an IV regional block
  Corticosteroids
Sympathetic blocks
  Lidocaine, mepivacaine, bupivacaine, etc., into sympathetic ganglion
  Bier block with IV bretylium, guanethidine or reserpine
  Oral α- and β-blockers
  Prazosin
  Sympathectomy
Depletion of substance P in peripheral nerves
  Topical capsaicin
Other treatments
  Tricyclic antidepressants
  Calcitonin
  Phenytoin
  Carbamazepine
  Calcium channel blockers
Psychological therapy
  Provide emotional support
  Assess for depression and treat with psychotherapy and medications if a problem
  Thermal biofeedback
  Relaxation training
  Stop alcohol and tobacco

BIBLIOGRAPHY

1. Amadio PC, Mackinnon SE, Merritt WH, et al: Reflex sympathetic dystrophy syndrome: Consensus report of an ad hoc committee of the American Association for Hand Surgery on the definition of reflex sympathetic dystrophy syndrome. Plast Reconstr Surg 87:371–375, 1991.
2. Awerbuch MS: Thermography—Its current diagnostic status in musculoskeletal medicine. Med J Aust 154:441–444, 1991.
3. Demangeat JL, Constantinesco A, Brunot B, et al: Three-phase bone scanning in reflex sympathetic dystrophy of the hand. J Nucl Med 29:26–32, 1988.
4. Genant HK, Kozin F, Bekerman C, et al: The reflex sympathetic dystrophy syndrome: A comprehensive analysis using fine-detail radiography, photon absorptiometry, and bone and joint scintigraphy. Radiology 117:21–32, 1975.
5. Jänig W, Stanton-Hicks M (eds): Reflex Sympathetic Dystrophy: A Reappraisal. Seattle, IASP Press, 1996.
6. Kleinert H, Cole NM, Wayne L, et al: Post-traumatic sympathetic dystrophy. Orthop Clin North Am 4:917–927, 1973.
7. Kozin F: Reflex sympathetic dystrophy syndrome: A review. Clin Exp Rheumatol 10:401–409, 1992.
8. Kozin F, Genant HK, Bekerman C, McCarty DJ: The reflex sympathetic dystrophy syndrome: II. Roentgenographic and scintigraphic evidence of bilaterality and of periarticular accentuation. Am J Med 60:332–338, 1976.
9. Kozin F, McCarty DJ, Sims J, Genant H: The reflex sympathetic dystrophy syndrome: I. Clinical and histologic studies: Evidence for bilaterality, response to corticosteroids and articular involvement. Am J Med 60:321–331, 1976.
10. Kozin F, Ryan LM, Carerra GF, et al: The reflex sympathetic dystrophy syndrome (RSDS): III. Scintigraphic studies, further evidence for the therapeutic efficacy of systemic corticosteroids, and proposed diagnostic criteria. Am J Med 70:23–30, 1981.
11. Pak TJ, Martin GM, Magness JL, Kavanaugh GJ: Reflex sympathetic dystrophy: Review of 140 cases. Minn Med 53:507–512, 1970.
12. Richards RL: Causalgia: A centennial review. Arch Neurol 16:339–350, 1967.
13. Silber TJ, Majd M: Reflex sympathetic dystrophy syndrome in children and adolescents: Report of 18 cases and review of the literature. Am J Dis Child 142:1325–1330, 1988.
14. Steinbrocker O: The shoulder-hand syndrome. Am J Med 3:402–407, 1947.
15. Subbarao J, Stillwell GK: Reflex sympathetic dystrophy syndrome of the upper extremity: Analysis of total outcome of management of 125 cases. Arch Phys Med Rehabil 62:549–554, 1981.

XII. Neoplasms and Tumor-like Lesions

While there are several chronic diseases more destructive to life than cancer, none is more feared.

Charles H. Mayo
(1865–1939), 1926

70. BENIGN AND MALIGNANT TUMORS OF JOINTS AND SYNOVIUM

Edmund H. Hornstein, D.O.

1. Why should practicing physicians be concerned with tumors that affect the joints and synovium?

Benign and malignant neoplasms affecting articular and periarticular structures may mimic inflammatory arthritis. Awareness of these conditions is crucial to prevent diagnostic delay and to avoid the initiation of ineffective and/or inappropriate therapy. Fortunately, primary neoplasms of the joint are rare.

2. A young adult presents with a solitary, painless mass adjacent to a finger joint which has been slowly enlarging. What tumor is suggested by this scenario?

This presentation would be typical for **pigmented villonodular synovitis** (PVNS). This benign condition, which occurs with a slightly increased predilection for females, is second only to the ganglion as a source of localized swelling in the hand and wrist. These nodular lesions may occur either in association with a tendon sheath (in which case it is called giant cell tumor of tendon sheath) or within the joint proper. It is most common in the fingers, followed by the knees, wrists, feet, and toes.

3. PVNS exists in two forms, localized and diffuse. How do these forms differ?

In **diffuse PVNS**, the entire synovium of an affected joint or structure is involved. Grossly, the synovium is prolific with coarse villi, finer fronds, and diffuse nodularity. It is often darkly pigmented, ranging from dark yellow to chocolate brown. **Localized PVNS** involves only a portion of a synovial surface, tends not to be as darkly pigmented and has less villous proliferation than is seen in the diffuse form. Diffuse PVNS is almost always monarticular, and the knee is the most common site. Swelling and effusion accompanied by moderate discomfort, decreased range of motion, and increased warmth to palpation are typical.

4. What does the synovial fluid analysis reveal in PVNS?

Typically, the fluid is grossly **hemorrhagic,** which should suggest the presence of this condition.

5. Describe the histologic characteristics of PVNS.

Microscopically, PVNS is distinctive. It is characterized by a dense cellular infiltrate composed of histiocytes, lipid-laden cells, hemosiderin-containing cells, and scattered, frequent, multinucleated giant cells. Controversy exists as to the nature of this condition. DNA analysis is supportive of a neoplastic etiology for diffuse PVNS but not for the localized form of the lesion.

6. How is PVNS treated?

Surgical treatment is standard, either via open or arthroscopic approaches. Recurrences, particularly in diffuse PVNS, are not uncommon.

7. Synovial chondromatosis is another benign lesion of joints. Does it represent neoplasia?

No. More appropriately considered a metaplastic lesion, this disorder is characterized by the development of multiple foci of cartilaginous metaplasia within the synovium. These foci form nodules which may calcify or ossify and which frequently are released as free bodies (**joint mice**) into the joint space.

8. How is synovial chondromatosis diagnosed?

Synovial chondromatosis is almost always monarticular. It usually occurs in the knee but can occur in the hip, ankle, elbow, or other joints. Clinically, there is increasingly compromised range of motion with crepitus and often with unexpected locking. Effusion may occur. The x-ray examination may be diagnostic if the chondroid bodies are calcified (see figure). If not, diagnosis may require arthroscopic biopsy.

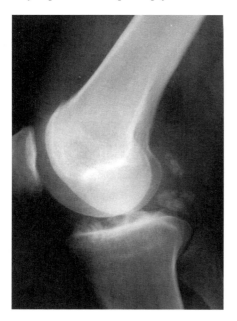

Synovial chondromatosis of the knee demonstrating multiple, calcified chondroid bodies.

9. How is synovial chondromatosis managed?

Treatment is via synovectomy. Though considered benign, this condition can result in extensive local joint destruction if left untreated. Occasionally, this lesion may be difficult to distinguish histologically from chondrosarcoma.

10. What other benign tumor-like lesions can involve the joints?

- **Lipomas** may occur within the joint capsule or synovium, but true intra-articular lesions are rare.
- **Chondroma** is an isolated mass of benign cartilage, usually in the knee.
- **Hemangiomas** are unusual intra-articular lesions that occur most frequently in the joints of children and young adults. The knee is the most common site. Recurrent hemarthrosis may occur. Diagnosis can be made by CT, MRI, or angiography.
- **Osteoid osteomas,** when occurring within the joint, have less of the "classic" pattern of nocturnal pain relieved by NSAIDs, and tend to involute spontaneously after 5–10 years.

12. What is the most common primary malignant neoplasm involving the joints?
Synovial sarcoma, which constitutes up to 10% of all soft-tissue sarcomas. It is a highly malignant neoplasm and generally occurs in the lower extremities of young people. The tumor usually arises in the periarticular tissue of the knee, though it may arise directly within the joint.

13. How does this tumor present clinically?
A slowly growing, often minimally symptomatic mass adjacent to the joint is the typical presentation. Pain is reported by about 50% of patients with this tumor. Soft-tissue calcification on plain x-ray occurs in 30% of the cases, and this finding serves to provide a clue as to the underlying diagnosis (see figure).

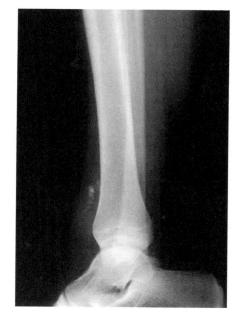

Synovial sarcoma adjacent to the ankle. Note the speckled calcifications.

14. What is the cell of origin for synovial sarcoma?
The histology of this tumor may be **biphasic**, in which epithelial cells arranged in clusters, tubules, and acini are interspersed in a spindle-cell stroma, or **monophasic**, in which either the epithelial or spindle cells predominate. Though this tumor is called synovial sarcoma, ultrastructural and immunohistochemical studies have implicated an epithelial origin.

15. How is synovial sarcoma treated? What is the prognosis?
Treatment is an aggressive combination of radical surgery, radiation therapy, and chemotherapy. Prognosis depends in large part on tumor size at the time of discovery. The cause of death in progressive disease is usually due to extensive pulmonary metastasis. Other common sites of metastasis include regional lymph nodes, bones, skin, and brain.

5-Year Survival in Synovial Sarcoma

All tumors	40%
Tumor < 5 cm	86%
Tumor > 10 cm	22%

16. Clear-cell sarcoma is a rare highly malignant tumor of tendons, ligaments, and fascial aponeuroses. It usually presents as a slowly growing mass about the foot. What is its association with a malignancy more commonly thought of as a skin cancer?

There are multiple lines of evidence suggesting, rather convincingly, that clear-cell sarcoma is a representation of **malignant melanoma.** This evidence includes an immunohistochemical staining pattern with S-100 and HMB-45 which are considered specific for melanoma, evidence of melanin by special staining, and the presence of characteristic pre-malanasomes by electron microscopy. Prognosis is generally poor.

17. Which primary malignant tumor of joints may be difficult to differentiate from the benign cartilaginous metaplasia of synovial chondromatosis?

Occasionally arising from synovial chondromatosis, **synovial chondrosarcoma** is an exceedingly rare malignancy that may be histologically difficult to differentiate from its benign cousin. Favoring a diagnosis of sarcoma is the loss of a differentiated clustering growth pattern, areas of necrosis, and spindling of cells in the periphery.

18. In which malignant diseases can joint involvement occur as a secondary feature?

Metastatic carcinoma
Lymphoma/myeloma
Leukemic infiltration
Contiguous spread of adjacent bone sarcomas

19. What is the "classic" presentation of carcinoma metastatic to a joint?

- Advanced lung or breast cancer is the most common etiology.
- Involvement is usually monarticular, with the knee the most common site.
- Effusion is often hemorrhagic.
- Synovial fluid cytology reveals the malignancy in approximately 50% of cases.

BIBLIOGRAPHY

1. Abraham JH, Canoso JJ: Tumors of soft tissue and bone. Curr Opin Rheumatol 5:193–198, 1993.
2. Bertoni F, Unni KK, Beabout JW, Sim FH: Chondrosarcomas of the synovium. Cancer 67:155–162, 1991.
3. Brodsky JT, Burt ME, Hajdu SI, et al: Tendosynovial sarcoma: Clinicopathologic features, treatment and prognosis. Cancer 70:484–489, 1992.
4. Burssens A, Dequeker J: Tumors of bone. In Klippel JH, Dieppe PA (eds): Slide Atlas of Rheumatology. St. Louis, Mosby, 1994: sect 7, unit 3, pp 43.1–43.14.
5. Caldwell DS: Musculoskeletal syndromes associated with malignancy. In Kelley WN, Harris ED, Ruddy S, Sledge CB (eds): Textbook of Rheumatology, 4th ed. Philadelphia, W.B. Saunders, 1993, pp 1552–1563.
6. Caldwell DS, McCallum RM: Rheumatologic manifestations of cancer. Med Clin North Am 70:385–417, 1986.
7. Docken WP: Pigmented villonodular synovitis: A review with illustrative case reports. Semin Arthritis Rheum 9:1–22, 1979.
8. Fam AG: Neoplasms of the joints. In Schumacher HR (ed): Primer on the Rheumatic Diseases, 10th ed. Atlanta, Arthritis Foundation, 1993, pp 238–241.
9. Gebhart MC, Ready JE, Mankin HJ: Tumors about the knee in children. Clin Orthopaed 255:86–110, 1990.
10. Nashitz JE, Rosner I, Rozenbaum M, et al: Cancer associated rheumatic disorders: Clues to occult neoplasia. Semin Arthritis Rheum 24:231–41, 1995.
11. Paley D, Jackson RW: Synovial haemangioma of the knee joint: Diagnosis by arthroscopy. Arthroscopy 2:174–177, 1986.
12. Ushijima M, Hashimoto H, Tsuneyoshi M, Enjoji M: Giant cell tumor of the tendon sheath (nodular tenosynovitis): A study of 207 cases to compare the large joint group with the common digit group. Cancer 57:875–884, 1986.
13. Young L, Bartell T, Logan SE: Ganglions of the hand and wrist. South Med J 81:751–760, 1988.

71. COMMON BONY LESIONS: RADIOGRAPHIC FEATURES

Luis Gonzalez, M.D.

1. What are the radiographic characteristics of a nonaggressive, histologically benign bone tumor?

1. **Geographic bone destruction.** A well-defined margin easily separated from normal surrounding bone is indicative of a slow-growing lesion. The zone of transition may be scalloped or sclerotic.

2. **Intact bony cortex.** The cortex usually provides an effective barrier to expansile growth, preventing penetration by nonaggressive, slow-growing lesions. While there may be cortical thinning or expansion, the cortex will remain intact and there will be no extension to the surrounding soft tissues.

3. **Lack of periosteal reaction.** If present, the periosteal response will be a singular, homogeneously expanding contour. Aggressive periosteal changes, such as the "onion-peel pattern" and the "radiating sunburst appearance" of Ewing's sarcoma and osteosarcoma, will not be seen.

4. **Slow growth over time.** Nonaggressive lesions are usually < 6 cm, with many being < 3 cm, and they show little change over a 6-month followup.

2. What are the types of tumor matrix?

1. Clear or cystic (Fig. 1)
2. Fibrous (Fig. 2)
3. Chondroid (Fig. 3)
4. Osteoid (Fig. 4)

The bony matrix refers to the internal architecture of the lesion. Tumors may be **clear or cystic,** or they can produce a matrix that calcifies or ossifies. Identifying the type of tumor matrix is extremely important to help differentiate lesions. **Fibrous** tumors demonstrate a uniform, homogeneous increase in radiodensity internally, known as a ground-glass appearance. **Chondroid** lesions frequently have a centrally located calcification described as ring-like, flocculent or fleck-like. **Osteoid** tumors have a radiodense collection of variable size that may be hetero- or homogeneous.

Types of Nonaggressive Primary Bone Tumors by Matrix Appearance

CLEAR	FIBROUS	CHONDROID	OSTEOID
Unicameral bone cyst	Fibroxanthoma	Enchondroma	Osteoma
Aneurysmal bone cyst	Fibrous dysplasia	Osteochondroma	Osteoid osteoma
Giant cell tumor		Chondroblastoma	Osteoblastoma
Eosinophilic granuloma		Chondromyxoid fibroma	

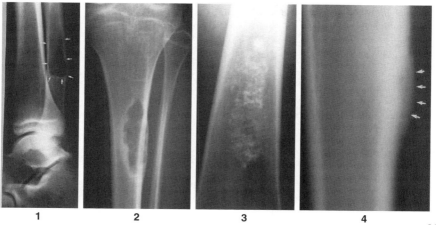

1   2   3   4

3. A 30-year-old man presents with rectal bleeding and a well-circumscribed, geographic area of increased bone density seen on skull films in the left frontal sinus. What bone lesion is this?

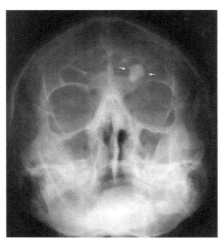

Osteoma. These tumors usually arise from areas of membranous bone formation such as the paranasal sinuses, skull, and mandible. The lesions are smooth, rounded, and often < 1 cm in size. Although they have no malignant potential, the tumors may become symptomatic according to their site of origin. Gardner's syndrome is a familial condition characterized by the triad of multiple osteomas, soft-tissue tumors, and colonic polyps.

4. A 20-year-old man with leg pain at night has a round, sharply delineated radiolucent tumor, covered with a wide zone of uniform reactive sclerosis, on his upper tibia. What might this lesion be?

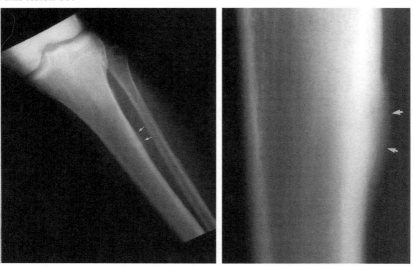

Osteoid osteoma. The round, sharply delineated radiolucent center or nidus measuring < 1 cm with a wide zone of uniform reactive sclerosis is characteristic of this lesion. Over 90% of patients with this lesion complain of nighttime pain relieved by aspirin. The area overlying the lesion is often tender to the touch. Tomography or CT scan may be helpful for demonstrating the nidus when it is obscured by the perilesional reactive zone. Because incomplete surgical excision of the nidus invites the recurrence of pain, radionuclide agents and the intraoperative use of a scintillation probe (Geiger counter) can help locate the intense focus of high radioactive counts associated with the nidus and guide the surgeon to complete removal of the lesion. Osteoid osteomas most frequently occur in the hip and occasionally the posterior spinous processes.

5. Describe the characteristics of a chondroblastoma.

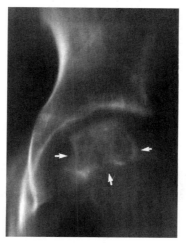

A chondroblastoma is an eccentric, lobulated lesion with a smooth geographic contour defined by a thin, discrete, marginal sclerosis. The internal matrix demonstrates flecks of stippled calcifications making this a chondroid lesion. Chondroblastomas are the only nonaggressive chondroid lesions that originate in the epiphysis. Other nonaggressive lesions that originate in the epiphysis or that cross the physis to involve the epiphysis include aneurysmal bone cysts and giant cell tumors.

6. A 31-year-old man with leg pain presented with an osseous tumor on the tibia, as seen in the following radiograph. What bone lesion does this represent?

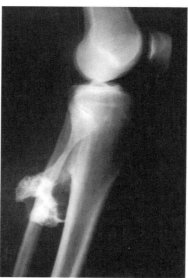

Osteochondroma. This osseous excrescence often arises from the metaphyseal region of a long tubular bone, such as the femur or tibia. The lesion is commonly pedunculated, directed away from the nearby joint along the path of ligamentous and tendinous insertion. The osteo-chondroma is continuous with the parent bone and contains both cortical and medullary ele-ments.

Variable calcification is associated with the cartilaginous cap. This cap is usually less than 1 cm in diameter. If the tip is enlarged or has poorly defined, irregular calcifications, malignant transformation should be suspected. MRI is an excellent modality for assessing the cartilaginous cap. This transformation should also be suspected with unexplained pain (i.e., lesional pain in the absence of pathologic fracture or impingement of nerves or vessels), the presence of a soft-tissue mass, or the continued growth of the lesion after physeal fusion around the time of puberty. The incidence of malignant transformation to chondrosarcoma ranges from 1–25%, depending on whether the lesion is solitary or multiple. Multiple hereditary osteochondromatosis or diaphyseal aclasis is an autosomal dominant disorder.

7. A 20-year-old woman has a painless soft-tissue swelling of the finger, as seen in the radiograph. What bone lesion is this?

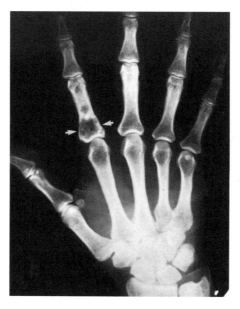

Enchondroma. This well-circumscribed, geographic lucency arises eccentrically within the diaphysis of the proximal phalanx. The lobulated contour is characteristic of cartilaginous lesions, as are the punctate, sharply defined calcifications. Endosteal erosion and bulging of the cortex are common.

Enchondromas are the most common, nonaggressive lesion of the hands. Greater than 50% of enchondromas occur in the diaphyses of the short, tubular bones of the hands and feet. The metaphysis is the site of origin when the long tubular bones are affected. Malignant transforma-tion occurs in 1% of solitary enchondromas, usually arising in lesions of the long, tubular or flat bones.

Enchondromatosis (Ollier's disease) is a rare, nonhereditary disorder consisting of wide-spread involvement of predominantly one side of the body with multiple, asymmetrically dis-tributed enchondromas. Often there is associated shortening and deformity of the long bones af-fected. Malignant transformation of an individual lesion in Ollier's disease is common, occurring in one-third to one-half of patients. Maffucci's syndrome is a rare, congenital disorder of meso-dermal dysplasia characterized by enchondromatosis and soft-tissue hemangiomas.

8. A 6-year-old boy with leg trauma presents with a 2-cm oval, geographic lesion on the lower tibia with erosion of the cortical surface and a sclerotic rim. What is it?

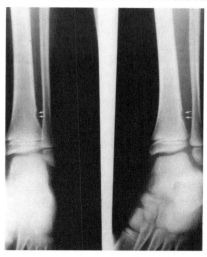

Fibrous cortical defect, or fibroxanthoma, is a common (30–40%) finding in children aged 2–8 years. These lesions occur predominantly in the lower extremities, especially within the metaphyseal region of the knee joint. The internal architecture, the matrix, is "ground glass," devoid of calcifications, and typical of a fibrous lesion. These lesions are usually asymptomatic, persist around 2 years, and then spontaneously regress.

Nonossifying fibromas are histologically identical, nonaggressive lesions. They tend also to occur about the knee but arise within the medullary cavity, unlike fibrous cortical defects which arise on the cortical surface. Nonossifying fibromas are far less common also. They occur in a slightly older population (6–10 year olds) and tend to be slightly larger ($\geq$ 4 cm). Some radiopathologists combine these similar lesions, referring to them as fibroxanthomas.

9. A 27-year-old woman with a previous history of precocious puberty presents with the bone lesions pictured in the radiograph. What does this bone lesion represent?

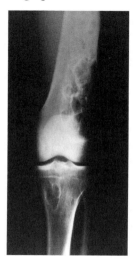

Fibrous dysplasia (FD). These large, geographic lesions with a homogeneous, ground-glass matrix and a thick rind of reactive bone are characteristic of this disease. As in this case, cortical expansion and deformities of bone, such as bowing or varus angulation (shepherd's crook deformity), are common. Histologically, FD represents a fibro-osseous lesion. Normal bone is replaced by abnormal fibrous tissue within an abnormally arranged trabecular pattern. This has led to speculation that FD may be a growth or developmental aberration rather than a true neoplasm. About 20–25% of patients with FD have multiple sites of involvement. The femur and tibia, skull and mandible, and ribs are commonly affected. McCune-Albright syndrome is identified by the triad of polyostotic, predominantly unilateral FD, café-au-lait macular lesions with irregular "coast of Maine" margins, and endocrine dysfunction, especially precocious puberty.

10. A 9-year-old boy was injured during soccer practice and presented with a radiolucent lesion with mild cortical thinning and expansion, proximal to the shoulder. What bone lesion is this?

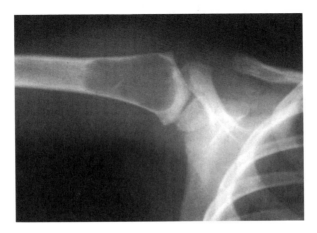

Unicameral (simple) bone cyst. On the radiograph, the short zone of transition of the lesion to normal bone is clearly defined by a thin, sclerotic margin. The internal matrix is clear or cystic. A vertical, bony density in the dependent portion of the lesion may represent a "fallen fragment" secondary to a pathologic fracture. Unicameral bone cysts generally occur in the long tubular bones, especially the proximal ends of the humerus and femur (up to 90%), and may represent a disturbance of growth at the physeal plate rather than a true neoplasm. Early intervention, either with surgical curettage and bone packing or steroid injection, is advocated to prevent a multiplicity of pathologic fractures and subsequent bone deformity and shortening. On radiographs, a favorable response is noted by a decrease in lesion size and an increase in radiodensity with adjacent cortical thickening.

11. A 32-year-old man presents with a tender wrist. Radiographs show an expansile, lytic lesion that extends to the articular surface, involving both the epiphysis and metaphysis of the distal radius. The cortex is thinned. The internal matrix is clear with a delicate trabecular pattern. Any ideas?
Giant cell tumor. These tumors may be differentiated from aneurysmal bone cysts because they tend to occur in the skeletally mature individual, after physeal closure, and involve the epiphysis extensively. Although soft-tissue involvement is suggested on plain films, CT or MRI is helpful to map the extent of bone and soft-tissue spread prior to resection. The prognosis with giant cell tumors is unpredictable: 50–60% recur; 10–15% undergo malignant transformation. Distal metastasis to remote sites such as the lungs has been reported.

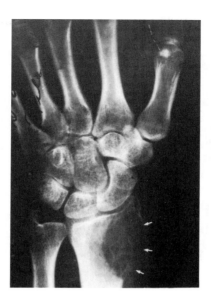

12. A 6-year-old boy presents with leg pain. A radiograph shows ballooning of the cortical surface of the fibular metaphysis. What bone lesion does this represent?

Aneurysmal bone cyst. This osteolytic lesion with occasional trabeculation arises from the fibular metaphysis. The cortical surface is markedly expanded or ballooned. The loss of cortical definition and suggestion of extension into the soft tissues are alarming features of a rapidly expansile lesion. Although histologically benign, aneurysmal bone cysts often simulate malignant tumors. They may be post-traumatic or reactive responses to preexisting bony lesions, possibly related to local alterations in hemodynamics (i.e., venous obstruction and arteriovenous fistulas). The blood-filled cavities of an aneurysmal bone cyst are exquisitely demonstrated by MRI which delineates the fluid–fluid levels caused by the settling of red blood cells from the fluid blood. About 60–70% of aneurysmal bone cysts occur within the long tubular bones, usually originating from the metaphysis. These cysts also have a predilection for the posterior elements of the vertebral bodies, where they can be difficult to distinguish from other nonaggressive lesions that occur in this location (e.g., osteoblastomas and giant cell tumors).

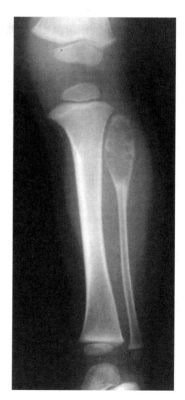

13. A 20-year-old man with head pain shows a single, lytic, "punched out" lesion on a skull film. What lesion is this?

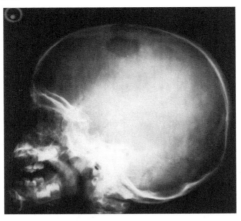

Eosinophilic granuloma (EG). The exquisitely well-circumscribed, "punched out" lesion in the skull with a clear matrix is characteristic of EG. Often, the margin appears beveled secondary to involvement of both the inner and outer tables of the calvarium. In the mandible, the loss of supporting bone results in the appearance of "floating teeth." When the metaphysis or diaphysis of the long bones is affected, the lesion is associated with both endosteal scalloping and extensive, thick, laminated periosteal reaction. EG is also one of the causes of complete collapse of a vertebral body, a condition known as vertebra plana.

Plain film remains the modality of choice for documentation of EG lesions, as 30–35% of lesions have no uptake of radionuclide and up to 10% result in "cold" areas of abnormally decreased uptake.

Letterer-Siwe and Hand-Christian-Schüller disease are EG syndromes reflecting a spectrum of bone and visceral involvement. Letterer-Siwe disease is an acute form of EG marked by rapid dissemination and poor prognosis. It tends to appear in children under 3-years-old, causing bone lesions, hepatosplenomegaly, and occasionally "honeycomb" interstitial lung disease. Death usually occurs within 1–2 years from hemorrhage or sepsis. Hand-Christian-Schüller disease is an extremely varied form of EG associated with the chronic dissemination of osseous lesions. When it appears in a child 5–10 years old, visceral involvement may result in diabetes insipidus and exophthalmos. Ten to 30% of cases are fatal.

BIBLIOGRAPHY

1. Hudson TM: Radiologic-Pathologic Correlation of Musculoskeletal Lesions. Baltimore, Williams & Wilkins, 1987.
2. Resnick D: Bone and Joint Imaging. Philadelphia, W.B. Saunders, 1989.
3. Resnick D, Niwayama G: Diagnosis of Bone and Joint Disorders. Philadelphia, W.B. Saunders, 1988.
4. Wilner D: Radiology of Bone Tumors and Allied Disorders. Philadelphia, W.B. Saunders, 1982.

XIII. Pediatric Rheumatic Diseases

Parents learn a lot from their children about coping with life.
Muriel Spark (1918–),
The Comforter

72. APPROACH TO THE CHILD WITH JOINT PAIN

Terri H. Finkel, M.D., Ph.D.

1. What is the differential diagnosis of joint pain in childhood?

The rheumatic diseases of childhood are not rare and include at least 110 illnesses associated with arthritis or related musculoskeletal syndromes. The differential diagnosis can be remembered with the well-worn mnemonic "De patient is DE VICTIM." For completeness, we will use DE VICTIMNS:

D—<u>D</u>rug
    Serum sickness
E—<u>E</u>ndocrine
    Hypercortisolism
    Hypothyroidism
V—<u>V</u>ascular/hematologic
    Vasculitis
    Sickle cell anemia
    Hemophilia
I—<u>I</u>nfectious/postinfectious
    Bacterial
        Osteomyelitis
        Discitis
        Septic arthritis
    Viral
        "Toxic" synovitis
        "Transient" synovitis
        Rubella vaccination
        HIV
C—<u>C</u>ollagen vascular
    Juvenile rheumatoid arthritis
    Juvenile psoriatic arthritis
    Reactive arthritis
    Inflammatory bowel disease
    Rheumatic fever
    Systemic lupus erythematosus
    Dermatomyositis
    Mixed connective tissue disease
    Vasculitis
    Scleroderma

C—<u>C</u>ollagen vascular (*continued*)
    Familial Mediterranean fever
    Sarcoidosis
T—<u>T</u>rauma/orthopedic/mechanical
    problems
    Chondromalacia patellae
    Osteochrondritis dissecans
    Osteoid osteoma
    Osgood-Schlatter disease
    Slipped capital femoral epiphysis
    Legg-Calvé-Perthes disease
    Hypermobility syndromes
I—<u>I</u>diopathic
    Reflex sympathetic dystrophy
    Fibromyalgia
    Growing pains
M—<u>M</u>etabolic
    Mucopolysaccharidoses
    Mucolipidoses
    Rickets (vitamin D)
N—<u>N</u>eoplastic
    Leukemia
    Neuroblastoma
    Bone tumors
    Synovial membrane tumors
    Metastases
S—P<u>S</u>ycho<u>S</u>omatic
    Hysteria/conversion reactions
    School phobia

2. What are the characteristics of an organic versus a nonorganic etiology for joint pain?

Organic	**Nonorganic**
Occurs day and night	Occurs only at night
Occurs during weekends and on vacation	Occurs primarily on school days
Severe enough to interrupt play and other pleasant activities	Child is able to carry out normal daily activities
Located in joint	Located between joints
Unilateral	Bilateral
Child limps or refuses to walk	Child is able to walk normally
Description fits with logical anatomic explanation	Description is illogical, often dramatically stated, and not consistent with known anatomic or physical process

3. What are the historical clues of an organic versus a nonorganic etiology for joint pain?
Organic: Signs of systemic illness, including weight loss, fever, night sweats, rash, diarrhea
Nonorganic: Otherwise healthy child, may have history of minor emotional disturbances

4. List the physical signs suggestive of an organic versus a nonorganic etiology for joint pain.

Organic	**Nonorganic**
Point tenderness	Normal exam or minor neurovascular changes, such as coolness or mottling of affected extremity
Redness	
Swelling	
Limitation of movement of affected extremity secondary to pain or anatomic restriction	
Objective muscle weakness or atrophy	
Signs of systemic illness: fever, rash, pallor, lymphadenopathy, and organomegaly	

5. Which laboratory tests are helpful in differentiating causes of joint pain?

TEST	CONDITIONS IN WHICH TEST MAY BE HELPFUL
CBC, differential, platelets	Leukemia
	Infections in bones, joints, muscles
	Systemic collagen vascular diseases
Sedimentation rate	Infections
	Collagen vascular diseases
	Inflammatory bowel disease
	Tumors
Radiographs	All bone tumors, malignant and benign
	Osteomyelitis (chronic)
	Discitis (late)
	Fractures
	Scoliosis
	Rickets
	Slipped capital femoral epiphysis
	Legg-Calvé-Perthes disease
	Leukemia
Bone scan	Osteomyelitis (acute and chronic)
	Discitis
	Osteoid osteoma
	Malignant bone tumors and metastases
	Infarction of bone
	Reflex sympathetic dystrophy
Muscle enzymes	Inflammatory muscle disease (idiopathic or viral)
	Muscular dystrophy
	Rhabdomyolysis

6. How does the number of affected joints help in sorting through the differential diagnosis of arthritis?

Factors helpful in assessing the etiology of arthritis are the duration of disease at the time the child is evaluated, the sex and age of the child, and the onset type and pattern of joint involvement. The differential diagnosis of polyarthritis is considerably different from that of monarthritis or oligoarthritis. Juvenile rheumatoid arthritis (JRA) is the most common cause of chronic monarthritis, especially in girls younger than 5 years of age.

MONARTHRITIS	POLYARTHRITIS
Acute onset of monarthritis	Seronegative spondyloarthropathy
Early rheumatic disease	Juvenile ankylosing spondylitis
Oligoarticular JRA	Juvenile psoriatic arthritis
Seronegative spondyloarthropathy	Arthritides of inflammatory bowel disease
Arthritis related to infection	Systemic lupus erythematosus
Septic arthritis	Polyarthritis related to infection
Reactive arthritis	Lyme disease
Malignancy	Reactive arthritis
Leukemia	Other
Neuroblastoma	Sarcoidosis
Hemophilia	Familial hypertrophic synovitis
Chronic monarthritis	Mucopolysaccharidoses
Oligoarticular JRA	
Juvenile ankylosing spondylitis	
Juvenile psoriatic arthritis	
Villonodular synovitis	
Sarcoidosis	

Adapted from Cassidy JT, Petty RE: Textbook of Pediatric Rheumatology, 3rd ed. Philadelphia, W.B. Saunders, 1995.

7. How does the diurnal variation in joint pain aid in diagnosis?

Stiffness and pain on range of motion (ROM) immediately upon arising in the morning (morning stiffness) and after periods of inactivity (gelling) are classic findings for the inflammatory arthritides. Morning stiffness will be relieved by heat and ROM exercises. The duration of morning stiffness is an excellent gauge of the severity of the arthritis and the efficacy of therapy. In contrast, mechanical joint pain will worsen over the course of the day and with activity. Finally, nighttime pain and/or awakening with pain are red flags for neoplasia or, on a less serious note, for "growing pains."

8. What are the features of synovitis?

The features of synovitis (joint inflammation) are the features of inflammation at any site:

Rubor (redness)
Calor (heat)
Tumor (swelling)
Dolor (pain, on ROM)

9. What are the characteristics of chronic inflammation?

- The process is characterized more by the infiltration of cells than by the accumulation of fluid.
- There is coexistent destruction and repair.
- The cellular infiltrate consists of polymorphonuclear (PMN) and mononuclear cells and their derivatives.

10. In which rheumatic conditions are the affected joints erythematous?

Septic arthritis, rheumatic fever, and neoplasia.

Red joints are very rare in JRA and in most other rheumatic conditions, and they should be a "red flag" for the above diagnoses. The arthritis of rheumatic fever is also characterized by its migratory nature and by pain often out of proportion to the apparent severity of findings on joint examination (e.g., degree of swelling, limitation of motion).

11. In a child with a swollen joint, how is joint fluid helpful in determining the etiology of joint pain?

GROUP/CONDITION	WBC COUNT (/μL)	PMN (%)	MISCELLANEOUS FINDINGS
Noninflammatory			
Normal	<200	<25	–
Traumatic arthritis	<2,000	<25	Debris
Osteoarthritis	1,000	<25	–
Inflammatory			
SLE	5,000	10	LE cells
Rheumatic fever	5,000	10–50	–
JRA	15,000–20,000	75	–
Reiter's syndrome	20,000	80	Reiter's cells
Pyogenic			
Tuberculous arthritis	25,000	50–60	Acid-fast bacteria
Septic arthritis	50,000–300,000	>75	Low glucose, bacteria

Adapted from Cassidy JT, Petty RE: Textbook of Pediatric Rheumatology, 3rd ed. Philadelphia, W.B. Saunders, 1995.

12. To make a definitive diagnosis of JRA, what duration of joint pain and other symptoms is required?
Six or more consecutive weeks of objective synovitis.

13. Describe the clinical characteristics of the three types of JRA.

	POLYARTHRITIS	OLIGOARTHRITIS (PAUCIARTICULAR DISEASE)	SYSTEMIC DISEASE (STILL'S DISEASE)
Frequency of cases	40%	50%	10%
Number of joints involved	>5	<4	Variable
Age of onset	Throughout childhood; peak at 1–3 yr	Early childhood; peak at 1–2 yr	Throughout childhood; no peak
Sex ration (F:M)	3:1	5:1	1:1
Systemic involvement	Moderate involvement	Not present	Prominent
Occurrence of chronic uveitis	5%	20%	Rare
Frequency of seropositivity			
Rheumatoid factors	10% (increases with age)	Rare	Rare
Antinuclear antibodies	40–50%	75–85%*	10%
Prognosis	Guarded to moderately good	Excellent except for eyesight	Moderate to poor

*In girls with uveitis.
Adapted from Cassidy JT, Petty RE: Textbook of Pediatric Rheumatology, 3rd ed. Philadelphia, W.B. Saunders, 1995.

14. How is leg length assessed in a child? Why is the affected leg often longer in a child with pauciarticular JRA?
Leg length is measured from the anterior superior iliac spine to the medial malleolus. In a child with a joint contracture, the functional leg length may be shorter than the actual leg length, and therefore both must be measured.

The affected leg is often longer in a child with pauciarticular JRA (in particular, that affecting the knee) due to increased blood flow to the joint in response to localized inflammation and cytokine release. This increased blood flow may also lead to development of "macroepiphysis." A leg-length discrepency may result in an abnormal gait, and correction with a lift on the bottom of the shoe of the shorter leg is recommended for a length discrepency > 2 cm. The shorter, unaffected leg will usually "catch up" to the affected leg, since the epiphysis of the inflamed joint will undergo accelerated fusion. Muscle bulk may also be affected in pauciarticular JRA. Interestingly, the muscles of the thigh *or* the calf may be affected in a particular patient with knee arthritis, and muscle bulk of the affected leg will rarely "catch up" to that of the unaffected leg, particularly if the arthritis has onset at <6 years of age.

15. What are "red flags" for neoplasia as the etiology of joint pain?
- Joint redness
- Night-time pain
- Associated bone pain (i.e., pain *between* joints and on direct palpation)

Malignancy *must* be considered in any child in whom a diagnosis of systemic JRA is entertained, since the classic features of systemic JRA (i.e., fever, rash, and arthritis) are also seen in malignancy. Malignant infiltration of bone or synovium may mimic polyarthritis. In addition, joint effusions occur in children with malignancy, possibly due to antigen–antibody complex deposition producing a serum sickness-like picture. This may also be responsible for the tremendous inflammatory response seen in some children with malignancy, again mimicking systemic JRA, with moderate to severe anemia, elevation of the ESR, and high platelet counts.

Radiographs of affected joints and/or whole body bone scans may be helpful in diagnosis. Bone marrow examination is recommended prior to initiation of high-dose corticosteroid therapy for systemic JRA, since inappropriate use of corticosteroids in malignancy can worsen prognosis.

16. What are the 6 criteria on physical examination for hypermobility syndrome?
1. Passive apposition of the thumb to the forearm
2. Hyperextension of the fingers parallel to the forearm
3. Elbow active hyperextension of $> 10°$
4. Knee active hyperextension of $> 10°$ (genu recurvatum)
5. Placing the palms on the floor with the knees fully extended
6. Ankle dorsiflexion $> 45°$

Hypermobility is defined as meeting 3 of these 6 criteria. Hypermobility is a common cause of arthralgias in adolescents and young adults. Diseases associated with hypermobility, such as Ehlers-Danlos, need to be ruled out.

17. Which children are at risk for HIV infection?
Children of HIV-infected mothers
Adolescents infected by sexual intercourse
Adolescents infected by intravenous drug abuse
Hemophiliacs

HIV infection can present as muscle, skin, or joint problems in children. In addition, children may present with FUO accompanied by organomegaly and other quasi-rheumatic complaints. Generalized lymphadenopathy and thrombocytopenia are other presenting manifestations.

18. Describe the characteristics of the childhood "pain amplification" syndromes: growing pains, primary fibromyalgia, and reflex sympathetic dystrophy (RSD).

	GROWING PAINS	PRIMARY FIBROMYALGIA	RSD
Age at onset	4–12 yrs	Adolescence to adulthood	Late childhood and adolescence to adulthood
Sex ratio	Equal	F>>M	F>>M
Symptoms	Deep aching, cramping pain in thigh or calf Usually in evening or during the night; never present in morning Bilateral Responds to massage and analgesia	Generalized fatigue, anxiety, depression Disturbed sleep patterns	Exquisite superficial and deep pain in the distal part of an extremity Exacerbated by passive or active movement
Signs	Physical exam normal	Tender points at characteristic sites (3 sites for 3 mos)	Diffuse swelling, tenderness, coolness and mottling Bizarre posturing of affected part
Investigations	Laboratory exam normal	Laboratory exam normal	Osteoporosis, bone scan abnormalities Laboratory exam normal

Adapted from Cassidy JT, Petty RE: Textbook of Pediatric Rheumatology, 3rd ed. Philadelphia, W.B. Saunders, 1995.

19. Describe the characteristics of the common non-rheumatic pain syndromes in childhood: patellofemoral pain syndrome (chondromalacia) and Osgood-Schlatter's disease.

	CHONDROMALACIA	OSGOOD-SCHLATTER'S
Age at onset	Adolescence to young adulthood	Athletic adolescents
Sex ratio	F>M	M>F
Symptoms	Insidious onset of exertional knee pain	Pain over tibial tubercle exacerbated by exercise
	Difficulty descending stairs; need to sit with legs straight	
Signs	Patellar tenderness on compression	Tenderness and swelling over attachment of
	Quadriceps weakness	patellar tendon
	Inhibition sign	
	Joint effusion	
Investigations	—	Radiograph shows soft tissue swelling, enlarged and sometimes fragmented tubercle

Adapted from Cassidy JT, Petty RE: Textbook of Pediatric Rheumatology, 3rd ed. Philadelphia, W.B. Saunders, 1995.

20. What are the causes of hip pain in childhood?

Transient synovitis
Bacterial infection
Avascular necrosis (Legg-Calvé-
    Perthes disease)
Slipped capital femoral epiphysis
Protrusio acetabuli
Arthritis
    B27 arthropathy
    JRA
    Rheumatic fever

Malignancy
Local
    Benign (e.g., osteoid osteoma)
    Malignant (e.g., Ewing's sarcoma)
Generalized
    Leukemia
    Neuroblastoma

Arthritis of the hip joint is rare at the onset of pauciarticular JRA. Onset of apparent arthritis in the hip in a very young child should be considered first to be a septic process or congenital dislocation. Transient synovitis of the hip may cause very severe pain, but the process is self-limited, lasting one to a few weeks, and all laboratory and radiologic studies are normal. In the older child and adolescent, avascular necrosis (Legg-Calvé-Perthes disease) and slipped capital femoral epiphysis should be considered. In older boys, juvenile ankylosing spondylitis may present with unilateral or bilateral hip involvement, although distal joints are affected more commonly than proximal joints. Be aware that hip pain may be referred to the knee. In particular, hip pain in the infant may be misinterpreted by parents and physicians as knee pain.

21. What causes back pain in childhood?

Back and neck pain are relatively rare complaints in young children (unlike the situation in adolescents and adults) and should be taken very seriously. Although infection of an intervertebral disc space is rare secondary to osteomyelitis of an adjoining vertebral body, acute discitis should be considered. Discitis is an inflammatory process that occurs throughout childhood, with a peak at age 1–3 years. It may be caused by pathogens of low virulence (e.g., viruses, *Staphylococcus aureus,* Enterobacteriaceae, or *Moraxella*), although bacteria or viruses are seldom recovered by aspiration. Fever, refusal to walk, unusual posturing, stiffness, and point tenderness over the lumbar region are characteristic. The ESR is usually moderately elevated. Plain radiographs may show disc-space narrowing, although often not until late in the disease. Earlier in the course, Tc-99m bone scan often shows increased uptake of isotope and is therefore valuable diagnostically at the time of presentation.

In addition, malignancy (e.g., metastases, primary bone tumors, or leukemia) should be considered, as well as juvenile ankylosing spondylitis (JAS). However, JAS generally presents as peripheral arthritis (75% of children at presentation), with back complaints (pain, stiffness, or limitation of motion of the lumbosacral spine or sacroiliac joints) only reported by 25% of affected children prior to the third decade. Back pain is uncommon in JRA. Spondylolysis, with or without spondylolisthesis, may cause chronic back pain. Scheuermann's disease or, rarely, herniation of an intervertebral disc results in pain in the lower thoracic or lumbar region.

22. What medications are used to treat inflammatory arthritis in childhood?

MEDICATION	DAILY DOSE (MG/KG/D)
NSAIDs	
Salicylate	< 25 kg: 80–100
	> 25 kg: 2.5gm/m^2/d
Ibuprofen	20–40
Naproxen	7–15
Indomethacin	0.5–3
Tolmetin	15–30
Sulindac	< 25 kg: 50 mg total
	> 25 kg: 75–100 mg total
Diclofenac	2–3
DMARDs	
Hydroxychloroquine	5–7
Auranofin	0.15–0.20
IM gold*	1 mg/kg/wk (max: 50 mg)
Penicillamine	10
Sulfasalazine	40
Methotrexate*	0.15–0.50 mg/kg/wk or 5–10 mg/m^2/wk (max: 15–20 mg/wk)
Corticosteroids	
Prednisone	1–2
Pulse methylprednisolone	15

*IM gold and methotrexate are given weekly, not daily. No dose should exceed the maximum dose recommended for adults. (DMARD, disease-modifying antirheumatic drugs.)

23. A child presents with a 1-week history of a single, hot, red, swollen, painful joint. The child is febrile and refuses to bear weight on the affected leg. Describe the work-up.

Immediate joint aspiration is always indicated in such a patient to exclude septic arthritis or osteomyelitis. Gram stain should be done; WBC and differential counts, glucose, and protein levels should be determined; and the synovial fluid should be cultured for *Haemophilus influenzae, Neisseria gonorrhoeae,* and gram-negative organisms. Special media and conditions are required if anaerobic organisms or mycobacteria are suspected. Cultures of blood and suspected sources of infection (e.g., cellulitis) are required in a child with suspected septic arthritis.

Although an organism can be identified in approximately two-thirds of children, no causative organism is identified in approximately one-third, with diagnosis being made on the basis of a consistent history and the presence of pus on arthrocentesis. However, synovial fluid WBC counts may be low (<25,000/mm^3) in up to one-third of patients with septic arthritis. Identification of an organism is particularly difficult in those patients who have received antibiotics. Supportive laboratory studies are an elevated WBC count with a predominance of PMNs and bands, and a markedly elevated ESR or C-reactive protein.

24. Another child has an 8-week history of a single warm, swollen joint that is not very painful, tender, or red. The child has been afebrile and, with the exception of a mild upper respiratory infection, has been otherwise well. Describe the work-up.

While any history of antecedent trauma should be elicited, trauma is very unlikely to cause a swollen joint persisting 8 weeks in the absence of significant pain. Interestingly, parents often date joint swelling to an acute event (such as a fall), although the event may serve only to bring their attention to an already swollen joint. The 8-week history of swelling meets the criteria of "> 6 weeks" required for a diagnosis of JRA. The first episode of JRA, and subsequent flares of arthritis are often precipitated by intercurrent illness, such as an upper respiratory infection.

The most useful finding on physical exam in this case would be the presence of a second (or more) affected joint(s), as this would argue strongly for a diagnosis of JRA. In particular, the small joints of the hands and feet should be examined carefully. If the knee is involved, a Baker's cyst would strongly indicate a diagnosis of JRA. Involvement of the wrists by JRA would be suggested if the child holds the hands still in the lap, supinated, with the wrists slightly flexed. Lack of neck movement, using only the eyes to follow the examiner, is a clue for neck involvement. Circumduction of the affected leg on gait examination may suggest a leg-length discrepency, indicating a longer duration of arthritis than 8 weeks. Similarly, the presence of joint contractures would suggest a longer duration of arthritis.

In pauciarticular JRA, the CBC and ESR are often entirely normal. Radiographs, other than confirming the presence of effusion, also are normal, without evidence of loss of joint space or bony erosion. This form of JRA does not generally lead to joint destruction, and even in the more destructive forms (e.g., a subgroup of polyarticular JRA), bony erosion is rarely seen until after 2 years of disease. The anti-nuclear antibody (ANA) will be the most helpful laboratory test in suspected pauciarticular JRA. One-half of children with this diagnosis have a positive ANA, and one-half of children with a positive ANA have chronic anterior uveitis, a potentially blinding (yet almost invariably asymptomatic) inflammation of the eyes. Children with JRA only rarely have positive rheumatoid factors.

BIBLIOGRAPHY

1. Ansell BM, Rudge S, Schaller JG: Color Atlas of Pediatric Rheumatology. St. Louis, Mosby Year Book, 1992.
2. Apley J: Limb pains with no organic disease. Clin Rheum Dis 2:487, 1976.
3. Cabral DA, Oen KG, Petty RE: SEA syndrome revisited: Long-term follow-up of children with a syndrome of seronegative enthesopathy and arthropathy. J Rheumatol 19:1282, 1992.
4. Cassidy JT, Levinson JE, Bass JC, et al: A study of classification criteria for a diagnosis of juvenile rheumatoid arthritis. Arthritis Rheum 29:274, 1986.
5. Cassidy JT, Petty RE: Textbook of Pediatric Rheumatology, 3rd ed. Philadelphia, W.B. Saunders, 1995.
6. Costello PB, Brecker ML, Starr JL, et al. A prospective analysis of the frequency, course, and possible prognostic significance of the joint manifestations of childhood leukemia. J Rheumatol 10:753, 1983.
7. Crawford AH, Kucharzyk DW, Ruda R, et al: Discitis in children. Clin Orthop 206:70, 1991.
8. Del Beccaro MA, Champoux AN, Bockers T, et al: Septic arthritis versus transient synovitis of the hip: The value of screening laboratory tests. Ann Emerg Med 21:1418, 1992.
9. Fink CW, Nelson JD: Septic arthritis and osteomyelitis in children. Clin Rheum Dis 12:423, 1986.
10. Fink CW, Windmiller J, Sartain P: Arthritis as the presenting feature of childhood leukemia. Arthritis Rheum 15:347, 1972.
11. Gedalia A, Person DA, Brewer EJ Jr, et al: Hypermobility of the joints in juvenile episodic arthritis/arthralgia. J Pediatr 107:873, 1985.
12. Kunnamo I, Kallio P, Pelkonen P, et al: Clinical signs and laboratory tests in the differential diagnosis of arthritis in children. Am J Dis Child 141:34, 1987.
13. Peterson H: Growing pains. Pediatr Clin North Am 33:1365, 1986.
14. Silber TJ, Majd M: Reflex sympathetic dystrophy syndrome in children and adolescents: Report of 18 cases and review of the literature. Am J Dis Child 142:1325, 1988.
15. Yates CK, Grana WA: Patellofemoral pain in children. Clin Orthop 255:36, 1990.

73. JUVENILE CHRONIC ARTHRITIS

Roger Hollister, M.D.

1. What are the main types of juvenile chronic arthritis?

1. **Polyarticular**, with involvement of many joints, large and small, in a symmetric fashion. Additionally, this type may be subgrouped on the basis of the presence or absence of rheumatoid factor in the blood. Rheumatoid factor positivity is a harbinger of a more-aggressive arthritis, with increased risk of joint damage, disability, and eventual need for surgery.

2. **Pauciarticular**, with one or a few (<5) large joints, frequently asymmetric. There are two subgroups:

     a. Peak age of onset at 2–5 years, with a 3:1 female predominance and a high frequency of positive antinuclear antibodies (ANA). This subtype has a relatively benign prognosis with remissions likely, but it runs the greatest risk of the associated chronic iridocyclitis (iritis).

     b. Older age of onset (>6 yrs), more often in males, and more often HLA B27 positive.

3. **Systemic onset**, which is characterized by high fevers, evanescent rash, polyarthralgia/arthritis, and extra-articular inflammation. Equal gender frequency and distribution throughout childhood characterize this type of juvenile chronic arthritis.

2. What types of anterior uveitis are associated with juvenile chronic arthritis (JRA)?

Anterior Uveitis in Juvenile Chronic Arthritis

	ACUTE UVEITIS	CHRONIC UVEITIS
Disease association	Spondyloarthropathy	Pauciarticular JRA
Lab markers	B27 antigen	Positive ANA
Symptoms	Hot, red, photophobic eye	None
Complications (if untreated)	Few	Synechiae, cataract, glaucoma, band keratopathy
Necessity of slit-lamp screening	No	Yes

3. Should ANA status affect the frequency of slit-lamp screening in pauciarticular JRA patients?

Yes. ANA-positive patients with pauciarticular JRA have a 33% risk of developing chronic, asymptomatic uveitis, whereas ANA-negative children have a 10% risk. Therefore, ANA-positive patients should be screened every 3 months, and ANA-negative patients can be seen every 6 months.

4. How long should slit-lamp screening be continued?

One-half of children who will develop chronic uveitis will have it present at the first eye appointment. Uveitis incidence diminishes with each subsequent year after joint swelling develops. Five years after joint swelling develops, the risk of new-onset uveitis is so low that screening is no longer cost-effective. However, slit-lamp screening is necessary within the first 5 years even when the joint disease is in remission.

5. In the differential diagnosis of arthritis in childhood, what is the significance of a migratory versus summating pattern of onset?

A **migratory pattern**—i.e., one joint is subsiding as another becomes inflamed—is seen in rheumatic fever, post-streptococcal arthritis, and gonococcal arthritis. A **summating pattern**—i.e., adding one inflamed joint to another—is characteristic of JRA, psoriatic arthritis, and spondyloarthropathy.

6. Two fever patterns are represented below which may aid in the diagnosis of a fever of unknown origin (FUO). Which is characteristic of systemic JRA?

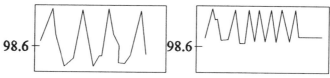

The fever pattern of systemic JRA is characterized by fever spikes occurring at the same time each day, with spontaneous difervescence to normal or subnormal levels. In contrast, the fever spikes of bacterial sepsis are hectic and occur on an elevated temperature base. Normal temperatures are not found until adequate antibacterial treatment is initiated.

7. In the diagnosis of FUO, what laboratory tests are specific for systemic JRA?
None. The laboratory tests demonstrate a chronic inflammatory process, and a normal sedimentation rate excludes the diagnosis of systemic JRA. The leukocyte count is often elevated to extraordinary, even leukemoid degrees, with a significant left shift. Platelet counts are often equally elevated, and thrombocytopenia is inconsistent with the diagnosis. A mild/moderate anemia of chronic disease is often present. Other acute-phase reactants, such as ferritin and C-reactive proteins are frequently increased. In perplexing cases, a normal lactate dehydrogenase level can add reassurance that a malignancy is not the cause of the FUO.

8. Which rashes are specific to causes of juvenile arthritis?
The rash of **erythema marginatum** is pathognomonic of acute rheumatic fever, a condition which has diminished in frequency over the past several decades for unknown reasons. This circinate rash with central clearing appears at the time of the migratory arthritis, heart murmur, and subcutaneous nodules. It is one of the five major criteria for diagnosis of rheumatic fever.

The **ecchymotic, lower-extremity rash** characteristic of Henoch-Schönlein purpura may start as a maculopapular or even urticarial lesion. The rash usually precedes joint swelling but may follow it by a few days. It leaves no residue and rarely needs treatment.

The **"Still's" rash** of systemic JRA is present in 90% of cases. The pink macules are very evanescent, most common on the trunk and proximal extremities and rarely pruritic. They are frequently present during fever spikes. If the lesions are present for 24 hours in a single location, they are *not* the lesions of Still's rash.

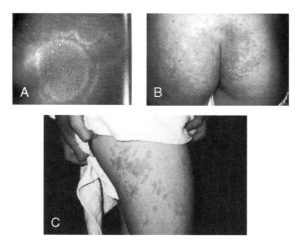

A, Erythema marginatum; *B*, Henoch-Schönlein purpura; *C*, Systemic JRA.

9. The child you are seeing with a single swollen knee has grandparents with what sounds to be rheumatoid arthritis. Is there a genetic relationship?
Little, if any. The histocompatibility gene linked to seropositive rheumatoid arthritis, DR4, is actually found less often in the JRA population than in normal children. In pauciarticular JRA, DR5 and DR8 show an association in several studies but certainly not to the degree of B27 and the spondyloarthropathies.

10. Which regions of the United States have the highest number of Lyme disease cases?
Over 80% of reported cases of Lyme disease are found in only 5 states: New York, Massachusetts, Connecticut, Minnesota, and Wisconsin.

11. In these regions, how does one clinically distinguish pauciarticular JRA from Lyme arthritis?

Lyme arthritis is an episodic inflammation with attacks lasting, on average, 2–5 weeks. The inflammation of **pauciarticular JRA** is chronic and must be present for at least 6 weeks before the diagnosis is certain.

12. A patient presents with poorly localized leg pain sufficient to interrupt sleep and cause a limp. Which malignancies must be considered in the differential diagnosis?

Leukemia and stage IV **neuroblastoma** are the two neoplasms that can involve bone and simulate arthritis, even to the point of producing joint swelling, elevated sedimentation rate, and increased platelet counts. If an isolated lactate dehydrogenase level is elevated while other liver functions tests are normal, additional tests such as bone scans, ultrasound, or bone marrow biopsy may be warranted to rule out malignancy.

13. A positive ANA is a prerequisite for the diagnosis of systemic lupus erythematosus (SLE) in childhood, and ANA is often seen in children with JRA. How specific is it to these diagnoses?

Not very. Autoantibodies can be seen in a variety of situations in which the common denominator is prolonged antigen stimulation. Rheumatoid factors can be produced in experimental animals with immunization with irrelevant antigens. Similarly, they are found in patients with subacute bacterial endocarditis. A positive ANA which does not match a patient's clinical presentation is seen in children with a recent history of recurrent streptococcal infection and elevated levels of anti-streptococcal antibodies (unpublished observation).

14. In a child with JRA, what is the risk that a sibling will develop the same illness?

In several published series, there is a remarkable agreement that the risk is 1 in 100. The prevalence of the disease in the normal population is 1 in 1000. Therefore, there may be a genetic predisposition, although it clearly is not as strong as that for diseases such as hemophilia, cystic fibrosis, or diabetes. These facts suggest that an unidentified environmental agent may also be necessary for disease expression.

15. The time-honored treatment for JRA was aspirin, but more recently, other nonsteroidal medications have supplanted aspirin. Why?

As an NSAID, aspirin is as effective as other agents; however, with the increased public awareness about Reye syndrome and the necessity of three or four doses a day, parents have become less accepting of this treatment. The relationship between Reye syndrome and salicylate treatment during chicken pox or Asian flu is statistically valid. With the use of acetaminophen as an antipyretic, the incidence of Reye syndrome has dropped dramatically.

In addition, NSAIDs are now available in liquid form (naproxen and ibuprofen), which are much easier to administer to children < 5 years of age. For older children, other NSAIDs allow once-daily administration (relafen and feldene), which has improved compliance.

16. Prednisone may be necessary for the treatment of systemic JRA, pericarditis, or refractory iritis, but the side effects of high-dose prednisone are well-known. Is it possible to avoid untoward effects by using low-dose prednisone therapy?

No. Osteoporosis and growth suppression can both be produced by as little as 5 mg of prednisone a day. The demineralization may be alleviated by a calcium intake of 1200 mg/day with 400 U of vitamin D.

Prednisone therapy has a profound effect on linear growth. However, alternate-day doses of prednisone up to 20 mg may still allow appropriate growth. Unfortunately, arthritis is more difficult to treat on an every-other-day basis in diseases such as SLE or dermatomyositis.

17. Injectable gold salts was formerly the second-line treatment of JRA. In one subgroup of JRA, however, this treatment is relatively contraindicated. Why?

In systemic JRA, a sufficient number of cases of disseminated intravascular coagulation have occurred with injectable gold salts (aurothioglucose or gold sodium thiomalate) to suggest a relative contraindication.

18. School-aged children with JRA have legal rights to therapeutic resources in school. What are they?
Under P.L. 94-142 (the Education for All Handicapped Act), children with arthritis are entitled to a free, public education which may require "special related services." These services may include physical and occupational therapy through the school system. This requirement depends on the financial status of the individual school district. However, if the school system provides such services for developmentally disabled children or those with cerebral palsy, then they must provide them to children with arthritis.

19. Advanced therapy for adult rheumatoid arthritis frequently includes low-dose weekly methotrexate therapy. Can this drug be used in children with JRA?
Yes. In fact. methotrexate has largely supplanted injectable gold as the second-line agent in the treatment of JRA. In numerous studies, methotrexate appears to be just as effective and safe in children as it is in adults. Furthermore, the injectable form of methotrexate (25 mg/ml), which is actually less expensive than the tablets, makes it easy to administer to children too young to swallow tablets. After 40 years of use, it is recognized that methotrexate carries very little oncologic risk and little to no risk to fertility. Liver function abnormalities and bone marrow side effects are similar to those in adults.

The starting dose should be 5 mg/wk in the smallest children and 7.5 mg/wk in older children. If no benefit is found after 3 weeks, the dose should be increased in 2.5-mg increments until a response is seen or the dose reaches 1 mg/kg/wk, at which point the patient should be considered a treatment failure. It is important to remind parents to continue to take their regular NSAID.

20. A 12-year-old boy develops knee pain during soccer season and is diagnosed with Osgood-Schlatter disease. Three months later, he is diagnosed with Achilles tendinitis. What form of juvenile chronic arthritis might he have?
Ankylosing spondylitis or another **spondyloarthropathy.** More than 50% of young patients with this disease present with peripheral lower-extremity symptoms, including arthritis or enthesopathy, as was the case with this patient. Enthesopathy refers to inflammation at the site of tendon insertion into the bone. The B27 antigen is found in >75% of patients. Long-term follow-up of these patients shows that about 30% will go on to develop sacroiliitis, the hallmark of the disease. Spondyloarthropathy is more episodic than JRA. Treatment with NSAIDs, especially indomethacin, permits most children to function quite normally.

21. Can corticosteroid injections be used in children?
Yes, particularly in older children who can understand the nature and reason for the injection. Published studies have shown good long-term results, especially with methylprednisolone acetate. However, if synovitis recurs in several weeks, steroid injections should not be repeated because of untoward effects on growing cartilage. In very young children, the use of Emla cream as a topical anesthetic may reduce the apprehension about the injection.

22. A 3-year-old presents with a 1-day history of fever, refusal to bear weight, and a hot, red, swollen knee. Besides coverage for gram-positive organisms, what other antibiotic coverage is warranted?
In children under age 5 years, *Haemophilus influenzae*, while not the major cause of septic arthritis, is nonetheless a significant intra-articular pathogen. Antibiotic coverage should be extended to include this organism until cultures are complete.

BIBLIOGRAPHY

1. Giannini EH, et al: Methotrexate in resistant juvenile rheumatoid arthritis: Results of the U.S.A.–U.S.S.R. double-blind, placebo-controlled trial. N Engl J Med 326:1043–1049, 1992.
2. Lang BA, Shore A: A review of current concepts on the pathogenesis of juvenile rheumatoid arthritis. J Rheumatol 17(suppl 21):1–13, 1990.
3. Prieur AM: HLA B-27 associated chronic arthritis in children: Review of 65 cases. Scand J Rheumatol (Suppl 66):51–56, 1987.

4. Rosenberg AM: Advanced drug therapy of juvenile rheumatoid arthritis. J Pediatr 114:171–178, 1989.
5. Schaller JG, Wedgewood RJ: Juvenile rheumatoid arthritis: A review. Pediatrics 50:940–953, 1972.
6. Steele RW, et al: Usefulness of scanning procedures for diagnosis of fever of unknown origin in children. J Pediatr 119:526–530, 1991.
7. Steere AC: Lyme disease. N Engl J Med 321:586–589, 1989.
8. Wallendahl M, Stark L, Hollister JR: The discriminating value of serum LDH values in children with malignancy presenting as joint pain. Arch Pedriatr Adol Med 150:70–73, 1996.

74. JUVENILE SYSTEMIC CONNECTIVE TISSUE DISEASES

Terri H. Finkel, M.D., Ph.D.

1. What are the juvenile systemic connective tissue diseases (CTDs)?

Systemic juvenile rheumatoid arthritis (see Chapter 73)

Systemic lupus erythematosus (SLE)

Overlap syndromes, including mixed CTD

Reactive arthritis, including Reiter's syndrome

Inflammatory bowel disease

Rheumatic fever

Dermatomyositis

Scleroderma

Vasculitis

2. Discuss the epidemiology of juvenile SLE.

Data on the incidence and prevalence of SLE in children are few. The proportion of all patients presenting with SLE in childhood is ~15%. In childhood, the disease generally presents in adolescence and rarely before age 5 years. The ratio of girls to boys is about 1:1 before age 10 years and then, in adolescents, is similar to the ratio of women to men (5:1 to 10:1). SLE appears to be more common in children of black, Asian, and Hispanic origin. About 10% have one or more affected relatives, including siblings and twins.

3. What are the criteria for the diagnosis of SLE in children?

The same as in adults. A person shall be said to have SLE if any 4 or more of 11 criteria are present:

1. Malar rash
2. Discoid rash
3. Photosensitivity
4. Oral ulcers
5. Arthritis
6. Serositis
   a. Pleuritis, or
   b. Pericarditis
7. Renal disorder
   a. Persistent proteinuria >0.5 gm/day, or
   b. Cellular casts
8. Neurologic disorder
   a. Seizures or
   b. Psychosis

9. Hematologic disorder
   a. Hemolytic anemia
   b. Leukopenia
   c. Lymphopenia or
   d. Thrombocytopenia
10. Immunologic disorder
    a. Positive LE cell preparation
    b. Anti-DNA antibody
    c. Anti-Sm antibody or
    d. False-positive serologic test for syphilis
11. Anti-nuclear antibody (ANA) in abnormal titer

Childhood-onset SLE is generally more severe than in adults, with a high incidence of nephritis, pericarditis, hepatosplenomegaly, and chorea.

4. What are the clinical manifestations of SLE?

SLE is characterized by multiple autoantibodies and multisystem involvement. An easy way to remember the complex array of systemic manifestations of SLE is to think from head to toe. Thus:

General	Malaise, weight loss, fever
Skin	Butterfly rash, discoid lupus, vasculitic skin lesions, alopecia, photosensitivity
Brain	Headache, blurred vision, psychosis, chorea, seizures, neuropathies, cerebrovascular accident, transverse myelitis
Eye	Cotton-wool spots, retinitis, episcleritis, iritis (rarely)
Mouth	Oral ulcers
Chest	Pleuritis, basilar pneumonitis, pulmonary hemorrhage
Heart	Pericarditis, myocarditis, Libman-Sacks endocarditis
Digestive system	Hepatosplenomegaly, mesenteric arteritis, colitis
Kidneys	Glomerulonephritis, nephrotic syndrome, hypertension
Extremities	Arthralgia or arthritis, myalgia or myositis, Raynaud's phenomenon, thrombophlebitis, aseptic necrosis

5. How does the ANA pattern and titer aid in the diagnosis and management of SLE?

ANAs are present in the sera of almost all children with active SLE. In fact, the absence of ANAs, particularly at the time of symptomatic disease, essentially eliminates SLE as a diagnostic consideration. The average ANA titer in individuals with SLE is 1:320, although in active disease it may be considerably higher. Changes in the ANA titer are not a useful indicator of disease activity and are not followed subsequent to diagnosis.

The "rim" pattern on the ANA, in which fluorescence is seen rimming the nuclear membrane, is pathognomonic of SLE, though rarely seen. The "homogeneous" pattern, in which fluorescence is seen uniformly over the nucleus, is the pattern most commonly seen in SLE, while the "speckled" pattern is the least specific.

The ANA is a highly subjective test, and the pattern and titer vary greatly among laboratories. False-positives are not uncommon. False-negatives are rare, but if you are convinced of the diagnosis of SLE in a patient, repeat of the ANA is indicated in a different laboratory and/or at a future date.

6. How does the ANA profile aid in the diagnosis and management of SLE and related juvenile systemic CTDs?

As detailed in the table, while a negative ANA profile does not rule out *any* of the juvenile systemic CTDs, a positive ANA profile can be extremely useful in making a specific diagnosis. In particular, anti-DNA and anti-Sm antibodies are specific for SLE; high titers of anti-RNP antibody are suggestive of mixed connective tissue disease (MCTD); and anti-Ro and/or anti-La antibodies are found in Sjögren's syndrome, although this syndrome and antibodies are most commonly seen as a part of SLE. In addition, anti-histone antibodies may be seen in SLE and in drug-induced lupus. These two diagnoses may be distinguished by the presence of antibodies to specific histones. Finally, a positive ANA is essentially never found in systemic juvenile rheumatoid arthritis (RA, Still's disease).

	ACTIVE SLE	MCTD	PSS	CREST	PRIMARY SJÖGREN'S	RA
ANA	>95%	>95%	70–90%	60–90%	>70%	40–50%
Anti-native DNA	60%	Neg	Neg	Neg	Neg	Neg
Anti-SM	30%	Neg	Neg	Neg	Neg	Neg
Anti-RNP	30%	>95% titer> 1:10,000	Common (low titer)	Neg	Rare (low titer)	Rare
Anti-centromere	Rare	Rare	10–15%	60–90%	Neg	Neg
Anti-Ro (SS-A)	30%	Rare	Rare	Neg	70%	Rare
Anti-La (SS-B)	15%	Rare	Rare	Neg	60%	Rare

PSS = progressive systemic sclerosis.

7. Which other autoantibodies (other than ANA and ANA profile) can be helpful in the diagnosis of systemic juvenile CTD?

Antibody reactive with Scl-70 is not typically measured in the standard ANA profile but is found in 15–20% of individuals with systemic sclerosis. Jo-1 and Mi-2 antibodies, while found in only a minority of children with juvenile dermatomyositis, may be useful in identifying those children at increased risk for complicating interstitial lung disease. Vasculitic syndromes associated with the presence of anti-neutrophil cytoplasmic antibodies (C-ANCA or P-ANCA) are Wegener's granulomatosis, polyarteritis nodosa, Churg-Strauss syndrome, leukocytoclastic angiitis, and crescentic glomerulonephritis.

8. How are autoantibodies related to the pathophysiology of SLE?

Autoantibodies to specific blood cells and vascular components are directly responsible for the hematologic manifestations of SLE, such as acute hemolytic anemia, thrombocytopenia, leukopenia, and coagulopathies. In addition, antigen–antibody complexes (in which the antigen is often an ANA) play a significant role in the pathogenesis of lupus vasculitis and nephritis. Lupus nephritis is caused by deposition of immune complexes composed of complement components, immunoglobulins, and DNA in the glomerular lesions. Elution techniques and fluorescence microscopy have demonstrated high titers of antibodies to native DNA in the renal glomeruli.

9. Describe the management of children with SLE.
- General
    Counseling, education
    Adequate rest
    Use of sunscreens
    Immunizations, especially pneumococcal
    Management of infection
- NSAIDs for musculoskeletal signs and symptoms
- Hydroxychloroquine for cutaneous disease and as adjunct to glucocorticoids for systemic disease
- Glucocorticoids
    Oral prednisone, 1–2 mg/kg/d
    IV methylprednisolone initially for severe disease and then monthly for maintenance therapy
- Immunosuppressives
    Azathioprine, 1–2 mg/kg/d
    Cyclophosphamide
        Oral 1–2 mg/kg/d
        IV 500–1000 mg/m^2/mo

10. Discuss the pathophysiology of neonatal lupus.

Neonatal lupus is associated with the transplacental passage of IgG antibody to Ro (SS-A) and with maternal lupus or Sjögren's syndrome. The most frequent abnormalities are rash (lesions of discoid lupus or subacute cutaneous lupus) and thrombocytopenia, although congenital heart block is of most concern. The cutaneous and hematologic manifestations are transient, generally resolving within 2–6 months, while heart block is frequently permanent and may require a pacemaker.

11. What is the differential diagnosis of Sjögren's syndrome in childhood?

Sjögren's syndrome is characterized by dry eyes (keratoconjunctivitis sicca), dry mouth and carious teeth, and parotitis. Differentiating children with **benign recurrent parotid swelling** or **AIDS** from children with Sjögren's syndrome is important. As in adults, salivary gland biopsy of the lip is often helpful to confirm a suspected diagnosis of Sjögren's syndrome. Sjögren's is rare in childhood and is usually found in association with other CTDs, such as **SLE** or mixed **CTD**.

12. What triad of signs and symptoms is associated with Henoch-Schönlein purpura (HSP) in children?
    Purpura
    Colicky abdominal pain
    Arthritis
HSP typically occurs in the spring, fall, or winter. The median age at presentation is 4 years,

and the female to male ratio is equal. About 50% of children have a history of preceding upper respiratory tract infection with a variety of organisms. 97% of children with HSP have a self-limited course, lasting 1–2 weeks. ~20% will recur during the first year. 3–5% of children will suffer persistent purpura with or without persistent renal disease. The purpura may be preceded by arthritis, edema, testicular swelling, and abdominal pain.

13. List the clinical manifestations of HSP.

HSP is a systemic vasculitis, and as a result, any organ may be affected.

	% AT ONSET	% POST ONSET	NOTES
Purpura	50	100	Normal platelet count
Edema	10–20	20–50	Painful
Arthritis	25	60–85	Large joints
GI	30	85	—
Renal	?	10–50	—
GU	?	2–35	Differential is torsion
Pulmonary	?	95 (by DL_{CO})	Abnormal CO diffusion
Hemorrhage	?	Rare	Fatal
CNS	?	Very rare	Headache, encephalitis, seizures

14. What are poor prognostic factors in HSP at onset?

Melena

Persistent rash for 2–3 mos

Hematuria with proteinuria 1 gm/day

Nephrosis with renal insufficiency,
>50% crescents

7.5-fold increase in renal disease

Associated with glomerulonephritis

15% progress to renal insufficiency

50% renal failure in 10 yrs

15. How should HSP be treated?

- Arthritis responds to NSAIDs
- Edema responds to steroids
- Abdominal pain resolves within 72 hrs with or without steroids
- Evaluate for and treat infection (e.g., group A β-hemolytic streptococci)
- Aggressive treatment for children with poor prognostic signs

16. Describe the physical exam of a child presenting with juvenile dermatomyositis (JDMS).

JDMS is a myositis with characteristic skin rash and vasculitis. Muscle weakness, in particular of the proximal musculature (limbs, girdle, neck), is prominent. The Gower's maneuver is abnormal, and the child will be unable to do a sit-up due to weakness. The head may hang back as the child is lifted from a lying position, due to weakness of the neck muscles. The eyelids and face are edematous, and a heliotrope or mauvish rash is noted around the eyes. Deep red patches, known as Gottron's papules, will be found over the extensor surfaces of the finger joints, as well as over the elbows, knees, and ankle joints. These patches may ulcerate due to vasculitis. Telangiectasias may be found around the eyelids and at the nailfolds. Arthralgia or arthritis may be found, sometimes with swelling and contractures of the fingers due to tenosynovitis. In severe chronic JDMS, nodules due to subcutaneous calcinosis may be found. Mobility may be impaired because of calcinotic lesions at the joints or to involvement of musculature.

17. How can the muscle weakness of JDMS be differentiated from that of other causes of weakness?

The muscle weakness of JDMS predominantly involves the proximal musculature, and in general, the involvement is symmetric. The child gives a history of difficulty in climbing stairs or riding a bicycle. Some of the maneuvers detailed in the previous question (e.g., Gower's maneuver) can discriminate true muscle weakness from, for example, inanition. The palate and swallowing musculature may be weak in JDMS and may lead to choking, cough, or aspiration pneumonia. Serum muscle enzymes are elevated, but not to the degree seen in the muscular dystrophies. Assays for all four muscle-derived enzymes are required (aldolase, creatine kinase, SGOT/AST, lactate dehydrogenase) because only one may be elevated. Electromyography will show denervation and inflammatory myopathy. Muscle biopsy will show inflammation and/or fiber necrosis and small vessel vasculitis.

18. How is JDMS distinguished from adult dermatomyositis or polymyositis?
In children, dermatomyositis is distinguished by a generalized vasculitis. Chronic polymyositis, in which the rash is absent, is exceedingly rare in childhood. The documented association of adult dermatomyositis or polymyositis with malignancy has not been found in children.

19. What forms of systemic vasculitis occur in childhood?
Vasculitis is a component of many of the juvenile systemic CTDs, including HSP, systemic juvenile rheumatoid arthritis, JDMS, and SLE. Five percent of cases of polyarteritis nodosa occur in childhood and, as in adults, are characterized by rash, fever, weight loss, myositis, and cutaneous nodules. Life-threatening renal, GI, cardiac, and CNS involvements are often seen. Large vessel vasculitis, such as Takayasu's, is exceedingly rare in childhood. Wegener's granulomatosis occurs in childhood and may present as HSP. The anti-neutrophil cytoplasmic antibodies (autoantibodies directed against enzymes in the neutrophil cytoplasmic granules) may be pathogenic and are of considerable use in the diagnosis and management of the childhood vasculitides.

20. What are the revised modified Jones criteria for the diagnosis of acute rheumatic fever?

Major Manifestations	Minor Manifestations
Carditis	Fever
Polyarthritis	Arthralgia
Chorea	Previous rheumatic carditis
Subcutaneous nodules	Prolonged PR interval
Erythema marginatum	Increased ESR or C-reactive protein

Diagnosis requires the presence of two major criteria, or one major and two minor criteria, supported by evidence of a preceding streptococcal infection (increased ASO titer, positive pharyngeal culture, recent scarlet fever).

21. When are each of the major manifestations of acute rheumatic fever seen?
In general, arthritis and carditis are manifestations of acute, early disease, while chorea is usually seen later and may occur in the absence of the other manifestations. Erythema marginatum and subcutaneous nodules are relatively infrequent in children.

22. An 8-year-old child has a history of 6 days of fever, migratory arthritis, and a throat culture positive for group A β-hemolytic streptococcus. He has a normal cardiac exam, EKG, and no other evidence for rheumatic fever. Laboratory evaluation, including CBC, ESR, C-reactive protein, and ANA, are negative. Discuss the diagnosis and management of this child.
This child has only one major and one minor criteria for acute rheumatic fever, although the clinical presentation makes a diagnosis of poststreptococcal arthritis likely. Similar to the arthritis of acute rheumatic fever, the symptoms of pain and limitation of motion are often out of proportion to the physical findings, and response to salicylates or NSAIDs is generally remarkable. Although controversial, an echocardiogram to rule out cardiac disease is not felt to be necessary in the face of a normal cardiac exam.

Therapy should include penicillin to eradicate any residual streptococcal infection and salicylate therapy. Few patients develop carditis on follow-up, and the course is usually benign, with resolution of arthritis/arthralgia within several weeks. In general, antibiotic prophylaxis is not recommended following a single episode of poststreptococcal arthritis, although carditis with repeat streptococcal infection has been reported.

23. What is Raynaud's?
In classic Raynaud's, a tricolor change of the fingers is seen, from white to blue to red. Only two colors, however, are required for diagnosis. Raynaud's involves the fingers only and not the whole hand. The thumb is frequently less involved.

24. Raynaud's may be seen as primary Raynaud's disease or as Raynaud's phenomenon secondary to another condition. How can these be distinguished?

Features of Raynaud's disease are:

Female sex

Symptoms for over 2 years

Normal physical exam including nailfold capillaries. No digital pits/ulcers.

Normal lab findings. In particular, absence of ANA or low-titer ANA, without centromere, nucleolar pattern, or specific antibody on ANA profile.

25. Compare the occurrence and frequency of Raynaud's phenomenon and Raynaud's disease in children and adults.

CATEGORY	CHILDREN	ADULTS
Raynaud's disease	5%	70%
Raynaud's phenomenon with		
Nonconnective tissue disease	1	15
Juvenile rheumatoid arthritis (or RA)	1	7
SLE	60	4
Scleroderma	30	3
Dermatomyositis	3	1

Adapted from Cassidy JT, Petty RE: Textbook of Pediatric Rheumatology, 3rd ed. Philadelphia, W.B. Saunders, 1995.

Raynaud's phenomenon should be distinguished from normal vasomotor instability, particularly in young girls. It should also be distinguished from acrocyanosis, a rare vasospastic disorder of persistent coldness and bluish discoloration of the hands and feet, which may follow a viral infection.

26. Describe the types of scleroderma that occur in childhood.

Scleroderma is characterized by abnormally increased collagen deposition in the skin and occasionally in the internal organs.

Localized scleroderma occurs most commonly in childhood. Localized scleroderma may take the form of *morphea,* with a single patch or multiple patches. *Linear* scleroderma may occur on the face, forehead and scalp (*en coup de sabre*), or on the limb (*en bande*).

Diffuse scleroderma (systemic sclerosis) may be limited in its involvement, with a prolonged interval before the appearance of visceral stigmata, or as part of the CREST syndrome (calcinosis, Raynaud's phenomenon, esophageal dysmotility, sclerodactyly, and telangectasias).

Fasciitis with eosinophilia

27. What laboratory abnormalities are seen in the juvenile systemic CTDs?

	SYSTEMIC JRA	SLE	JDMS	SCLERODERMA	VASCULITIS	ARF
Anemia	+ +	+ + +	+	+	+ +	+
Leukopenia	−	+ + +	−	−	−	−
Thrombocytopenia	−	+ +	−	−	−	−
Leukocytosis	+ + +	−	+	−	+ + +	+
Thrombocytosis	+ +	−	+	−	+	+
ANAs	−	+ + +	+	+ +	−	−
Anti-DNA antibodies	−	+ + +	−	−	−	−
Rheumatoid factors	−	+ +	−	+	+	−
Antistreptococcal antibodies	+	−	−	−	−	+ + +
Hypocomplementemia	−	+ + +	−	−	+ +	−
Elevated hepatic enzymes	+ +	+	+	+	+	−
Elevated muscle enzymes	−	+	+ + +	+ +	+	−
Abnormal urinalysis	+	+ + +	+	+	+ +	−

Adapted from Cassidy JT, Petty RE: Textbook of Pediatric Rheumatology, 3rd ed. Philadelphia, W.B. Saunders, 1995. JRA = juvenile rheumatoid arthritis, ARF = acute rheumatic fever.

28. What are general principles of therapy of the juvenile CTDs?

Although clearly therapy for the juvenile CTDs must be tailored to the specific diagnosis, certain therapeutic principles can be stressed. The principal drugs used are those that suppress the inflammatory and immune responses. The arachidonic acid metabolic pathways and the cells of the immune system are the primary targets of their therapeutic effects. An obvious difference in the use of these drugs in children, as compared to adults, is dosing on the basis of the weight of the child.

29. Which anti-inflammatory agents are used to treat children with juvenile CTDs?

NSAIDs. These agents have good analgesic and antipyretic properties, but are only weak anti-inflammatory agents. They are relatively safe when used long-term. Toxicities, particularly CNS and GI side effects, are less common than in adults and are seldom serious. There is considerable variation in patient response to the individual NSAIDs, and a trial of several may be necessary before finding one that is effective and well-tolerated.

Disease-modifying antirheumatic drugs (DMARDs), including the antimalarials, gold compounds, penicillamine, and sulfasalazine. Hydroxychloroquine is used in the management of SLE as well as in JRA. D-Pencillamine is used to treat scleroderma. Sulfasalazine is used to treat the seronegative spondyloarthropathies and inflammatory bowel disease. Gold compounds are generally reserved for JRA, but their use has been largely supplanted by methotrexate.

Glucocorticoids. Glucocorticoid drugs are the most potent of the anti-inflammatory agents in the treatment of the juvenile connective system disorders. However, the doses required (often upwards of 2 mg/kg/d) frequently result in substantial toxicity. In addition to the potentially life-threatening complications of hypertension, susceptibility to infection, impaired carbohydrate tolerance, GI bleeding, and osteoporosis, the marked growth suppression caused by prolonged use of high-dose glucocorticoids is particularly distressing in growing children. Even with cessation of therapy, catch-up growth often does not occur. In addition, the adverse cosmetic effects of glucocorticoids, including acne, hirsutism, obesity, and striae, negatively affect the already tenuous body image of the developing teenager. Thus, the goal of therapy is to use as little of these agents as possible and for as short a time as possible.

Cytotoxic or **immunosuppressive drugs,** including azathioprine, cyclophosphamide, methotrexate, and cyclosporine. Cytotoxic drugs prevent cell division or cause cell death of rapidly dividing cells, such as those of the immune system. Cytotoxic drugs have both anti-inflammatory effects, which act immediately, and immunosuppressive effects, which are delayed. Due to the oncogenic potential and other serious toxicities of these agents, they are, in general, reserved for children with severe, potentially life-threatening disease and with inadequate response to less toxic therapy. However, the remarkable efficacy and relative safety of at least one of these agents (methotrexate) and the effectiveness of these agents in "steroid-sparing" have argued for their use at earlier stages of disease.

30. Do biologic response modifiers have any role in the treatment of these children?

Although a number of these are in experimental use, the predominant biologic response modifier in use clinically is intravenous gammaglobulin (IVIG). This agent has demonstrated efficacy in at least one inflammatory disease, Kawasaki's disease, and has been tried in a number of the juvenile systemic CTDs. The mechanism of action is not understood, but possibilities include clearance of an etiologic infectious agent and antibodies to inflammatory mediators. Although because IVIG is a blood product, transmission of an infectious agent must be considered, in practice the long-term side effects of IVIG are rare, and the short-term side effects (including fever, headache and chills during the infusion) can be readily managed.

BIBLIOGRAPHY

1. American College of Rheumatology: Criteria for the classification of vasculitis. Arthritis Rheum 33:1065, 1990.
2. Ansell BM, Rudge S, Schaller JG: Color Atlas of Pediatric Rheumatology. St. Louis, Mosby, 1992.
3. Cassidy JT, Walker SE, Soderstrom SJ, et al: Diagnostic significance of antibody to native deoxyri-

bonucleic acid in children with juvenile rheumatoid arthritis and connective tissue diseases. J Pediatr 93:416, 1978.
4. Hagge WW, Burke EC, Stickler GB: Treatment of systemic lupus erythematosus complicated by nephritis in children. Pediatrics 40:822, 1967.
5. Kallenberg CGM: Early detection of connective tissue disease in patients with Raynaud's phenomenon. Rheum Dis Clinics North Am 16:11, 1990.
6. Lehman TJ, Hanson V, Zvaifler N, et al: Antibodies to nonhistone nuclear antigens and antilymphocyte antibodies among children and adults with systemic lupus erythematosus and their relatives. J Rheumatol 11:644, 1984.
7. Meislin AG, Rothfield NJ: Systemic lupus erythematosus in childhood. Pediatrics 42:37, 1968.
8. Pope RM: Rheumatic fever in the 1980's. Bull Rheum Dis 38(3):1, 1989.
9. Schumacher HR Jr (ed): Primer on the Rheumatic Diseases, 9th ed. Atlanta, Arthritis Foundation, 1988.
10. Singsen BH: Scleroderma in childhood. Pediatr Rheum 33:1119, 1986.
11. Singsen BH, Kornreich HK, Koster-King K, et al: Mixed connective tissue disease in children. Arthritis Rheum 20:355, 1977.
12. Stollerman CH, Markowitz M, Taranta A, et al: Jone's criteria (revised) for guidance in the diagnosis of rheumatic fever. Circulation 32:664, 1965.
13. Suarez-Almazor ME, Catoggio LJ, Maldonado-Cocco JA, et al: Juvenile progressive systemic sclerosis: Clinical and serologic findings. Arthritis Rheum 28:699, 1985.
14. Tan EM: Antinuclear antibodies: Diagnostic marker for autoimmune diseases and probes for cell biology. Adv Immunol 44:93, 1989.
15. Tan EM, Cohen AS, Fries JF, et al: The 1982 revised criteria for the classification of systemic lupus erythematosus. Arthritis Rheum 25:1127, 1982.

75. KAWASAKI'S DISEASE

Roger Hollister, MD

1. What are the diagnostic criteria for Kawasaki's disease?
1. Fever, usually high-grade for > 5 consecutive days, unresponsive to antibiotic treatment
2. Conjunctivitis, nonexudative often dramatic
3. Cracking and fissuring of lips, with inflammation of mucosal membranes; "strawberry" tongue
4. Cervical lymphadenopathy
5. Polymorphic rash involving trunk and extremities
6. Erythema of hands and feet, progressing to edema and finally desquamation

To meet the diagnosis, five of the above six criteria must be met, or four with echo-cardiographic demonstration of coronary artery dilatation.

2. What complications may be involved in the acute phase of the illness?
Cardiac—Myocarditis, pericarditis, and arteritis predispose to aneurysms in approximately 20% of patients.
Arthritis—Short-lived, may involve small joints of hands and feet
Uveitis—acute, anterior
Hydrops of gallbladder—Produces abdominal pain and jaundice
Gastrointestinal—Vomiting and diarrhea

3. Is there a diagnostic test for Kawasaki's disease?
No. Laboratory tests show the findings of acute inflammation. However, a progressive increase in the platelet count, often to thrombocytotic levels ($>10^6$/mm^3), is characteristic and is not seen in many other causes of fever of unknown origin.

4. Name three epidemiologic factors that adversely affect the prognosis in Kawasaki's disease.
Age < 1 year, male sex, oriental ancestry.

5. Name an illness in the differential diagnosis of Kawasaki's disease.

Scarlet fever shares many of the features, including fever, conjunctivitis, mucous membrane involvement, and desquamating skin rash. Some authorities suggest that scarlet fever must be ruled out by appropriate cultures for streptococci before concluding that the diagnosis is Kawasaki's disease.

6. What epidemiologic facts are known about Kawasaki's disease?

- It is a disease of young children:
  Peak incidence at 9–12 months of age
  50% cases in children < 2 years old
  80% in children < 4 years old
- There is a 1–2% incidence in siblings.
- There is a 3% recurrence rate.
- Epidemics appear to be cyclic, occurring at approximately 2–3 year intervals.

7. What symptoms and findings present in the acute phase of Kawasaki's disease suggest cardiac involvement?

Obviously, in preverbal children, it may be difficult to communicate ischemic myocardial pain. Symptoms that may be helpful include restlessness, pallor, weak pulse, abdominal pain, and vomiting. A gallop rhythm with a third heart sound may be heard in 70% of cases. Friction rubs indicative of pericarditis are much less common. Coronary artery aneurysms are more common in patients with pericarditis. In one series, palpable axillary artery aneurysms were highly predictive of coronary artery aneurysms.

8. What tests are helpful in assessing cardiac involvement?

Electrocardiograms may show ST-T wave changes indicative of pericarditis or myocarditis. Chest x-rays may show cardiomegaly. However, an echocardiogram is most useful to assess myocardial function, rarely valvular regurgitation, and most commonly coronary arterial dilatation and aneurysm formation (20% of all patients).

9. Besides the fact that "giant" coronary aneurysms sound bad, what is the significance of finding coronary artery dilatations > 8 mm on echocardiography?

"Giant" coronary artery aneurysms are the most prone to thrombosis and the least likely to regress with time. Their presence requires very close follow-up and perhaps longer term requirement for anticoagulation.

10. What is the natural history of these lesions?

From a peak incidence of 20% in the first 1–2 weeks of illness, most of the vascular dilatations will regress, so that only 2% can be found on echocardiography 1 year later. Antiplatelet therapy should begin with high-dose aspirin (80–100 mg/kg/day) split into three doses in the acute phase of the illness. This is followed by low-dose aspirin (10 mg/kg/d) once a day in the convalescent phase until aneurysms have regressed.

11. Is there an effective treatment for Kawasaki's disease?

Conclusive evidence from numerous multicenter, double-blinded, placebo-controlled series shows that intravenous immune globulin (IVIG) given within the first 10 days of illness is the treatment of choice in Kawasaki's disease. Two parameters have repeatedly been shown to be responsive to IVIG: resolution of the acute symptoms and prevention of coronary aneurysm formation. It is commonly observed that the fever lyses, the rash regresses, and the toxicity of the illness improves within 12 hours of IVIG administration.

12. How effective is IVIG in preventing aneurysm formation?

	ANEURYSM AT 14 DAYS	ANEURYSM AT 30 MOS
ASA alone	23%	11%
ASA and IVIG	8%	2%

13. What dose of IVIG should be used?

A single dose of 2 gm/kg of IVIG is as effective as various multiple-dose schemes that were previously employed. (The outcome measures were control of acute symptoms and prevention of aneurysm formation.)

14. IVIG is a very expensive medication. Is it cost-effective to use this medication on all patients with Kawasaki's disease?

Yes. In a comprehensive study, Klassen showed that the costs of acute care for Kawasaki's disease and the costs of the long-term sequelae of Kawasaki's disease (aneurysms, thromboses, etc.) were both significantly reduced by the administration of a single dose of 2 gm/kg of IVIG.

15. Does IVIG have any side effects?

The acute side effects include fever, chills, headache, and, rarely, aseptic meningitis. Most of these side effects respond to slowing the infusion. Fortunately, beyond the risk of all blood products, there are no long-term risks to IVIG.

16. What is unique about IVIG that might explain its usefulness in Kawasaki's disease?

IVIG is pooled material from 10,000 donors. When the antibody profile of IVIG was examined, it was found to have extraordinarily high titers of anti-staphylococcal, streptococcal, and toxic shock toxin antibodies. Many of the features of Kawasaki's disease (fever, rash, etc.) are reminiscent of toxin-mediated diseases.

BIBLIOGRAPHY

1. Dajani AS, Taubert KA, Takaheshi M, et al: Guidelines for long-term management of patients with Kawasaki disease. Circulation 89:916–922, 1994.
2. Klassen TP, Rowe PC, Gafri A: Economic evaluation of intravenous immune globulin therapy for Kawasaki sydrome. J Pediatr 122:538–542, 1993.
3. Newburger JW, Takahashi M, Burns JC, et al: The treatment of Kawasaki syndrome with intravenous gammaglobulin. N Engl J Med 315:341–347, 1986.
4. Rauch A, Hurwitz E: Centers for Disease Control case definition for Kawasaki syndrome. Pediatr Infect Dis 4:702–703, 1985.
5. Rosenfeld EA, Sheelman S, Corydon KE, et al: Comparative safety and efficacy of two immune globulin products in Kawasaki disease. J Pediatr 126:1000–1003, 1994.

XIV. Miscellaneous Rheumatic Disorders

Sickness is a place, more instructive than a long trip to Europe, and it is a place where there's no company, where nobody can follow.

Flannery O'Connor (1925–1963)

76. METABOLIC AND OTHER GENETIC MYOPATHIES

Ramon A. Arroyo, M.D.

1. What are metabolic myopathies?

Metabolic myopathies are conditions that share an underlying abnormality in muscle glycogen, lipid, or adenosine triphosphate (ATP) metabolism. These conditions must be considered in the differential diagnosis of persons with proximal muscle weakness, myoglobinuria, or exercise intolerance as a result of fatigue, myalgias, or cramps.

2. Which conditions are considered primary metabolic myopathies?

Defects of glycogen metabolism that affect muscle

Acid maltase deficiency (Pompe's disease)
Brancher enzyme deficiency (Andersen's disease)
Debrancher enzyme deficiency (Cori's-Forbes' disease)
Phosphorylase b kinase deficiency
Myophosphorylase deficiency (McArdle's disease)
Phosphofructokinase deficiency (Tauri disease)
Phosphoglycerate kinase deficiency
Phospholglyceromutase deficiency
Lactate dehydrogenase deficiency

Mitochondrial myopathies (diagnosed in adults)

Enzymes of β-oxidation deficiency
NADH-CoQ reductase deficiency
Cytochrome *b* deficiency
Cytochrome *bc*1 deficiency
Mitochondrial ATPase deficiency

Defects in lipid metabolism that affect muscle

Carnitine deficiency states (primary or secondary)
Carnitine palmitoyl transferase (CPT) deficiency
Fatty acid acylCoA dehydrogenase deficiency

Disorders of purine metabolism

Myoadenylate deaminase (MADA) deficiency

3. What are secondary causes of metabolic myopathies?

Endocrine myopathies

Acromegaly
Hyper- and hypothyroidism
Hyperparathyroidism

Cushing's and Addison's diseases
Hyperaldosteronism
Carcinoid syndrome

Metabolic-nutritional myopathies

Uremia   Vitamin D and E deficiencies
Hepatic failure   Malabsorption
Periodic paralysis

Electrolyte disorders

Elevated or decreased levels of   Hypophosphatemia
  sodium, potassium, or calcium   Hypomagnesemia

4. What is the source of energy for muscle contraction?

Hydrolysis of ATP. Intracellular concentrations of ATP are maintained by the action of enzymes such as creatine kinase, adenylate cyclase, and myoadenylate deaminase. The energy to replenish ATP after it is consumed during muscle contraction is provided by intermediary metabolism of carbohydrates and lipids by pathways of glycolysis, the Krebs' cycle, β-oxidation, and oxidative phosphorylation.

5. How does ATP provide the energy for muscle contraction?

The immediate source of energy for skeletal muscle during work is found in preformed organic compounds containing high-energy phosphates, such as ATP and creatine phosphate. Creatine (CK) helps maintain intracellular ATP concentrations by catalyzing the reversible transphorylation of creatine and adenine nucleotides and by modulating changes in cytosolic ATP concentrations.

At rest, when there is excess ATP, the terminal phosphate of ATP is transferred to creatine, forming creatine phosphate (CrP) and adenosine diphosphate (ADP) in a reaction catalyzed by CK. The CrP serves as a reservoir of high-energy phosphate. With muscle activity and ATP utilization, CK catalyzes the transfer of those phosphates from CrP to rapidly restore ATP levels to normal. The stores of CrP are sufficient to allow the rephosphorylation of ADP to ATP for only a few minutes of exercise.

Thus, CK along with its products, creatine and creatine phosphate, serve as a shuttle mechanism for energy transport between mitochondria, where ATP is generated by oxidative metabolism (Krebs' cycle and respiratory/cytochrome chain), and the myofibrils, where ATP is consumed during muscle contraction and relaxation.

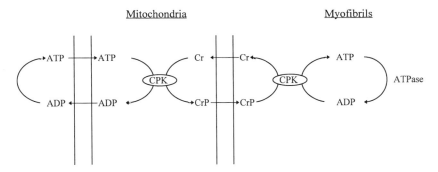

6. What is the purine nucleotide cycle?

When approximately 50% of creatine phosphate has been used during exercise, ATP levels in muscle begin to fall. When this occurs, the purine nucleotide cycle is activated.

During exercise, as ATP is hydrolyzed to ADP by ATPase and then to AMP by adenylate kinase, AMP accumulates. The first step of the purine nucleotide cycle is catalyzed by myoadenylate deaminase, which converts AMP to inosine monophosphate (IMP) with release of ammonia (NH_3). Both IMP and ammonia stimulate glycolytic activity in an attempt to generate more energy. As ATP levels fall, IMP levels rise until muscle activity decreases and recovery can occur. During recovery, oxidative pathways function and AMP is regenerated from IMP with the liberation of fumarate. Fumarate is converted to malate, which enters the mitochondria and participates in the tricarboxylic acid (Krebs') cycle. This helps to regenerate ATP by oxidative phosphorylation within the mitochondria.

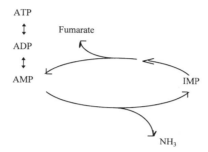

7. What is the role of carbohydrate metabolism during muscle work?

Glycogen, the major storage form of carbohydrate, is the major source of ATP generation when physical activity is of short duration and high intensity or when anaerobic conditions exist.

Glycogen is mobilized to form glucose-6-phosphate (G-6-P) by glycogenolysis in a process started by the enzyme myophosphorylase. Glucose and glucose-6-phosphate are metabolized through a series of reactions in the glycolytic pathway to pyruvate. Under aerobic conditions, pyruvate enters the Krebs' (TCA) cycle and is metabolized to carbon dioxide and water. The aerobic metabolism of 1 glucose molecule nets 38 molecules of ATP. However, under anaerobic conditions, pyruvate is converted to lactate and does not enter the Krebs' cycle. Under these conditions, only 2 molecules of ATP are generated for each glucose molecule. Anaerobic glycogenolysis can supply energy to muscle for only several minutes until the muscle fatigues, whereas there are sufficient muscle glycogen stores to supply energy for up to 90 minutes under aerobic conditions. At present, nine inborn errors of glycogen biochemistry that affect muscle function have been described.

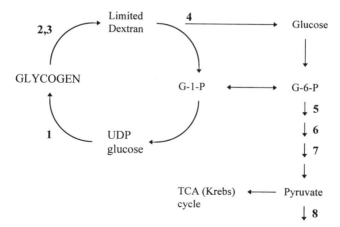

Catalyst enzymes: 1 = brancher enzyme, 2 = phosphorylase b kinase, 3 = myophosphorylase, 4 = debrancher enzyme, 5 = phosphofrutokinase, 6 = phophoglycerate kinase, 7 = phophoglycerate mutase, 8 = lactate dehydrogenase, 9 [not shown] = acid maltase, which catalyzes release of glucose from glycogen and maltase in lysosomes.

8. What is the role of lipid metabolism during muscle work?

Lipids, in the form of fatty acids, constitute the major substrate for energy production (ATP) during fasting intervals, at rest, and with muscular activities of low intensity and long duration.

Long-chain fatty acids (L-cFA) from adipose tissues move through the bloodstream bound to albumin. These, plus medium and small chain fatty acids, move across endothelial cells and into the muscle cells (called fibers), where they are available for energy production, storage, or synthesis into membrane components. To be processed for energy, the free fatty acid must enter the mitochondria. Long-chain fatty acids must combine with carnitine to enter the inner mitochondrial matrix. The combination of long-chain fatty acids with carnitine and their release into the mitochondrial matrix are catalyzed by carnitine palmitoyl transferase (CPT) I and CPT II, respectively, (1 and 2 in the diagram), which are located on the inner mitochondrial membrane (IM). Once in the mitochondria, the fatty acids are converted to their respective coenzyme A (CoA) esters and sequentially shortened by the process of β-oxidation, which release acetyl CoA which then enters the tricarboxylic acid (TCA, Krebs') cycle. For each molecule of long-chain fatty acid (palmitate), there is a net gain of 131 molecules of ATP. At present, carnitine deficiency, CPT deficiency, and acylCoA synthetase deficiency have been described in patients with abnormal muscle function. (OM = outer membrane; 3 = acylCoA synthetase.)

9. How do disorders of glycogen and glucose metabolism present clinically?

Persons with a glycogen storage disease are well at rest and perform mild exercise without difficulty, because free fatty acids are the major source of energy under these conditions. The enzymatic block that interferes with the use of carbohydrates to generate ATP causes problems only when exercise reaches a level that produces anaerobic conditions. Typically, the patient starts exercising and within a few minutes the muscle fatigues (patients describe this as "hitting the wall"). If they persist, the muscle becomes painful and may develop a firm indurated and painful contracture. This could result in severely damaged muscle. If the muscle damage is extensive, myoglobinuria may result and sometimes could be sufficient to compromise renal function.

10. Do all disorders of glycogen and glycolysis have the same clinical presentation?

No, even though exercise intolerance is the most common presentation, there are some differences in clinical features according to the specific enzyme deficiency.

11. Describe the clinical presentation seen in myophosphorylase deficiency (McArdle's disease).

Myophosphorylase degrades glycogen to glucose-1-phosphate and hence is important in calling up stored energy for muscle use. The cardinal manifestation of this deficiency is exercise intolerance associated with pain, fatigue, or weakness. The degree of intolerance varies among affected individuals. Symptoms can follow activities of high intensity and short duration or those that requires less intense effort for longer intervals, but always resolve with rest. In fact, at rest, affected individuals function well and adjust their activities to a level below their threshold for symptoms. Some individuals experience a "second wind" phenomenon; if they stop their activities at onset of symptoms and rest briefly, they can resume exercise with increased tolerance. For unknown reasons (possibly related to the presence of a fetal isoenzyme), severe cramps and myoglobinuria are rare before adolescence. Elevated CK is a common finding in this myopathy.

12. How do deficiencies of brancher and debrancher enzymes (Andersen's and Cori's-Forbes' disease) present clinically?

Brancher enzyme (UDP glucose to glycogen) deficiency causes fatal hepatic failure in childhood, which can be associated with hypotonia and contractures, or exercise intolerance and cardiomyopathy. In **debrancher enzyme** (limit dextran to glucose-1-phosphate) deficiency limit dextran accumulates in muscle, liver, and blood cells, causing hepatomegaly, fasting hypoglycemia, and failure to thrive in childhood. However, the first recognized manifestation of the disease may be slowly progressive muscle weakness beginning after age 20.

13. How does phosphofructokinase deficiency (Tauri's disease) present?

The clinical manifestations of phosphofructokinase (fructose-6-phosphate to fructose-1, 6-phosphate deficiency can be identical to those of McArdle's disease. The second wind phenomenon is less common, and the exercise intolerance is likely be associated with nausea and vomiting. About one-third of affected persons develop myoglobinuria, and most have elevated CK at rest. The disease can also cause hemolytic anemia.

14. And how does acid maltase deficiency present?

Acid maltase catalyzes the release of glucose from maltose, oligosaccharide, and glycogen in lysosomes. Its deficiency is transmitted by autosomal recessive inheritance and produces three different clinical syndromes.

1. The infantile form causes symptoms of muscle weakness, hypotonia, and congestive heart failure that begins shortly after birth and progress to death within the first 2 years of life.
2. The second form presents in early childhood with progressive proximal muscle weakness. Death is usually from respiratory failure and occurs before age 30.
3. The adult form presents in the third to fifth decades of life with insidous, painless limb-girdle weakness. The respiratory muscle can be affected. This form is frequently misdiagnosed as polymyositis, and a muscle biopsy is most helpful in differentiating them. Characteristically, there are muscle fibers with vacuoles filled with periodic acid–Schiff positive material with a prominent acid phosphatase activity.

15. How do disorders of lipid metabolism present clinically?

An increasing number of neurologic diseases have been associated with defects in fatty acid metabolism. Many of them cause abnormalities in the CNS. Few cases present as isolated instances of exercise intolerance. Abnormalities involving the processing of long-chain fatty acids for energy lead to lipid storage myopathies, conditions in which the predominant pathologic alteration is the accumulation of abnormal amounts of lipid droplets between myofibrils. Carnitine deficiency and carnitine palmitoyl transferase (CPT) deficiency are the classic examples.

16. What is the syndrome of carnitine deficiency?

The syndrome of myopathic carnitine deficiency is characterized by progressive muscle weakness that, with some exceptions, begins in childhood. The weakness is of the limb-girdle muscles, but facial and pharyngeal muscle involvement can be observed. Less common features are exertional myalgias, myoglobinuria, and cardiomyopathy. Half or more of the patients have high CK levels, and most have myopathic changes on electromyography. The diagnosis is made by biochemical analysis of muscle tissue.

17. How is it treated?

Treatment includes L-carnitine supplementation in the diet, but the response is variable. Attempts at treatment should include a diet rich in carbohydrates and medium-chain fatty acids and avoidance of fasting. During acute attacks, therapy should be designed to avoid hypoglycemia and correct any electrolyte and acid-base imbalances that develop. The dose of L-carnitine for children is 100 mg/kg/day, and for adults it is 2–4 gm in divided doses. The D-isomer of carnitine should not be used because it is not effective and can cause muscle weakness. Some patients benefit from corticosteroids and propranolol.

18. What is the syndrome of carnitine palmitoyl transferase (CPT) deficiency?

CPT deficiency is an autosomal recessive disorder characterized by attacks of exertional myalgias and myoglobinuria. Patients, most of whom are male, experience no difficulty with short bursts of strenuous activity. Indeed, the favorite recreational sport of the patient is often weightlifting. When prolonged exercise is demanded, particularly in the fasting state (when the body is dependent on fatty acid metabolism as a source of energy), muscle pain, fatigue, and myoglubinuria similar to that occurring in glycolytic disorders may ensue. The diagnosis is made by measuring CPT activity in biopsied muscle.

Treatment consists of education. Avoidance of prolonged strenuous exercise and fasting prevent most attacks. Myoglobinuria constitutes a medical emergency and should be treated as such. Interestingly, the development of renal failure does not correlate well with the amount of myoglobin in the urine.

19. How do you differentiate CPT deficiency from glycogen storage disease?

- CPT-deficient patients do not experience severe cramping, and fixed muscle weakness is rare.
- CPK is usually normal except during attacks or with prolonged fasting.
- Serum lactate levels, increase during exercise.
- Electromyographic findings are normal between attacks.

20. What are mitochondrial myopathies?

These are a clinically and biochemically heterogeneous group of disorders that have morphologic abnormalities in the number, size, and structure of the mitochondria. The most typical morphologic change is the **ragged red fiber**, a distorted-appearing fiber that contains large peripheral and intermyofibrillar aggregates of abnormal mitochondria. These appear as red deposits on modified Gomori staining.

The syndromes associated with abnormalities of mitochondria have a variety of clinical manifestations. Many present multisystem problems with involvement of the CNS heart, and skeletal muscle. The skeletal muscle involvement is manifested by progressive proximal muscle weakness, external ophthalmoplegia, inability to exercise, and severe fatigue.

21. Are disorders in purine metabolism associated with any problems besides gout?

Yes, myoadenylate deaminase (MADA), an isoenzyme found only in skeletal muscle, catalyzes the irreversible deamination of AMP to IMP and plays an important role in the purine nucleotide cycle. Individuals with MADA deficiency complain of exercise intolerance, postexertional cramps, and myalgias. MADA deficiency is probably the most common metabolic abnormality of muscle, but the precise relationship between MADA deficiency and muscular symptoms is controversial. ATP is rapidly consumed during exercise in these patients, and the time to replenish ATP to normal concentration is prolonged. The expected rise in lactate during exercise occurs, but the corresponding change in ammonia concentration does not. CK and aldolase are usually normal in MADA deficiency, as are the electromyographic and muscle biopsy findings. Histochemical techniques are useful in establishing this deficiency state.

22. How do you clinically evaluate patients with suspected metabolic muscle disease?

The evaluation begins with a careful history and thorough physical exam. The problem of diagnosing metabolic myopathies is confounded because at rest, patients are usually asymptomatic and have normal physical findings. The most significant complaints are severe prolonged cramps and **red-wine-colored urine**, indicating myoglobinuria. The physical findings may be entirely normal and at most may only show symmetrical proximal muscle weakness. The prime importance of the physical exam is to rule out other conditions that present with muscle weakness, especially those with a neurologic component.

23. How are the metabolic myopathies diagnosed?

Once a detailed history and physical examination are done, measurement of muscle enzymes and electrodiagnostic studies follow if complaints are suspicious for myopathy. Increased levels of CK, aldolase, aspartate aminotransferase (AST, SGOT), alanine aminotransferase (ALT, SGPT), or lactate dehydrogenase may be observed in the blood of patients with muscle disease. Of these, CK is the most sensitive. Levels are usually increased in patients with glycogen storage disease but are usually normal in diseases such as CPT or MADA deficiency.

The electromyogram (EMG) is useful in demonstrating myopathic changes and indicating a preferential site for muscle biopsy on the opposite side of the body. Elevated muscle enzymes and myopathic changes on EMG are variable and nondiagnostic. Measurement of venous lactate and ammonia before and after forearm ischemic exercise provides a useful tool for ruling out MADA deficiency and all myopathic forms of glycogen storage disease except acid maltase deficiency. A positive result should be confirmed by tissue analysis. A **muscle biopsy** provides the most important diagnostic information in the evaluation of a patient with a metabolic muscle disease.

24. What is the forearm ischemic test? How it is performed?

The forearm ischemic test is a nonspecific tool used in individuals suspected of having myophosphorylase deficiency or a block anywhere along the glycogenolytic or glycolytic pathway. This test exploits the abnormal biochemistry that results in the absence of those enzymes. Normal muscle generates lactate from the degradation of glycogen when it exercises under ischemic or anaerobic conditions. When these pathways are blocked, no lactate is released into the circulation. In addition, ammonia, inosine, and hypoxanthine concentrations increase significantly. A protocol for forearm ischemic testing follows:

1. A blood sample for analysis of baseline lactate and ammonia concentrations is drawn through an indwelling needle in an antecubital vein, preferably without use of a tourniquet.
2. A sphygmomanometer cuff is placed on the upper arm and inflated. It is maintained at least 20 mm Hg above systolic pressure while the subject squeezes a tennis ball, or similar object, at a rate one squeeze every 2 sec for 90 sec.
3. After 90 sec, the cuff is deflated and additional venous samples are obtained at 1, 3, 5, and 10 minutes thereafter.

In normal individuals, lactate and ammonia increase at least threefold from baseline values. The major reason for a false-positive result is insufficient work by the subject while exercising. This should be suspected if both lactate and ammonia fail to rise. If lactate does not rise but ammonia does, the patient may have a defect in glycolysis, such as McArdle's disease.

25. Why is muscle biopsy the most important diagnostic tool in the evaluation of metabolic myopathies?

Muscle biopsy for routine histologic, histochemical, and ultrastructural analysis (electron microscopy) is the most helpful tool in evaluating a suspected metabolic myopathy, primarily because it helps rule out other conditions that can cause muscle dysfunction and allows the specific enzyme defect to be determined. However, biopsy should be the final step in the clinical evaluation, done only after a preliminary diagnosis has been made. The most important histochemical studies are listed below:

STAIN	CONDITION
Periodic acid–Schiff	Glycogen storage diseases
Sudan or Oil red O	Lipid storage diseases
Gomori	Mitochondrial myopathy
Acid phosphatase	acid maltase deficiency
Histochemical for specific enzymes	Myophosphorylase, phosphofructokinase, lactate dehydrogenase, cytochromes, MADA

26. Describe the common muscular dystrophies that may be confused with childhood or adult polymyositis.

Duchenne dystrophy. X-linked disease. Onset of shoulder and pelvic girdle muscle weakness by age 5. Elevated CK, myopathic EMG, and abnormal muscle biopsy showing fat and occasionally inflammation. Pseudohypertrophy of calf muscles. Inability to walk by age 11 and death from respiratory failure by age 20. Abnormal gene on X chromosome coding for the myocyte membrane protein, dystrophin.

Becker dystrophy. X-linked disease. Similar to Duchenne dystrophy but milder, with patients able to walk beyond age 16 years.

Fascioscapulohumeral dystrophy. Autosomal dominant disease. Variable disease expression with disease onset between adolescence to middle-adult years. Presents with facial, shoulder, and proximal arm weakness. Lower extremities less involved. CK elevated up to 5 times normal, and inflammation can be seen on muscle biopsy.

Limb-girdle dystrophy. Autosomal recessive disease. Progressive upper and lower extremity proximal muscle weakness beginning in second to fourth decades. Facial muscles spared. This dystrophy is the one most readily confused with adult polymyositis.

Myotonic dystrophies. Autosomal dominant diseases. Facial weakness, ptosis, distal limb weakness, and systemic features (balding, cataracts, cardiorespiratory and gastrointestinal involvement). Characteristic physical finding is delayed relaxation and muscles stiffness (myotonia). Inability to relax handgrip when shaking hands and myotonic contraction of thumb when thenar eminence musculature is hit with a reflex hammer are commonly observed. EMG shows excessive insertional activity and a "dive bomber" sound with contraction of muscle. Ringed myofibers seen in 70% on muscle biopsy.

BIBLIOGRAPHY

1. Martin A, Haller RG, Barohn R: Metabolic myopathies. Curr Opin Rheumatol 6:552–558, 1994.
2. Plotz PH, Leff RL, Miller FW: Inflammatory and metabolic myopathies. In Schumacher HR Jr (ed): Primer on the Rheumatic Diseases, 10th ed. Atlanta, Arthritis Foundation, 1993, pp 127–131.
3. Wortmann RL: Metabolic diseases of muscle. In McCarty DJ, Koopman W (eds): Arthritis and Allied Conditions, 12th ed. Philadelphia, Lea & Febiger, 1993, pp 1895–1912.
4. Zeviani M, Amati P, Savoia A. Mitochrondrial myopathies. Curr Opin Rheumatol 6:559–567, 1994.

77. AMYLOIDOSIS

James D. Singleton, M.D.

1. What is amyloidosis?
Amyloidosis is a condition in which an insoluble proteinaceous material is deposited in the extracellular matrix of tissue. The deposits may be localized to one organ or may be systemic. Amyloid deposition may be subclinical or may produce a diverse array of clinical manifestations.

2. Why is it called amyloid? How does its deposition result in clinical disease?
In 1854, Rudolph Virchow coined the term *amyloid* (starch-like) due to the material's reaction with iodine and sulfuric acid. This designation has been retained despite the recognition of amyloid's proteinaceous nature. Amyloid deposits encroach on parenchymal tissues, compromising their function. Organ compromise is related to the location, quantity, and rate of deposition.

3. Why is knowledge of amyloidosis important?
Amyloidosis frequently mimics more common rheumatic diseases in its presentations. It also may occur as a potentially fatal sequela of long-standing inflammatory disease.

4. Describe the structure of amyloid.
All amyloid shares a unique ultrastructure as seen by electron microscopy. Thin, nonbranching protein fibrils constitute about 90% of amyloid deposits. Fibrils tend to aggregate laterally to form fibers. X-ray diffraction studies show that the polypeptide chains are oriented perpendicularly to the long axis of the fibril, forming a cross β-pleated sheet conformation. P-component, a protein composed of two pentagonal subunits forming a doughnut-like structure, makes up 5%. The remainder is composed of small amounts of carbohydrate and mucopolysaccharides.

5. Describe the light microscopic appearance of amyloid.
Without staining, amyloid appears as a homogeneous, amorphous, hyaline extracellular material. It is eosinophilic when stained with hematoxylin-eosin and metachromatic with crystal violet. Amyloid stains homogeneously with Congo red (congophilic) due to its β-pleated sheet configuration. Viewing of Congo red-stained tissue under polarized microscopy yields the pathognomonic apple-green birefringence.

6. So isn't all amyloid the same?
No. Although all amyloid shares a common structure and tinctorial properties, the major protein comprising the fibril varies from one disease to the next. Thus, there are many amyloidoses, each associated with a specific fibril protein. P-component is associated with all types of amyloid but is not essential for fibril formation.

7. Where do the amyloid proteins come from?
All fibrillar amyloid proteins are thought to derive from a larger serum precursor molecule. The amyloid protein is usually a fragment of the precursor molecule but may be an intact molecule (as it is with β_2-microglobulin). P-component is identical to a normal serum component, serum amyloid P (SAP). Although it is 50% homologous with C-reactive protein, an acute phase reactant, SAP is not an acute phase reactant.

8. How are the amyloidoses classified?
By the major protein component of the fibril. This also has become the basis for defining the clinical syndromes with certainty. However, routine stains do not identify the major fibril protein, and such testing is not used clinically.

CLINICAL CATEGORIES	MAJOR PROTEIN TYPES	RELATIVE FREQUENCIES
Primary amyloidosis	AL	56%
Myeloma-associated	AL	26%
Secondary (reactive) amyloidosis	AA	9%
Localized amyloidosis	Various	8%
Hereditary amyloidosis	ATTR and others	1%
Amyloidosis of dialysis	$A\beta_2M$	—

9. What is primary amyloidosis?

Formerly, systemic amyloidosis in the absence of multiple myeloma was called idiopathic or primary amyloidosis. It is now recognized that this amyloid, like that associated with myeloma, is composed of whole or fragments of immunoglobulin light chains. The designation AL was given to reflect the light chain source of this amyloid. AL amyloid appears to represent a spectrum of disease. At one end, the source of light chains is a malignant clone of plasma cells (myeloma-associated). At the other extreme, light chains are derived from a small, nonproliferative plasma cell population (immunocyte dyscrasia).

10. How then is primary amyloidosis distinguished from amyloidosis associated with myeloma?

The separation of AL amyloidosis into those with and without myeloma is not always clear-cut. Clinical judgment must play a role in distinguishing the two ends of the spectrum of one disease. Generally, multiple myeloma is considered to be absent when:

- There are no lytic bone lesions
- There is no hypercalcemia
- There is no anemia except that related to bleeding or renal insufficiency
- The serum or urine monoclonal component is small
- There are < 25% bone marrow plasma cells

These criteria have been applied in determining patient eligibility for participation in prospective treatment trials for amyloidosis. From a therapeutic standpoint, such distinction is not always necessary, as cytotoxic chemotherapy is used for both entities. However, treatment exclusively with noncytotoxic therapy should not be used for those with myeloma.

11. Describe the demographic features of primary amyloidosis.

AL occurs approximately twice as often in men as in women. The median age at diagnosis is 65 years, and 99% of patients are ≥40 years of age. Whites are more frequently affected than other races. AL has been very rarely described in children.

12. What are the most common initial symptoms in patients with primary amyloidosis?

Fatigue (54%)
Weight loss (42%)
Pain (15%)
Purpura (16%)
Gross bleeding (8%)

Weight loss can be striking, exceeding 40 lbs in some patients and prompting a search for occult malignancy. Pain is more common in those with myeloma (40%) than those without (8%). In those without myeloma, pain is frequently due to peripheral neuropathy and/or carpal tunnel syndrome. Other symptoms are often present in patients with specific organ involvement (dyspnea; pedal edema with congestive heart failure; paresthesias with peripheral neuropathy; orthostasis; syncope with autonomic neuropathy or low-output congestive heart failure).

13. What physical findings are common in patients with primary amyloidosis?

Edema (most common)
Palpable liver (34%)

Macroglossia (22%)
Purpura (16%)
Edema may occur due to nephrotic syndrome, congestive heart failure, and rarely, protein-losing enteropathy. Hepatomegaly is usually of only modest degree. Macroglossia and purpura should particularly raise suspicion of amyloidosis; both may be a source of patient complaints and are easily overlooked. Increased firmness of the tongue and dental indentations are helpful in determining the presence of macroglossia. Cutaneous purpura are generally localized to the upper chest, neck, and face. Purpura of the eyelids is a clue that is seen only when the patient's eyes are closed.

14. Since symptoms are nonspecific and physical findings insensitive, what clinical syndromes should suggest the presence of primary amyloidosis?

Nephrotic syndrome
Congestive heart failure (CHF)
Peripheral neuropathy
Autonomic neuropathy
Carpal tunnel syndrome
Hepatic disease

The most common initial clinical manifestation is nephrotic syndrome. The major sign distinguishing it from other causes of nephrosis is the finding of a monoclonal protein in the serum or urine (electrophoresis *and* immunofixation should be done). Although overt CHF can occur in up to one-third of patients, amyloid cardiomyopathy, as revealed by echocardiography, is even more common. Peripheral neuropathy clinically resembles the neuropathy seen in diabetes, including the chronic course. Autonomic neuropathy may be superimposed on peripheral neuropathy or occur alone. A history of carpal tunnel syndrome is a very important clue to the presence of amyloidosis. It is typically bilateral, and surgical release may not provide complete relief.

15. What clues should alert you to the presence of hepatic amyloidosis?
• Proteinuria—High association with nephrotic syndrome
• Monoclonal protein in serum
• Howell-Jolly bodies in the peripheral blood smear due to splenic infiltration
• Hepatomegaly out of proportion to liver function tests (one-third with hepatomegaly will have normal test results)

16. What are the echocardiographic findings in amyloid cardiomyopathy?
Two-dimensional echocardiography has a high sensitivity for detecting amyloid. Symmetric thickening of the left ventricular wall or thickening of the interventricular septum may lead to an erroneous diagnosis of concentric left ventricular hypertrophy or asymmetric septal hypertrophy. Hypokinesis may suggest prior "silent" infarction. The combination of increased myocardial echogenicity and increased atrial thickness is 60% sensitive and 100% specific for the diagnosis of amyloidosis.

17. So do most patients with primary amyloidosis display only one syndrome?
No. Most patients have widespread disease and more than one syndrome. Carpal tunnel syndrome is seen more often in those with peripheral neuropathy and cardiomyopathy than in other syndromes.

18. Name three presentations of amyloidosis that mimic other rheumatic diseases.
Vascular involvement by amyloid can lead to claudication of the extremities and jaw as seen in temporal arteritis. Amyloid arthropathy can mimic rheumatoid arthritis. Clues are the lack of inflammation and frequent hip and shoulder involvement with periarticular amyloid infiltration, which leads to enlargement of the pelvic or shoulder girdle (shoulder pad sign). Synovial fluid analysis can be helpful in detecting amyloid deposits. Infiltration of amyloid into muscle may lead to weakness or pain, simulating polymyositis. Enlargement of involved muscles (pseudohypertrophy) can be striking and may not be associated with other symptoms.

19. What is secondary (reactive) amyloidosis?
Secondary amyloidosis is due to deposition of amyloid A (AA) and can complicate any chronic inflammatory disorder, whether infectious, neoplastic, or rheumatic.

20. Name the infectious and neoplastic disorders most commonly associated with secondary amyloidosis.

Infections	Neoplasms
Tuberculosis	Hodgkin's disease
Leprosy	Non-Hodgkin's lymphoma
Chronic pyelonephritis	Renal cell carcinoma
Bronchiectasis	Melanoma
Osteomyelitis	Cancers of GI, GU tract, lung
Parenteral drug use	

21. What three rheumatic diseases are most commonly complicated by secondary amyloidosis?

Rheumatoid arthritis, juvenile rheumatoid arthritis, and ankylosing spondylitis.

There is a 5–15% overall incidence of amyloid in rheumatoid arthritis, with an average disease duration of 16 years before the onset of amyloidosis. A frequency of 0.14% for amyloidosis in juvenile rheumatoid arthritis in the United States compares with an overall frequency of about 10% in Europe. The reasons for this difference are unknown. Ankylosing spondylitis has also been associated with secondary amyloidosis. Amyloidosis has been cited as a relatively common cause of death in patients with ankylosing spondylitis, and this disease has been relatively over-represented in reports of secondary amyloidosis.

22. Amyloid may occur in localized deposits, resembling tumors. The lung, skin, larynx, eye, and bladder are common sites. Most patients with localized amyloid do not have systemic disease. What histopathologic finding prompts investigation for systemic disease?

Vascular involvement is common in primary and secondary amyloidosis, and if it is present in the biopsy of a localized form, further evaluation for widespread disease is required.

23. Name two forms of amyloid localized to the brain and three localized to endocrine tissue.

Aβ (β protein)—Alzheimer's disease, Down's syndrome
APrP (prion protein origin)—Creutzfeldt-Jakob disease, Gerstmann-Sträussler syndrome, kuru, scrapie
ACal (calcitonin)—medullary carcinoma of the thyroid
AANP (atrial natriuretic factor)—isolated atrial amyloid
AIAPP (islet amyloid polypeptide)—type II diabetes mellitus, insulinoma

24. Study of many types of hereditary amyloidosis have shown them to be due to single amino acid variants of transthyretin. What is their pattern of inheritance?

Autosomal dominant.

25. Describe the features of amyloidosis of chronic dialysis.

Serum β_2-microglobulin levels are elevated 50–100 times normal in patients on long-term dialysis. However, high levels alone do not predict the development of amyloid. Generally, patients with amyloidosis will have been on hemodialysis at least 5 years. Carpal tunnel syndrome is the most common clinical presentation. Chronic arthralgias, especially of the shoulders, may also occur. Cystic bone changes and a destructive arthropathy can develop. Rarely, other areas (skin, gastrointestinal tract) are involved.

26. How is the diagnosis of amyloidosis established?

Polarized light microscopy showing the characteristic apple-green birefringence of Congo red-stained tissue.

27. Which tissue should be biopsied?

A screening biopsy should be performed first, as the sensitivity is good and complications are few. Abdominal fat pad aspiration may be the most useful, as it has a sensitivity near 90%. Screening sites and their yields are:

Abdominal fat pat	90%
Bone marrow	30–50%
Rectal mucosa	73–84%
Gingiva	60%
Skin	50%

28. What if the screening biopsies are negative?

If screens are negative, biopsy of a clinically involved site may be undertaken, realizing that the risk of bleeding may be substantial. For this reason do *not* biopsy a liver that is grossly enlarged. Yields for clinically involved sites are:

Kidney	90–98%
Carpal ligament	90–95%
Liver	92–96%
Sural nerve	100%
Skin	45–83%

29. What laboratory studies should be performed?

All patients with systemic amyloidosis should be evaluated for evidence of an associated plasma cell dyscrasia using serum and urine protein electrophoresis *and* immunoelectrophoresis. Screening electrophoresis of serum and urine is insufficient to exclude the presence of a monoclonal band. Patients with amyloidosis associated with multiple myeloma will have a monoclonal protein in serum or urine. However, in up to 12% of patients with primary amyloidosis (not myeloma-associated), serum and urine studies will fail to show a monoclonal component.

30. Describe the pathogenesis of amyloidosis.

The pathogenesis is unknown, and there is no unified theory of pathogenesis. Little tissue reaction occurs around amyloid, and once deposited, amyloid resists proteolysis and phagocytosis. Features of the precursor proteins and/or host factors could result in abnormal processing by mononuclear phagocytic cells or ineffective degradation. Certain protein variants are "amyloidogenic," being more susceptible to the processing that leads to amyloidosis. The immunoglobulin light chain Vλ VI is highly associated with amyloidosis. Single amino acid variants of transthyretin are seen in many of the hereditary amyloidosis syndromes. Animal models suggest defective or inhibited enzymes may play a role in fibril deposition.

31. How is primary amyloidosis treated?

The control of light chain production by proliferating plasma cells has been the rationale for the use of cytotoxic agents. Melphalan-containing regimens have been shown to be superior to colchicine alone in the treatment of AL. However, melphalan-based therapy is not always effective and carries a risk of significant bone marrow damage. Noncytotoxic therapies (dimethyl sulfoxide [DMSO], vitamin E, and recombinant interferon α-2b) have no proven value.

32. Describe the treatment of secondary amyloidosis.

Mobilization and clearance of amyloid deposits are possible and are best recognized for patients with AA. A basic tenet is to control the underlying inflammatory disease. For example, treatment of osteomyelitis with amputation and aggressive surgical therapy for Crohn's disease have been reported to reverse or resolve nephrotic syndrome. Colchicine has also proved useful in treating renal amyloid complicating inflammatory bowel disease.

Most adults with AA suffer from rheumatoid arthritis or ankylosing spondylitis. The use of cytotoxic therapy in these patients remains controversial. Both DMSO and colchicine have been reported as useful. Chlorambucil is the most widely used therapy for amyloidosis complicating juvenile rheumatoid arthritis. Clinical remission of joint disease has been accompanied by lessened proteinuria and normal scan and plasma turnover studies of serum amyloid P, indicating regression of amyloid deposits. However, chlorambucil therapy carries a high incidence of azoospermia in males and risk of hematogenous malignancy in all patients.

33. How is the amyloidosis of familial Mediterranean fever (FMF) treated?

The excellent response of FMF to colchicine led to trials of colchicine in AL. Colchicine was first demonstrated to markedly decrease the attacks of polyserositis, in some patients completely suppressing attacks. Colchicine was then shown to be effective in the prevention of amyloidosis, decreasing the incidence of renal amyloidosis by two-thirds. In addition, colchicine can reverse the nephrotic syndrome in FMF patients and prevent recurrence of amyloid following renal transplantation in FMF patients who develop end-stage renal disease.

34. What factors are prognostic in AL amyloidosis?

The presence of multiple myeloma reduces the median survival from 13 months to 5 months and the 5-year survival from 20% to 0. Grouping of patients by clinical manifestation (heart failure, nephrotic syndrome, peripheral neuropathy, and other) is a useful guide to long-term prognosis. The presence of heart failure is associated with the worst prognosis (median survival, 7.7 months). The best prognosis has long been associated with peripheral neuropathy when it occurs as the sole manifestation (median survival, 56 months). Although the 24-hour urinary total protein excretion does not affect survival, the presence of urinary free light chains and increased serum creatine are powerful prognostic indicators. A trend has been noted for superior survival in female patients.

BIBLIOGRAPHY

1. Buxbaum J: Mechanisms of disease: Monoclonal immunoglobulin deposition. Hematol Oncol Clin North Am 6:323–346, 1992.
2. Buxbaum J: The amyloidoses. In Schumacher HR Jr (ed): Primer on the Rheumatic Diseases, 10th ed. Atlanta, Arthritis Foundation, 1993, pp 234–237.
3. Cohen AS: Amyloidosis. Bull Rheum Dis 40:1–12, 1991.
4. Cohen AS, et al: Survival of patients with primary (AL) amyloidosis. Am J Med 82:1182–1190, 1987.
5. Cornelis F, et al: Rheumatic syndromes and β_2-microglobulin amyloidosis in patients receiving long-term peritoneal dialysis. Arthritis Rheum 32:785–788, 1989.
6. Dhillon V, Woo P, Isenberg D: Amyloidosis in the rheumatic diseases. Ann Rheum Dis 48:696–701, 1989.
7. Duston MA: Diagnosis of amyloidosis by abdominal fat aspiration. Am J Med 82:412–414, 1987.
8. Gertz M, Kyle R: Primary systemic amyloidosis—A diagnostic primer. Mayo Clin Proc 64:1505–1519, 1989.
9. Gertz MA, Kyle RA: Amyloidosis: Prognosis and treatment. Semin Arthritis Rheum 24:124–138, 1994.
10. Glenner GG: Amyloid deposits and amyloidosis: The β fibrilloses. N Engl J Med 302:1283–1292, 1333–1343, 1980.
11. Kyle R, Greipp P: Amyloidosis (AL): Clinical and laboratory features in 229 cases. Mayo Clin Proc 58:665–683, 1983.

78. RAYNAUD'S PHENOMENON

Steven A. Older, M.D.

1. What is Raynaud's phenomenon (RP)?

Raynaud's phenomenon is a vasospastic disorder characterized by episodic attacks of well-demarcated color changes with numbness and pain of the digits on exposure to cold. It may be primary (idiopathic) or secondary to an underlying condition.

2. How common is RP? Who gets it?

The prevalence of RP is approximately 3–4% in most studies, although it may be higher (up to 30%) in colder climates. The true prevalence may never be established because many people with mild or infrequent attacks do not seek medical attention. Primary RP is a predominantly female disorder, with female:male ratios ranging from 4:1 to 9:1. From the data currently available, RP appears to be equally distributed among different ethnic groups.

3. Which conditions are associated with secondary RP?
Conditions associated with secondary RP may be grouped into six broad categories: systemic rheumatic disorders, occupational (vibration) injury, drugs or chemicals, occlusive arterial disease, hyperviscosity syndromes, and miscellaneous causes (see table).

Causes of Secondary Raynaud's Phenomenon

CATEGORY	CONDITION
Systemic rheumatic disorders	Systemic sclerosis, systemic lupus erythematosus, polymyositis–dermatomyositis, Sjögren's syndrome, rheumatoid arthritis, vasculitis, chronic active hepatitis, primary pulmonary hypertension
Occupations	Rock drillers, lumberjacks, grinders, riveters, pneumatic hammer operators
Drugs or chemicals	Beta-blockers, ergot, methysergide, vinblastine, bleomycin, imipramine, bromocriptine, clonidine, cyclosporine, vinyl chloride
Occlusive arterial disease	Postembolic/thrombotic arterial occlusion, carpal tunnel syndrome, thoracic outlet syndromes
Hyperviscosity diseases	Polycythemia, cryoglobulinemia, paraproteinemia, thrombocytosis, leukemia
Miscellaneous	Infections (bacterial endocarditis, Lyme borreliosis, infectious mononucleosis, viral hepatitis), reflex sympathetic dystrophy, fibromyalgia, peripheral arteriovenous fistula, carcinoma

From Klippel JH: Raynaud's phenomenon: The French tricolor. Arch Intern Med 151:2389–2393, 1991, with permission.

4. Discuss the relevant pathophysiology of RP.
Digital artery blood flow is dependent on a pressure gradient that, in turn, is dependent on vessel length, blood viscosity, and vessel radius. The radius of a vessel is most subject to change and may be altered by variations in wall thickness, intrinsic smooth muscle tone, and sympathetic nervous system activity. A given reduction in radius results in a fourfold decrease in blood flow (Law of Poiseuille).

In both primary and secondary RP, the mechanisms that cause acute vasospasm are unclear. Current leading hypotheses derive from two earlier theories:
- Hyperactivity of the sympathetic nervous system—Maurice Raynaud, 1862
- Local dysregulation of vascular tone ("local fault")—Thomas Lewis, 1929
    Increased peripheral alpha-adrenergic responsiveness
    Deficiency of calcitionin gene-related peptide, a vasodilatory neuropeptide
    High levels of endothelin, a potent vasoconstrictor

In secondary RP, intrinsic vascular abnormalities may predispose to digital artery closure. Proximal vascular obstruction or occlusion (e.g., thoracic outlet syndromes) or rheologic abnormalities (e.g., hyperviscosity or polycythemia) may also facilitate digital artery closure.

5. Describe the triphasic color response of RP and briefly explain the pathophysiology of each phase.
The sequential color changes of RP have been likened to the colors of the French flag ("the French Tricolor"):[9] a white to blue to red. Initial digital artery vasospasm causes a **pallor** (blanching) of the digit (see following figure), which gives way to **cyanosis** as static venous blood deoxygenates. Reactive hyperemia causes the final stage, **rubor**.

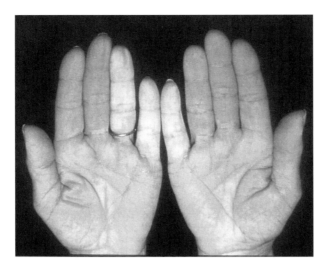

The pallor (blanching) stage of Raynaud's phenomenon. (From the Revised Clinical Slide Collection of the Rheumatic Diseases, copyright 1991. Used by permission of the American College of Rheumatology.)

6. Contrast the clinical presentations of primary and secondary RP.

The onset of primary RP usually occurs in women between the ages of 15 and 45 years. The fingers are most commonly affected, but 40% of patients have attacks in the toes as well. Ears, nose, tongue, and lips may also be involved. For reasons unexplained, the thumbs are usually spared. Patients will describe well-demarcated color changes involving part or all of one or more digits (never the "whole hand") on exposure to cold. The color changes are accompanied by numbness during the ischemic phase and by a throbbing pain during the reactive hyperemic phase. The frequency, duration, and severity of attacks vary widely, with some patients having several attacks per day and others having two or three per winter. Rarely in primary RP do trophic complications such as digital ulceration, pitting, fissuring, and gangrene arise as a result of recurrent attacks.

The onset of secondary RP is usually in the third and fourth decades and may be seen in either men or women depending on the underlying condition. The symptoms of digital vasospasm are the same as those of primary RP; however, secondary RP patients are more prone to trophic complications. Signs and symptoms related to an underlying condition are usually obvious by careful history and physical examination.

7. Are all three color changes required for the diagnosis of RP?

No. The full triphasic response is infrequently seen. Most authorities agree that pallor is the most characteristic feature and should be required for the diagnosis. The significance of cyanosis alone is unclear; it has been noted in healthy individuals in the absence of vasospasm. Recent studies suggest that at least two color changes be present to establish a definitive diagnosis of RP.

8. Is cold the only precipitant of RP?

Cold exposure is by far the most common precipitating cause of RP, especially when accompanied by pressure. Typical examples would be the gripping of a cold steering wheel, holding a cold soft drink can, or grasping items in the frozen food section of a grocery store. Other stimuli include emotion, trauma, hormones, and certain chemicals such as those found in cigarette smoke. Additional "causes," like vibration injury, are more correctly attributed to the associated conditions of secondary RP.

9. Is the vasospasm of RP restricted to digital vessels?

A large case control study has demonstrated an increased frequency of migraine headaches and chest pain in patients with primary RP. Other studies have implicated vasospasm of the myocardium, lungs, kidneys, esophagus, and placenta. Although definitive proof is lacking, most authorities support the contention that RP is a systemic vasospastic disorder.

10. In the evaluation of a patient with RP, what abnormalities may be noted on physical examination?

Patients may occasionally present to the clinic with an ongoing attack of RP, thereby allowing a definitive diagnosis. Induction of an attack in the physician's office by submergence of hands in an ice water bath is frequently unsuccessful, seldom necessary, and sometimes dangerous.

The physical examination in primary RP is normal. The real goal in patients with RP is to discern the presence or absence of findings attributable to an underlying condition of secondary RP. A careful search for evidence of collagen vascular disease is required. Allen's and Adson's tests as well as nailfold capillary microscopy (see below) should be performed on all patients.

11. Describe the technique, clinical findings, and prognostic value of nailfold capillary microscopy (NCM).

Along with the retina, the nailfold represents one of the only sites in the body where direct visualization of the vasculature may be readily accomplished. The technique of NCM involves the placement of a drop of immersion oil on the cuticle of one or more digits (usually the ring or middle fingers), and visualization of the capillaries through an ophthalmoscope set at +40 diopters. One focuses the ophthalmoscope to within millimeters of the oil until the nailbed capillaries come into focus.

The normal nailbed will demonstrate a confluent distribution of fine capillary loops (see following figure). Dilated tortuous capillary loops and areas of avascularity ("dropout") are often demonstrated in patients with underlying collagen vascular diseases, especially systemic sclerosis, dermatomyositis, and mixed connective tissue disease.

In RP patients without clinical evidence of an underlying condition (primary RP), normal NCM connotes an excellent prognosis. Collagen vascular disease rarely develops in these patients. A small percentage of primary RP patients who demonstrate abnormal NCM may eventually develop a collagen vascular disease, typically limited systemic sclerosis.

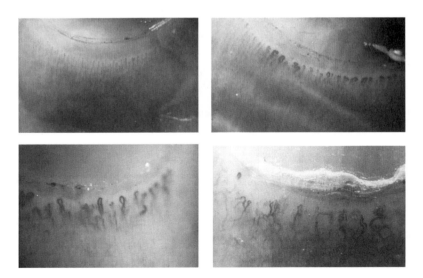

Nailfold capillary microscopy. *Upper left,* Normal pattern. *Upper right,* Dilated capillary loops in systemic sclerosis. *Lower left,* Dilated loops and avascularity in adult dermatomyositis. *Lower right,* Childhood dermatomyositis. (From the Revised Clinical Slide Collection on the Rheumatic Diseases, copyright 1991. Used by permission of the American College of Rheumatology.)

12. Which laboratory studies are worthwhile in the evaluation of a patient with RP?
To date, no laboratory test is pathognomonic of RP. In primary RP, laboratory tests should be normal or negative, although up to one third of patients will exhibit low titer antinuclear antibodies in their serum. Less than 25% of these patients develop an autoimmune disorder. In patients with clinical evidence suggestive of an underlying collagen vascular disease, appropriate studies should be obtained.

13. List the "red flags" that would be worrisome for the potential presence or later development of secondary RP.
- Onset of digital vasospasm after age 30
- RP in a man
- Unilateral involvement or color changes involving the whole hand
- Trophic changes of the digits (ulcers, pits, gangrene)
- Abnormal nailfold microscopy
- Sclerodactyly, rashes, or other obvious evidence of an underlying condition
- Serologic presence of autoantibodies, especially anticentromere antibodies, ANA with a nucleolar pattern, or antinuclear antibodies against a specific antigen (SCL-70, RNP, Sm, SS-A, SS-B).

14. Which general measures are important in the treatment of patients with RP?
The majority of RP patients respond best to simple prevention measures. Careful planning of one's activities of daily living minimizes unnecessary exposure to cold. Because reductions in core temperature as well as peripheral temperature may induce digital vasospasm, it is important to promote "total body" heat conservation. Loose-fitting, layered clothing, warm socks, hats, and scarves should be worn in addition to gloves or mittens. Chemical or battery hand and foot warmers are useful. Tobacco must be avoided. Nonpharmacologic treatments that have shown some benefit include temperature biofeedback, autogenic training (similar to self-hypnosis), and Pavlovian conditioning.

15. When is pharmacologic intervention indicated in the management of RP?
Most patients with primary RP will not require pharmacologic therapy. Those with secondary RP frequently require (but less often respond) to medication. In general, pharmacologic intervention is indicated in patients who suffer frequent, prolonged, and/or severe episodes of RP in the setting of adequate preventative measures or with minimal provocation. Patients who manifest evidence of ischemic injury (digital pitting, etc.) should definitely be considered for medical management. Many patients who do require medication may only need it during the colder months of the year.

16. Which medications have been useful in the management of RP?
At the present time, no drug has been approved in the United States for the treatment of RP; however, several have demonstrated utility. Calcium channel blockers, especially nifedipine, isradipine, and amlodipine, are best tolerated and most efficacious. Slow-release preparations are unproven in controlled studies but commonly used. Sympatholytic agents like prazosin or phenoxybenzamine have been beneficial, as have direct vasodilators such as topical nitrates and hydralazine.

Several other drugs are currently under evaluation. Of particular interest are ketanserin, a serotonin receptor antagonist that blocks serotonin-mediated vasoconstriction and platelet aggregation, and iloprost, a prostaglandin analogue that is thought to cause direct vasodilation and inhibition of platelet aggregation.

17. What can be done for patients who are refractory to standard therapy?
Surgical sympathectomy may be considered in patients who have failed more conservative measures and who present with impending digital necrosis or evidence of recurrent ischemic complications. It can be performed at the cervical, lumbar, or digital levels.

Permanent surgical ablation should be preceded by demonstrated efficacy using a bipuvicaine stellate ganglion block or epidural infusion. If temporary sympathetic block results in clear clinical improvement, one may either proceed with surgical sympathectomy or attempt a trial of oral vasodilators as maintenance therapy. As with the pharmacologic modalities, sympathectomies have not achieved proven efficacy status in controlled RP treatment trials.

18. What is the prognosis for patients with RP?

The prognosis for patients with primary RP is excellent. In 10% of patients, attacks disappear completely. One third report a decrease in the number and severity of attacks over time and more than one third report no change in symptoms. Digital vascular complications occur rarely. The vast majority of patients with primary RP never develop an underlying condition associated with secondary RP. This is especially true if nailfold capillary microscopy and autoantibody testing are negative.

The prognosis for patients with secondary RP is generally dependent on the underlying condition. Intrinsic vascular disease is often present. Complications arising from vasospasm (see question 6) are far more prevalent. Elimination of offending agents or correction of anatomic, rheologic, or metabolic abnormalities when possible often results in a resolution or reduction of symptoms.

BIBLIOGRAPHY

1. Belch JJF: Raynaud's phenomenon. Curr Opin Rheumatol 3:960–966,1991.
2. Belch JJF: The clinical assessment of the scleroderma spectrum disorders. Br J Rheumatol 32:353–356, 1993.
3. Brennan P, Silman A, Black C, et al: Validity and reliability of three methods used in the diagnosis of Raynaud's phenomenon. Br J Rheumatol 32:357–361, 1993.
4. Campbell PM, LeRoy EC: Raynaud phenomenon. Semin Arthritis Rheum 16:92–103, 1986.
5. Coffman JD: Raynaud's Phenomenon. New York, Oxford University Press, 1989.
6. Coffman JD: The diagnosis of Raynaud's phenomenon. Clin Dermatol 12:283–289. 1994.
7. Kahaleh B, Matucci-Cerinic M: Raynaud's phenomenon and scleroderma: Dysregulated neuroendothelial control of vascular tone. Arthritis Rheum 38:1–4, 1995.
8. Kallenberg CGM: Early detection of connective tissue disease in patients with Raynaud's phenomenon. Rheum Dis Clin 16:11–30, 1990.
9. Klippel JH: Raynaud's phenomenon: The French tricolor. Arch Intern Med 151:2389–2393, 1991.
10. LeRoy EC, Medsger TA Jr: Raynaud's phenomenon: A proposal for classification. Clin Exp Rheumatol 10:485–488, 1992.
11. Maricq HR, Carpentier PH, Weinrich MC, et al: Geographic variation in the prevalence of Raynaud's phenomenon: Charleston, SC, USA, vs Tarentaise, Savoie, France. J Rheumatol 20:70–76, 1993.
12. O'Keeffe ST, Tsapatsaris NP, Beetham WP Jr: Increased prevalence of migraine and chest pain in patients with primary Raynaud's disease. Ann Intern Med 116:985–989, 1992.
13. Seibold JR, Allegar NE: The treatment of Raynaud's phenomenon. Clin Dermatol 12:317–321. 1994.
14. Taylor W: The hand-arm vibration syndrome—diagnosis, assessment and objective tests: A review. J R Soc Med 86:101–103, 1993.
15. Toumbis-Ioannou E, Cohen PR: Chemotherapy-induced Raynaud's phenomenon. Cleve Clin J Med 61:195–199, 1994.
16. Wigley FM: Raynaud's Phenomenon. Curr Opin Rheumatol 5:773–784, 1993.
17. Wigley FM, Matsumoto AK: Raynaud's phenomenon. In Weisman MH, Weinblatt ME (eds) : Treatment of the Rheumatic Diseases. Philadelphia, W.B. Saunders, 1995.

79. UVEITIS

Raymond J. Enzenauer, M.D.

1. What is uveitis?

The diagnostic term *uveitis* indicates the presence of inflammation in the uveal tract, which includes the iris, ciliary body, and choroid (see figure). Like arthritis, uveitis may be caused by many different diseases.

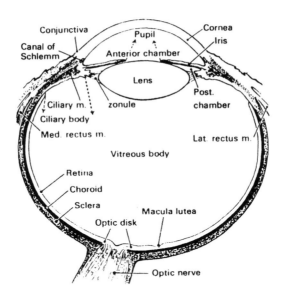

Diagram of a human eyeball. (From Stedman's Medical Dictionary, 23rd ed. Baltimore, Williams & Wilkins, 1976, p 500, with permission.)

2. List the four primary parameters used to characterize subsets of uveitis.
1. Anatomic location of inflammation (anterior, intermediate, posterior, panuveitis)
2. Laterality (unilateral, bilateral)
3. Onset (acute, insidious)
4. Duration (self-limited, chronic, recurrent)

The location, laterality, and onset of uveitis can assist in identifying a specific etiology of the uveitis. For example, HLA-B27-associated uveitis is almost always acute, anterior, and unilateral, while the uveitis associated with sarcoidosis may be a chronic, bilateral panuveitis.

3. Which laboratory tests are of diagnostic value for a patient with unclassified uveitis?
Chest roentgenogram and **fluorescent treponomal antibody absorption** (FTA-ABS). Because sarcoidosis and syphilis may have ocular inflammation without clinically apparent systemic disease, tests for these two entities are indicated in *all* patients with uveitis of unknown etiology. Specifically, one should obtain a serologic test for syphilis (FTA) and a chest roentgenogram to screen for sarcoidosis. Other laboratory tests should be ordered depending on the nature and setting of the uveitis.

Antinuclear antibody (ANA) testing is indicated only in the evaluation of pediatric patients with bilateral, chronic iritis, as this test is positive in up to 88% of patients with juvenile rheumatoid arthritis and iritis. It is not indicated for routine screening of adult patients with unclassified uveitis because a patient with uveitis and a positive ANA has a <1% chance of having systemic lupus erythematosus.

Similarly, a patient with uveitis and a positive **purified protein derivative** (PPD) test has only a 1% likelihood of having tuberculosis. PPD testing in uveitis should be limited to patients having an appropriate exposure history or an abnormal chest roentgenogram suggestive of tuberculosis.

HLA-B27 testing is only appropriate for patients presenting with acute, anterior uveitis. It is not helpful in the evaluation of patients with chronic, intermediate or posterior uveitis.

4. What percentage of acute anterior uveitis (AAU) is associated with HLA-B27? How does HLA-B27 affect presentation and outcome?
In a white population, AAU is associated with HLA-B27 in 50% of cases. Of patients with HLA-B27-positive AAU, more than half suffer from an associated seronegative spondyloarthropathy

(ankylosing spondylitis, Reiter's syndrome, psoriatic arthritis, or inflammatory bowel disease). Patients positive for HLA-B27 are often younger, are predominantly men, and have more frequent recurrences of AAU than patients negative for HLA-B27.

5. List a differential diagnosis of anterior uveitis. Which is the most common cause?

Idiopathic	52%
HLA-B27 (ocular only)	36%
Ankylosing spondylitis	8%
Reiter's syndrome	3%
Juvenile rheumatoid arthritis	<1%
Fuchs' iridocyclitis	<1%
Psoriatic arthritis	<1%
Inflammatory bowel disease	<1%
Acute interstitial nephritis	<1%
Kawasaki's disease	<1%
Posner-Schlossman syndrome (glaucomatocyclic crisis)	<1%

Idiopathic anterior uveitis is probably the most common form of anterior segment inflammation, accounting for >50% of cases.

6. Define intermediate uveitis and pars planitis.

Intermediate uveitis refers to an anatomic distribution of ocular inflammation primarily in the vitreous and peripheral retina just behind the lens. The condition is sometimes referred to as **peripheral uveitis** because the inflammation involves, or is adjacent to, the peripheral retina in the area of the pars plana. When there is a large white opacity, or "snowbank," over the pars plana and ora serrata, this subset of intermediate uveitis is termed **pars planitis.**

7. Define chronic uveitis. Describe the location of ocular inflammation and its etiology.

Chronic uveitis is defined as intraocular inflammation persisting for 3 months or more. Most patients have chronic anterior uveitis (46%), with panuveitis in 25%, intermediate uveitis in 15%, and isolated posterior uveitis in 14%. An associated condition can be found in 60% of cases, with Behçet's disease being the most common etiology, particularly in panuveitis patients.

8. What systemic diseases have been associated with intermediate uveitis?

Although most cases are idiopathic, underlying systemic disease may occasionally be found to include **sarcoidosis** (2–10%), **multiple sclerosis** (10%), or **infection** (syphilis, Lyme disease, tuberculosis).

9. List the rheumatic diseases most likely to be associated with uveitis. Compare their onset, laterality, and location.

RHEUMATIC DISEASE	ONSET	LATERALITY	LOCATION
Ankylosing spondylitis	Acute	Unilateral	Anterior
Juvenile rheumatoid arthritis	Insidious	Bilateral	Anterior
Psoriatic arthritis	Acute	Unilateral	Anterior
Reiter's syndrome	Acute	Unilateral	Anterior
Sjögren's syndrome	Insidious	Bilateral	Panuveitis

Adult rheumatoid arthritis is *not* associated with uveitis. Early literature that described ankylosing spondylitis as "rheumatoid spondylitis" contributed to the mistaken impression that patients with rheumatoid arthritis are at increased risk for uveitis.

10. How is the uveitis of juvenile rheumatoid arthritis (JRA) unique from all other causes of anterior uveitis?

Unlike patients with almost all other causes of anterior uveitis, JRA patients with anterior uveitis usually are asymptomatic, and the involved eye is often white, without obvious evidence of inflammation. As a result, complications of uveitis may develop before the inflammation is detected.

11. How do the typical presenting symptoms differ among anterior, intermediate, and posterior uveitis?

Anterior uveitis. Patients usually present with complaints of **pain, redness, and photophobia.** Most cases are **unilateral,** but bilateral disease can be seen in patients with interstitial nephritis or Sjögren's syndrome.

Intermediate uveitis. Patients usually complain of the insidious onset of **floaters** or **mild haziness** of vision. Typically, the external eye is quiet, and there is no pain or photophobia. Although initial complaints are usually limited to **one eye,** evidence of mild inflammation in the contralateral eye is common.

Posterior uveitis. Patients usually complain of the insidious onset of **blurred vision, floaters, and scotomata.** As in intermediate uveitis, the external eye is quiet and there is no pain or photophobia.

12. Define posterior uveitis. List the differential diagnosis of inflammation of the posterior uveal tract.

Posterior uveitis describes inflammation that involves the retina and vitreous near the optic nerve and macula.

Differential diagnosis of posterior uveitis[*]

Idiopathic retinal vasculitis (Eale's disease)	Acute posterior multifocal placoid pigment epitheliopathy
Sarcoidosis	Infectious posterior uveitis
Birdshot choroidoretinopathy	Herpes simplex-induced acute retinal necrosis
Behçet's disease	Cytomegalovirus retinitis
Vogt-Koyanagi-Harada syndrome	Toxoplasmosis retinochoroiditis[†]
Sympathetic ophthalmia	Syphilis
Serpiginous choroiditis	Histoplasmosis
	Tuberculosis

[*]An etiology (other than infection) is more often found in patients with panuveitis than isolated posterior uveitis.
[†]Toxoplasmosis is now thought to account for 30–50% of all granulomatous inflammations of the posterior segment of the eye and is the leading cause of posterior uveitis.

13. Which causes of uveitis have been associated with specific HLA types?

Reiter's syndrome	HLA-B27
Behçet disease	HLA-B51
Birdshot retinochoroidopathy	HLA-A29
Pars planitis	HLA-DR2

14. What are the indications for systemic corticosteroids in the management of uveitis?

Bilateral moderate to severe ocular inflammation *or* vision-threatening anterior- or posterior-segment inflammation unresponsive to topically or periocularly administered corticosteroids. Systemic therapy is generally reserved for patients whose visual acuity has declined to 20/40 or worse because of an inflammatory condition and in whom recovery of vision is thought to be possible.

Usually, the initial dosage is 60 mg or 1–1.5 mg/kg/day, which is subsequently tapered slowly. A good approach is to taper the dosage to 15–20 mg over 3–4 weeks and to observe the patient carefully for any recurrence of symptoms. If the patient's condition remains stable, a slow taper off the medication may then be attempted.

15. Discuss the indications and contraindications for cytotoxic therapy for uveitis.

Indications: Sight-threatening uveitis unresponsive to corticosteroids or patients intolerant of corticosteroids because of side effects. Forms of uveitis commonly requiring cytotoxic therapy include sympathetic ophthalmia, posterior segment Behçet's disease, and ocular Wegener's granulomatosis.

Contraindications: Any uveitis of infectious origin.

16. What is the drug of choice for uveitis associated with various etiologies?

Wegener's granulomatosis	Oral cyclophosphamide
Behçet disease	Oral chlorambucil
Reiter's syndrome	Topical corticosteroids
Vogt-Koyanagi-Harada syndrome	Oral corticosteroids
Sarcoidosis	Topical/oral corticosteroids

17. Which immunosuppressive drugs are reported to be effective in the treatment of uveitis?

Cyclophosphamide	po	1–2 mg/kg/day
	iv	500–1000 mg/M²/mo
Chlorambucil	po	0.1 mg/kg/day
Methotrexate	po/im	10–25 mg/wk
Cyclosporine	po	5–7 mg/kg/day
Bromocriptine	po	2.5 mg 3–4 times daily
Dapsone	po	25–50 mg 2–3 times daily
Colchicine	po	0.65 mg 2–3 times daily

18. List the frequency of the common ocular presentations of sarcoidosis.

Anterior uveitis 54%	Posterior uveitis 15%
Panuveitis 27%	Intermediate uveitis 4%

19. What masquerade syndromes mimic uveitis? How can they be distinguished clinically?

Masquerade syndromes include leukemia, lymphoma, retinitis pigmentosa, malignant melanoma, antiphospholipid antibody syndrome, and retinoblastoma. The diagnosis of a masquerade syndrome may be suggested by the appearance of the eye alone, age of the patient, or lack of response to standard uveitis therapy.

20. What are some causes of an elevated serum angiotensin-converting enzyme (ACE) level in a patient with uveitis?

Sarcoidosis, liver disease (primary biliary cirrhosis, granulomatous hepatitis, alcoholic liver disease), diabetes mellitus (especially with retinopathy), granulomatous infections (tuberculosis, coccidioidomycosis, leprosy, HIV), Wegener's granulomatosis, pneumoconioses (berylliosis, asbestosis, silicosis), Gaucher's disease, Hodgkin's disease, hyperthyroidism.

BIBLIOGRAPHY

1. Bloom JN: Uveitis in childhood. Opthalmol Clin North Am 3:163–176, 1990.
2. Forrester JV: Endogenous posterior uveitis. Br J Ophthalmol 74:620–623, 1990.
3. Hemedy R, Tauber J, Foster CS: Immunosuppressive drugs in immune and inflammatory ocular disease. Surv Ophthalmol 35:369–385, 1991.
4. Herman DC: Endogenous uveitis: Current concepts of treatment. Mayo Clin Proc 65:671–683, 1990.
5. Malinowski SM, Folk JC, Pulido JS: Pars planitis. Curr Opin Ophthalmol 5:72–82, 1994.
6. Nussenblatt RB, Palestine AG (eds): Uveitis: Fundamentals and Clinical Practice. Chicago, Yearbook, 1989.
7. Rosenbaum JT: Characterization of uveitis associated with spondyloarthritis. J Rheumatol 16:792–796, 1989.
8. Rosenbaum JT: An algorithm for the systemic evaluation of patients with uveitis: Guidelines for the consultant. Semin Arthritis Rheum 19:248–257, 1990.
9. Rosenbaum JT, Wernick R: The utility of routine screening of patients with uveitis for systemic lupus erythematosus or tuberculosis. Arch Ophthalmol 108:1291–1293, 1990.
10. Rothova A, van Veenendaal WG, Linssen A, et al: Clinical features of acute anterior uveitis. Am J Ophthalmol 103:137–145, 1987.
11. Studdy PR, Lapworth R, Bird R: Angiotensin-converting enzyme and its clinical significance—a review. J Clin Pathol 36:938–947, 1983.
12. Weiner A, BenEzra D: Clinical patterns and associated conditions in chronic uveitis. Am J Ophthalmol 112:151–158, 1991.

80. RHEUMATIC SYNDROMES ASSOCIATED WITH SARCOIDOSIS

Daniel F. Battafarano, D.O.

1. What is sarcoidosis?
Sarcoidosis is a multisystem disorder of unknown etiology characterized by **noncaseating granulomas** in biopsy specimens from clinically involved or uninvolved organs.

2. Who is affected by sarcoidosis?
Primarily young adults in the third or fourth decade of life, with a slight female predominance. Sarcoidosis occurs most frequently in African-Americans and northern European whites.

3. What are the immunologic features of sarcoidosis?
In the peripheral blood, there is evidence of depressed cellular immunity and enhanced humoral immunity. The depressed cellular immunity is manifested by lymphopenia, a low CD4/CD8 T-cell ratio (0.8/1), and cutaneous anergy. (In contrast, the pulmonary lesion in sarcoidosis is characterized by CD4+ T-cell infiltration.) Increased humoral immunity is noted by the presence of a polyclonal gammopathy and autoantibody production. Antinuclear antibodies, rheumatoid factor, antilymphocyte antibodies, and circulating immune complexes are often present in sarcoid patients.

4. What is the typical clinical presentation of sarcoidosis?
Sarcoidosis typically presents asymptomatically with an abnormal chest roentgenogram that shows hilar and paratracheal adenopathy, evidence of parenchymal infiltrate, or both.

5. Describe the stages of sarcoidosis and their prognosis.

STAGE	CHEST RADIOGRAPHIC FINDINGS	REMISSION RATE (%)
0	Normal	—
1	Bilateral hilar adenopathy	60–80
2	Bilateral hilar adenopathy with parenchymal infiltrate	30–50
3	Parenchymal infiltrates without hilar adenopathy	< 20

6. What are the extrathoracic clinical manifestations of sarcoidosis?
The most common extrathoracic manifestations are **cutaneous** and **ocular involvement.** Cutaneous involvement occurs in one-third of patients and may be manifest as erythema nodosum in early sarcoidosis or as subcutaneous nodules, papules, plaques, and lupus pernio in chronic disease. Eye involvement can be seen in 20% and typically involves the conjunctiva, lacrimal gland, or uveal tract. Arthralgias and arthritis are present in up to 50%.

Hepatomegaly (30%) and splenomegaly (10%) are common findings but rarely cause significant complications. Bilateral parotid enlargement is seen in <10% and is associated with xerostomia. Neurologic findings are observed in 5%, with unilateral facial nerve palsy being most common. Heart involvement (5%) presents with arrhythmias, left ventricular dysfunction, and pericarditis. The hypothalamic-pituitary axis may be involved and classically presents as diabetes insipidus. Kidney and gastrointestinal organs are rarely affected.

7. Where are granulomas most commonly found on biopsy in sarcoidosis?
Noncaseating granulomas are widely distributed and have been reported in many organs. They are most commonly found in the lung (86%), lymph nodes (86%), liver (86%), muscle (75%),

spleen (63%), heart (20%), kidney (19%), bone marrow (17%), and pancreas (6%). Granulomas may produce elevated serum angiotensin-converting enzyme (ACE) levels and may secrete 1,25-dihydrocholecalciferol responsible for clinical hypercalcemia.

8. Is the serum ACE level useful for the diagnosis of sarcoidosis?

No. The ACE level is elevated in only 60–80% of all patients with sarcoidosis. It is also elevated in various other diseases, including miliary tuberculosis, histoplasmosis, Gaucher's disease, silicosis, asbestosis, leprosy, HIV infection, hepatitis, hyperthyroidism, and diabetes. The ACE levels can be useful in individual patients if elevated at the time of diagnosis. Serial levels in these patients tend to correlate with disease activity and will normalize in response to effective medical treatment.

9. How do acute and chronic sarcoid arthritis differ clinically?

FEATURES	ACUTE	CHRONIC
Initial clinical manifestation	Common	Not seen
Joint involvement	Symmetrical; ankles, knees, wrists, PIP joints	Same as acute + dactylitis
Hilar adenopathy	Common, no parenchymal disease	May be seen with parenchymal disease
HLA association	B8, DR3, in whites of Northern European ancestry	Not known
Synovial fluid	Mildly inflammatory; 3000 cells (80% mononuclear)	Inflammatory; 25,000 cells (90% neutrophil)
Synovial biopsy	Synovial hyperplasia, no inflammatory infiltrate	Sarcoid granuloma
Destructive bony lesions	Absent	Present
Clinical course	Benign, self-limited	Chronic

Modified from Mathur A, Kremer JM: Immunology, rheumatic features, and therapy of sarcoidosis. Curr Opin Rheumatol 4:76–80, 1992.

10. What is Lofgren's syndrome?

This is a triad of acute arthritis, erythema nodosum, and bilateral hilar adenopathy in a patient with sarcoidosis. The arthritis typically involves the ankles, knees and/or wrists. These patients respond very well to corticosteroid therapy and have an excellent prognosis with a >90% remission rate.

11. What are the rheumatic manifestations of sarcoidosis?

MANIFESTATION	FREQUENCY IN SARCOIDOSIS (% OF PATIENTS)	DIFFERENTIAL DIAGNOSIS
Arthritis	15%	Rheumatoid arthritis, gonoccocal arthritis, rheumatic fever, SLE, gout, spondyloarthropathies
Parotid gland enlargement	5	Sjögren's syndrome
Upper airway disease (sinusitis, laryngeal inflammation, saddle nose deformity)	3	Wegener's granulomatosis
Uveitis	19	
Anterior	18	Spondyloarthropathies
Posterior	7	Behçet's
Keratoconjunctivitis	5	Sjögren's syndrome
Proptosis	1	Wegener's granulomatosis
Myositis	4	Polymyositis
Mononeuritis multiplex	1	Systemic vasculitis
Facial nerve palsy	2	Lyme disease

Modified from Hellman DB: Sarcoidosis. In Schumacher HR, et al (eds): Primer on the Rheumatic Diseases, 10th ed. Atlanta, Arthritis Foundation, 1993.

12. How does muscular sarcoidosis present clinically?

Muscle involvement in sarcoidosis is usually asymptomatic. There are three clinical presentations that are well-recognized: nodular, acute myositic, and chronic myopathic. The nodular presentation is the least common type, involving the musculotendinous junctions. Acute inflammatory myositis is rare and is seen more commonly in women. Chronic myopathy is the most common form and is manifested by an insidious onset of proximal symmetrical muscle weakness. Muscle enzyme levels, electromyography, and muscle biopsies are necessary to differentiate the types of muscle involvement.

13. What osseous changes occur in patients with sarcoidosis?

The overall incidence of osseous sarcoid varies between 1–13%. The phalanges of the hands are most commonly involved. The metacarpophalangeal joints, metacarpals, and wrists are usually spared. Radiographic findings include soft tissue swelling, periarticular osteopenia, joint-space narrowing, cyst formation, eccentric/punched-out erosions, trabecular changes, pathologic fractures, and phalangeal fragmentation.

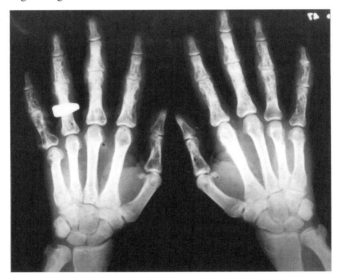

Osseous sarcoidosis involving the hands. The phalanges demonstrate a coarsened, reticulated or lacelike trabecular pattern that can be seen in chronic sarcoid arthritis.

14. Can sarcoidosis and other connective tissue diseases coexist?

Yes. Several reports have described sarcoidosis in patients with other rheumatic diseases, including systemic lupus erythematosus, rheumatoid arthritis, Sjögren's syndrome, and spondyloarthropathies. This occurrence is felt to be a coincidence since there is not a known common etiopathogenesis.

15. How is sarcoidosis usually treated?

Corticosteroids (30–60 mg) are considered the most effective treatment for sarcoidosis. Significant impairment of vital organs (lung, heart, eye, kidney, or brain) or hypercalcemia is a clear indication for corticosteroid therapy. NSAIDs and/or corticosteroids (15–40 mg) are used for joint and muscle involvement. Colchicine can be effective for acute arthritis. Chloroquine/hydroxychloroquine and low-dose methotrexate have been effective for long-term management of musculoskeletal involvement in selected patients. Cutaneous disease is typically treated with corticosteroids (topical or oral), but antimalarials and low-dose methotrexate have been useful for chronic lesions.

BIBLIOGRAPHY

1. Bascom RA, Johns CJ: The natural history and management of sarcoidosis. Adv Intern Med 31: 1986.
2. Chapelon C, Ziza JM, Piette JC, et al: Neurosarcoidosis: Signs, course and treatment in 35 confirmed cases. Medicine 69:261–276, 1990.
3. Douglas AC, Macleod JG, Matthews JD: Symptomatic sarcoidosis of skeletal muscle. J Neurol Neurosurg Psychiatry 36:1034–1040, 1973.
4. Enzenauer RJ, West SG: Sarcoidosis in autoimmune disease. Semin Arthritis Rheum 22:1–17, 1992.
5. Hellman DB: Sarcoidosis. In Schumacher HR, Klippel JH, Koopman WJ (eds): Primer on the Rheumatic Diseases, 10th ed. Atlanta, Arthritis Foundation, 1993.
6. Longscope WT, Frieman DG: A study of sarcoidosis: Based on a combined investigation of 160 cases including 30 autopsies from the John Hopkins Hospital and Massachusetts General Hospital. Medicine 31:1–132, 1952.
7. Mathur A, Kremer JM: Immunopathology, rheumatic features, and therapy of sarcoidosis. Curr Opin Rheumatol 4:76–80, 1992.
8. Mitchell DN, Scadding JG, Heard BE, Hinson KF: Sarcoidosis: Histopathological definition and clinical diagnosis. J Clin Pathol 30:395, 1977.
9. Murray JF, Nadel JA (eds): Textbook of Respiratory Medicine, 2nd ed. Philadelphia, W.B. Saunders, 1994, pp 1873–1888.
10. Myers GB, Gottlieb AM, Mattman PE, et al: Joint and muscle manifestations in sarcoidosis. Am J Med 12:161–169, 1952.
11. Sartoris DJ, Resnick D, Resnick C, Yaghmai I: Musculoskeletal manifestations of sarcoidosis. Semin Roentgenol 20:376–386, 1990.
12. Schumacher HR: Sarcoidosis. In McCarty DJ, Koopman WJ (eds): Arthritis and Allied Conditions, 12th ed. Philadelphia, Lea & Febiger, 1993, pp 1449–1455.
13. Silverstein A, Siltzbach LE: Muscle involvement in sarcoidosis: Asymptomatic myositis, and myopathy. Arch Neurol 21:235–241, 1969.
14. Spilberg I, Siltzbach LE, McEwen C: The arthritis of sarcoidosis. Arthritis Rheum 12:126–137, 1969.
15. Stobo JD, Hellman DB: Sarcoidosis. In Cohen AS, Bennet JD (eds): Rheumatology and Immunology, 2nd ed. Orlando, Grune & Stratton, 1986, pp 301–309.

81. RHEUMATIC DISORDERS IN THE DIALYSIS PATIENT

Mark Jarek, M.D.

1. What is renal osteodystrophy?

The term *renal osteodystrophy,* which was introduced by Liu and Chu in 1943, refers to the full spectrum of musculoskeletal disorders associated with renal failure. Because the kidney plays a critical role in the overall regulation of mineral homeostasis, the development of renal failure has widespread consequences for the skeleton. Some of the musculoskeletal disorders that develop in chronic renal failure and dialysis can be recalled with the mnemonic **VITAMINS ABCDE:**

    V – **V**ascular calcification
    I – **I**nfections (osteomyelitis, septic arthritis)
    T – **T**umoral calcifications
    A – **A**myloid arthropathy (β_2-microglobulin)
    M – **M**etabolic bone disease (osteomalacia, osteoporosis)
    I – **I**nfarction (osteonecrosis)
    N – **N**odules (tophi)
    S – **S**econdary hyperparathyroidism

    A – **A**luminum toxicity
    B – **B**ursitis (olecranon)
    C – **C**rystal arthropathy (gout, CPDD, hydroxyapatite)
    D – **D**igital clubbing
    E – **E**rosive spondyloarthropathy

2. Why does secondary hyperparathyroidism develop in chronic renal failure? How does this lead to bone disease?

Secondary hyperparathyroidism starts relatively early, when the glomerular filtration rate is in the range of 60–90 ml/min, as evidenced by increased levels of parathyroid hormone (PTH) and histologic changes in bone. As renal function deteriorates, these changes become more dramatic. Several factors in patients with chronic renal failure contribute to the sustained increases in PTH secretion and, ultimately, to parathyroid gland hyperplasia.

- Hyperphosphatemia due to impaired renal excretion
- Impaired renal hydroxylation of 25-hydroxyvitamin D to 1,25-dihydroxyvitamin D
- Low calcium intake and absorption
- Insensitivity of the parathyroid gland to the suppressive effects of calcium on PTH secretion

The end result of each of these defects is a sustained increase in PTH release, which stimulates osteoclast activation and rapid bone resorption. Secondary hyperparathyroidism is usually asymptomatic but may cause bone pain and polyarthralgias.

3. List the characteristic radiographic features of secondary hyperparathyroidism.
Early
Subperiosteal resorption in the hands, wrists, feet, and medial tibia, particularly on the
    radial side of the middle phalanx of the index and middle fingers (See Chapter 52).
Osteoporosis
Intermediate
Subchondral resorption of sternoclavicular, acromioclavicular, discovertebral, and
    sacroiliac joints and symphysis pubis
Loss of the lamina dura around teeth
Acro-osteolysis of the phalangeal tufts
Chondrocalcinosis of knees, wrists, and symphysis pubis (see Chapter 50)
Periarticular and soft tissue calcification
Late
Bone cysts (single or multiple) (see figure)
Subligamentous bone resorption of trochanters, ischial tuberosities, humeral tuberosities,
    and calcanei

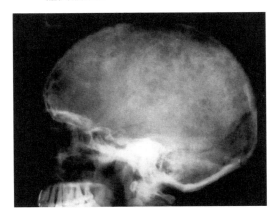

Skull radiograph of a patient with renal failure and secondary hyperparathyroidism. Note the bone cysts ("brown tumors") superimposed on a "salt and pepper" skull.

4. What is a "salt and pepper" skull? "Rugger-jersey spine?"
Both terms are descriptions of radiographic findings seen in hyperparathyroidism. Trabecular bone resorption creates a characteristic mottling of the cranial vault with alternating areas of lucency and sclerosis, producing the **salt and pepper** radiographic appearance. **Rugger-jersey spine** refers to band-like osteosclerosis of the superior and inferior margins of the vertebral bodies (see figure next page).

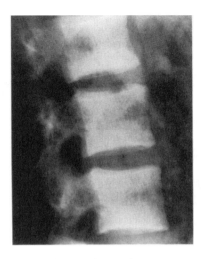

Rugger-jersey spine.

5. How can you distinguish primary from secondary hyperparathyroidism on radiographs?

Osteitis fibrosa cystica was the term applied to the characteristic subperiosteal erosions that were originally identified on radiographs in primary hyperparathyroidism. Today, routine serum chemistry screening provides for early detection of primary hyperparathyroidism in the asymptomatic stage, prior to the development of the characteristic bony findings. Therefore, osteitis fibrosa cystica has all but disappeared in primary hyperparathyroidism and is now seen only in renal osteodystrophy with secondary hyperparathyroidism.

Primary Versus Secondary Hyperparathyroidism

FINDING	PRIMARY HYPERPARATHYROIDISM	SECONDARY HYPERPARATHYROIDISM*
Brown tumors	Common	Less common
Osteosclerosis	Rare	Common
Chondrocalcinosis	Not infrequent	Rare
Periostitis	Rare	Not infrequent

Adapted from Resnick D, Niwayama G: Parathyroid disorders and renal osteodystrophy. Resnick D, Niwayama G (eds): Diagnosis of Bone and Joint Disorders, 2nd ed. Philadelphia, W.B. Saunders, 1988, pp 2219–2285.

Additional findings of renal osteodystrophy are observed in secondary hyperparathyroidism, including osteomalacia and soft tissue and vascular calcification.

6. What dietary modifications decrease PTH secretion and help to prevent the development of secondary hyperparathyroidism in chronic renal failure?

Phosphate restriction
Calcium supplementation (calcium carbonate)
Adequate 1,25-dihydroxyvitamin D intake

Once hyperparathyroidism is advanced, it may be refractory to these dietary interventions, at which time high-dose intravenous 1,25-dihydroxyvitamin D may be beneficial. If these measures fail, subtotal parathyroidectomy is indicated to correct symptomatic hyperparathyroidism.

7. What is amyloid arthropathy of renal failure?

β_2-Microglobulin is an endogenous structural protein that is poorly cleared by standard dialysis membranes and accumulates to extremely high levels in patients on long-term hemodialysis.

It is deposited in and around joints, leading to chronic arthralgias and carpal tunnel syndrome. This chronic arthropathy most commonly involves the shoulder, hip, wrist and finger tendon sheaths, and rarely the spine. Rotator cuff and subacromial bursae deposition leads to impingement syndrome.

Synovial fluid is noninflammatory but may be hemorrhagic due to anticoagulation use during dialysis. Synovial fluid or biopsy will identify amyloid fibrils when stained with Congo red. Radiographs are notable for large subchondral bony cysts and erosions. The use of more permeable membranes may delay the onset of disease but does not prevent disease development.

8. What role does aluminum play in renal osteodystrophy?

In renal failure or hemodialysis, dietary aluminum is not adequately cleared and deposits in the osteoid lamellae of newly formed bone, inhibiting mineralization which leads to osteomalacia. Clinically, osteomalacia presents as diffuse bone pain and predisposes to insufficiency fractures. Radiographic findings are osteopenia and Looser's zones. Deferoxamine chelation therapy is beneficial. Other common causes of osteomalacia, such as vitamin D deficiency, need to be considered, although this is now uncommon with the routine supplementation of vitamin D in dialysis patients. Secondary hyperparathyroidism, if present, needs to be treated aggressively to prevent concomitant osteoporosis.

9. How can you prevent aluminum-induced osteomalacia in renal failure?

1. Avoid all aluminum-containing compounds (most phosphate binders, antacids).
2. Ensure adequate vitamin D intake.
3. Maintain normal plasma 25-dihydroxyvitamin D levels.
4. Maintain dialysate aluminum content <20 mg/ml
5. Measure plasma aluminum levels frequently.

10. A patient who is 3 months' post-renal transplant develops an acute knee arthritis. His current medications include cyclosporine, azathioprine, and prednisone. What is the most likely etiology for the knee pain?

This is a common presentation of **acute gouty arthritis** associated with **cyclosporine** use. Cyclosporine blocks renal uric acid clearance, leading to marked hyperuricemia and gout. Polarized microscopy of the synovial fluid may identify numerous intracellular, negatively birefrigent, needle-shaped crystals, confirming the diagnosis of gout. Positive birefrigent rhomboid crystals of pseudogout also may be seen because of the association of secondary hyperparathyroidism and calcium pyrophosphate deposition (CPDD) disease. Septic arthritis needs to be considered in the differential diagnosis because of the potent immunosuppressive therapy used in this post-transplant patient. Therefore, joint fluid should be sent for Gram stain and cultures to include fungi and tuberculosis. Listeriosis also occurs in this setting.

11. How do you treat a patient who has acute gouty arthritis following renal transplant?

The usual treatment for acute gouty arthritis and hyperuricemia needs to be modified in this instance:

1. NSAIDs can increase cyclosporine renal toxicity and therefore should be avoided.

2. Colchicine has a very narrow therapeutic index when used in renal insufficiency and should be used with extreme caution.

3. Azathioprine is metabolized hepatically by the enzyme xanthine oxidase. Allopurinol is a xanthine oxidase inhibitor and therefore leads to markedly elevates serum azathioprine levels, with marrow suppression and cytopenias. To avoid this, the dose of azathioprine needs to be reduced by 75% if it is used in combination with allopurinol.

4. Systemic corticosteroids will add to the ongoing immunosuppression, and therefore close monitoring is necessary.

5. Intra-articular corticosteroid injections are the best option in this case once an infection has definitely been ruled out.

12. Which spondyloarthropathy is unique to dialysis patients?

A **destructive spondyloarthropathy** (DSA) is found only in long-term dialysis patients and is defined by its radiologic picture. There is multilevel disc-space narrowing with erosions and cysts of adjacent vertebral endplates without significant osteophytosis or sclerosis. Calcification of surrounding vertebral discs is common. The cervical and lumbar spine are most frequently involved. The erosions progress radiographically over a few weeks or more, followed by reactive endplate sclerosis. Diffuse spinal involvement is unusual, although multisegment involvement has been described.

This entity has been reported occasionally in uremic patients prior to dialysis but has not been reported following renal transplantation. Most patients are asymptomatic, which accounts for the rarity of its description. Neck pain or cervical radiculopathy are the most common complaints in symptomatic patients. Despite the severe radiologic picture, medullary compression has been reported only once. Biopsies reveal calcium crystals (CPDD or hydroxyapatite) or β_2-microglobulin. Hyperparathyroidism is usually also present and appears to play a role in the pathogenesis of DSA. Control of hyperparathyroidism, including subtotal parathyroidectomy, appears to prevent progression of DSA.

13. What is tertiary hyperparathyroidism?

Under normal homeostasis, a normal or elevated serum calcium level feeds back to inhibit PTH release, maintaining normal calcium levels. Tertiary hyperparathyroidism is the loss of this feedback inhibition on PTH release which develops in long-standing secondary hyperparathyroidism. Renal transplantation often unmasks tertiary hyperparathyroidism, when PTH secretion remains elevated despite normalization of serum calcium with the improved renal function. This PTH release results in further bone resorption and hypercalcemia. In general, surgical treatment is indicated in symptomatic patients with nonsuppressible serum PTH levels. Symptoms may include those related to hypercalcemia, hyperparathyroidism, nephrocalcinosis, or nephrolithiasis. A subtotal parathyroidectomy is the treatment of choice.

14. Where do soft tissue calcifications occur in renal osteodystrophy?

Soft-tissue calcification is common in renal osteodystrophy. Sites of soft-tissue deposition are multiple, including the cornea and conjunctiva, viscera, vasculature, and subcutaneous and periarticular tissues. Calcification occurs in chronic renal failure when the concentration (mg/dl) product of plasma calcium and phosphorus exceeds 70. Periarticular and subcutaneous deposits may become quite large, particularly around the hips, knees, shoulders, and wrists, where they may cause pain, reduce range of motion, and predispose to infection. Vascular calcification may compromise blood flow leading to skin ulceration or tissue infarction. The chemical composition of the calcium depends on the site of deposition. In subcutaneous, vascular, and periarticular sites, hydroxyapatite is observed, while in viscera, magnesium Whitlokite-like material is found.

15. What types of crystal deposition diseases occur in patients with renal disease?

- Monosodium urate arthritis (**gouty arthritis**) occurs occasionally, although less frequently than one would expect considering how comon hyperuricemia is in patients with chronic renal failure.
- **Calcium pyrophosphate deposition disease** (CPDD) is seen occasionally in secondary hyperparathyroidism (although less common than in primary hyperparathyroidism). CPDD is manifested by chondrocalcinosis (knee, wrist, symphysis pubis), acute pseudogout, and/or a degenerative arthritis.
- **Secondary oxalosis** rarely develops in long-standing renal failure. It is marked by oxalate deposition in visceral organs, blood vessels, bones, and articular cartilage, where it may contribute to chronic polyarthralgias. Oxalate is produced from ascorbic acid and is cleared very poorly in chronic renal failure and dialysis. Most cases of oxalosis can be prevented by limiting ascorbic acid intake. Treatment of established calcium oxalate arthropathy with NSAIDs, colchicine, intra-articular corticosteroids, or increased dialysis has produced only slight improvement.

16. Describe what happens to the serum calcium, phosphate, 25-hydroxyvitamin D, and 1,25-dihydroxyvitamin D levels in osteomalacia and the hyperparathyroidism syndrome.

	Ca	PO$_4$	25-VIT D	1,25-VIT D	iPTH	AlkPhos
Renal osteomalacia	↓	↓	↔	↓	↔↓	↔↓
Primary hyperparathyroidism	↑	↓↔	↔	↑↓	↑	↑
Secondary hyperparathyroidism	↓↔	↓↔	↔	↓	↑	↑↔
Tertiary hyperparathyroidism	↑	↑	↔	↓	↑↑	↑

↓, decreased; ↑, increased; ↔, normal. Ca, calcium; PO$_4$, phosphate; 25-Vit D, 25-hydroxyvitamin D; 1,25-Vit D, 1,25-dihydroxyvitamin D; iPTH, immunoreactive parathyroid hormone; AlkPhos, alkaline phosphatase.

17. What dose adjustments are needed for antirheumatic drugs when used in patients with renal failure or insufficiency?

NSAIDs: Ibuprofen, diclofenac, naproxen, fenoprofen, indomethacin, ketoprofen, meclofenamate, tolmetin, piroxicam, salsalate are primarily eliminated and metabolized by the liver and require no dose adjustment in endstage renal disease (ESRD). Diflunisal and sulindac require 50% dose reduction when the glomerular filtration rate (GFR) is <10 ml/min (i.e., ESRD). NSAIDs as a group can cause increased renal insufficiency secondary to prostaglandin inhibition.

Disease-modifying antirheumatic drugs: *Antimalarials* require a 25% dose reduction with GFR <10 ml/min (i.e., ESRD). *Dapsone* should be given every other day instead of daily if the GFR is <50 ml/min. *Sulfasalazine* and *oral gold* require no dose change in patients with renal insufficiency. Oral gold should be avoided in ESRD. Intramuscular gold should be avoided in patients with GFR <50 ml/min. *Penicillamine* dose should be reduced 25–50% for GFR <50 ml/min and by 75% or avoided in ESRD.

Immunosuppressive agents: *Corticosteroids* require no dose adjustments. *Azathioprine* dose should be reduced by 25% in ESRD. *Cyclophosphamide* dose should be reduced 50% in ESRD. *Cyclosporine* requires no dose adjustment but may cause worsening renal insufficiency. *Methotrexate* dose should be reduced by 50% if GFR <50 ml/min. It should be used with extreme caution in anyone with renal insufficiency. Many physicians avoid using methotrexate entirely in patients with renal insufficiency.

Anti-gout and other medications: *Colchicine* dose should be reduced 50% in ESRD. Prolonged colchicine use should be avoided when GFR is <50 ml/min. *Allopurinol* dose should be reduced by 50% if GFR <50 ml/min and by 50–75% in ESRD. *Probenecid* and *sulfinpyrazone* lose their uricosuric effect with GFR <50 ml/min and should be avoided if GFR is low. *Bisphosphonates* should be avoided in ESRD.

BIBLIOGRAPHY

1. Bardin T, Kuntz D: Dialysis arthropathy. In Klippel JH, Dieppe PA (eds): Rheumatology. London, Mosby, 1994, pp 7.26.
2. Bindi P, Chanard J: Destructive spondyloarthropathy in dialysis patients: An overview. Nephron 55:104–109, 1990.
3. Bland JH, Frymoyer JW, Newberg AH, et al: Rheumatic syndromes in endocrine disease. Semin Arthritis Rheum 9:23–61, 1979.
4. Bywaters EG, Dixon AS, Scott JT: Joint lesions of hyperparathyroidism. Ann Rheum Dis 22:171–187, 1963.
5. Eastwood JB, Pazianas M: Renal bone disease. In Klippel JH, Dieppe PA (eds): Rheumatology. London, Mosby, 1994, pp 7.36.1–7.36.4.
6. Galbraith SC, Quarles LD: Tertiary hyperparathyroidism and refractory secondary hyperparathyroidism. In Favus MJ (ed): Primer on the Metabolic Bone Diseases and Disorders of Mineral Metabolism, 2nd ed. New York, Raven Press, 1993, pp 159–163.
7. Goodman WG, Coburn JW, Ramirez JA, et al: Renal osteodystrophy in adults and children. In Favus MJ (ed): Primer on the Metabolic Bone Diseases and Disorders of Mineral Metabolism, 2nd ed. New York, Raven Press, 1993, pp 304–323.
8. McGuire JL: The endocrine system and connective tissue disorders. Bull Rheum Dis 39:1–8, 1990.
9. McGuire JL, Lambert RE: Arthropathies associated with endocrine disorders. In Kelley WN, Harris ED,

Ruddy S, Sledge CB (eds): Textbook of Rheumatology, 4th ed. Philadelphia, W.B. Saunders, 1993, pp 1527–1544.
10. Ott SM: Metabolic bone disease. In Schumacher HR, Klippel JH, Koopman WJ (eds): Primer on the Rheumatic Diseases, 10th ed. Atlanta, Arthritis Foundation, 1993, pp 290–293.
11. Rafto SE, Dalinka MK, Schieber ML, et al: Spondyloarthropathy of the cervical spine in long-term hemodialysis. Radiology 166:201–204, 1988.
12. Resnick D, Niwayama G: Parathyroid disorders and renal osteodystrophy. In Resnick D, Niwayama G (eds): Diagnosis of Bone and Joint Disorders, 2nd ed. Philadelphia, W.B. Saunders, 1988, pp 2219–2285.

82. RHEUMATIC DISEASE AND THE PREGNANT PATIENT

Mark Jarek, M.D.

1. A young patient with recently-diagnosed SLE is currently being treated with low-dose prednisone, naproxen, and hydroxychloroquine with good disease control. She is considering pregnancy and asks about the optimal timing of a pregnancy and the potential maternal and fetal complications. What advice do you give her?

Patients with systemic lupus erythematosus (SLE) should be advised to conceive while SLE is quiescent or at least under good control. Patients who conceive with inactive SLE still are at increased risk for intrauterine growth retardation (IUGR), prematurity, and toxemia of pregnancy. There is a 20–50% likelihood of stable SLE relapsing during pregnancy, although the long-term disease outcome in these patients probably is not altered since most exacerbations are mild. Therefore, such patients need to be followed closely by a rheumatologist during pregnancy.

Patients with severe SLE, particularly active lupus nephritis, are at particularly high risk for maternal and fetal complications and should be cautioned strongly against conception. Fetal mortality in this group is increased at least 3-fold, and prematurity occurs in most of the successful pregnancies. In some studies, the fetal mortality rate did not improve even when the SLE nephritis was inactive. There is no increased rate of infertility for patients with SLE as long as the disease is under control.

2. How can you distinguish lupus nephritis from toxemia of pregnancy?

The **toxemia** syndrome (preeclampsia-eclampsia) usually occurs in the third trimester of primigravidas. It is manifested in mild cases by hypertension, proteinuria, and edema, with a consumptive coagulopathy, microangiopathic hemolytic anemia, and convulsions occurring in severe cases. The distinction between eclampsia and active **lupus nephritis** can be difficult since both diseases can cause thrombocytopenia, hemolytic anemia, hypertension, and renal insufficiency with proteinuria. The absence of other clinical manifestations of SLE, such as arthritis, rash, and cytopenias, as well as the lack of red cell casts and stable anti-DNA antibodies, make the diagnosis of eclampsia more likely.

Complement values usually rise during a normal pregnancy but have been reported to decrease in SLE patients during pregnancy independent of a lupus relapse, and therefore complement values may not be helpful in distinguishing the two diseases. The ESR is of no value since it is elevated in both normal pregnancy and SLE. Proteinuria can occur during a normal pregnancy due to the physiologic increased renal blood flow but should be accompanied by a normal, pregnancy-associated rise in creatine clearance and a corresponding fall in serum creatinine. Toxemia of pregnancy remits immediately following delivery and therefore requires no further therapy, whereas lupus nephritis usually requires high-dose corticosteroids frequently in combination with azathioprine during pregnancy or cyclophosphamide after completion of pregnancy.

Clinical Findings Distinguishing Proteinuria Due to Pregnancy-induced
Hypertension (PIH) and Active Lupus Glomerulonephritis

ABNORMALITY	PIH	SLE
Blood pressure	High	Normal or high
Platelets	Low or normal	Low or normal
Complement	Elevated or normal	Normal or low
Uric acid	High	High or normal
Proteinuria	High	High
Hematuria	Macroscopic, no casts	Microscopic, with casts
Anti-DNA antibody	Normal or stable	Rising or high
Other SLE symptoms	Absent	Present

3. What is the significance of SLE developing during pregnancy?

Fetal outcome is very poor when SLE develops during pregnancy, with a fetal death rate as high as 45%. In addition, the maternal course is frequently severe if lupus nephritis occurs for the first time during pregnancy.

4. A patient whose SLE is well controlled on prednisone (5 mg/day), naproxen (500 mg/day), and hydroxychloroquine (400 mg/day) informs you that she is pregnant. What should you recommend regarding the current medications?

Low doses of prednisone (5–10 mg/day) are generally well tolerated during pregnancy and probably are protective against a flare of SLE during pregnancy or postpartum. NSAIDs have been used widely in pregnancy for preterm labor and have not demonstrated major adverse outcomes (although there are a few reports of premature ductus arteriosus closure, oligohydramnios, respiratory distress syndrome, pulmonary hypertension, and fetal death associated with indomethacin). Although congenital malformations, particularly cleft lip and palate, have been seen in animal studies, there is no evidence to suggest that aspirin, indomethacin, diclofenac, diflunisal, or sulindac cause human fetal abnormalities; phenylbutazone has been associated with chromosomal abnormalities.

Low-dose aspirin (80 mg/day) is safe and may be effective prophylaxis for preeclampsia and IUGR. Full-dose aspirin use at the time of delivery is associated with prolonged labor, anemia, and increased maternal blood loss, along with a possible increased risk of neonatal hemorrhage in premature infants. Because of these concerns regarding aspirin and other NSAID use late in pregnancy, the First International Conference on Rheumatic Diseases in Pregnancy recommended switching to low doses of prednisone (<20 mg/day) at least 2 months before delivery for management of most rheumatic complaints occurring during pregnancy. Chloroquine and hydroxychloroquine are contraindicated during pregnancy because of the possible increased risk of miscarriages, retinal damage, ototoxicity, and congenital birth defects (although multiple normal births have been reported).

5. Can aspirin, NSAIDs, corticosteroids, and antimalarial medications be used during breast-feeding?

- **Aspirin** in doses greater than one 325-mg tablet result in high infant plasma salicylate levels and should be used cautiously during breast-feeding.
- **NSAIDs** can be used during breast-feeding.
- **Corticosteroids** are excreted in the breast milk at a rate of 10–20% of the maternal dose. Patients on corticosteroids can breastfeed but should wait at least 4 hours if the prednisone dose is >20 mg.
- **Antimalarials** (chloroquine/hydroxychloroquine) are contraindicated during breast-feeding due to potential accumulation in the infant and retinal toxicity.

6. Which disease-modifying antirheumatic drugs (DMARDs) can be used safely during pregnancy and lactation?

Sulfasalazine has been used safely throughout pregnancy and lactation in the treatment of inflammatory bowel disease. Therefore, although its safety in pregnant patients with rheumatic diseases has not been established, it is probably safe and can be used with caution during pregnancy and lactation. Folate supplementation is recommended.

Gold salts, although associated with teratogenesis in animals, have only rarely been associated with congenital anomalies in humans. Nonetheless, the small number of patients with long-term exposure and the potential toxicities of the drug preclude recommendation of its use in pregnancy. Gold is excreted in breast milk (20% of dose) and should be used cautiously if at all during breast-feeding.

Azathioprine has been used in patients with renal transplants, hematologic malignancies, inflammatory bowel disease, and lupus nephritis during pregnancy. Although placental metabolism may offer some protection to the fetus, various adverse effects including fetal growth retardation, cytopenias, and opportunistic infections have been described. Therefore, azathioprine should be reserved for patients whose rheumatic disease is severe and life-threatening (such as lupus nephritis). Close prenatal monitoring and long-term evaluation of the offspring are essential. Azathioprine has been detected in breast milk and therefore is not safe for use during breast-feeding.

7. Which ones can't?

Penicillamine has been used in patients with Wilson's disease and cystinuria, during which adverse effects on the fetus, such as serious connective tissue disorders, have occasionally been identified.

Methotrexate is associated with increased spontaneous abortions and birth anomalies. Breast milk appears to be a minor route of excretion of methotrexate, but most physicians would recommend against breast-feeding if a patient is on methotrexate.

Cyclophosphamide and **chlorambucil** are generally contraindicated during pregnancy because of the risks of teratogenicity during the first trimester and concerns about neonatal bone marrow suppression, infection, and hemorrhage in later pregnancy. Cyclophosphamide induces age-dependent gonadal toxicity. Chlorambucil has not been shown to pass into breast milk, but data are insufficient to recommend its use during lactation.

Cyclosporine crosses the placenta and has been associated with IUGR and prematurity. It is probably not teratogenic but is probably contraindicated in pregnancy and breast-feeding.

8. Do oral contraceptives influence the activity of SLE?

For many years there has been indirect evidence suggesting that sex hormones play a role in SLE activity:

- Women in child-bearing years are generally the most severely affected with SLE.
- Disease severity often varies with the menstrual cycle.
- SLE relapse during pregnancy occurs commonly.
- Klinefelter patients with SLE have elevated female hormone levels.

Despite these associations, the effects of oral contraceptive therapy on SLE activity remains controversial. There may be a slight increased risk of SLE relapse with low-dose oral contraceptive therapy, particularly when lupus nephritis is present, and therefore other methods of contraception are recommended in patients with active SLE. **Progesterone-only** contraceptive therapy is not associated with increased relapses in SLE patients. The lower doses of estrogens used as **hormone replacement therapy** in postmenopausal women have not been proved to exacerbate SLE. Although there may be a small risk of inducing a SLE relapse with hormone replacement therapy, this risk is offset by many beneficial effects of estrogens in this group of patients.

9. Describe the typical laboratory findings and clinical presentation of infants with neonatal lupus erythematosus (NLE).

The major clinical manifestations are dermatologic, cardiac, and hepatic. Hemolytic anemia and thrombocytopenia are less common manifestations. The skin rash is quite similar to that of subacute cutaneous lupus erythematosus. Congenital heart block is the most common cardiac manifestation, but congestive heart failure can also be seen in the neonatal period. The major morbidity and mortality of NLE is from congenital heart block which, unlike the other disease manifestations, is irreversible in most cases; permanent pacemaker therapy is required in about one-half of cases. Mortality in this subset is 20–30%, including death from pacemaker failure. Anti-Ro (SS-A) and anti-La (SS-B) maternal autoantibodies cross the placenta and bind to fetal heart conducting cells, eliciting an inflammatory injury during the second trimester of pregnancy. Clinical disease occurs in 5% of offspring of mothers with high circulating levels of these antibodies.

When NLE is suspected, fetal echocardiography should be performed, and if fetal heart block or congestive heart failure is documented, close monitoring of the fetus and elective delivery at deterioration or maturity is indicated. Successful intrauterine therapy with dexamethasone or betamethasone for fetal myocarditis and heart block has been reported. Dexamethasone and betamethasone are the corticosteroids of choice because they are not inactivated by the placenta and therefore will be active in the fetal circulation. Potential postnatal therapies include pulse steroids, exchange transfusions, and intravenous gammaglobulin although none has been thoroughly evaluated. No prophylactic treatment in subsequent pregnancies has yet been proven effective. The predominant autoimmune disorder in mothers of children with NLE is subclinical primary Sjögrens syndrome.

10. How does rheumatoid arthritis (RA) usually react during pregnancy?

Rheumatoid arthritis improves in approximately 75% of patients during pregnancy, with most occurring in the first trimester. This improvement recurs with subsequent pregnancies. This improvement is unfortunately short-lived, as 90% develop a relapse by 6 months postpartum. Two percent of RA patients have initial onset of disease during pregnancy, and 10% have initial onset within 6 months postpartum.

The relationship between RA and pregnancy, along with the female predominance of the disease during reproductive years (4:1), suggests a hormonal influence. Multiple clinical studies have examined the effects of oral contraceptive therapy on the incidence and severity of RA, but their results to date are contradictory and have failed to consistently support a beneficial effect of oral contraceptives in the prevention or treatment of RA.

11. Does the presence of RA have an effect on fertility or pregnancy complications?

Infertility is not increased in RA patients, and there is no increase in fetal or maternal complications.

12. How does systemic sclerosis affect fertility and pregnancy complications?

There is a 2- to 3-fold increased rate of infertility in systemic sclerosis. Infertility is also increased to a lesser degree in primary Raynaud's disease and in patients with Raynaud's phenomenon who are destined to develop systemic sclerosis. Fetal complications, such as prematurity and small-for-gestational-age growth, are increased in systemic sclerosis. A small percentage of women experience a worsening of their disease during pregnancy. The most feared complication is the development of scleroderma renal crisis during pregnancy, which is associated with very high fetal and maternal morbidity and mortality.

13. What are some practical considerations for the pregnant scleroderma patient?

Patients with systemic sclerosis need to be monitored closely for problems arising during pregnancy. Although successful pregnancies are common, the involvement of multiple organ systems by systemic sclerosis can greatly influence the postpartum course and subsequent child care.

Difficulties of Pregnancy in Systemic Sclerosis

ORGAN INVOLVEMENT	DIFFICULTIES
Skin	Tight abdominal wall, venous/arterial access, oximetry, problems holding baby
Keratoconjunctivitis	Keratitis
Microstomia	Oral intubation
Nasal telangiectasias	Bleeding
Skeletal muscle	Weakness, prolonged motor blockade with regional anesthetic
Heart	Cardiac failure
Lungs	Dyspnea, pulmonary hypertension
Kidneys	Renal failure, hypertension
Esophagus	Worsening dysphagia, aspiration risk
Small bowel	Malnutrition
Large bowel	Constipation, incontinence

14. What are the clinical features of the anti-phospholipid antibody (aPLA) syndrome?

aPLA syndrome is clinically associated with thrombocytopenia, recurrent arterial and/or venous thrombosis, and recurrent fetal wastage. It can occur as a primary disorder (see Chapter 27) or occur in association with SLE or another rheumatic disorder. The syndrome is characterized by the production of autoantibodies against negatively charged phospholipids. These antibodies can be detected by different laboratory assays and may reflect different antibody activity and specificity:

- IgG or IgM anti-cardiolipin antibodies (aCL) detected by ELISA
- Prolonged activated partial thromboplastin time that does not correct with a mixing study with normal plasma (lupus anticoagulant)
- False-positive rapid plasma reagin (RPR)
- Dilute Russell viper venom time (dRVVT) prolongation

15. How does the aPLA syndrome affect pregnancies?

A recent prospective study found at least one aPLA present in 24% of low-risk patients at the first prenatal visit. However, only the presence of IgG aCL, which was present in 5% of mothers, was significantly associated with fetal loss (fetal loss 28%, RR 3.5). There was no increase in maternal complications, low birth weight, or low Apgar scores in mothers with IgG aCL. Therefore, routine screening in asymptomatic patients is currently not recommended. Primiparas and women with prior liveborns who are found to have aPLA need not be treated prophylactically, but the progress of their pregnancies (fetal growth and activity) should be monitored closely. Slowing of fetal growth or reduction in amniotic fluid volume would be warning signs. Though its prognostic value is less certain, a falling platelet count is taken by some authorities to indicate fetal involvement. In the presence of slow fetal growth or thrombocytopenia not explained by toxemia or SLE or a history of prior fetal deaths, prophylaxis treatment with aspirin (85 mg/day) or subcutaneous heparin (10,000–20,000 units twice daily) is recommended. High dose (>40 mg/day) prednisone is less beneficial for aPLA syndrome uncomplicated by active SLE.

16. A 35-year-old woman in her third trimester complains of unilateral hip pain that began 1 month ago. The pain is constant, dull, and unrelieved by rest or recumbancy. Physical examination reveals an antalgic gait with normal range of motion, except for minimal pain with full flexion and internal rotation. The reflexes and sensory and motor examinations are unremarkable. Routine laboratory studies are normal, except for an ESR of 50 mm/hour. How do you proceed with your evaluation, and what is the most likely diagnosis?

Although the ESR is elevated, this is a normal phenomenon of the third trimester of pregnancy and is not supportive of an infection in the hip. Septic hip arthritis is unlikely in this case because of the chronicity of the pain, presence of full range of motion, and a normal WBC count; arthrocentesis therefore is unnecessary. Plain radiographs with fetal shielding can be performed and would be diagnostic in this case. They probably would reveal marked unilateral osteopenia of the femoral head and acetabulum, indicating the diagnosis of **transient osteoporosis of pregnancy** (TOP).

TOP is a rare condition of unknown etiology that most commonly affects the hips (left more often than right) but can be seen in the knees or shoulders. It is more commonly seen in young women. Protected weight-bearing, rest, and acetaminophen offer some temporary benefit. The pain and osteopenia usually resolve after delivery. Isotope scans, CT, and MRI are all more sensitive than plain radiographs early in the disease process but are contraindicated in pregnancy. Additionally, these studies may be helpful in excluding osteonecrosis of the femoral head, which may have a similar clinical presentation.

BIBLIOGRAPHY

1. Bobrie G: Pregnancy in lupus nephritis and related disorders. Am J Kidney Dis 4:339–343, 1987.
2. Brooks PM, Needs CJ: Antirheumatic drugs in pregnancy and lactation. Bailliere's Clin Rheumatol 4:156–169, 1990.
3. Buyon JP, Yaron M, Lockshin MD: First International Conference on Rheumatic Diseases in Pregnancy. Arthritis Rheum 36:59–64, 1993.

4. Carreira PE, Gutierrez-Larraya F, Gomez-Reino JJ: Successful intrauterine therapy with dexamethasone for fetal myocarditis and heart block in a woman with systemic lupus erythematosus. J Rheumatol 20:1204–1207, 1993.
5. Floyd RC: Autoimmune diseases in pregnancy. Obstet Gynecol Clin North Am 4:719–732, 1992.
6. Groff GD: Hip pain during pregnancy. In Klippel JH, Dieppe PA (eds): Rheumatology. London, Mosby Europe, 1994, pp 5.15.6–5.15.7.
7. Julkunen HA: Oral contraceptives in systemic lupus erythematosus: Side-effects and influence on the activity of SLE. Scand J Rheumatol 20:427–433, 1991.
8. Lockshin MD: Pregnancy in a patient with systemic lupus erythematosus. In Klippel JH, Dieppe PA (eds): Rheumatology. London, Mosby Europe, 1994.
9. Lynch A, Marlar R, Murphy J, et al: Antiphospholipid antibodies in predicting adverse pregnancy outcome—A prospective study. Ann Intern Med 120:470–475, 1994.
10. Ostensen M: Treatment with immunosuppressive and disease modifying drugs during pregnancy and lactation. Am J Reprod Immunol 28:148–152, 1992.
11. Rider LG, Buyon JP, Rutledge J, Sherry DD: Treatment of neonatal lupus: Case report and review of the literature. J Rheumatol 20:1208–1211, 1993.
12. Rubbert A: Pregnancy course and complications in patients with systemic lupus erythematosus. Am J Reprod Immunol 28:205–207, 1992.
13. Silman AJ: Pregnancy and scleroderma. Am J Reprod Immunol 28:238–240, 1992.
14. Soscia PN, Zurier RB: Drug therapy of rheumatic diseases during pregnancy. Bull Rheum Dis 41:12–13, 1992.
15. Waltuck J, Buyon JP: Autoantibody-associated congenital heart block: Outcome in mother and children. Ann Intern Med 120:544–551, 1994.
16. Wong KL, Chan FY, Lee CP: Outcomes of pregnancy in patients with systemic lupus erythematosus—A prospective study. Arch Intern Med 151:269–273, 1991.

83. ODDS AND ENDS

James D. Singleton, M.D.

1. Name the periodic syndromes. Why are they grouped together?

Intermittent hydrarthrosis
Palindromic rheumatism
Familial Mediterranean fever (FMF)
Tietze's syndrome

These syndromes are grouped because they share the four features: (1) intermittent arthritis followed by periods of remission; (2) complete resolution between attacks; (3) only rare development of joint damage; and (4) unknown cause.

2. Are all disorders with intermittent arthritis encompassed by the periodic syndromes?

No. Many other disorders may include intermittent joint swelling and other characteristics of the periodic syndromes. Among these are mechanical and inflammatory disorders. Thus, a broad differential should be kept in mind in patients presenting with intermittent arthritis.

Periodic syndromes	Spondyloarthropathies
Intermittent hydrarthrosis	Reactive arthritis
Palindromic rheumatism	Enteropathic arthritis
FMF	Infections
Crystalline arthropathies	Lyme disease
Gout	Whipple's disease
CPPD/pseudogout	Mechanical
Hydroxyapatite	Loose bodies
Sarcoidosis	Meniscal tears

3. Describe the typical clinical features of intermittent hydrarthrosis.

Recurrent joint effusions occur at regular intervals, frequently paralleling menses in females. The knee or another large joint develops an effusion over 12–24 hours, with no or minimal discomfort or signs of inflammation. There are no systemic symptoms, no treatment is proven to prevent or abort attacks, and episodes may occur lifelong.

4. What do laboratory studies and joint radiographs show in intermittent hydrarthrosis?

Laboratory tests, including the ESR, are normal, even during an attack. Synovial fluid is normal or mildly inflammatory with a slight increase in polymorphonuclear leukocytes. An effusion may be seen on radiographs, but no other abnormalities are seen even after years of attacks.

5. What is palindromic rheumatism? What does it mean?

Palindromic rheumatism is a recurrent syndrome of acute arthritis and periarthritis. *Palindromic* means "recurring" and is derived from a Greek word which literally means "to run back." The term *palindromic* was introduced by Hench and Rosenberg in 1944 as descriptive of the syndrome. They preferred *rheumatism* to *arthritis* due to the frequent involvement of periarticular structures and occasional presence of subcutaneous nodules.

6. How do the clinical features of palindromic rheumatism (PR) differ from those of intermittent hydrarthrosis?

PR, like intermittent hydrarthrosis, affects both men and women, often begins in the third to fifth decade, and frequently affects the knees. Constitutional symptoms are uncommon in PR. However, attacks occur irregularly and may involve more than one joint (usually 2–5). The pattern of joint attacks tends to be characteristic in an individual patient. Symptoms may begin in one joint while waning in another. Attacks are sudden and pain may be intense, often reaching a peak within a few hours. Signs of joint inflammation (swelling, warmth, redness) can be noted soon after pain begins. Small joints of the hands and feet may be affected, and occasionally also the spine and temporomandibular joints. Also, unlike intermittent hydrarthrosis, periarticular attacks (occurring in one-third) and transient subcutaneous nodules may be seen.

7. What do laboratory studies and joint radiographs show in PR?

The ESR and other acute-phase reactants may be elevated during attacks but are normal between them. Serum complement levels are normal. There have been few studies of synovial fluid in PR. Leukocytes may vary from a few hundred to several thousand, with the magnitude poorly correlated with symptom severity. Radiographs show only soft-tissue swelling.

8. How is PR treated?

NSAIDs may provide some relief from joint symptoms but do not reliably prevent attacks. A variety of other agents have been used, with injectable gold salts being reported as the most consistently successful. Good clinical responses have also been reported with antimalarial agents, colchicine, sulfasalazine, and penicillamine.

9. Describe the course of PR.

Although the course is variable, fewer than 10% of patients experience a spontaneous remission. Some patients continue to have the disease for many years. However, 30–50% evolve into a chronic inflammatory arthritis, usually rheumatoid arthritis. Less commonly, a diagnosis of SLE or other connective tissue disease is eventually made, or an appropriate diagnosis of crystal disease (gout, pseudogout, apatite) is established.

10. What features are predictive of a patient with PR later developing rheumatoid arthritis (RA)?

The presence of serum rheumatoid factor, persistent rheumatoid nodules, and HLA-DR4 positivity increase the likelihood of evolution to RA. Other factors that may be predictive are significant constitutional symptoms, persistently elevated ESR, and a family history of RA. No synovial fluid feature is predictive.

11. What is familial Mediterranean fever (FMF)?
FMF is an autosomal recessively inherited disorder (FMF gene on chromosome 16) characterized by irregular attacks of fever and one or more inflammatory manifestations. FMF usually has its onset in childhood and is seen primarily in ethnic groups of east Mediterranean origin. Men seem to be affected more commonly than women. Amyloidosis is very prevalent in several ethnic groups with FMF and may be the sole phenotypic expression of the disease. Before the use of colchicine, amyloidosis was the cause of death in 99% of >500 patients in one study—90% of these deaths occurred before age 40.

12. What are the clinical features of FMF?
Fever	100%
Peritonitis	85–97%
Arthritis	50–77%
Pleuritis	33–66%
Erysipelas-like rash	46%
Lymphadenopathy	1–6%

Aseptic meningitis has been stressed as a clinical manifestation of FMF. Splenomegaly (33%) is felt to be largely due to amyloidosis.

13. Describe the arthritis of FMF.
Intermittent monarticular attacks of the knee or other large joint are most typical. Polyarthritis occurs in 20%. Arthritic episodes may be prolonged, lasting weeks or months in about 8% of patients, and subsequent attacks tend to follow the established pattern. Localized pain, exquisite tenderness, and joint dysfunction out of proportion to the degree of swelling should suggest the diagnosis of FMF. Joint erythema and warmth are notably absent.

14. How is the arthritis of FMF treated?
Recovery of joint function between attacks is the rule, and joint destruction is rare. However, in prolonged episodes involving the hip, functional recovery is less likely, and joint damage requiring surgical therapy may be needed. Temporary relief of joint pain may be achieved with analgesic therapy, but due to the recurrent nature of FMF, narcotics should be avoided. Glucocorticoids are ineffective, a feature that may assist in the differential diagnosis. Physical therapy is used to avoid muscle atrophy due to disuse.

15. How does Tietze's syndrome differ from costochondritis?
Tietze's syndrome is a syndrome of pain, tenderness, and swelling of joints of the chest wall, usually the costochrondral joints. Costochondritis is a much more common syndrome of costochondral joint pain and tenderness without objective signs of inflammation. Tietze's syndrome is more common in women, usually (80%) involves a single joint, and is rarely bilateral, affecting neighboring articulations on the same side of the sternum when polyarticular.

16. What causes Tietze's syndrome? What is the treatment of choice?
Tietze's syndrome is *not* caused by the bite of the "Tietze fly." The cause is unknown, although in one series, 90% of cases followed episodes of coughing. The differential diagnosis includes myocardial pain; post-tussive rib fracture; pulmonary embolism and pneumothorax; rheumatoid, septic, and other arthritides; and tumors of the bone and soft tissue. The treatment of choice is local glucocorticoid injection.

17. Define foreign-body synovitis.
It is the inflammatory reaction of synovium (from either joint, bursa, or tendon sheath) to the introduction of a foreign material. Most commonly, this results from a traumatic event, but it may also follow surgical introduction of foreign material.

18. Name the foreign bodies most commonly associated with foreign-body synovitis.

Plant thorns, wood splinters, and sea urchin spines are the most common. Some other recognized materials include fish bones, chitin fragments, stones, gravel, brick fragments, lead, glass, fiberglass, plastic, and rubber. Surgically implanted materials include metallic fragments, cement (methylmethacrylate), and silicone.

19. Name five activities that are risk factors for foreign-body synovitis.

Professional fishing, professional diving, marine recreational activities, farming, and gardening.

20. Describe the clinical, laboratory, and radiographic features of foreign-body synovitis.

The joints of the hands and knees are most commonly affected. There is sudden onset of pain at the site of injury, but this may be forgotten by the patient or overlooked by the physician. The patient may be seen with acute synovitis several days after the injury, ranging to months to years later, with a chronic synovitis (this is particularly true of the knee). The ESR is usually normal, and synovial fluid is inflammatory with a predominance of neutrophils. Radiographs may show soft-tissue swelling only and can be useful to detect radiodense particles (metal, fish bones, sea urchin spines) but not wood, plastic, or plant thorns. Chronic changes of periarticular osteoporosis, osteolysis, osteosclerosis, and periosteal new bone formation can mimic osteomyelitis or bone tumors.

21. How is foreign-body synovitis diagnosed and treated?

In the approximately two-third of patients with foreign-body synovitis due to exogenous particles who develop a chronic or relapsing course, diagnosis and treatment usually necessitate excisional biopsy with synovectomy. Ultrasound, CT, and MRI may be helpful in detecting particles that are small or radiolucent with conventional radiography. Bacteriologic studies (including mycobacterial studies) and histopathologic examination of tissue are essential. Polarized microscopy is useful in detecting birefringent fragments of plant origin, sea urchin spines, and polymethylmethacrylate.

22. Multicentric reticulohistiocytosis (MRH) is a rare disease affecting the skin and joints. Describe its cutaneous features.

Firm papulonodules, reddish-brown or yellow in color, occur most commonly on the face, hands, ears, arms, scalp, neck, and chest. These nodules may wax and wane and even disappear completely. A classic finding is "coral beads" around the nailbeds. In two-thirds of patients, the nodular skin eruption follows the onset of arthritis by months to years.

23. How does the arthritis of MRH resemble that of RA? How does it differ?

Like RA, the arthritis of MRH is inflammatory, usually chronic, symmetric, and polyarticular; it affects the joints of the hands and cervical spine; and it is destructive. Women are affected more frequently than men, and the onset is usually in middle age. However, unlike in RA, distal interphalangeal joint synovitis and destruction may be prominent, and severely deforming arthritis mutilans occurs in one-half of patients. Glucocorticoid therapy has little, if any, effect on the arthritis. Also in contrast to the case with RA, radiographs in MRH feature well-circumscribed erosions, widened joint spaces, and absent or disproportionately mild periarticular osteopenia for the degree of erosive change.

24. Several disorders have been associated with MRH. Name them.
- Tuberculin skin test positivity is seen in about 50%, but only two patients have been reported to have active **tuberculosis.**
- **Xanthelasma** occurs in one-third of patients.
- **Malignant disease** of various types has been reported in approximately 25%.

The cancer may precede, be concurrent with, or follow the development of MRH. Treatment of the malignancy has led to improvement of the MRH in some.

25. What are the typical histologic findings of MRH on biopsy of skin or synovium?

The characteristic finding is aggregates of multinucleated giant cells and histiocytes having a granular, ground-glass appearance. This ground-glass cytoplasm contains a periodic acid–Schiff-reactive material thought to be due to a mucoprotein or glycoprotein. This cellular tissue reaction has prompted the idea that MRH represents a histiocytic granulomatous reaction to an as-yet unidentified stimulus. Fat stains, such as Sudan black, are also positive. MRH was once thought to represent a lipid storage disease, but no consistent abnormalities of lipids, serum or intracellular, have been discovered.

26. How is MRH treated?

No treatment has consistently shown benefit, and the rarity of this disease precludes a good prospective study. In patients with mild disease, symptomatic therapy with NSAIDs or nonnarcotic analgesics should be tried. Unfortunately, the arthritis in 40–50% of patients progresses to an arthritis mutilans. Cytotoxic therapy (cyclophosphamide, chlorambucil) has been reported to achieve partial and complete remissions. Topical nitrogen mustard therapy led to marked improvement in skin lesions in one patient.

BIBLIOGRAPHY

1. Ben-Chetrit E, Levy M: Colchicine prophylaxis in familial Mediterranean fever: Reappraisal after 15 years. Semin Arthritis Rheum 20:241–246, 1991.
2. Ferriero-Seoane JL: Foreign body synovitis. In Schumacher HR (ed): Primer on the Rheumatic Diseases, 10th ed. Atlanta, Arthritis Foundation, 1993, pp 294–295.
3. Ginsburg WW, O'Duffy JD: Multicentric reticulohistiocytosis. In Kelley WK, Harris ED, Ruddy S, Sledge CB (eds): Textbook of Rheumatology, 4th ed. Philadelphia, W.B. Saunders, 1993, pp 1444–1447.
4. Hench PS, Rosenberg EF: Palindromic rheumatism. Arch Intern Med 73:293–321, 1944.
5. Lightfoot RW: Intermittent and periodic arthritic syndromes. In McCarty DJ, Koopman WJ (eds): Arthritis and Allied Conditions, 12th ed. Philadelphia, Lea & Febiger, 1993, pp 1121–1137.
6. Pinals RS: Periodic syndromes. In Schumacher HR (ed): Primer on the Rheumatic Diseases, 10th ed. Atlanta, Arthritis Foundation, 1993, pp 208–209.
7. Reginato AJ, Ferreiro JL, O'Connor CR, et al: Clinical and pathologic studies of twenty-six patients with penetrating foreign body injury to the joint, bursae, and tendon sheaths. Arthritis Rheum 33:1753–1762, 1990.
8. Schumacher HR: Palindromic onset of rheumatoid arthritis. Arthritis Rheum 25:361–369, 1982.

XV. Management of the Rheumatic Diseases

As to diseases, make a habit of two things—to help, or at least to do no harm.
Hippocrates
(c 460–377 BC)

84. NONSTEROIDAL ANTI-INFLAMMATORY DRUGS (NSAIDs)

David H. Collier, M.D.

1. Describe the general properties of the NSAIDs.

The NSAIDs are weak organic acids that bind avidly to serum proteins (mainly albumin). The vast majority have ionization constants (*pKa*) ranging from 3–5, meaning that in the acidic environment of the stomach, NSAIDs are un-ionized which can lead to local mucosal damage. Beneficially, acidic NSAIDs may become sequestered preferentially in inflamed joints, giving the NSAID a longer synovial half-life than plasma half-life. NSAIDs generally have anti-inflammatory properties, probably by inhibiting prostaglandin production but also by a number of other mechanisms.

2. When were NSAIDs first used?

Salicylates have probably been used for centuries. Hippocrates, Celsus, Galen, and many medieval herbalists recorded the use of willow bark and other plants known to contain salicylates to treat fever and pain. In more recent history:

1826—Salicylin, the active principle of salicylates, isolated from willow bark.
1838—Salicylic acid derived from salicylin.
1853—Acetylsalicylate (**aspirin**) first synthesized.
1899—Aspirin introduced in the United States.
1949—Phenylbutazone, the first alternative to salicylates, introduced.
1965—Idomethacin introduced.

Although it was first synthesized in 1853, aspirin was not used until late in the 19th century, when F. Hoffman of Bayer Company gave it to his arthritic father and it helped his arthritis. (This was essentially stage 1, 2, and 3 testing of this drug, which for new drugs today, takes many millions of dollars and an average of 10 years.) Since the 1960s, a proliferation of NSAIDs has occurred. In some countries, there is a selection of up to 40 NSAIDs from which to choose.

3. How often are NSAIDs used?

It is estimated that > 100 million prescriptions for non-salicylate NSAIDs, costing > $1 billion, were dispensed in the United States in 1993.

4. What are the beneficial effects of NSAIDs?

Analgesia—These drugs are as analgesic as narcotics (in therapeutic doses) in acute pain.
Antipyresis—NSAIDs inhibit prostaglandins in the CNS, which reduces fever.
Anti-inflammatory—These effects are achieved by a number of mechanisms.
Antiplatelet—NSAIDs decrease platelet aggregation by preventing thromboxane A_2 production, which is important in activating platelets, and thus preventing the first step in coagulation.

5. What is the structural classification of NSAIDs?

Salicylates
    Acetylated—aspirin
    Nonacetylated—sodium salicylate, choline salicylate, magnesium salicylate, salsalate,
        salicylamide, diflunisal
Acetic acids
    Indole derivatives—indomethacin, tolmetin, sulindac
    Phenylacetic acid—diclofenac
    Pyranocarboxylic acid—etodolac
Propionic acids—ibuprofen, naproxen, fenoprofen, ketoprofen, flurbiprofen, oxaprozin
Fenamic acids—mefenamic acid, meclofenamic acid
Enolic acids
    Oxicams—piroxicam
    Pyrazolones—phenylbutazone
Nonacidic compounds
    Naphthylalkanone—nabumetone

6. Why should you know the structural classification of the NSAIDs?

The drugs in each class tend to have similar **side effects.** For example, the pyrazolones that were available in the United States at one time included oxyphenbutazone and phenylbutazone. Because of idiosyncratic aplastic anemia, oxyphenbutazone was taken off the market, and phenylbutazone was discontinued by its major manufacturer. The salicylates tend to have tinnitus as a consistent side effect. The propionic acid derivatives are generally a very safe group of drugs, and three of them are now available over-the-counter, ibuprofen, naproxen sodium, and ketoprofen.

The second, and controversial, reason to know the structural classifications might be to select alternative treatments. If a drug in one classification is ineffective, then you might try a different structural compound instead of repeatedly using drugs from one structural group.

7. Describe the mechanism of action of the NSAIDs.

The major mechanism of action is thought to be the inhibition of cyclo-oxygenase, causing a decrease in prostaglandin production. Other mechanisms have been defined for various specific NSAIDs, including:
    Inhibitory effects on lipoxygenase products (sulindac, meclofenamate, diclofenac)
    Inhibition of superoxide formation (indomethacin, piroxicam)
    Inhibition of neutrophil aggregation, adhesion, and enzyme release (salicylates,
        indomethacin)
    Depression of lymphocyte transformation (salicylates)
    Inhibition of rheumatoid factor production (piroxicam)
    Inhibition of acidic and neutral degradative enzymes
    Inhibition of cytokine production
    Suppression of proteoglycan production in cartilage (salicylates, piroxicam,
        ibuprofen, fenoprofen, tolmetin)

8. What factors affect the choice of NSAIDs?

Properties of the drug	Properties of the patient
Efficacy	Individual variation
Tolerance	Disease being treated
Safety	Age
Convenience of dosage	Other diseases
Formulation	Other drugs
Cost	

9. What have efficacy studies of NSAIDs found?

The effects of most NSAIDs are compared to aspirin and, more recently, naproxen. In general, there are no important differences among the various NSAIDs, although there are clear individual variations in response. In certain arthritic diseases, one structural group of NSAIDs may be tried initially over another. For example, in gout and the seronegative spondyloarthropathies, indomethacin or tolmetin are usually the initial drugs of choice. There is no clear relationship between the amount of cyclo-oxygenase inhibition and activity in arthritis. Although the pharmacodynamics of the drug are important in a given individual, there is no good correlation between the plasma level of the drug and efficacy except for salicylates.

10. Who is at risk for a hypersensitivity reaction to NSAIDs?
The patient most at risk is a severe asthmatic with nasal polyps; up to 78% may react to aspirin. Patients with nasal polyps, asthma, or chronic urticaria are also mildly at risk to react to NSAIDs usually with acute bronchospasm and shortness of breath. It is important to note that this is a sensitivity and not an allergy, because it is not IgE-mediated.

11. Discuss the hepatotoxicity of the NSAIDs.
The clearance of NSAIDs is predominantly by hepatic metabolism, with the production of inactive metabolites that are excreted in urine. An elevation of liver enzymes, especially the aminotransferases (AST and ALT), is seen with all NSAIDs to some extent. This was first noticed with the use of aspirin in patients with systemic lupus erythematosus and juvenile rheumatoid arthritis. **Idiosyncratic severe hepatitis** has been reported with indomethacin, diclofenac, sulindac, and phenylbutazone. **Fatal hepatotoxicity** in children using indomethacin has been noted, prompting the recommendation that children under age 11 should not be given indomethacin for arthritis. **Cholestasis** has also been described. The NSAID-induced hepatotoxicity is usually evident during the first 6 months of use. Liver function studies should be obtained during the first month of use and every 3–6 months thereafter.

12. Which NSAIDs are inactive drugs that must be metabolized by the liver to become the active metabolite?
Sulindac and **nabumetone** are prodrugs. Sulindac is reversibly metabolized to sulindac sulfide, a potent cyclo-oxygenase inhibitor, and then converted back to the parent compound in the gut and kidney. Sulindac and its metabolites undergo extensive enterohepatic recirculation, which contributes to its long half-life of 16–18 hours. Nabumetone is a not acidic and is a poor inhibitor of prostaglandin production. It is metabolized to 6-methoxy-2-naphthylacetic acid, which is a potent inhibitor of prostaglandin synthesis. Nabumetone is hepatically, not renally, cleared and does not undergo enterohepatic circulation.

13. What are the gastrointestinal (GI) side effects of NSAIDs?
> Dyspepsia, indigestion and vomiting
> Gastroesophageal reflux
> Gastric erosions
> Peptic ulcers
> Gastrointestinal hemorrhage and perforation
> Small and large bowel ulceration
> Diarrhea (especially with meclofenamate)

Although NSAIDs commonly cause GI symptoms, about one-half of all patients who develop significant peptic ulcers do not develop symptoms.

14. How common are NSAID-induced gastritis and peptic ulcers?
Gastritis and peptic ulcers are among the most common side effects of these drugs. NSAID injury to the GI tract is responsible for an estimated 70,000 hospitalizations and 7,000 deaths annually in the United States. Approximately 2% of patients treated with NSAIDs develop clinically significant, chronic peptic ulceration. Meta-analysis of pooled data suggests a threefold increased risk of adverse GI events among NSAID users as compared to nonusers. The most common area for NSAID-induced ulcers to develop is the stomach, usually the antrum. Unfortunately, routine stool guaiac testing for blood is insensitive in detecting these lesions. The medical costs of GI complications from NSAIDs have been estimated to be $3.9 billion per year.

15. Who is at risk for NSAID-induced gastroduodenal ulcer disease?
Elderly people (>60 yrs old)
History of peptic ulcer disease, with or without NSAIDs
Higher dosage of NSAIDs
Previous use of antacids, H_2-blockers, or omeprazole for GI symptoms,
    with or without NSAIDs
History of abdominal pain of unclear etiology, with or without NSAIDs
Extent of inflammatory disease for which NSAIDs are prescribed
Concomitant corticosteroid use
Controversial
Existing infection with *Helicobacter pylori*
Tobacco use
Alcohol use

16. How do prostaglandins protect the gastric mucosa? What are the effects of NSAIDs on the stomach?
Prostaglandin E_1 and E_2 effect on gastric mucosa
• Induce protective superficial mucous barrier
• Induce bicarbonate output
• Increase mucosal blood flow in the superficial gastric cell layer
• Inhibit gastric acid synthesis
Effects of NSAIDs on the stomach
• Decrease mucous secretion
• Decrease bicarbonate synthesis
• Decrease mucosal blood flow
• Increase gastric acid secretion
• Decrease glutathione synthesis, thus decreasing superoxide scavenging

17. How can you decrease the incidence of NSAID-induced gastric and duodenal ulcers?
1. When appropriate, use alternative analgesics.
2. Use the lowest dose of NSAID possible.
3. If NSAIDs are required, choose a nonacetylated salicylate (which are poor prostaglandin inhibitors).
4. If treating a high-risk patient, consider using misoprostol (a prostaglandin E_1 analog).
5. If misoprostol cannot be used, prescribe an H_2-antagonist or omeprazole to decrease the risk for a duodenal ulcer in the high-risk patient group.
6. If the patient is symptomatic, treat with antacids, H_2 antagonist, or omeprazole.

18. How nephrotoxic are the NSAIDs?
Prostaglandins have relatively little effect on the normal kidney in the euvolemic person. However, in renal insufficiency or hypovolemic states, prostaglandins are important in maintaining adequate glomeruler flow and pressure. Thus, prostaglandins can vasodilate renal arteries, increase sodium loss and increase renin release. Nephrotoxic effects of NSAIDs include:
• Vasoconstriction decreasing glomerular filtration rate and increasing creatinine
• Increase sodium retention and blood volume (this can be important in patients with borderline congestive heart failure)
• Papillary necrosis
• Hyperkalemia
• Hyponatremia
• Acute allergic interstitial nephritis associated with fenoprofen
• Acute tubular necrosis with phenylbutazone

- Interstitial nephritis with aspirin and phenacetin (aspirin alone and other NSAIDs have been associated with interstitial nephritis in a few case reports)

19. What NSAIDs would you use in a patient with mild renal compromise?

The **nonacetylated salicylates** are poor prostaglandin inhibitors and may have less effect on glomerular filtration rate. **Sulindac** has been described as having less renal effects. The rationale for the use of sulindac is that this drug is a prodrug which gets activated to sulindac sulfide, the active compound; the kidney then can revert the active compound back to sulindac and thus not compromise the beneficial effects of prostaglandins. Studies have shown that, empirically, sulindac behaves similarly to other NSAIDs in the patient with renal insufficiency and offers no advantage. Thus sulindac should not be used preferentially in patients with renal compromise.

20. What auditory complications can NSAIDs cause?

Tinnitus is a relatively common complication of salicylates. Although tinnitus has been associated with a wide range of plasma levels of salicylates, it usually indicates that the plasma level is above the therapeutic range. Thus, tinnitus has been used as a "poor man's" way of monitoring salicylate levels. High levels of salicylates in children and the elderly may not induce tinnitus but instead may cause a reversible **hearing deficit.**

21. Do NSAIDs cause any central nervous system problems?

Headaches, dizziness, loss of concentration, depersonalization, tremor, and psychosis have been described in patients taking indomethacin and, to a lesser extent, tolmetin. Ibuprofen has been associated with aseptic meningitis, especially in patients with systemic lupus erythematosus.

22. Your patient responds well to indomethacin but develops headaches. How can you decrease this side effect?

Probenecid is a uricosuric and renal tubular blocking agent. Its co-administration increases the mean plasma elimination half-life of indomethacin, naproxen, ketoprofen, and meclofenamate. It may also interfere with indomethacin's passage through the blood-brain barrier. Thus, with the concomitant use of probenecid, you may be able to reduce the dose of indomethacin by as much as half and still get a good response without CNS side effects.

23. List some rare adverse reactions to NSAIDs.

1. Febrile reactions—ibuprofen
2. Drug-induced lupus—phenylbutazone, ibuprofen
3. Vasculitis—indomethacin, naproxen
4. Mediastinal lymphadenopathy—sulindac
5. Pericarditis, myocarditis—phenylbutazone
6. Aplastic anemia—most NSAIDs, but most significantly phenylbutazone
7. Pure red cell aplasia—phenylbutazone, indomethacin, fenoprofen
8. Thrombocytopenia—most NSAIDs
9. Neutropenia—most NSAIDs
10. Hemolytic anemia—mefenamic acid, ibuprofen, naproxen
11. Stomatitis—most NSAIDs
12. Cutaneous effects (photosensitivity, erythema multiform, urticaria, toxic epidermal necrolysis)—most NSAIDs, especially piroxicam.
13. Aseptic meningitis (especially SLE patients)—ibuprofen, other NSAIDs less commonly

24. Which of the NSAIDs have short plasma elimination half-lives and which have long half-lives?

DRUG	HALF-LIFE (HRS)	DOSAGE
Short half-life (< 6 hrs)		
Aspirin	0.25	
Diclofenac	1.1	25–50 mg bid–tid
		75 mg bid
Etodolac	3.0/6.5*	200 mg tid-qid
		400 mg tid
Fenoprofen	2.5	200–600 mg tid-qid
Flurbiprofen	3.8	50–100 mg bid-tid
Ibuprofen	2.1	300–800 mg tid-qid
Indomethacin	4.7	25 mg tid-qid
		50 mg tid
		75 mg SR bid
Ketoprofen	1.8	50 mg qid
		75 mg tid
		200 mg ER qd
Tolmetin	1.0/6.8*	400–600 mg tid
Long half-life (> 10 hrs)		
Diflunisal	13	250–500 mg bid
Nabumetone	26	500–1000 mg bid
		1000–2000 mg qd
Naproxen	14	250–500 mg bid
Oxaprozin	58	600–1200 mg qd
Phenylbutazone	68	100–400 mg qd
		100 mg tid–qid
Piroxicam	57	10–20 mg qd
Salicylate	2–15†	
Sulindac	14	150–200 mg bid

*Elimination of this drug occurs in two phases, of which the first is generally more important.
†Elimination of this drug is dose-dependent. SR, sustained release; ER, extended release.

Patients are more compliant with single and twice-a-day regimens. The longer half-life drugs may have advantages in patients with morning pain and stiffness.

25. What are some different formulations of NSAIDs?
1. **Enteric-coated tablets**. Enteric-coated aspirin are supposed to have less GI symptoms than regular aspirin, but there is no evidence that the enteric coating decreases gastritis or peptic ulcers.
2. **Liquid formulations**. Ibuprofen, naproxen, choline magnesium trisalicylate, and indomethacin are available in liquid formulations that are designed for patients who have difficulty swallowing pills and for children.
3. **Slow release**. The slow-release formulation is designed to give a short-acting drug a longer half-life so that the drug can be taken only twice a day (indomethacin SR) or once a day (ketoprofen ER).

26. Which NSAIDs can be used in children?
Salicylates, ibuprofen, naproxen, and tolmetin are FDA-approved for use in children.

27. Are precautions needed when using NSAIDs in the elderly?
Rheumatic diseases are common in the elderly, and this group of patients frequently use NSAIDs. The elderly realize more complications from these drugs than any other group of patients, because of:
- Altered drug absorption. The gastric pH rises with age. Active absorption and transport of drugs may be altered.
- Reduced drug distribution
- Decreased protein-binding. Plasma albumin decreases with aging, decreasing protein-binding sites.
- Hepatic metabolism and renal excretion may be altered.

- Polypharmacy. Some patient's medications may have drug interactions with NSAIDs.
Thus, to reduce the risk of NSAIDs in the elderly:
  - Do not prescribe NSAIDs when they are not necessary. Do not continue treatment longer than necessary.
  - Start at the lowest dose and follow up within a month for toxicity and therapeutic benefit.
  - Increase the dose cautiously.
  - Beware of high-risk drugs.
  - Beware of high-risk patients.
  - Maintain close supervision.

28. List some drug–drug interactions involving NSAIDs.

NSAIDs Affecting Other Drugs

DRUG AFFECTED	NSAID IMPLICATED	EFFECT
Warfarin	Phenylbutazone	Inhibits metabolism of warfarin, increasing anti-coagulent effect
	All NSAIDs	Increases risk of bleeding owing to inhibition of platelet function and gastric mucosal damage
Sulfonylurea	Phenylbutazone	Inhibits sulfonylurea metabolism, increasing risk of hypoglycemia
	High-dose salicylate	Potentiates hypoglycemia by different mechanism
Beta-blocker	All PG-inhibiting NSAIDs	Blunts hypotensive but not negative chronotropic or inotropic effect
Hydralazine Prazosin ACE-inhibitor	All PG-inhibiting NSAIDs	Loss of hypotensive effects
Diuretics	All PG-inhibiting NSAIDs	Loss of natriuretic, diuretic, hypotensive effects of furosemide
		Loss of natriuretic effect of spironolactone
		Loss of hypotensive but not natriurectic or diuretic effects of thiazide
Phenytoin	Phenylbutazone	Inhibits metabolism, increasing plasma concentration and thereby risk of toxicity
	Other NSAIDs	Displaces phenytoin from plasma protein, reducing total concentration for the same active concentration
Lithium	Most NSAIDs	Increases plasma lithium level
Digoxin	Most NSAIDs	May increase digoxin levels
Aminoglycosides	Most NSAIDs	May increase aminoglycoside level
Methotrexate	Most NSAIDs	May increase methotrexate plasma concentration
Sodium valproate	Aspirin	Inhibits valproate metabolism, increasing plasma valproate concentration

Other Drugs Affecting NSAIDs

DRUG-IMPLICATED	NSAID AFFECTED	EFFECT
Antacids	Indomethacin Salicylates	Aluminum-containing antacids reduce rate and extent of absorption
	Other NSAIDs?	Sodium bicarbonate increases rate and extent of absorption
Cimetidine	Piroxicam	Increases plasma concentrations and half-life of piroxicam
Probenecid	Most NSAIDs	Reduces metabolism and renal clearance of NSAIDs
Cholestyramine	Naproxen Probably others	Anion exchange resin binds NSAIDs in gut, reducing rate (and extent?) of absorption
Caffeine	Aspirin	Increases rate of absorption of aspirin
Metoclopramide	Aspirin and probably others	Increases rate and extent of absorption in patients with migraines

29. Future NSAIDs may have benefits over present NSAIDs. Discuss this considering our recent understanding of prostaglandin synthase H (cyclooxygenase) regulation.

There are at least two isoforms of the cyclooxygenase enzyme. These two isoforms are regulated and expressed differently. The prostaglandin H synthase 1 (PGHS-1) or cyclooxygenase 1 (COX-1) products are constitutively made and involved in normal cellular processes or "housekeeping" functions. COX-1 products are stimulated by hormones or growth factors and are important in protecting gastric mucosa. Prostaglandin H synthase 2 (PGHS-2) or cyclooxygenase 2 (COX-2) products are stimulated in white blood cells and fibroblasts by an inflammatory process. These products are usually undetected unless stimulated by inflammation. Future NSAIDs will selectively inhibit COX-2 products while not inhibiting COX-1 products. Thus, the beneficial anti-inflammatory effects will occur with future NSAIDs without the serious side effects.

BIBLIOGRAPHY

1. Clements PJ, Paulus HE: Nonsteroidal anti-inflammatory drugs (NSAIDs). In Kelly WN, Harris ED, Ruddy S, Sledge CB (eds): Textbook of Rheumatology, 4th ed. Philadelphia, W.B. Saunders, 1993, pp 700–730.
2. Huskisson EC: How to choose a non-steroidal anti-inflammatory drug. Rheum Dis Clin North Am 10:313–323, 1984.
3. Brooks PM, Day RO: Nonsteroidal antiinflammatory drugs—Differences and similarities. N Engl J Med 324:1716–1725, 1991.
4. Simon LS, Goodman T: NSAID-induced gastrointestinal toxicity. Bull Rheum Dis 44:1–5, 1995.
5. Hollander D: Gastrointestinal complications of nonsteroidal anti-inflammatory drugs: Prophylactic and therapeutic strategies. Am J Med 96:274–281, 1994.
6. Tolman KG: Hepatotoxicity of antirheumatic drugs. J Rheumatol 17:6–11, 1990.
7. Rodriguez LAG, Williams R, Derby LE, et al: Acute liver injury associated with nonsteroidal anti-inflammatory drugs and the role of risk factors. Arch Intern Med 154:311–316, 1994.
8. Scheiman JM: Pathogenesis of gastroduodenal injury due to nonsteroidal antiinflammatory drugs. Implications for prevention and therapy. Semin Arthritis Rheum 21:201–210, 1992.
9. Webster J: Interactions of NSAIDs with diuretics and beta-blockers: Mechanisms and clinical implications. Drugs 30:32–41, 1985.
10. O'Brien WM, Bagby GF: Rare adverse reactions to nonsteroidal antiinflammatory drugs [pts I and II]. J Rheumatol 12:13–20, 347–353, 1985.
11. Clive DM, Stoff JS: Renal syndromes associated with nonsteroidal antiinflammatory drugs. N Engl J Med 310:563–572, 1984.
12. Garella S, Matarese RA: Renal effects of prostaglandins and clinical adverse effects of nonsteroidal anti-inflammatory agents. Medicine 63:165–181, 1984.
13. Abramson SB, Weissmann G: The mechanisms of action of nonsteroidal antiinflammatory drugs. Arthritis Rheum 32:1–9, 1989.
14. Morgan J, Furst DE: Implications of drug therapy in the elderly. Rheum Dis Clin North Am 12:227–244, 1986.

85. GLUCOCORTICOIDS—SYSTEMIC AND INJECTABLE

Gregory J. Dennis, M.D.

1. List some general indications for implementation of glucocorticoid therapy.

Glucocorticoids or corticosteroids are potent medications commonly used for a variety of medical reasons. For rheumatic disorders, there are two main general indications for the use of corticosteroids:

    1. To suppress the inflammatory cascade
    2. To modify the immune response

2. Which modes of administration of corticosteroids are effective in the treatment of rheumatic disease?

While certain modes of administration clearly modify immune function and inflammatory reactions more rapidly, some conditions respond similarly to multiple modes of administration. Common effective modes of corticosteroid therapy for rheumatic disorders include:

    a. Intrasynovial therapy (needle injection into joint, bursa, or tendon sheath) is generally used to control inflammatory reactions involving the synovial lining of articular surfaces.

    b. Oral or alimentary therapy

    c. Parenteral: intramuscular and intravenous

3. List some important factors to consider prior to beginning corticosteroid therapy.

Historical factors to consider include:

    Chronic infection

    Glucose intolerance or a history of familial diabetes

    Osteoporosis

    Peptic ulcer disease, gastritis, or esophagitis

    Cardiovascular disease or hypertension

    Mental disturbance

These factors do not preclude the use of steroids but may serve to heighten one's awareness of the possibility for specific adverse consequences.

4. How can the physician establish a baseline for each of these historical factors before instituting corticosteroid therapy?

Some **chronic infections** which may not be immediately apparent on the initial physical examination are primarily opportunistic and will progress when corticosteroid therapy is implemented. Examples include tuberculosis and fungal disorders that commonly cause pulmonary infections in immunocompromised hosts. For a baseline, obtain a **chest x-ray** and a **tuberculin skin test.**

A predisposition to **glucose intolerance** is an important clue to the likelihood of diabetes occurring in association with steroid therapy. Performing a baseline **fasting glucose** is sufficient prior to the implementation of therapy, with periodic monitoring, especially with longer courses of therapy.

Adverse problems related to **osteoporosis** may occur surprisingly soon after the implementation of corticosteroid therapy. To assess one's risk for osteoporosis-related problems, a **spinal x-ray** should be performed in all postmenopausal patients. Bone mineral densitometry and the institution of prophylactic therapy should be considered in those with abnormal findings.

The activity of **gastrointestinal erosive disease** may be further aggravated by corticosteroid medications. A **stool guaiac** test and a **complete blood count** with mean cell volume should be performed prior to beginning therapy.

Since both **cardiovascular disease** and **hypertension** may be aggravated by corticosteroid medications, particular attention should be given toward **blood pressure determination** as well as the presence of peripheral edema on physical examination, with periodic reevaluation.

Finally, performing a **MiniMental status examination,** especially in those with a history of mental disturbance, will provide an objective baseline to which the patient may be compared on future evaluations.

5. Is corticosteroid therapy ever considered to be the cornerstone of therapy for a rheumatic disease?

Yes, for several rheumatic diseases. In general, the rheumatic diseases for which steroids are primarily used are classified as **connective tissue diseases.** Among these disorders are:

- Polymyalgia rheumatica
- Polymyositis/dermatomyositis
- Vasculitic disorders
- Selective complications associated with the connective tissue diseases (rheumatoid arthritis, systemic lupus erythematosus, Sjögren's, others)

6. Does dosage scheduling influence the potency of corticosteroid therapy?
Yes. The potency of corticosteroid therapy clinically correlates with the duration of hypothala-mic-pituitary axis suppression. From the least to the most suppressive, these are:

> Intermittent oral dosing
> Alternate day
> Single daily AM dose
> Intermittent intravenous pulse therapy
> Multiple daily dosing

7. Are corticosteroid medications ever used in rheumatic diseases other than connective tissue diseases?
Yes, but primarily in the form of local therapy. A variety of therapeutic modalities have been used for the local administration of corticosteroids; however, needle injection remains the most effective means of delivering medication to the musculoskeletal structures. Specific conditions for which corticosteroid injections are particularly effective include:

> a. Intrabursal treatment of bursitis
> b. Tendon sheath injection for tendinitis
> c. Intra-articular injection for synovitis
> d. Soft-tissue trigger point injection

8. How are the corticosteroids grouped in terms of biologic activity?
The corticosteroids may be divided into three main groups according to their duration of biologic activity.

> **Short-acting** (half-life <12 hrs)   **Long-acting** (half-life >48 hrs)
> Hydrocortisone   Paramethasone
> Cortisone   Betamethasone
> **Intermediate-Acting** (half-life of 12–36 hrs)   Dexamethasone
> Prednisone
> Prednisolone
> Methylprednisolone
> Triamcinolone

9. What additional characteristic of the corticosteroid preparation is important to consider when determining which to use for injection therapy? Why?
Solubility of the corticosteroid preparation is an important factor when considering injection therapy. Reducing the solubility of a compound increases the duration of the local effect, since slower diffusion of the medication will occur. Thus, more insoluble preparations have greater potency but are also more likely to result in adverse consequences.

10. List some important drug properties to consider when deciding which corticosteroid preparation to use.

> Biological half-life
> Mineralocorticoid effects
> Need for conversion to biologically active equivalents
> Formulation of the preparation
> Cost of the medication

11. Which group of corticosteroid medications results in the least amount of sodium retention?
Sodium retention is dependent on the mineralocorticoid effect of the preparation. It is insignificant in the usual doses of methylprednisolone, triamcinolone, paramethasone, betamethasone, and dexamethasone.

Mineralocorticoid Properties of Glucocorticoid Preparations

GLUCOCORTICOID	MINERALOCORTICOID POTENCY*
Short-Acting	
Hydrocortisone	1
Cortisone	0.8
Intermediate-Acting	
Prednisone	0.25
Prednisolone	0.25
Methylprednisolone	±
Triamcinolone	±
Long-acting	
Paramethasone	±
Betamethasone	±
Dexamethasone	±

*Potency is expressed in milligram comparisons to cortisol (reference value of 1).

12. How do the glucocorticoid properties of the corticosteroids compare with cortisol?

The glucocorticoid potency of medications correlates in part with the duration of biologic activity.

Glucocorticoid Properties of Corticosteroid Preparations

GLUCOCORTICOID	GLUCOCORTICOID POTENCY*
Short-acting	
Hydrocortisone	1
Cortisone	0.8
Intermediate-acting	
Prednisone	4
Prednisolone	4
Methylprednisolone	5
Triamcinolone	5
Long-acting	
Paramethasone	10
Betamethasone	25
Dexamethasone	30–40

*Potency is determined with cortisol as a reference (1).

13. What are some of the adverse consequences of corticosteroid therapy?

Glucose intolerance

Muscle weakness

Skin disorders (bruising, striae, delayed wound repair)

Obesity

Peptic ulcer disease

Osteoporosis

Growth suppression

Cataract formation

Hirsuitism

Infection

Abnormal menstruation

Mental disturbance

14. When establishing the patient's tuberculin reactivity status, why is it important to obtain skin testing before implementing corticosteroid therapy?

Continuous administration of pharmacologic doses of corticosteroid is likely to result in suppression of the cellular response to skin testing within 2 weeks of therapy. Furthermore, the altered cellular response may selectively affect tuberculin reactivity. Thus, negative skin test results obtained after starting glucocorticoid medications are unreliable, even when control skin testing is positive.

15. How common is adrenal atrophy in patients taking glucocorticoids?

Exogenous administration of glucocorticoids is the most common cause of adrenal insufficiency, resulting from suppression of ACTH. In the complete absence of ACTH, the human adrenal cortex begins to atrophy in 1 week. The recognition that treatment with ACTH-suppressive doses may lead to functional adrenocortical atrophy is important, because when such patients are stressed by infection, trauma, or surgery, they are unable to respond with the usual cortisol output (up to 200–300 mg/day). Proper management during periods of physiologic stress aims to mimic the normal cortisol response.

16. In the treatment of rheumatic disease, what is considered to be low-, medium-, and high-dose daily prednisone therapy?

Low dose	<15 mg/d
Medium dose	15 – < 40 mg/d
High dose	> 40 mg/d

17. To minimize the risk of hypothalamic-pituitary-adrenal (HPA) axis suppression, when should patients take their daily dose of corticosteroid medication?

Because natural cortisol secretion in humans has a circadian rhythm with the peak level in the morning, taking the corticosteroid at that time will have less of a suppressive effect on the release of cortisol-releasing factor. As such, taking the supplemental corticosteroid before approximately 10:00 AM will result in less suppression of the HPA axis.

18. What are the major benefits of intrasynovial corticosteroid injections?
- Alleviate inflammation in a joint, bursa, or tendon sheath
- Avoid institution of systemic therapy

19. List some of the general indications for corticosteroid injection therapy in rheumatic conditions.

  1. Isolated joint inflammation in patients with polyarticular disease out of proportion to other joints (after joint infection is ruled out)
  2. Recurrent joint effusion
  3. Tendon sheath inflammation
  4. Bursitis or tendinitis refractory to NSAIDs
  5. Noninfectious monarthritis

20. What disease processes have an indication at some time in their clinical course for corticosteroid injection therapy?

Rheumatoid arthritis	Osteoarthritis
Crystal deposition disease	Shoulder tendinitis/bursitis
Systemic lupus erythematosus	Tietze's syndrome
Acute traumatic arthritis	Seronegative spondyloarthropathies

21. What corticosteroid preparations are available for injection into a joint, bursa, or tendon sheath?

Corticosteroid Preparations Suitable for Joint or Other Injection

PREPARATION	STRENGTHS (MG/ML)	PREDNISONE EQUIVALENT (MG)*
Short-acting, soluble		
Dexamethasone sodium phosphate (Decadron, Hexadrol)	4	40
Hydrocortisone acetate (Hydrocortone)	25	5
Long-acting, less soluble		
Prednisolone tebutate (Hydeltra-TBA)	20	20
Methylprednisolone acetate (Depo-Medrol)	20, 40, 80	25, 50, 100
Dexamethasone acetate (Decadron-LA)	8	80
Longest-acting, least soluble		
Triamcinolone acetonide (Kenalog, Aristocort)	10, 40	12.5, 50
Triamcinolone hexacetonide (Aristospan)	20	25
Betamethasone sodium phosphate/acetate (Celestone, Soluspan)	6	50

*Of 1 ml of injected steroid preparation.

22. What volume of corticosteroid can be safely injected into a joint?
The volume of corticosteroid that can be safely injected depends on the size of the joint. The physician must be aware of the volume to be injected into the joint, and all attempts should be made to avoid overdistention of the surrounding joint capsule.

SIZE OF JOINT	VOLUME (ML)
Large (Knees, ankles, shoulders)	1–2
Medium (Elbows, wrists)	0.5–1
Small (Interphalangeal, metaphalangeal)	0.1–0.5

23. Is there an optimal dose of corticosteroid to be injected into synovial-lined spaces?
The dose of corticosteroid to be injected into synovial-lined cavities depends on the:
  a. Size of the joint
  b. Degree of inflammation
  c. Amount of fluid present
  d. Concentration of corticosteroid used

24. What type and amount of corticosteroid should be injected into a joint, bursa, or tendon sheath? (*Controversial*)
It is generally recommended that short-acting or long-acting corticosteroid be injected into tendon sheaths since they are more soluble and cause less soft tissue atrophy or chance of tendon rupture. The longest-acting, least-soluble corticosteroid preparations are typically injected into inflamed joints since they tend to be more efficacious.

Guidelines for the Appropriate Dose of Corticosteroid to be Injected

SITE	PREDNISONE EQUIVALENT DOSE (MG)
Bursa	10–20
Tendon sheath	10–20
Small joints of hands and feet	5–15
Medium-sized joints (wrist, elbow)	15–25
Large joints (knee, shoulder, ankle)	20–50

25. How often can a joint or tendon sheath be injected with corticosteroid medications?
The main concern with frequent injections is accelerated deterioration of the joint due to cartilage breakdown or weakening of the tendon with tendon rupture. The longer the interval between injections, the better. A minimum of 4–6 weeks between injections is recommended. Weight-bearing joints should not be injected more frequently than every 6–12 weeks. The same joint or tendon sheath should not be injected more than 3 times yearly.

26. Can the corticosteroid for injection be combined with anesthetic to minimize the number of needlesticks to the patient?
Yes, anesthetic preparations can be safely combined or mixed with the corticosteroid preparation. However, if the corticosteroid preparation contains a paraben compound as a preservative, flocculation of the suspension is likely to occur.

27. What are the potential complications and sequelae of corticosteroid injections?

1. Infection
2. Steroid crystal-induced synovitis (postinjection flare)
3. Hypopigmentation
4. Subcutaneous tissue atrophy
5. Tendon rupture

28. Are there any contraindications to intrasynovial corticosteroid injections?
The physician must be aware of the contraindications to corticosteroid injection (whether relative or absolute) in order to decide if the injection is truly in the best interests of the patient. The following situations require serious consideration before injecting corticosteroid:

Periarticular and articular sepsis   Lack of response to previous injections
Bacteremia   Blood clotting disorders
Joint instability   Intra-articular fracture
Inaccessible joints

29. How are the anti-inflammatory effects of corticosteroids mediated?

Steroids have beneficial anti-inflammatory effects through numerous mechanisms. Some of the most important are:

- Decrease in neutrophil margination, migration, and accumulation at inflammatory sites
- Inhibition of neutrophil and macrophage phagocytosis, enzyme release, and pro-inflammatory cytokine production (especially interleukin-1 and tumor necrosis factor)
- Induction of lipocortin and lipomodulin, which decrease arachidonic acid synthesis with a corresponding decrease in prostaglandin and leukotriene production
- Decrease T-cell proliferation and interleukin-2 synthesis and secretion

BIBLIOGRAPHY

1. Axelrod L: Glucocorticoid therapy. Medicine 55:39, 1976.
2. Baxter JD: The effects of glucocorticoid therapy. Hosp Pract 27:111–134, 1992.
3. Chrousos GP: The hypothalamic pituitary-adrenal axis and immune-mediated inflammation. N Engl J Med 332:1351–1362, 1995.
4. Cupps TR: Therapeutic use. In Boumpas DT (moderator): Glucocorticoid therapy for immune-mediated diseases: Basic and clinical correlates. Ann Intern Med 119:1198–1208, 1993.
5. Fauci AS, Dale DC, Balow JE: Glucocorticoid therapy: Mechanisms of action and clinical considerations. Ann Intern Med 44:304–315, 1976.
6. Paulus HE, Bulpitt KJ: Nonsteroidal antiinflammatory agents and corticosteroids. In Schumacher HR Jr (ed): Primer on the Rheumatic Diseases, 10th ed. Atlanta, Arthritis Foundation, 1993, pp 300–304, 310–311.

86. SYSTEMIC ANTIRHEUMATIC DRUGS

James O'Dell, M.D.

If many drugs are used for a disease, all are insufficient.

—Sir William Osler

1. What is meant by a disease-modifying drug or remission-inducing drug in rheumatoid arthritis?

Because there is no cure for rheumatoid arthritis (RA), the goal of treatment is to put the disease in remission. Different names have been used to describe a category of drugs with at least some ability to do this:

Disease-modifying antirheumatic drugs (DMARDs)
Remission-inducing drugs
Second-level drugs
Slow-acting antirheumatic drugs (SAARDs)

All of these designations are unsatisfactory for one reason or another. *Disease-modifying drugs* is a misnomer, as these drugs do not always modify the disease, at least not in all patients. *Remission-inducing drugs* suffers from the obvious problem that drug-induced remissions in RA are rare. *Second-level drugs* may imply that these drugs are used later in the course of treatment. *Slow-acting drugs* is descriptive in that most of these drugs do take months to work, but this name does not instill a lot of confidence in patients or physicians.

None of the drugs in this category is consistently able to produce a complete remission in patients with RA. However, most are able to modify the course of the disease.

2. List the drugs felt to be in the disease-modifying category for the treatment of RA.
Intramuscular (IM) gold (Solganal, Myochrysine)
Antimalarials (hydroxychloroquine [Plaquenil], chloroquine [Aralen])
Sulfasalazine (Azulfidine)
D-Penicillamine (Cupramine, DePen)
Oral gold/auranofin (Ridaura)
Methotrexate (Rheumatrex)
Azathioprine (Imuran)
Cyclosporine (Sandimmune, Neoral)

3. Which DMARDs are most effective against RA?

Most	Methotrexate
	IM gold
	Sulfasalazine
	D-Penicillamine
	Azathioprine
Mid	Antimalarials (hydroxychloroquine, chloroquine)
Least	Oral gold

Meta-analysis has shown rather similar efficacies for most DMARDs over the short-term. Antimalarials and oral gold are weaker than the others but are clearly better than placebos. The overall efficacy of oral gold is about 40% and antimalarials about 55%. Methotrexate has been placed at the top of this list because studies have shown that its beneficial effects last significantly longer than those of the other DMARDs.

4. Which DMARDs are most toxic?
In order from most to least, they are:
IM gold
Sulfasalazine
D-Penicillamine
Methotrexate
Oral gold
Antimalarials

Almost all of the side effects from sulfasalazine are minor GI tract problems. Therefore, it could be placed after oral gold on this list if severity of side effects is considered.

5. What are the objectives of therapy when treating RA?
1. To do everything possible to allow the patient to *function* as normally as possible in the *short-term*.
2. To make sure that the therapy we prescribe today is as effective as possible in arresting or delaying the joint damage and destruction so that joints will *continue to function* well for many years to come.

6. When should a patient with RA be started on a DMARD?

Indications for DMARD Therapy in Rheumatoid Arthritis

Evidence of active disease (synovitis, morning stiffness, etc.)
Evidence of progressive bony erosions or deformities
Extra-articular manifestations

Once erosions and/or deformities occur, they are generally *irreversible;* therefore, it is clearly important that therapy is instituted early to prevent these. Once the diagnosis of RA is established (generally after 6 weeks to 6 months of symptoms), most rheumatologists would start DMARD therapy for the indications listed.

7. How quickly can DMARDs be expected to work?
When these drugs are started, it is important to educate the patient about the time frame of response. Most of the disease-modifying therapies in RA take several months to achieve a significant response. If the patients expect that the pills you gave them today will make them better tomorrow, they are going to be very disappointed (and they will let you know it).

8. What are the common side effects of IM gold?
Nitritoid reaction (10–15%)
Skin rash (10–15%)
Proteinuria (3–4%)
Hematologic reactions (1–2%)
The nitritoid reaction is flushing and hypotension, which occurs within 15–30 minutes of receiving IM gold (usually myochrysine).

9. Describe the standard protocol for administration of IM gold.
IM gold therapy is most commonly initiated with a test dose of 10 mg intramuscularly. If no untoward reactions occur, this is followed 1 week later by 25–50 mg (most patients are placed on 50 mg). Weekly injections of 50 mg are then given until the patient has a significant response, or until 1 gm of gold has been given. If 1 gm of gold has been given without improvement, therapy is usually abandoned for lack of efficacy. If the patient improves, the frequency of the gold injections is commonly decreased to every 2–3 weeks, and occasionally to monthly intervals. Once the gold injections are spaced out, it is common for the patient to have a flare of disease, which generally means the gold shots need to be given at closer intervals.

10. What laboratory follow-up is necessary for patients on gold therapy?
The standard recommendations are to do a **CBC** with **platelet count** and a **dipstick urinalysis** looking for proteinuria prior to each gold injection. If a significant decline in the WBC count, platelets, or significant proteinuria (generally > 2+ on the dipstick) is found, therapy may need to be discontinued.

11. How is *oral* gold used in the treatment of RA? Does it differ from IM gold?
How supplied: 3-mg capsules
Side effects: Diarrhea, rashes, proteinuria, bone marrow depression
Dosage: 3–9 mg orally per day
Follow-up: Monthly CBC, platelet count, and dipstick urinalysis
The major problem with administering oral gold, besides its lower efficacy, is **GI intolerance,** predominantly **diarrhea,** which occurs in at least 5% of the patients. Oral gold is similar to IM gold in its potential to cause rashes, proteinuria, or bone marrow depression, but all of these are significantly less common with oral gold.

12. How are the antimalarial drugs used in the treatment of RA?
How supplied: Hydroxychloroquine, 200-mg tablets
              Chloroquine, 250- and 500-mg tablets
Side effects: Nausea, vomiting, rashes, ophthalmologic problems (rare)
Dosage: Hydroxychloroquine, 200–400 mg/day;
          Chloroquine, 250 mg/day
Follow-up: Ophthalmologist visit every 6 months
The antimalarials are clearly the **least toxic** of all the DMARDs used in the treatment of RA.

The major toxicity of these drugs is on the retina, but at the doses currently recommended, retinal toxicity that threatens vision is extremely uncommon (< 0.2%). Antimalarials may cause GI problems, including nausea and vomiting, in approximately 3% of patients, and skin rashes may occur in approximately 2%. In this country, the current recommendation is that patients see an ophthalmologist every 6 months so that any retinal toxicity can be detected early.

13. Discuss the use of D-penicillamine in the treatment of RA.

> How supplied: 125-mg and 250-mg tablets or capsules
> Side effects: Skin rash, proteinuria, hematologic (thrombocytopenia)
> Dosage: 125–250 mg/day for 2–3 mos, increased stepwise to 750–1000 mg/day to maximum response
> Follow-up: Monthly CBC, platelet count, and dipstick urinalysis

D-Penicillamine has fallen out of favor with many rheumatologists because it often takes 6 or more months to get any significant response and because its side effects include some fairly rare but serious autoimmune diseases.

14. Tell me more. What autoimmune syndromes have been attributed to D-penicillamine?

> Drug-induced lupus
> Goodpasture's syndrome
> Myasthenia gravis (up to 3% of patients)
> Pemphigus
> Polymyositis
> Red cell aplasia or aplastic anemia

15. Discuss the use of sulfasalazine in the treatment of RA.

> How supplied: 500-mg tablets (regular or enteric-coated)
> Side effects: Nausea, vomiting, skin rashes, hepatic enzyme elevation, neutropenia, azoospermia (reversible)
> Dosage: 1–3 gm a day
> Follow-up: CBC, platelet count, and liver function tests monthly for 3 mos, then every 3 months

Even though sulfasalazine is the only DMARD that was originally developed as an antirheumatic drug, it is not formally approved by the FDA for the treatment of RA. Nonetheless, since its potential for significant toxicity is very low, and its efficacy compares favorably with that of other DMARDs, its use in the treatment of RA is currently increasing. Sulfasalazine is a two-component drug, made up of sulfapyridine and 5-aminosalicylic acid (5-ASA).

16. When should DMARDs be stopped in an RA patient who is doing well?

In most cases, DMARD therapy should be *continued indefinitely* in patients who are doing well. Spontaneous remissions in RA patients who have required DMARD therapy are very uncommon, and continued efficacy of all currently available DMARDs requires maintenance therapy. Flares that are severe may occur with discontinuation of most of these drugs.

17. Can combinations of two or more DMARDs be used in therapy for RA?

There is currently much enthusiasm for the simultaneous use of two or more DMARDs in the treatment of RA patients. This enthusiasm may result from the success of this approach in a variety of patients with infectious diseases and cancer. Some surveys have suggested that one-third to one-half of rheumatoid arthritis patients may be on combination therapy. Unfortunately, very little data available in RA support this practice.

Most of the studies have not used full therapeutic doses when DMARDs have been combined. A recent study has reported that the combination of methotrexate, sulfasalazine, and hydroxychloroquine is significantly more effective than methotrexate alone in the treatment of RA. Another study has shown the combination of methotrexate and cyclosporine to be effective in RA. These studies await further confirmation.

18. RA commonly occurs in women of child-bearing age. How safe are the DMARDs in pregnancy?
All the currently available disease-modifying drugs should be considered **contraindicated** in pregnant women. The teratogenic risk appears to be greatest with methotrexate. Fortunately, pregnancy has a dramatic ameliorating effect on the activity of RA in most patients. If therapy for RA is needed during pregnancy, steroids can be used without fetal toxicity.

19. What manifestations of SLE are most amenable to antimalarial therapy?
    Skin manifestations
    Joint disease
    ± Constitutional symptoms (fatigue, fever, etc.)
    ± Serositis
Antimalarial therapy is very useful in treating patients with SLE in general. However, most clinicians do not find it useful in the acute treatment of patients with nephritis, pneumonitis, CNS problems, or hematologic problems (hemolytic anemias, thrombocytopenias, etc.).

20. Are there other indications for the use of antimalarial therapy in SLE?
Convincing data are now available that antimalarial therapy is extremely useful in **maintaining remissions** or **preventing flares** in patients with SLE. Lupus patients who are on chronic antimalarial therapy are less likely to have flares of their disease, including flares of nephritis and CNS manifestations. Therefore, almost all patients who have demonstrated a significant tendency toward organ involvement from their lupus should be maintained on antimalarial therapy while they are felt to be at high risk for flares of their disease.

21. Although NSAIDs are often used to treat minor manifestations of psoriatic arthritis, which drugs are useful in treatment of more severe disease?
    IM gold, sulfasalazine, methotrexate, hydroxychloroquine, and azathioprine.
    Both IM gold and methotrexate, given as for RA, have been effective in treating psoriatic arthritis. Methotrexate has the added advantage of being very beneficial for the skin lesions of psoriasis. Unfortunately, the liver toxicity of methotrexate, when used in the treatment of psoriatic arthritis, appears to be more of a problem than in RA. Sulfasalazine also has been used successfully to treat patients with psoriatic arthritis. Azathioprine and cyclosporine have been used in limited numbers of patients. Significant flares of skin disease have been reported with hydroxychloroquine.

22. What can be used to treat Reiter's syndrome that is refractory to NSAIDs?
Reiter's syndrome may respond to sulfasalazine, methotrexate, or azathioprine. Caution should be used before immunosuppressive therapy is given to patients with Reiter's syndrome to make sure that they are not HIV-positive. The onset of AIDS has been precipitated by immunosuppressive therapy. This has also been reported in HIV-positive patients with psoriasis.

23. In which rheumatic syndromes is treatment with hydroxychloroquine (Plaquenil) indicated?
Rheumatoid arthritis, SLE, palindromic rheumatism, psoriatic arthritis, and Sjögren's syndrome (possibly). The efficacy of hydroxychloroquine in psoriatic arthritis has been reported, but so have significant flares of skin disease.

24. What rheumatic syndromes might respond to sulfasalazine?
    Rheumatoid arthritis
    Reiter's syndrome
    Psoriatic arthritis
    Ankylosing spondylitis (peripheral manifestations)
    Enteropathic arthritis

25. In which syndromes might treatment with gold be indicated?
Rheumatoid arthritis
Psoriatic arthritis
Palindromic rheumatism
Reiter's syndrome (maybe)

26. List the diseases commonly treated with D-penicillamine.
Rheumatoid arthritis
Systemic sclerosis (controversial)
Wilson's disease
Cystinuria
Primary biliary cirrhosis (controversial)

Systemic sclerosis is commonly treated with D-penicillamine because fairly large retrospective studies showed a decreased progression of skin involvement with long-term therapy. Because of the lack of prospective data and the potential side effects, however, some rheumatologists are reluctant to use D-pencillamine in this condition. (The use of D-penicillamine in the treatment of RA has been discussed in Question 13.)

BIBLIOGRAPHY

1. Canadian Hydroxychloroquine Study Group: A randomized study of the effect of withdrawing hydroxychloroquine sulfate in systemic lupus erythematosus. N Engl J Med 324:150, 1991.
2. Cash JM, Klippel JH: Second-line drug therapy for rheumatoid arthritis. N Engl J Med 330:1368, 1994.
3. Dougados M, van der Linden S, Leirisalo-Repo M, et al: Sulfasalazine in the treatment of spondyloarthropathy: A randomized, multicentre, double-blind, placebo-controlled study. Arthritis Rheum 38:618–27, 1995.
4. Felson DT, Anderson JJ, Meenan RF: The comparative efficacy and toxicity of second-line drugs in rheumatoid arthritis. Arthritis Rheum 33:1449, 1990.
5. Felson DT, Anderson JJ, Meenan RF: Use of short-term efficacy/toxicity tradeoffs to select second-line drugs in rheumatoid arthritis: A metaanalysis of published clinical trials. Arthritis Rheum 35:1117, 1992.
6. Harris ED: Treatment of rheumatoid arthritis. In Kelley WN, Harris ED Jr, Ruddy S, Sledge CB (eds): Textbook of Rheumatology, 4th ed. Philadelphia, W.B. Saunders, 1993, pp 912–923.
7. Klippel JH, Dieppe PA: Rheumatology. London, Mosby Europe 1994.
8. McCarty DJ, Koopman WJ: Arthritis and Allied Conditions, 12th ed. Philadelphia, Lea & Febiger, 1993.
9. O'Dell J, Haire C, Erikson N, et al: Treatment of rheumatoid arthritis with methotrexate, sulfasalazine, and hydroxychloroquine, or a combination of these medications. N Engl J Med 334:1287–1291, 1996.
10. Situnayake RD, Grindulis KA, McConkey B: Long term treatment of rheumatoid arthritis with sulphasalazine, gold, or penicillamine: A comparison using life-table methods. Ann Rheum Dis 46:177, 1987.
11. Williams HJ: Rheumatoid arthritis. In Schumacher HR (ed): Primer on the Rheumatic Diseases, 10th ed. Atlanta, Arthritis Foundation, 1993, pp 86–99.

87. CYTOTOXIC DRUGS AND IMMUNOMODULATORS

James O'Dell, M.D.

The physician without physiology and chemistry practices a sort of popgun pharmacy, hitting now the malady and again the patient, he himself not knowing which.

—Sir William Osler

1. What is the place of methotrexate relative to other DMARDs in the overall treatment of rheumatoid arthritis?
Methotrexate (Rheumatrex, Immunex) is widely considered to be the *most effective* DMARD currently available for the treatment of rheumatoid arthritis (RA). This is particularly true if we examine the percentage of patients who remain on a DMARD after 3–5 years of therapy. This 3–5-year time period is much more indicative of a drug's long-term usefulness in RA than most available data which look at 6-month to 1-year periods. However, with long-term therapy, significant concerns about methotrexate hepatotoxicity arise. Fortunately, in RA patients, cirrhosis from methotrexate has been extremely uncommon. Acute pneumonitis, while a rare occurrence, is troublesome because it is difficult or impossible to predict which patients may develop it.

2. How is methotrexate used in the treatment of RA?
How supplied: 2.5-mg tablets, 25 mg/ml vials
Side effects: Oral ulcers, nausea, bone marrow depression, cirrhosis, pneumonitis
Dosage: 7.5–20 mg orally, subcutaneously, or IM *weekly*
Follow-up: CBC, AST (SGOT), ALT (SGPT), and albumin every 4–6 weeks
Precautions: Abstain from alcohol consumption, avoid with renal insufficiency, avoid in pregnancy, avoid with trimethoprim-sulfamethoxazole
When starting methotrexate, one should evaluate renal function closely because toxicity correlates with renal insufficiency. *In patients with renal insufficiency, methotrexate should be avoided entirely or given with extreme caution.* Additionally, patients who have histories of alcoholism, are diabetic, or are obese may be at increased risk for hepatic toxicity, and a pretreatment liver biopsy should be considered. Some clinicians believe that a chest x-ray should be done prior to methotrexate therapy and, if there is evidence of rheumatoid lung, that methotrexate should be avoided (controversial). Hepatitis B and C serologies should be obtained prior to methotrexate therapy and a baseline liver biopsy obtained if positive.

3. What can be done if patients develop minor side effects from methotrexate, such as mouth ulcers or nausea?
There are now convincing data that folic acid, usually in a dose of 1 mg/day (occasionally as high as 3 mg/day), significantly decreases these particular side effects in patients taking methotrexate without decreasing the efficacy of the methotrexate against RA. Some clinicians start all methotrexate patients on concomitant folic acid, while most reserve this therapy for patients who develop these side effects.

4. When should a liver biopsy be done on patients receiving methotrexate?
Although routine liver biopsies in RA patients receiving methotrexate are not currently recommended, many clinicians recommend liver biopsies for patients who have:
1. Risk factors for cirrhosis, such as prior alcoholism or hepatitis;

2. Persistent elevations of aspartate aminotransferase (AST or SGOT), usually defined as elevations of over 50% of the determinations done within 1 year;

3. Decreasing albumin level; or

4. Psoriasis (controversial)

The recommendations for liver biopsies in patients with psoriasis treated with methotrexate are more controversial, since methotrexate appears to be more hepatotoxic in these individuals. Many clinicians would perform routine liver biopsies on psoriatic patients after a cumulative dose of 1.5–2.5 gm of methotrexate.

5. Methotrexate is currently an accepted treatment of which rheumatic diseases?

Rheumatoid arthritis	Systemic lupus erythematosus
Psoriatic arthritis	Systemic sclerosis
Reiter's syndrome	Wegener's granulomatosis
Polymyositis/dermatomyositis	Takayasu's arteritis

Studies are currently underway to assess methotrexate's efficacy in SLE, systemic sclerosis, and Wegener's. Many physicians also use methotrexate in giant cell arteritis.

6. How is azathioprine (Imuran) supplied and used?

How supplied: 50-mg tablet, 100 mg/20 ml vial

Side effects: Bone marrow depression, nausea, vomiting, skin rash, malignancy, hepatotoxicity, infections (herpes zoster)

Dosage: 50–200 mg/day (1–2.5 mg/kg/day)

Follow-up: Monthly CBC and liver enzymes

Precautions: Avoid in pregnancy, avoid concomitant use of angiotensin-converting enzyme inhibitors, drastically reduce dose with allopurinol (reduce azathioprine dose by 75%)

7. What rheumatic diseases are commonly treated with azathioprine?

Rheumatoid arthritis

Systemic lupus erythematosus (particularly lupus nephritis)

Polymyositis/dermatomyositis

Reiter's syndrome

Many other rheumatic diseases in an attempt to decrease corticosteroid dosage

8. Discuss the use of cyclophosphamide in the rheumatic diseases.

How supplied: 25- and 50-mg tablets; 100-, 200-, 500-, and 1000-mg vials

Dosage: Daily oral, 50–150 mg (0.7–3 mg/kg/day)

Monthly IV, 0.5–1 gm/m^2 body surface area

Follow-up: Daily dosing: CBC every 1–2 weeks until stable dose, then monthly; urinalysis monthly

Monthly dosing: CBC and urinalysis before each dose, CBC 10–14 days after each dose

9. What precautions are necessary when using cyclophosphamide in RA?

- Maintain WBC count > 3000/mm^3. If nadir WBC count falls below this level, decrease dose by 25%.
- With IV administration, many physicians use Mesna in a dose of 1 mg for each 1 mg of cyclophosphamide, given in 4 divided doses over 24 hours. Vigorous IV and oral hydration is also done to decrease the risk of hemorrhagic cystitis.
- Premedicate with antiemetics before giving IV cyclophosphamide.

10. In which rheumatic diseases is cyclophosphamide therapy indicated? How effective is it in these disease processes?

Wegener's granulomatosis

Systemic lupus erythematosus (particularly lupus nephritis)

Rheumatoid arthritis

Other systemic vasculitis syndromes
Other rheumatic diseases refractory to conventional therapy

Cyclophosphamide (Cytoxan) is widely considered to be one of the *most potent* immunosuppressive drugs available. Its use has succeeded in almost all rheumatic diseases, particularly when other less-potent and usually less-toxic forms of therapy have not. When preservation of renal function in patients with lupus nephritis is the desired result, cyclophosphamide has superior efficacy. However, because of its potentially severe toxicity, overall improvements in mortality have been more difficult to demonstrate.

Cyclophosphamide has also been shown to be an effective disease-modifying drug in patients with RA refractory to other forms of therapy. While there are no controlled studies available on the treatment of Wegener's granulomatosis, cyclophosphamide therapy is universally considered to be the cornerstone of therapy for these individuals, who otherwise have a fatal disease process.

11. What are the major side effects of cyclophosphamide?
- Alopecia
- Nausea
- Infections (especially herpes zoster)
- Non-Hodgkin's lymphoma
- Hemorrhagic cystitis
- Bladder carcinoma
- Gonadal failure

The biggest worry of most clinicians when giving cyclophosphamide, or other alkylating agents, is the long-term risk for development of **malignancies,** particularly non-Hodgkin's lymphomas and bladder cancer. This is a well-documented risk and should always be kept in mind. Additionally, with the degree of immunosuppression that is occurring, the risk of infection is markedly increased, particularly herpes zoster. Cyclophosphamide is very toxic to the bladder and not uncommonly causes hemorrhagic cystitis and may lead to bladder cancer. The risk of bladder complications can be decreased by the use of monthly IV cyclophosphamide protocols.

Bone marrow depression occurs in a dose-dependent fashion when using cyclophosphamide, and as a result, the dose needs to be adjusted constantly. Suppression of gonadal function occurs in both men and women, and the harvesting of eggs or the banking of sperm should be considered before patients are put on these drugs.

Recent protocols for the treatment of lupus nephritis, Wegener's granulomatosis, and RA have looked at the use of monthly IV cyclophosphamide therapy to replace conventional daily oral therapy. These protocols are effective in most cases, and clearly decrease some of the toxicities of cyclophosphamide, particularly the hemorrhagic cystitis.

12. What other alkylating agents have been used to treat rheumatic diseases?
Nitrogen mustard and **chlorambucil** both have been used to treat several rheumatic diseases. Of these, chlorambucil is the more commonly used. The usual dose is 0.1 mg/kg/day (2–8 mg/day). It has been used primarily to treat the eye and neuropsychiatric complications of Behçet's disease. It has also been used in cryoglobulinemia, refractory polymyositis, lupus nephritis, and amyloidosis secondary to chronic inflammatory arthritis (RA, juvenile RA, ankylosing spondylitis). Major toxicities are myelosuppression and induction of leukemia and other malignancies.

13. Discuss the use of cyclosporine in the treatment of rheumatic diseases.
How supplied: 25- and 100-mg capsules; oral solution 100 mg/ml; IV solution 50 mg/ml
Dosage: < 5 mg/kg for most rheumatic diseases
Follow-up: Monthly creatinine, blood pressure, cyclosporine levels (controversial)
Precautions: Concurrent use of NSAIDs may contribute to renal insufficiency
　　　　　Diltiazem increases cyclosporine levels causing toxicity
　　　　　Cyclosporine is stopped if creatinine increases 30% over baseline

Cyclosporine is a potent immunomodulating agent that was originally developed as an antifungal agent. Its primary use has been to suppress the immune system to prevent organ transplant rejection, but due to its potent immunosuppressive properties, it recently has been used to treat various rheumatic diseases that are refractory to other therapies.

14. What is FK506?

FK506 is a macrolide produced by a fungus. It has immunosuppressive effects similar to cyclosporine but at a dose 10–100 times lower. It may replace cyclosporine in the future. Both cyclosporine A and FK506 are potent inhibitors of T-cell activation and inhibit transcription of early T-cell activation genes, such as *IL-2* (interleukin-2). It does this by interfering with the binding of the nuclear regulatory factor, NF-AT, to its target region in the enhancer region of these inducible genes.

15. What rheumatic syndromes have been treated with cyclosporine?

Rheumatoid arthritis
Polymyositis/dermatomyositis
Psoriatic arthritis
Systemic lupus erythematosus
Uveitis

Studies have shown that cyclosporine is more effective in treating RA then placebo and has similar efficacy to that of some other disease-modifying drugs. Patients with many other rheumatic disease syndromes have been treated with cyclosporine with improvement reported, but without good studies to confirm this improvement. Cyclosporine currently seems to hold promise in treating patients with refractory polymyositis/dermatomyositis and uveitis.

16. What are the major toxicities of cyclosporine?

Decreased renal function (usually reversible)   Hirsutism, gum hypertrophy
Infections   Malignancies
Hypertension   Hyperuricemia and gout
Hyperpigmentation   Headaches

The renal toxicity of cyclosporine has been particularly troublesome when treating patients with rheumatic diseases, many of whom already have renal problems. Of lupus patients, often we would most like to treat those with lupus nephritis with this drug but are limited by its renal toxicity. In the case of RA, the renal toxicity of cyclosporine has been heightened because many of these patients are on concomitant NSAIDs. Recently, in protocols in which cyclosporine has been used without NSAIDs in RA patients, the renal toxicity has been more manageable. A further significant consideration when prescribing cyclosporine is its cost, especially if the patient's medical insurance does not cover this cost.

17. How significant is the risk of potential malignancies after use of methotrexate, azathioprine, cyclophosphamide, or cyclosporine?

The possible induction of malignancies in patients by these treatments should always be a major concern. Therefore, many clinicians have been reluctant to treat patients having so-called nonmalignant diseases with therapies that can induce malignancies. The risk/benefit ratio always needs to be kept in mind, but few can argue against use of cyclophosphamide therapy, which is life-saving for most patients with Wegener's granulomatosis, even if a small percentage of these patients develop non-Hodgkin's lymphomas after this therapy.

The risk of malignancy after treatment with immunosuppressive drugs is clearly greatest when using an alkylating agent, such as cyclophosphamide and chlorambucil, the two that are used most commonly in treatment of rheumatic diseases. The use of azathioprine clearly increases (2–5 times) the risk for induction of malignancies, but this risk appears to be a much more significant problem in organ transplant patients than in RA patients. The risk of malignancy induction with methotrexate appears to be extremely small, despite some reports of lymphomas in patients treated with methotrexate for RA. Studies have implicated cyclosporine in causing lymphomas in some patients. Some lymphomas induced by these immunosuppressive therapies regress when the immunosuppressive therapy (i.e., methotrexate and cyclosporine) is stopped.

18. Which cytotoxic drugs can be used safely in pregnancy?

All cytotoxic or immunomodulatory drugs should be considered **contraindicated in pregnancy.** However, their relative toxicities are probably different. Methotrexate and cyclophosphamide clearly cause substantial teratogenicity and should be considered absolutely contraindicated in all but the most extreme of circumstances. Some lupus patients have taken azathioprine successfully, but concern exists for its potential teratogenicity as well. Cyclosporine is both embryo- and fetotoxic when given to rats and rabbits in doses 2–5 times the human dose. At conventional doses, several pregnancies have been reported to be carried successfully to term on cyclosporine.

19. What kinds of biologic agents are being studied for use in the treatment of inflammatory rheumatic diseases?

With our increasing understanding of the pathogenesis of autoimmune rheumatic diseases, several biologic agents are being developed for treatment, especially for RA. These can be classified as follows:

Monoclonal antibodies
  Against T-cell surface molecules: Pan T-cell antigens (CAMPATH 1H [anti-CD52]);
    (anti-CD5); CD4 antigen (anti-CD4);
    activation antigens (anti-TAC [CD25])
  Against cytokines: TNF-α (anti-TNF-α[CA2])
  Against adhesion molecules: ICAM-1/LFA-1 interaction (anti-ICAM-1 [CD54])
Biologics targeting T-cell activation antigens (DAB IL-2 fusion toxin)
Biologics targeting T/B-cell collaboration molecules
  CD28/B7 interaction (CTLA-4 Ig)
  Cytokine inhibitors and soluble receptors
  Cytokine receptor antagonist proteins (IRAP, IL-1Ra)
  Soluble receptors (IL-1R, TNF-α receptor)
Methods targeting antigen–MHC-TcR interaction
  Oral tolerance (Type II collagen in RA)
  TcR Vβ peptide use
  MHC peptide use
Other
  Antisense oligonucleotides
  T-cell vaccination
  Gene therapy

20. How is intravenous gammaglobulin used as an immunomodulator in the rheumatic diseases?

How supplied: Multiple suppliers; solution varies from 3–12%; cost is \$25–\$60/gm
Dosage: 1–2 gm/kg administered over 1–5 days
Side effects: Headache (2–20%), flushing, chest tightness, back pain/myalgias, fever, chills, nausea, diaphoresis, hypotension, aseptic meningitis
Follow-up: Creatinine 24 hrs after infusion
Precautions: Anaphylactic reaction in patients with IgA deficiency; transmission of infectious agents (rare)

Side effects of gammaglobulin are avoided by premedicating patients with acetaminophen and diphenhydramine hydrochloride (Benadryl) or hydrocortisone sodium succinate (Solu-Cortef) and by slowing the rate of infusion. Infusion is started at 30 ml/hr and increased to a maximum of 250 ml/hr (sometimes higher).

21. In which rheumatic diseases is IV gammaglobulin indicated? How does it work in these?

Autoimmune thrombocytopenia
Kawasaki's disease
Dermatomyositis
Wegener's granulomatosis (controversial)

The mechanisms by which IV immunoglobulin causes clinical improvement are debated. In autoimmune thrombocytopenia, IV immunoglobulin acts by Fc receptor blockade, reducing the efficacy of the reticuloendothelial system to remove antibody-coated platelets. Other effects include a reduction of autoantibody production and decreased autoantibody binding to platelets.

In Kawasaki's disease, IV immunoglobulin may work by reducing expression of adhesion molecules on endothelial cells, binding cytokines that can cause inflammation, reducing the number of activated T cells, and binding staphylococcal toxin superantigens. In Wegener's, it may reduce the level of ANCA autoantibodies. Clearly, other mechanisms of action may play a role.

22. When is plasmapheresis used in the treatment of rheumatic diseases?

Theoretically, plasmapheresis should remove immune complexes and autoantibodies that contribute to the pathogenesis of some of the rheumatic diseases. There is good evidence for a beneficial effect of plasmapheresis combined with alpha-interferon (or other antiviral agent) in the treatment of hepatitis B-associated polyarteritis nodosa and hepatitis B- or C-associated cryoglobulinemia. Anecdotally, plasmapheresis has been a useful therapy when used in conjunction with corticosteroids and cytotoxic medications in the treatment of severe lupus pneumonitis and neuropsychiatric lupus with coma. Plasmapheresis is usually used in combination with corticosteroids and/or cytotoxic therapy to decrease the risk of a rebound flare of the underlying immunologic disease once the pheresis is stopped. To date, there is little evidence to support its routine use in other rheumatic diseases.

Most plasma exchange protocols remove 2–4 liters of plasma over a 2-hour period daily. Replacement fluid is generally albumin-saline or another protein-containing solution. To decrease the risk of infection and bleeding, 1–2 units of fresh-frozen plasma are included as part of the replacement solution. If not, monitoring of coagulation studies and immunoglobulin levels are important. If the patient develops hypogammaglobulinemia, intravenous gammaglobulin needs to be given.

23. Discuss the dosing of corticosteroids in the treatment of severe rheumatic diseases.

The typical approach to treating severe presentations of rheumatic diseases is to give **prednisone** orally in doses of 1–2 mg/kg/day in divided doses. The reason for divided dosing is that the immunologic effects of prednisone typically last 8–12 hours before dissipating. Theoretically, prednisone given as a single daily dose would not be as immunomodulating as divided doses. Consequently, many clinicians start with divided dosing for the first 2–4 weeks, until the rheumatic disease is brought under control, and then consolidate the prednisone to a single daily dose before starting a taper schedule. There is no role for every-other-day corticosteroids in the initial treatment of severe rheumatic diseases.

24. What about "pulse" corticosteroids? Are they used?

Many clinicians use intravenous "pulse" corticosteroids as the initial treatment of **severe life-threatening** or **organ-threatening presentations** of rheumatic diseases. This is typically **methylprednisolone** given in doses of 1 g/day for 3 consecutive days. This regimen of corticosteroid administration is felt to have more immunomodulating effects than high-dose daily oral corticosteroids (controversial). As the sole therapeutic intervention, pulse steroids probably have no role in **long-term therapy.** However, in combination therapy with a cytotoxic agent, pulse steroids may provide time for a second agent to achieve its therapeutic effect.

The effect of pulse steroids usually lasts 3–4 weeks. It has been used most often in the treatment of severe vasculitis, lupus nephritis, and neuropsychiatric lupus. Side effects include psychosis, arrhythmias, and, rarely, sudden death. The risk of these adverse effects may be lessened by using a slow rate of infusion and ensuring that the serum potassium level is normal.

BIBLIOGRAPHY

1. Dalakas MC, Illa I, Dambrosia JM, et al: A controlled trial of high-dose intravenous immune globulin infusions as treatment for dermatomyositis. N Engl J Med 329:1993–2000, 1993.
2. Fauci A, Young K Jr: Immunoregulatory agents. In Kelley WN, Harris ED Jr, Ruddy S, Sledge CB (eds): Textbook of Rheumatology, 4th ed. Philadelphia, W.B. Saunders, 1993, pp 797–821.

3. Felson DT, Anderson JJ, Meenan RF: The comparative efficacy and toxicity of second-line drugs in rheumatoid arthritis. Arthritis Rheum 33:1449, 1990.
4. Klassen LW, Calabrese LH, Laxer RM: Intravenous immunoglobulin in rheumatic disease. Rheum Dis Clin North Am 22:155–174, 1996.
5. Klippel JH, Dieppe PA (eds): Rheumatology. London, Mosby Europe, 1994, pp 14.1–4.
6. Kremer JM, Alarcon GS, Lightfoot RW Jr, et al. Methotrexate for rheumatoid arthritis: Suggested guidelines for monitoring liver toxicity. Arthritis Rheum 37:316, 1994.
7. Landewe RBM, Goei The HS, van Rijthoven AWAM, et al: A randomized, double-blind, 24-week controlled study of low dose cyclosporine versus chloroquine for early rheumatoid arthritis. Arthritis Rheum 37:637, 1994.
8. Lewis EJ, Hunsicker LG, Lan SP, et al: A controlled trial of plasmapheresis therapy in severe lupus nephritis. N Engl J Med 326:1373–1379, 1992.
9. McCarty DJ, Koopman WJ (eds): Arthritis and Allied Conditions, 12 ed. Philadelphia, Lea & Febiger, 1993, pp 645–664.
10. Morgan SL, Baggott JE, Vaughn WH, et al: The effect of folic acid supplementation on the toxicity of low-dose methotrexate in patients with rheumatoid arthritis. Arthritis Rheum 33:9, 1990.
11. Ratko TA, Burnett DA, Foulke GE, et al: Recommendations for off-label use of intravenously administered immunoglobulin preparations. JAMA 273:1865–1870, 1995.
12. Schumacher HR (ed): Primer on the Rheumatic Diseases, 10th ed. Atlanta, Arthritis Foundation, 1993.
13. Situnayake RD, Grindulis KA, McConkey B: Long-term treatment of rheumatoid arthritis with sulphasalazine, gold, or penicillamine: A comparison using life-table methods. Ann Rheum Dis 46:177, 1987.
14. Strand V, Keystone E, Breedveld F: Biologic agents for treatment of rheumatoid arthritis. Rheum Dis Clin North Am 22:117–132, 1996.
15. Tugwell P, Pincus T, Yocum D, et al: Combination therapy with cyclosporine and methotrexate in severe rheumatoid arthritis. N Engl J Med 333:137–141, 1995.

88. HYPOURICEMIC AGENTS AND COLCHICINE

David R. Finger, M.D.

1. Identify the goals in the treatment of gout.
The first goal is safe and rapid treatment of acute gouty attacks so as to alleviate pain and restore joint function. This is usually done with NSAIDs or colchicine. Once this is accomplished, the next goal is to prevent recurrent attacks and the future development of destructive arthropathy, tophi formation, and nephrolithiasis.

2. What is colchicine?
Colchicine, an alkaloid derivative from the plant *Colchicum autumnale,* has been used in the treatment of acute gout for nearly 2 centuries and for joint pain since the 6th century. It has long been felt that the clinical response of acute arthritis to colchicine was diagnostic for gout, though a few other inflammatory arthropathies (pseudogout, acute sarcoidosis) respond as well. Garrod stated over a century ago that "colchicine possesses as specific a control over the gouty inflammation as cinchona barks over intermittent fever. . . . We may sometimes diagnose gouty from any other sort of inflammation by noting the influence of colchicine on its progress."

3. When is colchicine therapy indicated? What are the correct dosages?
Colchicine can be used in the treatment of acute gouty attacks and as prophylaxis against future attacks, especially when hypouricemic therapy is initiated. Colchicine is available orally in 0.5- and 0.6-mg tablets and in a parenteral solution of 0.5 mg/ml.

The average dose for **prophylaxis** is 0.5 mg twice daily. This dosage either completely prevents attacks or significantly lowers their frequency in > 90% of patients followed long-term, with minimal toxicity. Prophylaxis doses usually do not cause gastrointestinal side effects and should be continued until the patient is without symptoms of gout for several months.

For **acute attacks**, colchicine is most effective if given in the first few hours. The dosage can be as high as 0.5 mg/hr orally until relief or side effects occur, not to exceed 12 tablets (except in the elderly and those with renal insufficiency, who should receive fewer tablets). Pain is usually gone within 24 hours in 90% of patients, but many will experience diarrhea with this regimen.

4. What are the contraindications to the use of parenteral colchicine?

Parenteral therapy has less gastrointestinal side effects than oral administration but is otherwise much more toxic. Many countries, including Great Britain, along with many hospitals in the United States, have removed parenteral colchicine due to reports of death from bone marrow suppression. For this reason it is more likely to be considered in postoperative patients who cannot take oral medications. Intraveneous colchicine may soon not be manufactured due to its toxicity.

Contraindications to the Use of Intravenous Colchicine

ABSOLUTE	RELATIVE
Preexisting bone marrow depression	Prior use of colchicine
Creatinine clearance < 10 ml/min	Hepatic or renal insufficiency
Extrahepatic biliary obstruction	Advanced age
Sepsis	Localized infection

5. Discuss other concerns regarding the dosage and administration of parenteral colchicine.

- No more than 2 mg of colchicine should be given in any single dose, and the total 24-hour dosage should not exceed 4 mg. Use a dose 50% lower in patients with decreased renal or hepatic function and in the elderly. Do not use colchicine if a patient has both renal and hepatic dysfunction.
- Colchicine can cause local tissue necrosis; so it should be given by a separate intravenous line to minimize the risk of extravasation.
- No additional colchicine should be prescribed for 7 days following parenteral administration.

6. Discuss the mechanism of action and pharmacokinetics of colchicine.

Colchicine has no effect on the serum urate concentration or on urate metabolism. It functions as an anti-inflammatory agent primarily by binding irreversibly to tubulin dimers, preventing their assembly into microtubules (which interferes with neutrophil chemotaxis). Colchicine also interferes with membrane-dependent functions of neutrophils, such as phagocytosis, and inhibits phospholipase A_2, which can lead to lower levels of inflammatory prostaglandins and leukotrienes. Colchicine is not bound to plasma proteins and is highly lipid-soluble, readily passing into all tissues. The half-life is 4 hours following oral administration and < 1 hour parenterally. It can be detected in neutrophils up to 10 days after a single dose. It is hepatically metabolized and excreted principally in the bile, with 20% excreted unchanged in urine.

7. Describe the different manifestations of colchicine toxicity.

Most adverse effects of colchicine are dose-related and more likely to be observed following intravenous rather than oral administration (except for gastrointestinal side effects). There are no antidotes to overdose, and hemodialysis is ineffective. Potential side effects include:

Gatrointestinal effects (diarrhea, nausea, vomiting, rarely malabsorption syndrome and hemorrhagic gastroenteritis)—usually seen following oral administration
Bone marrow suppression (thrombocytopenia, leukopenia)
Neuromyopathy (elevated creatine kinase, proximal weakness, peripheral neuropathy, lysosomal vacuoles on biopsy)—usually seen in renal insufficiency with chronic dosing
Alopecia
Shock, disseminated intravascular coagulation (parenteral)
CNS dysfunction
Cellulitis or thrombophlebitis (parenteral)

8. What antihyperuricemic agents are available?

Antihyperuricemic agents include **uricosurics** (probenecid and sulfinpyrazone), which reduce the serum urate concentration by enhancing renal excretion of uric acid, and **xanthine oxidase inhibitors** (allopurinol), which inhibit uric acid synthesis by inhibiting xanthine oxidase, the final enzyme involved in the production of uric acid. These agents should be initiated only after an acute attack of gout has resolved entirely.

The risk of acute gouty attacks following the initiation of antihyperuricemic therapy can be minimized by gradual dose increases and by prophylaxis with colchicine or NSAIDs. The decision to use uric acid-lowering therapy is usually a lifelong commitment, so it is essential that these agents are only initiated when they are truly indicated. Uricosurics can be safely used along with allopurinol in some patients with severe tophaceous gout.

9. Which gouty patients are candidates for uricosuric therapy?

- Hyperuricemia secondary to underexcretion of uric acid (< 800 mg of uric acid in a 24-hour urine collection, while on a regular diet)
- Age < 60 yrs
- Creatinine clearance > 50 ml/min
- No history of nephrolithiasis

10. Identify some uricosuric agents and describe their mechanism of action.

Many drugs have uricosuric properties, including high-dose aspirin or salicylates, but the two most common agents used clinically are **probenecid** and **sulfinpyrazone**. Uricosuric agents are weak organic acids, like uric acid, and they increase urinary excretion of uric acid by competitively inhibiting tubular reabsorption of urate. These agents are successful in lowering the serum uric acid to < 6.7 mg/dl in 75% of patients. Low doses of aspirin or salicylates should be avoided since they inhibit urate secretion. Uricosurics work better when there is good urine alkalinization and flow (> 1500 ml/day) to minimize the risk of uric acid nephropathy and nephrolithiasis.

11. How are probenecid and sulfinpyrazone dosed? How do these drugs differ?

Sulfinpyrazone is an analogue of a phenylbutazone metabolite but possesses no anti-inflammatory properties. This drug is 98% bound to plasma proteins and has a half-life of 1–3 hours. Twenty to 45% is excreted unchanged in the urine, with most as a uricosuric metabolite. Unlike probenecid, sulfinpyrazone has antiplatelet activity through inhibition of thromboxane synthesis. It is available in 100-mg and 200-mg oral preparations, and is dosed initially at 50 mg twice daily but increased gradually to maintenance levels of 300–400 mg/day in 3 or 4 divided doses. Sulfinpyrazone is more effective than probenecid in patients with renal insufficiency and is 3–6 times more potent.

Probenecid has a longer half-life (6–12 hours) and is more extensively metabolized than sulfinpyrazone. Allopurinol prolongs the half-life of probenecid, while probenecid prolongs the half-life of penicillin, ampicillin, dapsone, indomethacin, and sulfinpyrazone by decreasing their renal excretion and prolongs the metabolism of heparin. Probenecid is available in 500-mg tablets. It is dosed initially at 250 mg twice daily but can be increased gradually up to 3 gm daily (average dose 1 gm/day) in 2–3 divided doses.

12. What are the side effects of uricosuric therapy?

Uricosuric therapy is generally well tolerated by > 90% of patients, with serious side effects occurring rarely.

Preventable	Rare
Acute gouty attacks	Hemolytic anemia
Urate nephropathy	Aplastic anemia
Urate nephrolithiasis	Nephrotic syndrome
Relatively common	Hepatic necrosis
Gastrointestinal symptoms (10%)	Anaphylaxis
Dermatitis (5%)	
Headache	
Drug fever	

13. Which inhibitors of uric acid synthesis are available?

Allopurinol, a hypoxanthine analogue, is the most commonly used inhibitor of uric acid synthesis. **Oxypurinol**, a xanthine analogue and the major metabolite of allopurinol, is not available in the United States and has poor gastrointestinal absorption, but it has been used in Europe in patients who are allergic to allopurinol.

14. What are the indications for use of allopurinol?

Indications for allopurinol use in patients with gout include:
1. Urate overproduction (uric acid > 800 mg in 24-hr urine collection on a regular diet)
2. Nephrolithiasis
3. Renal insufficiency (creatinine in clearance < 50 ml/min)
4. Tophi (may take 6–12 months to resolve)
5. Failure or intolerance of uricosuric agents

Other indications for allopurinol include:
1. Hyperuricemia with nephrolithiasis of any type
2. Prophylaxis against tumor lysis syndrome
3. Hypoxanthine phosphoribosyltransferase (HPRT) deficiency (Lesch-Nyhan syndrome)
4. Hyperuricemia due to myeloproliferative disorders
5. Serum urate > 12.0 mg/dl or 24-hr urine uric acid > 1100 mg

15. Describe the mechanism of action and pharmacokinetic properties of allopurinol.

Allopurinol lowers blood and urine urate concentrations by inhibiting the enzyme xanthine oxidase, thus leading to increases in the precursors xanthine and hypoxanthine. Allopurinol itself is metabolized by xanthine oxidase to the active metabolite, oxypurinol, which can be measured to assess compliance. Drugs that depend on this enzyme for their metabolism, such as 6-mercaptopurine and azathioprine, require a 50–75% dosage reduction if they are given concomitantly with allopurinol. Allopurinol is well absorbed from the gastrointestinal tract and has a half-life of 40 minutes, while oxypurinol is poorly absorbed and has a much longer half-life (14–28 hours). The dosage of allopurinol must be lowered in the presence of renal insufficiency. The maximum antihyperuricemic effect is seen 4–14 days after starting allopurinol.

16. How is allopurinol dosed?

Allopurinol is available orally in 100- and 300-mg tablets, usually given in once-daily doses, to lower the serum urate < 6.7 mg/dl. The average dose needed to accomplish this is 300 mg/day but can be as high as 600 mg. One should investigate other correctable factors leading to hyperuricemia if it requires > 300 mg/day to achieve adequate uric acid levels. The dose should be reduced in the presence of renal insufficiency because oxypurinol is renally excreted. The dose should be lowered to 200 mg/day when the glomerular filtration rate approaches 60 ml/min and to 100 mg/day when it reaches 20 ml/min.

17. List the major toxicities of allopurinol.

The overall incidence of side effects is around 20%, but only 5% of all patients discontinue therapy due to drug toxicity. Desensitization with low oral doses has been successful in some patients with less serious reactions to allopurinol.

Common (rarely serious)
    Acute gouty arthritis
    Maculopapular erythema (3–10%; risk 3 times higher with ampicillin)
    Nausea
    Diarrhea
    Abnormal liver-associated enzymes
    Headache

Uncommon (potentially serious)
    Toxic epidermal necrolysis, exfoliative dermatitis   Oxypurinol or xanthine nephrolithiasis
    Allopurinol hypersensitivity syndrome   Cataracts

Bone marrow suppression	Sarcoid-like reaction
Hepatitis	Alopecia
Vasculitis	Lymphadenopathy
Peripheral neuropathy	Fever
Renal failure (interstitial nephritis)	Death

18. What is the allopurinol hypersensitivity syndrome?

The allopurinol hypersensitivity syndrome occurs in approximately 10% of patients who experience an allopurinol rash. These patients usually have associated renal insufficiency (75%) and are on diuretic therapy (50%). This syndrome typically occurs 2–4 weeks following initiation of therapy, with a 25% mortality and significant morbidity. Clinical manifestations include skin rash, fever, eosinophilia, hepatic necrosis, leukocytosis, and worsening renal function in most patients. Treatment with high-dose prednisone and hemodialysis (to remove oxypurinol) has been successful.

19. Identify the sites of action for drugs that are used to treat acute gout and to lower serum urate levels.

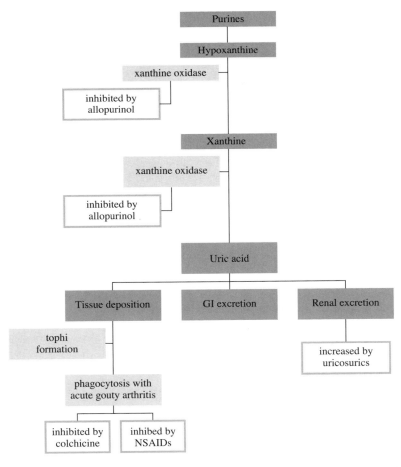

Drugs used in the treatment of gout and their sites of action. (Adapted from Klippel JH, Dieppe PA [eds]: Rheumatology. London, Mosby, 1994; with permission.)

BIBLIOGRAPHY

1. Emmerson BT: Antihyperuricemics. In Klippel JH, Dieppe PA (eds): Rheumatology, London, Mosby, 1994, pp 8:15.1–15.6.
2. Fam AG, Lewtas J, Stein J, Paton TW: Desensitization to allopurinol in patients with gout and cutaneous reactions. Am J Med 93:299–302, 1992.
3. Fox IH: Antihyperuricemic drugs. In Kelly WN, Harris ED, Ruddy S, Sledge CB (eds): Textbook of Rheumatology, 4th ed. Philadelphia, W.B. Saunders, 1993, pp 822–831.
4. Hande KR, Noone RM, Stone WJ: Severe allopurinol toxicity: Description and guidelines for prevention in patients with renal insufficiency. Am J Med 76:47–56, 1984.
5. Hardin JG, Longenecker GL: Drugs used in the treatment of gout and pseudogout. In Hardin JG, Longenecker GL (eds): Handbook of Drug Therapy in Rheumatic Disease. Boston, Little, Brown & Co, 1992, pp 146–174.
6. Hartung EF: History of the use of colchicine and related medicaments in gout. Ann Rheum Dis 13:190–200, 1954.
7. Roberts WN, Liang MH, Stern SH: Colchicine in acute gout: Reassessment of risks and benefits, JAMA 257:1920–1922, 1987.
8. Singer JZ, Wallace SL: The allopurinol hypersensitivity syndrome: Unnecessary morbidity and mortality. Arthritis Rheum 29:82–87, 1986.
9. Terkeltaub RA: Pathogenesis and treatment of crystal-induced inflammation. In McCarty DJ, Koopman WJ (eds): Arthritis and Allied Conditions, 12th ed. Philadelphia, Lea & Febiger, 1993, pp 1819–1833.
10. Wallace SL, Bernstein D, Diamond H: Diagnostic value of the colchicine therapeutic trial. JAMA 199:525–528, 1967.
11. Wallace SL, Singer JZ: Systemic toxicity associated with the intravenous administration of colchicine—Guidelines for use. J. Rheumatol 15:495–499, 1988.
12. Wortmann RL: Management of hyperuricemia. In McCarty DJ, Koopman WJ (eds): Arthritis and Allied Conditions, 12th ed. Philadelphia, Lea & Febiger, 1993, pp 1807–1818.

89. BONE-STRENGTHENING AGENTS

Michael T. McDermott, M.D.

1. Define bone remodeling.

This is the process by which osteoclasts resorb old bone and osteoblasts secrete osteoid, which subsequently becomes mineralized with hydroxyapatite crystals to form new bone. Bone remodeling ensures that weak, older bone is removed and strong, new bone is formed in skeletal areas subject to the greatest mechanical stress.

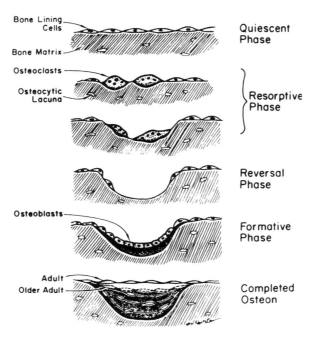

Bone remodeling. Osteoclasts resorb old bone, leaving an empty resorption pit. Osteoblasts then fill the pit by secreting osteoid, which is subsequently mineralized by calcium and phosphate from the extracellular fluid, forming new bone. (From Peck WA, ed: Bone and Mineral Research Annual 2. New York, Elsevier, 1984; with permission.)

2. How does bone resorption occur?

Bone resorption occurs when hematopoietic stem cells are recruited to form new osteoclasts. These multinucleated giant cells attach to bone surfaces by their ruffled border and secrete acid and enzymes that degrade bone. Osteoclastic bone resorption is stimulated primarily by circulating parathyroid hormone and by locally produced cytokines, such as interleukin-6. It is inhibited by calcitonin, sex steroids, and other cytokines.

3. How is bone formation regulated?

Bone formation occurs when osteoblasts secrete osteoid that is subsequently mineralized by the deposition of hydroxyapatite (calcium phosphate) crystals. Bone formation is stimulated by parathyroid hormone, sex steroids, insulin-like growth factor 1, and locally produced cytokines.

4. How do high-turnover and low-turnover osteoporosis differ?

High-turnover osteoporosis presents with rapid bone loss due to a high rate of bone resorption associated with normal or moderately increased bone formation. This form typically occurs in the early postmenopausal years and accounts for < 30% of all cases of osteoporosis. Urinary excretion of pyridinoline crosslinks, a marker of resorption, and serum osteocalcin, which reflects bone formation, are characteristically high-normal or elevated. Treatment is with an antiresorptive agent.

Low-turnover osteoporosis presents with a low rate of bone resorption and a very low rate of new bone formation. This form usually occurs in patients ≥10 years after menopause. Urinary pyridinoline crosslinks and serum osteocalcin levels tend to be low. A bone-formation–stimulating agent is the treatment of choice.

5. What therapeutic interventions effectively alter bone remodeling?

BONE-RESORPTION–INHIBITING AGENTS	BONE-FORMATION–STIMULATING AGENTS
Calcium	Fluoride
Vitamin D	Calcitriol
Estrogen	Androgens
Calcitonin	Growth hormone
Bisphosphonates	Parathyroid hormone

6. How do antiresorptive and formation-stimulating agents affect bone mass?

Bone-formation–stimulating agents typically bring about a progressive linear increase in bone mass in most treated patients. In contrast, antiresorptive drugs characteristically increase bone mass by 0–4% in low-turnover osteoporosis and by 5–20% in high-turnover osteoporosis during the first 6–18 months of treatment and then stabilize it at a constant level.

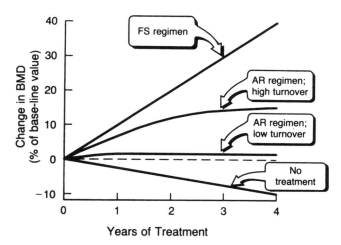

Bone mineral density (BMD) response to therapeutic interventions. Formation-stimulating (FS) agents produce a progressive linear increase in BMD. Antiresorptive (AR) agents transiently increase BMD 5–20% in high-turnover osteoporosis and 0–4% in low-turnover osteoporosis, after which they maintain BMD at a stable level. (From Riggs BL, Melton III LJ: The prevention and treatment of osteoporosis. N Engl J Med 327:620–627, 1992, with permission.)

7. How do antiresorptive agents increase bone mass?

These drugs significantly reduce bone resorption while formation remains unaffected so that, at least temporarily, formation exceeds resorption and bone mass increases. This phenomenon is referred to as **bone remodeling transients.** After 6–18 months, formation gradually declines to the level of resorption, and bone mass no longer increases.

8. Why are antiresorptive medications the primary approach to osteoporosis prevention and treatment?

Antiresorptive drugs are generally safe, effective, and affordable. Formation-stimulating agents, on the other hand, are largely of unproven efficacy, have significant side effects, and/or are expensive. Most are therefore still considered investigational.

9. What are the best sources of dietary calcium?

Dairy products and calcium-fortified citrus juices. Patients should be asked about their use of these foods. If dietary calcium consumption is inadequate, calcium supplements should be added to achieve the desired intake.

Dietary Sources of Calcium

SOURCE	APPROXIMATE CALCIUM CONTENT
Milk	300 mg/cup
Cheese	200 mg/oz
Yogurt	350 mg/cup
Citrus juice with calcium	300 mg/cup

10. Give the current recommendations for oral calcium intake.

Men and premenopausal women 1000 mg Ca/day. Postmenopausal women and patients with osteoporosis 1500 mg Ca/day.

11. What is the role of vitamin D therapy?

Vitamin D promotes intestinal calcium absorption. The recommended daily allowance of vitamin D is 400 U. Intakes of 400–800 U/day ensure optimal calcium absorption and reduce bone loss, particularly in the winter months when sunlight exposure significantly declines. Calcitriol in physiologic doses of 0.25–1.0 µg/day has similar effects but is considerably more expensive.

12. What is the role of estrogen replacement therapy in osteoporosis?

Estrogens inhibit bone resorption. They increase bone mass moderately and reduce the risk of spine, hip, and wrist fractures. Estrogens are the most effective means of preventing postmenopausal osteoporosis, and recent studies indicate that they are also useful in treating established osteoporosis. Women with an intact uterus must also take **progesterone** to prevent estrogen-induced endometrial hyperplasia and carcinoma. The main drawback of cyclic hormonal replacement is monthly withdrawal bleeding, which can be significantly reduced or eliminated by continuous (daily) regimens.

Common Estrogen-Replacement Regimens

		REGIMEN	
	DOSE	CYCLIC	DAILY
Estrogen replacement			
Conjugated estrogens (Premarin)	0.625–1.25 mg	Day 1–25	Daily
Ethinyl estradiol	50 mg	Day 1–25	Daily
Estrogen patch (Estraderm)	0.05–0.1 mg	Every 3 days, Day 1–25	Every 3 days
Progesterone replacement			
Medroxyprogesterone (Provera)	10 mg	Day 13–25	
	2.5 mg		Daily

13. How effective is calcitonin in the management of osteoporosis?

Calcitonin directly inhibits osteoclasts. Treated patients show a slight gain in bone mass similar to that seen with estrogens. Calcitonin also reduces pain significantly in 80% of patients with fractures. The mechanism appears to be CNS opioid release. The most common preparation currently in use is salmon calcitonin, which is given subcutaneously in a dose ranging from 50 units three times weekly to 100 units/day. A calcitonin nasal spray (Miacalcin, 200 units/spray) is available. Dosage is one spray in one nostril each day. Nostrils should be alternated daily.

14. Are bisphosphonates effective agents for osteoporosis?

Bisphosphonates have been shown to increase bone mass modestly and to reduce the incidence of subsequent fractures. Concern about their longer-term effects exists, but results thus far appear promising. **Etidronate** is given cyclically in an oral dose of 200 mg twice daily for the first 14 days of each 90-day cycle; calcium supplements, which impair bisphosphonate absorption from the intestine, are not given during these 14 days but must be used during the subsequent 76 days of the cycle. **Alendronate,** a newer, more potent agent, is given continuously as 10 mg orally every morning, with calcium supplements being administered at bedtime.

15. What is the role of exercise?

Exercise stimulates bone formation and inhibits resorption. It may also reduce the incidence and severity of falls by improving muscular strength and coordination. Both aerobic and weight-training are beneficial.

16. What are the skeletal effects of sodium fluoride?

Sodium fluoride stimulates osteoblastic bone formation by as-yet-uncertain mechanisms. When given to osteoporotic patients in oral doses of 50–75 mg/day, it produces significant progressive increases in bone mass. However, histologically, the bone is disorganized, and clinically, there is no reduction in fracture incidence, indicating that the new bone is not structurally or mechanically normal.

17. Are there adverse effects with sodium fluoride administration?

Symptomatic **gastritis** develops in 20–30% of patients on 50-mg/day dosages and in up to 50% of patients on 75-mg/day dosages.

A **painful lower-extremity syndrome,** consisting of acute pain, tenderness, and swelling in the lower extremities, particularly the heels and ankles, occurs in many patients. The disorder appears to be due to the development of stress fractures, probably related to rapid bone turnover. With rest and analgesia, resolution usually occurs in 6–8 weeks after the medication is discontinued. This syndrome tends not to recur if sodium fluoride is later reinstituted.

18. Should we give up on sodium fluoride as a therapeutic agent?

Not at all. Most experts agree that we just have not yet discovered the best way to give this drug. Results from a recent study reveal that intermittent administration of a slow-release sodium fluoride preparation increases bone mass and reduces new vertebral fractures, with a low incidence of side effects.

19. How does calcitriol (1,25-dihydroxyvitamin D) therapy affect skeletal integrity?

By stimulating intestinal calcium absorption, physiologic doses (0.5 μg/day) of calcitriol promote positive calcium balance and reduce the incidence of fractures. High-dose calcitriol (2.0 μg/day) additionally stimulates bone formation, resulting in an increase of bone density. High-dose calcitriol must be coupled with a low to moderate calcium intake to avoid toxicity.

20. How do you monitor for calcitriol toxicity?

Vitamin D and its analogues are fat-soluble and can therefore accumulate to toxic levels in the body. Vitamin D toxicity results initially in hypercalciuria, which predisposes to nephrolithiasis and eventually to hypercalcemia. Patients on supraphysiologic doses of vitamin D or calcitriol should be monitored every 6 months with measurement of **24-hour urinary calcium excretion** and a **serum calcium level.**

21. Are androgens useful for increasing bone mass?

Androgens are anabolic agents that stimulate bone formation. In hypogonadal males, testosterone replacement therapy significantly increases skeletal mass. Similar results are seen with a variety of androgens in postmenopausal women, but side effects such as hirsutism, acne, temporal balding, and other signs of virilization limit their use.

22. How effective are growth hormone and insulin-like growth factor 1 therapy?

Growth hormone (GH) is another anabolic agent that may promote bone formation. Although potentially useful in adults with GH deficiency, its effects in postmenopausal and senile osteoporosis have been moderate at best. GH therapy is also costly and may cause complications, such as acral enlargement, hyperglycemia, and hypertension. Studies with IGF-1 have only recently begun but its effects on bone remodeling appear to be beneficial.

23. Parathyroid hormone (PTH) treatment also increases bone mass. How does this occur?

Osteoblasts have surface receptors for PTH; osteoclasts do not. PTH initially stimulates osteoblasts, which secrete cytokines and other factors that in turn stimulate osteoclasts. When given as daily subcutaneous injections, PTH promotes bone formation more than resorption, resulting in progressive increases in bone mass. Although expensive at present, this promising therapy is under active investigation.

24. What is the principle behind the use of oral phosphate therapy?

Oral phosphate administration stimulates intermittent endogenous PTH secretion which, like PTH injections, may stimulate bone formation in excess of resorption. There is no evidence that phosphate alone is beneficial, but it may be useful when given in combination with an antiresorptive agent. Studies are currently in progress.

25. What is coherence therapy?

Coherence therapy, also known as ADFR (activate, depress, free, repeat), is a program in which antiresorptive medications are used in conjunction with or in alternation with bone-formation–stimulating agents. The best studied regimens have been growth hormone combined with calcitonin and oral phosphate alternating with etidronate. For both programs, the combination has proved to be minimally to no better than the antiresorption agent alone. Thus, while this remains an attractive concept, further work is needed before coherence therapy gains widespread acceptance.

BIBLIOGRAPHY

1. Brixen K, et al: A short course of recombinant human growth hormone treatment stimulates osteoblasts and activates bone remodeling in normal human volunteers. J Bone Min Res 5:609–618, 1990.
2. Chapuy MC, Arlot ME, Duboeuf F, et al: Vitamin D_3 and calcium to prevent hip fractures in elderly women. N Engl J Med 327:1637–1642, 1992.
3. Chestnut III CH, Ivey JL, Gruber HE, et al: Stanozolol in postmenopausal osteoporosis: Therapeutic efficacy and possible mechanisms of action. Metabolism 32:571–580, 1983.
4. Civitelli R, Gonnelli S, Zacchel F, et al: Bone turnover in postmenopausal osteoporosis: Effect of calcitonin treatment. J Clin Invest 82:1268–1274, 1988.
5. Dawson-Hughes B, Dallal GE, Krall EA, et al: Effect of vitamin D supplementation on wintertime and overall bone loss in healthy postmenopausal women. Ann Intern Med 115:505–512, 1991.
6. Degerblad M, Elgindy N, Hall K, et al: Potent effect of recombinant growth hormone on bone mineral density and body composition in adults with panhypopituitarism. Acta Endocrinol 126:387–393, 1992.
7. Ebeling PR, Jones JD, O'Fallon WM, et al: Short-term effects of recombinant human insulin-like growth factor I on bone turnover in normal women. J Clin Endocrinol Metab 77:1384–1387, 1993.
8. Finkelstein JS, Klibanski A, Neer RM, et al: Increases in bone density during treatment of men with idiopathic hypogonadotropic hypogonadism. J Clin Endocrinol Metab 69:776–782, 1989.
9. Gallagher JC, Goldgar D: Treatment of postmenopausal osteoporosis with high doses of synthetic calcitriol. Ann Intern Med 113:649–655, 1992.
10. Harris ST, Watts NB, Jackson RD, et al: Four-year study of intermittent cyclic etidronate treatment of

postmenopausal osteoporosis: Three years of blinded therapy followed by one year of open therapy. Am J Med 95:557–567, 1993.

11. Hock JM, Gera I: Effects of continuous and intermittent administration and inhibition of resorption on the anabolic response of bone to parathyroid hormone. J Bone Min Res 7:65–72, 1992.

12. Johnston CC Jr, Miller JZ, Slemenda CW, et al: Calcium supplementation and increases in bone mineral density in children. N Engl J Med 327:82–87, 1992.

13. Kleerekoper M, Mendlovic DB: Sodium fluoride therapy of postmenopausal osteoporosis. Endocr Rev 14:312–323, 1993.

14. Lufkin EG, Wahner HW, O'Fallow WM, et al: Treatment of postmenopausal osteoporosis with transdermal estrogen. Ann Intern Med 117:1–9, 1992.

15. Marx CW, Dailey GE III, Chemey C, et al: Do estrogens improve bone mineral density in osteoporotic women over age 65? J Bone Min Res 7:1275–1279, 1992.

16. Overgaard K, Hansen MA, Jensen SB, Christiansen C: Effect of salcatonin given intranasally on bone mass and fracture rates in established osteoporosis: A dose-response study. BMJ 305:556–561, 1992.

17. Pak CYC, Sakhaee K, Adams-Huet MS, et al: Treatment of postmenopausal osteoporosis with slow-release sodium fluoride. Ann Intern Med 123:401–408, 1995.

18. Reis IR, Ames RW, Evans MC, Gamble GD, Sharpe SJ: Effect of calcium supplementation on bone loss in postmenopausal women. N Engl J Med 328:460–464, 1993.

19. Riggs BL, Melton III LJ: The prevention and treatment of osteoporosis. N Engl J Med 327:620–627, 1992.

20. Silverberg SJ, Shane E, Clemens TL, et al: The effect of oral phosphate administration on major indices of skeletal metabolism in normal subjects. J Bone Min Res 1:383–388, 1986.

21. Slovik DM, Rosenthal DL, Doppelt SH, et al: Restoration of spinal bone in osteoporotic men by treatment with human parathyroid hormone (1–34) and 1,25-dihydroxyvitamin D. J Bone Min Res 1:377–381, 1986.

22. Watts NB, Harris ST, Genant HK, et al: Intermittent cyclical etidronate treatment of postmenopausal osteoporosis. N Engl J Med 323:73–79, 1990.

90. REHABILITATIVE TECHNIQUES

Douglas E. Hemler, M.D.

1. What is the goal of rehabilitation for patients with rheumatic disease?

The goal of rehabilitation is to maintain or restore the individual's ability to function successfully in personal, family, and community life by developing that person to the fullest physical, psychological, social, vocational, avocational, and educational potential consistent with his or her physiologic or anatomic impairment and environmental limitations.

2. Which functional areas may need to be assessed in a patient with a rheumatic disease?

Physical function assessment

History: pain and fatigue (can use visual analogue scales)

Physical examination

    Manual muscle strength testing

    Range of motion (ROM, can use goniometers)

    Transfers and ambulation

Ability to perform activities of daily living (ADLs)

Recreational (avocational) or leisure activities

Occupational (vocational) activities including job, housework, and schoolwork

Sexual activities

Sleep history

Psychological/cognitive function assessment

Affective function (depression, anxiety, mood)

Coping skills

Cognitive function

Compliance with treatment plan

Social function assessment (family, friends, community)

Social support systems

Interpersonal relationships

Social integration

Ability to fulfill social roles

Family functioning

Socioeconomic/financial

3. A quick screen of a rheumatic disease patient's functional abilities should include which areas?

The most critical functional areas to be reviewed when time is limited can be remembered by using the mnemonic ADEPTTS—how well does the patient "adapt" to his/her physical disability:

- A—Ambulation
- D—Dressing
- E—Eating
- P—Personal hygiene
- T—Transfers
- T—Toileting
- S—Sleeping/Sexual activities

4. What health care personnel are available to help rehabilitate patients with rheumatic diseases? What rehab techniques does each use?

Physical therapist—administers and instructs patients in the use of various therapeutic and pain-relieving techniques, including heat, cold, traction, diathermy, electrically stimulation, therapeutic exercise, stretching, transfer skills, ambulation methods, and joint ROM/function/strength.

Occupational therapist (OT)—responsible for optimizing function by instruction in joint protection and energy conservation. In addition, OTs provide or fabricate adaptive equipment and splinting, especially for upper-extremity functional activities. Some OTs, but usually **podiatrists**, provide orthotics for lower-extremity problems.

Social workers and **rehabilitation counselors**—assist in the management of social, economic, and psychologic problems that creates stress for the patient and family. This can include assistance in recreational activities as well as interpersonal and sexual relationships.

Psychotherapists—assist the patient with the psychologic problems that arise from dealing with pain and loss of function.

Vocational counselors—can mobilize community resources to retrain and restore the patient to the workplace.

Arthritis rehabilitation nurses and **patient educators**—assist in instruction about the rheumatic disease and its therapy. Provide information, monitor compliance, and give emotional support to the patient and family.

EXERCISE AND REST

5. Name three forms of rest.

Rest in an arthritic person may be done specifically to benefit an inflamed joint, to provide energy conservation, or, in specific disorders, to affect sedimentation rate and creatine kinare levels.

- **Local rest** is performed in a specific joint utilizing splinting techniques to reduce pain, inflammation, or to prevent contracture.
- **Systemic rest** is used for a period of up to 4 weeks if appropriate anti-inflammatory medication and outpatient rehabilitation management are ineffective in alleviating the manifestations of rheumatoid arthritis or polymyositis.
- **Short rest periods** are becoming increasingly popular, particularly in patients with rheumatoid arthritis. These are a preventive and proactive means of managing inflammation and fatigue. The patient interrupts daily activities of longer than 30 continuous minutes to take short breaks.

6. How does exercise benefit a patient with arthritis?

Fatigue, weakness, and decreased stamina or endurance are common symptoms in patients with rheumatic disease. Disuse or excessive rest and inactivity can be a major cause of lost muscle strength. Up to 30% of a muscle's bulk and 5–10% of its strength can be lost within a week if a joint is immobilized. In addition, joint immobility can lead to contractures with loss of ROM. Therapeutic exercise has the following goals and benefits in a patient with arthritis:

Maintaining or improving ROM

Preventing or reducing contractures

Increasing strength

Enhancing endurance

Preserving bone mineralization

Improving the ability for functional activities

Improving patient's overall feeling of well-being

7. Which factors need to be considered in prescribing an exercise program for a patient with a rheumatic disease?

Stage of disease

Extent of inflammation and deformity

Patient's general medical condition

Types of activities the patient enjoys (to improve compliance)

8. Name three types of ROM exercise.

1. **Passive ROM** — Motion is performed by the therapist or mechanical device without help of the patient.
2. **Active ROM** — The patient performs the movement.
3. **Active-assisted ROM** — The patient moves the limb with the assistance of the therapist.

9. What is the minimum ROM of each joint that allows adequate function to perform activities of daily living?

JOINT	ROM
TMJ	2.5 cm of jaw opening
Shoulder	Flexion 45°, abduction 90°, external rotation 20°
Elbow	Flexion 70°
Wrist	Dorsiflexion 5–10°, supination 10–15°
MCP	Flexion >30°
PIP	Flexion >30°
DIP	Flexion >30°
CMC	Internal rotation >30°
Hip	Extension 0° to flexion 30°
Knee	Neutral to 60° flexion
Ankle	Plantar flexion 20° to 10° of dorsiflexion

TMJ = temporomandibular joint. (Adapted from Hicks JE: Exercise in patients with inflammatory arthritis and connective tissue disease. Rheum Dis Clin North Am 16:845, 1990.)

10. What types of active exercise are used to increase muscle strength and endurance in a patient with arthritis?

1. **Isometric training.** A static muscle contraction in which the muscle length does not change and the limb does not move through ROM. Two to six contractions of each muscle are recommended, with each contraction held for 3–6 sec with 20–60 sec rest periods between contractions. This form of exercise is particularly good to maintain or increase muscle bulk and strength without increasing joint inflammation in a patient with active arthritis.

2. **Isotonic exercise.** A dynamic muscle contraction with movement through an arc of motion against a fixed resistance. It should be done when joint inflammation is under control. Isotonic training begins with 1–2-lb weights. Before increasing weight, patients should comfortably perform 12 repetitions.

3. **Isokinetic exercise.** The rate of movement is held constant, but the force produced by the individual may vary through the arc of motion. This form of exercise is rarely used in rehabilitation of arthritic patients.

4. **Aerobic and aquatic exercise programs.**

11. How does strength training differ from endurance training?
Strength is increased by isometric exercises and by isotonic exercises with increased resistance, resulting in fewer repetitions (7–10 repetitions). Endurance is increased by isotonic exercises with low resistance, enabling multiple repetitions (3 sets of 10 repetitions).

12. What aerobic activities can a rheumatic disease patient participate in to increase cardiovascular fitness?
Swimming, walking, stationary bicycling, and treadmill walking are recommended to increase cardiovascular fitness. The intensity should be sufficient to elevate the heart rate to 75% of maximum (220 − age) for 20–40 minutes.

13. How often should a patient with arthritis exercise?
All patients with arthritis should perform stretching for 10 minutes and ROM exercises daily. A patient with active joint inflammation or those with Class III or IV functional capacity should also do isometric exercises and aquatic therapy for 30 minutes, 3–4 times a week. A patient whose disease is controlled and is functional Class I or II should do isotonic exercises and aerobic exercises for 30 minutes, 3–4 times a week. Particular attention should be given to strengthening the shoulder and knee musculature.

14. How can a patient with arthritis determine if they have done too much exercise?
- Excessive pain during the exercise session
- Postexercise fatigue lasting >1 hour
- Postexercise soreness lasting >2 hours
- Increased joint pain or swelling the day following exercise

15. What precautions should be taken before advising a patient to perform isometric exercise training?
Isometric exercises, particularly of the upper extremities, increase systemic peripheral vascular resistance. These exercises are relatively contraindicated in patients with severe hypertension or a history of significant cardiovascular or cerebrovascular disease.

PHYSICAL MODALITIES

16. Which physical modalities are available for management of musculoskeletal pain?

Thermal agents	**Electrotherapy**
Superficial moist or dry heart	TENS
Deep heat with ultrasound or diathermy	Iontophoresis
Cryotherapy	**Traction**

17. What is the main purpose of physical modalities in a patient with arthritis?
To decrease pain so that the patient can participate in therapeutic exercises.

18. How are superficial and deep heat used in the treatment of musculoskeletal problems?
   Superficial heat includes moist heat delivered by hot packs, whirlpool, paraffin baths, or aqua therapy and dry heat delivered by fluidotherapy. This heat only penetrates tissue to a depth of 1–1.5 cm, and its effects last for 30–45 minutes.
   Deep heat is delivered by ultrasound or short-wave diathermy. Tissues at a depth of 3–6 cm can be heated to 41°C. The effect lasts for 30–45 minutes, during which time exercises should be done.

19. What are some of the therapeutic effects of heat treatments?
By warming tissue, several effects occur simultaneously: increased tendon and joint capsule extensibility, reduction in muscle spasm, production of analgesia, increased tissue blood flow, and increased tissue metabolism. Superficial joints are typically easier to heat by techniques such as

hot packs, paraffin wax, fluidotherapy, hydrotherapy, and radiant heat. Heat treatments can be used palliatively to reduce pain and spasm, particularly in subacute and chronic conditions. To restore function, heat, both superficial and deep, is used in conjunction with formal therapy and therapeutic exercise; this improves joint ROM by way of reduction in tendon and joint capsule tightness and reduction of contracture.

20. Are there contraindications to treating with heat?

Tissue pain and damage commence with tissue temperatures of 113° (45°C). Increased collagenolysis has been found to occur with increased intra-articular temperatures. While there are potentially adverse implications for using heat in inflammatory conditions, such as rheumatoid arthritis, investigators have not found increased joint destruction to occur when heat is used.

Because pain is a critical warning sign of tissue injury, desensitized areas or patients with a reduction in mental status are contraindications to the use of heat. Other common contraindications include bleeding diathesis, malignancy, and tumor. Also, heat applications to the gonads or to a fetus should be avoided. Areas with inadequate vascular supply should not be heated because of their inability to dissipate heat appropriately or to meet the increased metabolic demands caused by the increased temperature. Deep heat should not be used if metal is in the area being treated.

21. How is cryotherapy applied?

Cold application can be very specific, as in the use of vapocoolant sprays, localized massage, or locally applied cold pack. Or it can be very generally applied, as in ice water immersion, refillable bladders, thermal blankets, or contrast baths. For subacute pain and spinal muscle spasm, it is typically applied as ice massage or cold pack. Cryotherapy is the treatment of choice following acute injury, particularly when combined with compression.

22. Both superficial heat and cryotherapy reduce muscle spasm. How does the mechanism of cold differ from that of heat?

Cold has its effect directly on the muscle, the intrafusal fibers of the muscle spindle mechanism, and sensory wrappings of the muscle spindles. **Heat** primarily affects muscle spasm indirectly by slowing the firing rate of secondary afferents, increasing the firing rate of Golgi tendon organs, and decreasing the firing rate of efferent fibers to the muscle spindle (gamma fibers).

23. What is iontophoresis?

It is the use of DC current to induce topically applied medications to migrate into soft tissues and nerves up to 3–5 mm deep. Common topical medications applied include lidocaine gel, dexamethasone gel, and analgesics. This therapy has been used in tendinitis (especially Achilles tendinitis), bursitis, and neuritis.

24. When is traction useful for the management of cervical and lumbar spinal disorders?

Traction involves applying force in a manner to distract the cervical or lumbar vertebral bodies. This increases the intervertebral foraminal area, allowing more space for the exiting nerve root. Cervical traction is set up in a specific position with weight from 10–15 lbs or more. Lumbar traction is applied with the patient supine and both hips and knees flexed to 90°. The traction is 40–80 lbs. Both cervical and lumbar traction work best if applied two or three times a day until pain relief occurs. Failure to improve pain within 2–4 weeks or exacerbation of pain during traction are indications to stop this therapy.

ORTHOSES, JOINT PROTECTION, AND ASSISTIVE DEVICES

25. Why are splints and orthotics used in arthritis patients?

Splints and orthotics are used in the treatment of inflammatory and degenerative arthritis to unweight joints, create stability in selected joints, decrease joint motion, increase joint motion, or support the joint in the position of maximal function. They can either be purchased over-the-counter or custom-formed to fit the individual patient.

26. Name the major factor in patient noncompliance in the use of splints and orthotics.
The **cosmetic appearance** of the splint is a major factor in nonuse. Fear of public attention to the device, including discrimination at work and in other environments, adds to a patient's unwillingness to use the device. Compliance with splints is increased when the splints significantly improve pain or function and when family or support groups reinforce the need to use the splint regularly. Cosmetic splints, particularly for the small digits of the hand, can be constructed of precious metals, and semiprecious stones.

27. What are joint protection techniques?
Techniques for joint protection and energy conservation include task modification, environmental design/modification, and adaptation. By reducing mechanical stress, joint integrity is preserved and inflammation is reduced. Minimizing static positions while emphasizing proper posture reduces stress on individual joints. Joint protection includes maintaining ROM, unloading painful joints, and adequate rest periods throughout the day.

28. How can the use of adaptive devices and mobility aids benefit a patient with arthritis?
Assistive devices which substitute for deficient function help a patient with arthritis conserve energy, decrease stress on joints, relieve pain, and be more functionally independent. Adaptive devices for kitchen, bathroom, and self-care are readily available and listed in many patient manuals. Mobility aids include canes, crutches, and wheelchairs.

29. In which hand should a cane be placed to provide weight-bearing relief for a diseased hip?
The cane is placed in the hand of the contralateral arm. This creates a moment arm which counteracts the patient's weight and significantly reduces the amount of force applied to the hip joint. Placing the cane on the same side as the involved hip actually increases loading on the hip joint and potentially exacerbates the discomfort, pain, or joint dysfunction. Note that with walking, the stress across the hip joint is equal to two to three times body weight.

30. For an involved knee or ankle, which hand should hold the cane?
Below the level of the hip, ground reactive force to an individual joint is relieved most effectively when the cane is held on the **ipsilateral side** as the involved joint. This position can be advantageous for climbing and descending stairs but can be disruptive to the normal rhythm of gait because of the reversal of the natural swing of the arm. The patient may find that the cane works well when held in the contralateral hand during normal ambulation, but then can change it to the ipsilateral side for specific actions or activities requiring direct force on the ankle and knee. With walking, the normal stress across the knee is 3–4 times body weight, whereas stress across the ankle can be as high as 4–5 times body weight.

31. How can you tell if a cane or crutch has been properly fitted to the patient?
A properly fitted cane or crutch should reach 8 inches lateral to the front of the foot when the patient is standing and holding the cane or crutch handle with the elbow flexed 15–30°. This position permits stability on standing and an easy reach to the ground ahead during walking.

SPECIFIC DISEASE REHABILITATION

32. Name some general goals of therapeutic exercise for osteoarthritis.
In addition to localized involvement of the joint and weakness of the directly associated muscles, patients with osteoarthritis who become inactive lose cardiovascular fitness and functional independence, and gain weight. The patients also progressively deteriorate in the performance of their ac-

tivities of daily living and progressively lose independence. Exercise, as a part of treatment of osteoarthritis, attempts to counter this general decline. The general goals of an exercise program are to increase or maintain joint motion, normalize gait, build muscular strength and endurance, improve aerobic capacity, facilitate weight loss, improve functional capacity, and provide an opportunity for socialization.

33. What kinds of exercise are available for a patient with osteoarthritis?
Based on the general degree of dysfunction and specific involvement of individual joints, a physician may prescribe exercise that includes isometric, isotonic, aerobic, or aquatic exercise. The type of program should be individualized to the patient's interests, ability, and tolerance for exercise. The patient's compliance improves with his or her understanding of the exercise program and encouragement from physical therapists, group leaders, other patients, and family. Consistency in attendance to an exercise program is far more important than the intensity when the goals are more specifically directed to functional well-being than to increased performance.

34. Describe a sample physical and occupational therapy prescription for a patient with rheumatoid arthritis who has recently recovered after an exacerbation requiring 2 weeks of bedrest.
Physical therapy: Assess current function and commence progressive remobilization, including passive and active techniques, gait training, instruction in joint protective techniques, with goals of improved endurance, mobility, and reduction in pain. Three times per week for 4–6 weeks, 1–2 hours per session. Include aquatics therapy to enhance posture, gait, and strength 2 times per week. Transition this to a self-managed program.
Occupational therapy: Assess current functional activities and provide instruction for self-care activities, dressing, grooming, and hygiene. Progress to household activities as tolerated.
Contraindications: Avoid excessive stress to joints with residual inflammation, reduce activities if pain or fatigue occurs, provide adequate periods of rest, and avoid severe discomfort and pain.

35. Can patients with rheumatoid arthritis benefit from a regular exercise program?
Regular exercise can increase their functional levels, including endurance, activities of daily living, and mobility. Exercise programs must be adjusted specifically for the disease process. Patients benefit from low-repetition, low-resistance isotonic exercises, frequently undertaken through short arcs as compared to the entire arc of motion. The addition of swimming, bicycling, gardening, and other activities helps preserve and develop both type I and type II muscle fibers.

36. What rehabilitative techniques can be used for some other rheumatic diseases?
- Ankylosing spondylitis—spinal extension and hip and shoulder ROM exercises. Deep breathing exercises.
- Polymyositis/dermatomyositis—isometric exercises 3 times a week after inflammation is under control. ROM exercises to prevent contractures daily.
- Steroid-induced myopathy—active isometric and isotonic exercise program delay and decrease the severity of steroid myopathy.
- Systemic sclerosis—ROM exercises and splinting to decrease contractures. Finger flexion and extension exercises.
- Reflex sympathetic dystrophy—ROM exercises must be part of any program. Often, exercises must be performed after stellate ganglion blocks have been done to reduce the pain.

BIBLIOGRAPHY

1. Blount WP: Don't throw away the cane. J Bone Joint Surg 38A:695–708, 1956.
2. Feinburg J, Brandt K: Use of resting splints by patients with rheumatoid arthritis. J Occup Ther 35:173–178, 1978.
3. Guide to Independent Living for People with Arthritis. Atlanta, Arthritis Foundation, 1988.

4. Hicks JE: Exercise in patients with inflammatory arthritis and connective tissue disease. Rheum Dis Clin North 16:845–870, 1990.
5. Hicks JE: Exercise and rheumatoid arthritis. Phys Med Rehabil Clin North Am 5:701–728, 1994.
6. Hicks JE, Gerber LH: Rehabilitation of patients with arthritis and connective tissue disease. In DeLisa JA (ed): Rehabilitation Medicine: Principles and Practice, 2nd ed. Philadelphia, J.B. Lippincott, 1993.
7. Kaul MP, Herring SA: Superficial heat and cold: How to maximize benefits. Phys Sportsmed 22(12):65–74, 1994.
8. Melvin JL: Rheumatic Disease: Occupational Therapy and Rehabilitation, 3d ed. Philadelphia, F.A. Davis, 1982.
9. Nicholas JJ, Gwen H: Splinting and rheumatoid arthritis: I. Factors affecting patient compliance. Arch Phys Med Rehabil 63:92–94, 1982.
10. Norden DK, Leventhal LJ, Schumacher HR: Prescribing exercise for osteoarthritis of the knee. J Musculoskel Med 11(9):14–12, 1994.
11. Oosterveld FGJ, Rasker JJ: Treating arthritis with locally applied heat or cold. Semin Arthritis Rheum 24:82–90, 1994.
12. Semble EL, Loeser RF, Wise CM: Therapeutic exercise for rheumatoid arthritis and osteoarthritis. Semin Arthritis Rheum 20:32–40, 1990.
13. Swezey RL: Rehabilitation medicine and arthritis. In McCarty DJ, Koopman WJ (eds): Arthritis and Allied Conditions, 12th ed., Philadelphia, Lea & Febiger, 1993, pp 887–917.

91. PSYCHOSOCIAL ASPECTS OF RHEUMATIC DISEASES

Elizabeth Kozora, Ph.D.

1. Name the most common psychosocial problems in rheumatic diseases.

Depression and anxiety

Uncertainty and loss of control regarding the disease process

Altered body image and reduced physical ability

Decreased self-esteem and self-confidence

Fear of becoming physically dependent and disabled

Loss of independence and security in career and personal roles

Increased stress related to social changes and disability limitations

2. Is there a relationship between psychological factors and the onset of illness?

Con: In some studies, psychosocial stress has been associated with disease onset, but the mechanisms underlying this association are unclear. It is likely that there are multiple etiologies, and under heightened stress, disease activity may increase.

Pro: Studies to date suggest that stress can precede flare-ups of rheumatic disorders, such as systemic lupus erythematosus and rheumatoid arthritis. Psychosocial stressors, such as disrupted or conflictual relationships or lack of social support, have been associated with exacerbations. There is also evidence suggesting that stress can lower a patient's pain threshold in certain medical disorders.

3. Can features of the history identify psychosocial problems in rheumatic patients?

- History of psychological problems prior to the illness
- Patient's self-report of significant emotional or social decline lasting > 2 weeks
- Prolonged negative and pessimistic attitude by the patient regarding his or her medical diagnosis
- Abrupt change in patient compliance toward medical treatment

4. What factors are associated with depressive symptoms in rheumatic diseases?

1. Increased disease severity and disability have been associated with increased depressive symptoms.

2. The secondary consequences of severe medical disease may increase depression by perpetuating losses (i.e., career or social roles), increasing financial difficulties, and reducing access to social support.

3. Patients with lower socioeconomic status and education may be more susceptible to depression associated with medical disease.

4. Increased age is associated with increased depression in physically ill patients.

5. Although not consistently reported, female patients may experience greater depression.

5. What are the most important symptoms associated with depression in rheumatic disease patients?

Somatic symptoms that represent diagnostic criteria for major depression (e.g., fatigue, anorexia, weight loss, insomnia, sleep disturbance, loss of sexual interest) are common in both depressed and nondepressed medical patients. Thus, they may be less useful in identifying depression in rheumatic disease patients.

Some studies suggest that irritability, crying, sadness, dissatisfaction, discouragement about the future, and difficulty with decisions might be considered normal psychological reactions to illness. However, prolonged periods of these emotional states may signify depression.

Additional symptoms that help identify depression in rheumatic patients include:

Guilt	Low self-esteem
Pessimism	Feelings of worthlessness
Sense of failure	Feelings of being punished
Poor body image	Suicidal ideation

6. Are there risk factors for developing depressive symptoms in rheumatic diseases?

- Personal history or family history of depression prior to diagnosis of rheumatic illness
- Increased pain and physical discomfort
- Lack of satisfaction with current lifestyle
- Rapid decline in functional ability
- Loss of ability to participate in valued activities

7. What can the physician do to decrease psychological problems in rheumatic disease patients?

- Be honest about the nature of the illness, provide information to demystify the illness, and discuss treatment options openly.
- Any change in compliance should be directly addressed with the patient. For example, if the patient has not been taking prescribed medications, ask about the patient's perception of the medications and side effects.
- Know what is meaningful in a patient's life and how his or her self-esteem might be challenged. For example, if work is a primary source of identity for the patient, then loss of work may require increased sensitivity and additional intervention.
- Overmanaging these patients and making them more dependent may be detrimental to their overall development of adaptive coping styles.

8. Do any individual psychological techniques appear most useful in treating psychological problems in patients with rheumatic diseases?

Psychiatric consultation and possible **medication** should be considered in patients who demonstrate prolonged emotional distress that interferes with everyday functioning or full participation in treatment. **Individual, family,** or **group therapy** might be considered for mild psychological distress. The following techniques are commonly used in medical groups:

a. **Behavior therapy** focuses on modifying behavior-mediated aspects of illness. Therapy may be designed to alter personal or family behaviors that contribute to poor health habits.

   b. **Cognitive therapy** focuses on changing faulty and distorted perceptions and thoughts that interfere with healthy adjustment.

   c. **Relaxation therapies** (i.e., biofeedback, progressive muscle relaxation and imagery) have been useful in decreasing pain and depression.

   d. **Coping skills training** provides adaptive coping styles to improve problem-solving.

   e. **Supportive therapy** can reduce feelings of isolation and helplessness and encourage expression of emotions related to illness.

   f. **Educational** and **skills training** focuses on information and strategies for increasing patient involvement in treatment.

9. What factors facilitate psychological adjustment to rheumatic diseases?

   1. Adequate social support, satisfaction in the quality of interaction with others, and the ability to overcome devaluating social attitudes

   2. Constructive cognitive appraisal of illness and the ability to restructure long-term goals toward realistic outcomes

   3. Using active coping strategies which include seeking information about disease, focusing on positive thoughts, and deriving personal meaning from illness experiences

   4. Perseverance, independence, intelligence, internal control, creativity, aggressiveness, and moral stamina

   5. Developing a broader scope of values with physical attributes subordinate to other values

   6. Obtaining alternate financial resources and maintaining a flexible work schedule

10. How do social factors influence the rehabilitation process associated with disability and pain in rheumatic diseases?

Higher levels of education may benefit some patients in allowing them to have greater flexibility in their employment opportunities.

The loss of income associated with disability can dramatically affect family patterns as well as rehabilitation and therapeutic options. Social service agencies may be required for less economically advantaged.

Married patients may adjust better to disability by limiting the negative effects of social deprivation.

The age of disease onset may be associated with specific developmental phases which significantly impact the patient's life and choices.

Slowly progressing chronic illness is different than acute trauma. In general, the more responsibility a person had for the event, the better the adjustment. A degenerative prognosis requires continued reassessment and readjustment to conditions.

For many rheumatic disorders, the disability is invisible (i.e., pain and stiffness in rheumatoid arthritis) which may adversely affect rehabilitation and social awareness. The better the individual is able to integrate their disability into their lifestyle and self-concept, the greater their acceptance of limitations.

11. What are the estimates of medical compliance in rheumatic disorders?

Long-term compliance to therapeutic treatment in rheumatic disorders is about 50%, a rate consistent with other chronic illnesses. Estimates of noncompliance to **medications** in rheumatic disease range from 22–67%. Noncompliance to **physical therapy** ranges from 33–66%.

12. What factors are related to compliance with medical treatment in the rheumatic disorders?

Adherence declines when patients have significant **side effects** to medications or take medications that require **multiple dosages.** Compliance also declines when the patient doubts the effectiveness of the treatment.

Compliance increases when:

• The patient and physician agree on the problem, model of the disease, and goals of treatment. Shared information and decision-making, with the patient participating as a "co-manager" of his treatment, probably improves patient motivation and the patient–physician relationship.

- The patient is threatened by the disease symptoms and believes an effective treatment exists. The caregivers should inform patients about all aspects of the disease and its treatment. This facilitates the patients' ability to plan their lives efficiently, ease uncertainties, make wise use of available resources, and create better arrangements for a possible decrease in the ability to care for themselves.
- Simple self-monitoring techniques are used, and social reinforcement is appropriate. Encourage cooperation from patient and family members.
- The disease has a more recent onset, and the prescribed regimen is not disruptive to normal patterns of daily living.

13. Do rheumatic diseases affect sexuality? How might that impact psychological function?
In many rheumatic diseases, sexuality may be impaired due to the disease itself or the medications prescribed. Sexuality may be problematic when accompanied by pain, discomfort, fatigue, poor self-image, or side effects from medication. The partner of a rheumatic disease patient may also develop fears about sex (i.e., being too demanding of a sick person, causing pain), and changes in sexual functioning are likely to contribute to emotional distress. The physician should assess changes in sexuality by directly raising the issue and offering appropriate referrals (i.e., psychotherapy) if necessary.

14. Can medications administered in rheumatic diseases affect psychological functioning?
Corticosteroids are the most frequently reported medications associated with psychological abnormalities, which include psychosis, euphoria, and depression. They have also been correlated with cognitive difficulties. Group studies have not consistently reported dose-response associations, and individual differences have been strongly noted. In patients undergoing significant changes (increase or decrease) in prednisone, possible psychiatric and cognitive dysfunction should be monitored.

Psychological changes associated with other common antirheumatic medications are fairly infrequent, although there have been some documented changes. For example, **NSAIDs** have been associated with dizziness, vertigo, headaches, paranoia, depression, and hostility; **gold** and **choroquine** have been previously associated with confusion, hallucinations, delirium, and nightmares; and **methotrexate** is known to cause behavioral abnormalities in high doses.

BIBLIOGRAPHY

1. Ahles TA, Khan S, Yunus MB, et al: Psychiatric status of patients with primary fibromyalgia, patients with rheumatoid arthritis, and subjects without pain: A blind comparison of DSM-III diagnosis. Am J Psychiatry 148:1721–1726, 1991.
2. Bauman A, Barnes C, Schrieber L, et al: The unmet needs of patients with systemic lupus erythematosus: Planning for patient education. Patient Educ Counseling 14:235–242, 1989.
3. Burckhardt CS, Archenholtz B, Bjelle A: Quality of life of women with systemic lupus erythematosus: A comparison with woman with rheumatoid arthritis. J Rheumatol 20:977–981, 1993.
4. Feinblatt A, Anderson FS, Gordon W: Psychosocial and vocational considerations. In Leek JC, Gershwin ME, Fowler WM (eds): Principles of Physical Medicine and Rehabilitation in the Musculoskeletal Diseases. Orlando, FL, Grune & Stratton, 1986, pp 217–234.
5. Hudson JI, Goldenberg DL, Pope HG, et al: Comorbidity of fibromyalgia with medical and psychiatric disorders. Am J Med 92:363–367, 1992.
6. Katz D, Yelin EH: The development of depressive symptoms among women with rheumatoid arthritis. Arthritis Rheum 38:49–56, 1995.
7. Liang MH, Rogers M, Larsen M, et al: The psychosocial impact of systemic lupus erthematosus and rheumatoid arthritis. Arthritis Rheum 27:13–19, 1984.
8. Liang MH: Psychosocial management of rheumatic diseases. In Kelly WM, Harris ED, Ruddy S, Sledge CB (eds): Textbook of Rheumatology, 4th ed. Philadelphia, W.B. Saunders, 1993.
9. Milgrom H, Bender BG: Psychological side effects of therapy with corticosteroids. Am Rev Respir Dis 147:471–472, 1993.
10. Moran MG: Psychological factors affecting pulmonary and rheumatological diseases. Psychosomatics 32:14–23, 1991.
11. Rodin G, Graven J, Littlefield C: Depression in the Medically Ill. New York, Brunner/Mazel, 1991.
12. Young LD: Psychological factors in rheumatoid arthritis. J Consult Clin Psychol 60:619–627, 1992.

92. SURGICAL TREATMENT AND RHEUMATIC DISEASES

John A. Reister, M.D.

1. What are the major indications for joint replacement surgery in patients with arthritis?

Pain and/or loss of function that have failed to respond to medical therapy. Pain relief is the most attainable result of surgery. Restoration of motion and function is less predictable.

2. What medical factors require preoperative attention in patients undergoing total joint arthroplasty (TJA)?

All surgical candidates for orthopedic reconstructive procedures require a comprehensive history and physical examination to assess the overall general operative risks. Patients should be examined for carious teeth, skin ulcerations (especially around the feet), and symptoms of urinary tract infection or prostatism, as these could increase the risk of postoperative infections. Women should have a urine culture to rule out asymptomatic bacteriuria. If patients are receiving NSAIDs, these medications should be stopped several days (at least five halflives) before surgery to prevent bleeding due to their antiplatelet effects.

3. What other factors must be addressed preoperatively in patients with rheumatoid arthritis (RA)?

Cervical spine—An unstable cervical spine due to arthritic involvement places the patient at risk for catastrophic neurologic loss when the neck is manipulated during intubation. Preoperative lateral flexion and extension radiographs of the cervical spine are mandatory.

Temporomandibular arthritis (especially juvenile RA patients) and cricoarytenoid arthritis—May make intubations more difficult.

Immune status—Infection rates are significantly higher in RA patients, partly because of the disease process and partly because of the immunosuppressive drugs used to control it. Patients should be on the lowest corticosteroid dosage possible. It is recommended that methotrexate be withheld for the week of surgery and the week after surgery (controversial).

Nutritional status—RA patients may be relatively malnourished, which predisposes them to infection. Patients with a total lymphocyte count >1500/mm³ and albumin level >3.5 gm/dl are less prone to infections.

Hypothalamic-pituitary-adrenal axis—Patients on chronic corticosteroid therapy are unable to respond normally to surgical stress. They must receive increased corticosteroids immediately preoperatively, intraoperatively, and postoperatively.

4. Patients with RA frequently have multiple joints involved. What is the recommended sequence for reconstructive surgery?

Lower-extremity surgery is done before upper-extremity surgery, since crutch use postoperatively would place excessive demands on any upper-extremity reconstructive surgery.

In the multiply involved lower-extremity, the hip is reconstructed before the knee to get the best possible alignment of the knee. Also, rehabilitation from hip surgery is less demanding than from knee TJA.

In the upper extremity, the preferred order is controversial. Usually proximal joints, nerve, and tendon problems are addressed before the hand and wrist. The wrist is done before the hand joints to help with alignment. For the shoulder and elbow, the most symptomatic joint is usually done first.

5. What additional intraoperative and postoperative medical procedures are done to prevent postoperative complications following TJA of the hip or knee?

Intraoperative **prophylactic antibiotics** are given to decrease the chance of infection. For lower-extremity TJA (hip, knee), compression stockings, early ambulation, and **anticoagulation** are done to prevent postoperative deep venous thrombosis. Deep venous thrombosis occurs in 50–60% of patients with a 1–3% prevalence of fatal pulmonary embolus if postoperative anticoagulation (usually for 3–6 weeks) is not done.

6. What is Steel's rule of thirds?

At the level of the first cervical vertebra (C1), the antero-posterior diameter is divided into thirds, allowing ⅓ for the dens, ⅓ for the spinal cord, and ⅓ for free space. Because there is significant free space at this level, small degrees of C1–2 subluxation (3–8 mm) usually do not compromise the cord. However, when the *anterior* atlanto-dens interval (measured from posterior part of anterior arch of C1 to the anterior aspect of odontoid) becomes >10–12 mm, all the atlantoaxial ligamentous complex has usually been destroyed, and the space available for the spinal cord is usually compromised. Likewise, when the *posterior* atlanto-dens interval (measured from posterior aspect of the odontoid to the anterior aspect of the posterior arch of C1) is <14 mm, the spinal cord is usually compressed. (See also Chapter 18.)

7. When should the cervical spine (C1–2) be fused in patients with RA?

This is an area of significant controversy. The presence of severe pain, myelopathic symptoms or signs, and/or basilar invagination >5 mm seen on a lateral radiograph of the cervical spine are indications for surgical fusion. Recently, prophylactic arthrodesis regardless of symptoms and neurologic findings has been recommended for patients with anterior instability of C1–2 and a posterior atlanto-dens interval of 14 mm or less.

8. Give the potential intraoperative and postoperative complication rates following cervical spine fusion in an RA patient.

• Postoperative mortality: 0–10%. Has been as high as 33% for patients with severe neurologic compromise.
• Wound infections and dehiscence: up to 25% in older reports. Significantly less today.
• Nonunion rates: 0–50%. Average 20%.
• Late subaxial subluxation below previous fusion due to transfer of increased stresses.

9. What surgical procedures are available for RA patients with shoulder involvement?

Surgical procedures of the shoulder are performed predominantly for pain control. An increase in range of motion usually does not occur. Replacement arthroplasty can include the entire joint, termed total **shoulder arthroplasty,** or only the humeral head, termed **hemiarthroplasty.** The principal factor in choosing between the two is the status of the rotator cuff. For maximal functional use and stability of a total shoulder arthroplasty, soft-tissue tension from an intact rotator cuff plays an integral role. If the rotator cuff is not intact and cannot be repaired, then a constrained arthroplasty or an oversized hemiarthroplasty is chosen.

10. What are the surgical options for management of arthritis involving the elbow joint?

In **inflammatory arthritis** not responsive to medical management, synovectomy will temporarily control the disease and reliably decrease pain, but it infrequently has any positive effect on joint motion. Open synovectomy may also include excision of the radial head if significantly involved.

In **osteoarthritis of the elbow,** the ulnohumeral articulation is predominantly affected, usually by osteophytes that develop on the coronoid process or olecranon. Surgically, these osteophytes are removed through an osteotomy in the distal humerus (Outerbridge-Kashiwagi). When the articular cartilage is lost, the joint surface can be resurfaced with autologous tissue, fascia lata most commonly.

In **post-traumatic arthritis** involving the radiohumeral or proximal radioulnar joint, a radial head excision can be performed with predictably good results, as long as the medical collateral ligament of the elbow is intact. Total elbow arthroplasty is becoming the surgical option of choice for most arthritic conditions of the elbow. This is due to the increasing reliability of the current prostheses and the magnitude of functional improvement for the patient.

Elbow arthrodesis should be a very last resort, as this procedure makes it impossible to position the hand for functional use. It is reserved for a septic elbow that has not responded to other treatments and when total elbow replacement is not feasible. Arthroscopy is used for diagnostic purposes, removal of loose bodies, and synovectomy for both biopsy and treatment purposes.

11. How are the common problems of the wrist in RA managed surgically?

RA has a predilection for the small joints of the hand and wrist. The wrist is almost universally involved and usually presents predictable patterns of involvement and resultant deformities. The goal of medical management lies in control of the inflammatory synovitis to prevent destruction of bony and soft-tissue structures. When this fails, surgery can be used to remove inflammatory synovium or correct deformity.

The dorsal wrist capsule and dorsal tendon sheath are commonly involved with synovitis and tenosynovitis that often lead to extensor tendon rupture. Prevention of tendon rupture is far better than tendon transfer, and therefore, if medical control is inadequate, early surgical synovectomy and tenosynovectomy are warranted. The term **Vaughn-Jackson syndrome** is applied when the extensor tendons of the ring and small finger have ruptured. Primary tendon repair is usually not possible, especially if the rupture occurred longer than a few days previously. Tendon transfer surgery is then required to restore function.

On the volar aspect of the wrist, tenosynovitis of the flexor tendons can cause compression of the median nerve in the carpal canal, leading to carpal tunnel syndrome. It can also lead to rupture of the flexor pollicis longus tendon, leading to inadequate thumb flexion and resting hyperextension at the interphalageal joint. This is called the **Mannerfelt syndrome.** It usually requires tendon transfer or arthrodesis of the interphalangeal joint of the thumb.

The distal radioulnar joint is commonly involved by synovitis, which leads to laxity of this joint, osseous destruction of the ulnar head, and pain with forearm rotation. The ulnar head becomes dorsally prominent and adds to stress on the ulnar extensor tendons. This constellation of findings is called the **caput ulna syndrome.** Its surgical management entails aggressive synovectomy, ulnar head excision, capsulorrhaphy, and lateral tenodesis using a portion of the extensor carpal ulnaris tendon.

When the true wrist joint (radiocarpal joint) is involved, the deformity usually involves five components: radial translation, ulnar deviation, volar subluxation, intercarpal supination, and carpal collapse. Early on, reconstruction using an extensor carpi ulnaris tenodesis can be beneficial. With advanced changes, total wrist arthroplasty or wrist arthrodesis can be used to control pain and improve function.

12. What are the surgical options for basilar thumb osteoarthritis?

The carpometacarpal joint of the thumb, also known as the trapeziometacarpal or basilar thumb joint, is a saddle-shaped articulation with a high propensity for degenerative change. The older middle-aged to elderly woman is most at risk for degenerative arthritis in this region.

Surgical procedures include implant arthroplasty, tendon interposition arthroplasty, tendon suspension arthroplasty, and arthrodesis. Implants have a high rate of failure, and work continues on a better prosthetic design. Tendon interposition entails placing a wad of tendon into the cavity created by removal of some or all of the trapezium. Tendon suspension is similar, except after the trapezium is removed, a weave of tendon is created that supports the thumb metacarpal base like a sling. Arthrodesis is probably the best procedure for longevity of the reconstruction, but it does restrict metacarpal motion somewhat and it requires very precise positioning or function will not be optimal.

13. How is a mucous cyst and osteroarthritis of the distal interphalangeal (DIP) joint managed?

Mucous cysts are commonly associated with osteoarthritis of the DIP joints of the fingers. They present as a clear mucin-filled cystic mass, usually between the DIP joint and the proximal aspect of the nail. Historically, they may have had a number of spontaneous ruptures, resolution, and recurrences. This cycle may lead to thinning of the overlying skin, making surgical correction more risky.

Pathophysiologically, the mucous cyst results from chronic inflammation secondary to a dorsal osteophyte of the DIP joint. Therefore, appropriate evaluation includes an x-ray, and definitive management must be directed at removal of the osteophyte. If the DIP joint is significantly painful or unstable, fusion of the DIP joint in mild flexion becomes the treatment of choice.

14. How are deformities of the proximal interphalangeal joints (PIP) surgically managed in RA patients?

Boutonniere deformities result from synovitis within the PIP joints, causing extensor tendon elongation and rupture and leading to progressive flexion contactures. During early stages, synovectomy may be helpful.

Swan-neck deformities progress through four stages of deformity. During the first three stages, splinting, synovectomy, and surgical release of intrinsic muscle tightness and tendon adhesions are used. In the last stage, when the PIP joint is destroyed, surgical options include joint replacement or fusion.

15. Describe the results of metacarpophalangeal (MCP) joint surgery in RA patients.

Synovitis of the MCP joints ultimately leads to joint destruction, MCP subluxation, and ulnar deviation of the fingers. Early in the disease course, before significant radiographic joint destruction or deformity, synovectomy may be performed for pain relief if medical therapy has failed. There is little evidence that prophylactic synovectomy slows joint destruction, but it may postpone the need for joint replacement surgery.

MCP arthroplasty is indicated when synovitis has resulted in cartilage destruction, decreased motion, pain, ulnar drift, deformity, and loss of function. The most commonly used arthroplasty is made of silicone rubber (Swanson's implants). Common problems include breakage, stiffness, instability, and reactive synovitis to silicone debris. MCP arthroplasties, irrespective of design, result in 60° of motion which may decrease to 30° over time. Postoperative splinting and hand rehabilitation are extensive and last for several months. Consequently, a compliant and cooperative patient is necessary for optimal results.

Arthrodesis is not done except for the thumb MCP joint. This is because the thumb needs strength for pinch, whereas motion is less important.

16. Name three symptoms that are indications for joint replacement surgery in a patient with arthritis of the hip or knee.
1. Inability to walk more than one block due to pain.
2. Inability to stand in one place for longer than 20–30 minutes due to pain.
3. Inability to obtain restful sleep due to pain when rolling in bed at night.

17. What does the term "low friction arthroplasty" mean?
Sir John Charnley, a pioneer in total joint replacement, coined this term in 1979 when describing his prosthesis for total hip arthroplasty. It refers to the small size (22 mm) of the head of the femoral component. Because of the small surface area, friction between the prosthetic head and polyethylene socket was minimized. This reduced friction lead to less shear forces imparted to the acetabular cup, which decreased the rate of loosening and less volumetric wear on the polyethylene, which in turn decreased the amount of particulate debris created over time. However, the small femoral head concentrated the joint reactive force and over time produced an increase

in creep deformation of the polyethylene. Therefore, today's prosthetic head sizes range between 26–28 mm in an effort to reduce both forms of wear.

18. How do cemented, cementless, and hybrid prostheses differ?

The terms cemented and cementless refer to methods of fixation of total joint arthroplasty prostheses for the hip and knee. Most experience is with **cemented** prostheses where a self-curing acrylic cement, polymethylmethacrylate, is used to improve fixation between the prosthetic component and bone. Advances in cementing techniques over the years have lead to less problems with aseptic loosening.

Cementless prostheses include press fit and porous ingrowth prostheses. Press fit relies on a snug fit between prosthesis and bone without the use of cement. Porous ingrowth prostheses contain pores located on the proximal portion of the femoral component and acetabulum that allow ingrowth of bone. Hydroxyapatite or growth factors may be incorporated into the porous coating to stimulate bone ingrowth and better fixation. Overall, there is bone ingrowth into about 10% of the porous-coated surface.

Cementless acetabular components have demonstrated the best bony ingrowth into the porous-coated areas. Consequently, many centers use a cementless acetabular component with a cemented femoral component. This is termed a **hybrid** hip replacement.

19. Who should get a cemented total hip arthropathy (THA) and who should get a cementless prosthesis?

This is an area of controversy. Younger, active patients with good bone quality in whom intimate apposition of prosthesis to bone can be achieved intraoperatively are the best candidates for cementless THA. This is usually a patient <50–60 years old with osteoarthritis of the hip. Cemented prostheses usually are used in RA patients with poor bone stock and in the elderly with low activity levels. Rehabilitation postoperatively is easier for cemented than cementless THA.

20. How commonly does aseptic loosening occur in THA? What causes this loosening?

In cemented THA done using older techniques, the rate of aseptic loosening requiring revision was 10–15% at 10–15 years of follow-up (1% per year). Radiographic loosening of the femoral prosthetic component was as high as 30–40%. With modern surgical techniques, there is now < 3% loosening at 10 years, a rate that compares to the degree of loosening (3% at 10 years) occurring in porous-coated cementless prostheses. Patients who are young (< age 50), and heavy (>200 lbs) have the highest incidence of loosening.

Today, the cause of loosening is not primary cement failure. Most loosening is caused by particulate debris (polyethylene, methylmethacrylate, or metal) from the prosthetic joint. This debris stimulates macrophages in the membrane lining the bone-cement interface to produce prostaglandins and cytokines, such as interleukin-1 and tumor necrosis factor, which leads to endosteal bone resorption and a loose prosthesis.

21. What unique postoperative complication occurs in patients receiving cementless THA?

Mild to moderate **thigh pain** occurs in approximately 20% of patients receiving the porous-coated THA. This pain is due to a bony stress reaction occurring at the tip of the femoral stem. It usually does not require medication and resolves in 12–18 months.

22. Discuss the problems that can occur with a revision THA.

Revision THA is technically more challenging than primary arthroplasty, and the outcome (longevity) of the revision is significantly shorter and attendant complications higher. One of the significant problems encountered during revision is loss of bone stock. Loss of bone stock is greater if cement was used initially. To avoid this problem, the current recommendations are to perform a hybrid THA initially. However, in a younger, more active adult (usually < 60 years old), press fit of both the acetabulum and femur is recommended to minimize loss of bone stock since a revision arthroplasty will probably have to be done in the future.

23. How is arthroscopy used in the management of knee osteoarthritis?
Arthroscopic debridement of the knee is indicated in early osteoarthritis if some of the patient's symptoms are due to an internal derangement, such as a meniscal tear. Arthroscopic debridement and/or lavage can provide several months of lessened pain in some patients with more advanced degenerative arthritic changes (controversial).

24. When should osteotomy about the knee be chosen over total knee replacement?
In the young, active patient with unicompartmental arthritis. The high tibial osteotomy is the most commonly performed realignment procedure for the knee with degenerative changes limited to either the medial or lateral compartment. Involvement of the patellofemoral compartment, inflammatory arthritis, marked loss of motion, and older age are contraindications. This procedure is usually intended to relieve pain, preserve functional status, and delay the need for a total knee replacement. It is performed by realigning the mechanical axis (center of femoral head to center of the ankle mortise). The axis is moved from the involved to the uninvolved compartment by a wedge-shaped osteotomy of the tibia most commonly. If correction of the mechanical axis requires >12° wedge, then the osteotomy should be performed in the distal femur to prevent the production of a laterally sloped joint line. The most common complications include under correction and peroneal nerve injury.

25. What are the indications for unicompartmental arthroplasty of the knee?
This is an area of some controversy, and many surgeons are opposed to unicompartmental arthroplasty. It is indicated in the older, thinner, sedentary patient with at least 90° of flexion arc and arthritic involvement of only one compartment of the knee. It is contraindicated in inflammatory arthritis, obesity, young age, <90° arc of motion or 15° flexion contracture, and involvement of the patellofemoral compartment. It is accomplished by resurfacing the femoral and tibial joint surface in the involved compartment. Revision to total knee replacement is possible, but this is technically more difficult and has higher complication and failure rates than primary arthroplasty.

26. Who should get a cemented total knee arthroplasty and who should get a cementless prosthesis?
The cemented posterior stabilized condylar prosthesis and the total condylar prosthesis demonstrated 90–95% satisfactory results at 5–10 years for both RA and osteoarthritis patients. Cementless prostheses have not been as successful due to poor bone ingrowth and tibial component subsidence. At present cementless total knee arthroplasties usually are not used.

27. How frequently does infection complicate total hip and total knee arthroplasties?
Early postoperative infection rates are typically <0.5% with use of perioperative antibiotics and clean-air operating suites. late infections (>1 year postoperatively) occur in 1% of RA patients and fewer patients with osteoarthritis.

28. Should patients with total joint arthroplasties receive prophylactic antibiotics prior to having dental work done?
Yes. Amoxicillin, erthromycin, cephalexin, or cephadrine, 1000 mg orally 1 hour before and 500 mg 4 hours after the procedure.

29. How is an infected joint prosthesis managed?
Early infections (≤ 2weeks postoperatively) can be managed with antibiotics and open synovectomy, thorough debridement, and retention of the prosthesis. Multiple surgical debridements are usually necessary.

Late infections usually present with only pain but can present with obvious sepsis of the involved joint. Once the diagnosis is made, treatment is removal of prosthetic components, thorough debridement, and intravenous antibiotics for 6 weeks. If a low virulence organism is cultured, replantation with antibiotic-impregnated cement can be performed at 6 weeks. If gram-negative organisms are cultured, a longer duration of resection arthroplasty is required, with occasionally 12 months needed to reduce the reinfection rate.

30. Name the two most common etiologies of ankle arthritis. How are they managed surgically?

Post-traumatic arthritis and RA. The ankle joint very rarely becomes arthritic compared to the hip and knee, but when it does, it is most commonly related to post-traumatic changes. Fractures that result in minimal amounts (1–2 mm) of lateral talar subluxation will produce degenerative changes in a relatively short time because of decreased surface area contact and increased joint reactive forces.

Regardless of the etiology, functional bracing should be pursued until the patient can no longer tolerate this form of management. Total ankle replacement arthroplasty has historically had a high failure rate from infection and prosthetic loosening and cannot be recommended as a procedure of choice. Ankle arthrodesis is currently the best salvage procedure for the end-stage arthritic ankle. The success rate of arthrodesis is better in post-traumatic arthritis than in RA, where the rates of both infection and failure of fusion are significant. Technically, positioning of the talus properly under the tibia to facilitate walking is the key point of the surgical procedure to allow a relatively normal gait and prevent lateral metatarsal stress fractures.

31. Which joints are fused in a triple arthrodesis?

The subtalar calcaneocuboid, and talonavicular joints. Both RA and juvenile RA affect the subtalar and transtarsal joints. These joint involvements can be isolated or combined, and there has been a trend toward isolated arthrodesis of involved joints rather than triple arthrodesis when possible. Particularly common is isolated talonavicular joint destruction. If this presents in an adult with RA, then isolated fusion is recommended. Conversely, if the involvement occurs at a young age secondary to juvenile RA, then the entire transtarsal joint (talonavicular, calcaneocuboid) should be arthrodesed because this will provide a longer term satisfactory result.

Isolated subtalar arthrodesis is commonly performed when the remaining articulations of the triple joint are uninvolved and supple. Triple arthrodesis requires similar precision in positioning as does ankle arthrodesis to maximize walking biomechanics. In general, asensate feet (usually secondary to diabetes) are a contraindication to bony fusion due to the high likelihood of skin ulceration and subsequent infection.

32. What are the surgical indications for correction of the bunion deformity?

Pain and/or skin breakdown that is unresponsive to conservative measures. Bunion is the prominence on the medial aspect of the foot at the level of the first metatarsal head. Hallux valgus describes excessive lateral deviation of the great toe distal to the metatarso phalangeal (MTP) joint.

On initial presentation, all patients should be managed conservatively. This includes wider toebox shoes or pressure-relieving alterations in existing shoe wear. If this fails to provide relief after 2–3 months, surgery is planned. There are a number of surgical options, depending on the degree of deformity, congruence of the first MTP joint, and whether or not degenerative changes are present in the joint. In RA patients, arthrodesis is favored over soft-tissue reconstruction or osteotomy. Implant arthroplasty, once common, does not provide a reliable long-term result. Juvenile bunions, unfortunately not rare, have a >50% recurrence rate after surgery.

33. What is a Clayton-Hoffman procedure?

A commonly performed salvage procedure for advanced rheumatoid forefoot deformity. The rheumatoid forefoot pattern of involvement usually includes degeneration and instability at the first MTP joint, leading to hallux valgus and bunion deformity. The lesser toes are also involved with synovitis, leading to subluxation and eventual dislocation at the remaining MTP joints. This results in prominent metatarsal heads on the plantar surface and the development of intractable plantar keratoses. This progressive deformation commonly involves all the MTP joints to some degree.

The Clayton-Hoffman procedure entails resection of all the metatarsal heads through either a plantar or dorsal approach. Rarely, only two metatarsal joints will be involved, and the procedure can be performed only on the involved joints. However, it is not recommended to remove only one or three involved metatarsal heads. Fusion of the first MTP joint is often done concurrently with the Clayton-Hoffman procedure.

34. Differentiate between hammer toe, claw toe, and mallet toe.

FLEXIBLE TOE DEFORMITY	JOINT POSITION			SURGICAL MANAGEMENT
	MTP	PIP	DIP	
Hammer toe	Uninvolved, neutral	Flexion	Uninvolved, neutral	Flexible—flexor to extensor transfer. Fixed—hemiresection arthroplasty excision of distal portion of proximal phalanx
Claw toe	Fixed, extension	Fixed, flexion	Uninvolved, neutral or flexion	Resection of both sides of the PIP joint; joint dorsal capsulotomy and extensor tenotomy; flexor to extensor transfer
Mallet toe	Uninvolved, neutral	Uninvolved, neutral	Fixed, flexion	Excision of middle phalanx and/or flexor tenotomy if flexible

35. Discuss the indications for surgery in a patient with symptomatic disc herniation.

Overall, about 1% of patients with herniated discs eventually require surgery. Absolute indications include disc herniation causing cauda equina syndrome, progressive spinal stenosis, or marked muscular weakness and progressive neurologic deficit despite conservative management. Controversy arises over indications for surgery in patients with less severe symptoms and signs. Relative indications for laminectomy and disc removal include intolerable pain with sciatica symptoms unrelieved by nonsurgical treatment and recurrent back pain and sciatica that fail to improve significantly so that the patient can participate in activities of daily living after 6–12 weeks of conservative nonsurgical therapy.

Overall, long-term relief of sciatica has been shown to be the same in operative versus nonoperative patients, although the operative patients achieve their degree of relief more rapidly. The best results from surgery are obtained in the emotionally stable patient who has unequivocal disc herniation documented by consistent symptoms, appropriate tension sign, and MRI of the spine or myelogram. The most common cause for surgical failure is poor initial patient selection.

BIBLIOGRAPHY

1. Ayers DC, Short WH: Arthritis surgery. Clin Exp Rheumatol 11:75–84, 1993.
2. Ballard WT, Callaghan JJ, Sullivan PM, Johnston RC: The results of improved cementing techniques for total hip arthroplasty in patients less than 50 years old: A ten year follow-up study. J Bone Joint Surg 76(A):959–964, 1994.
3. Blackburn WD, Alarcon GS: Prosthetic joint infections: A role for prophylaxis. Arthritis Rheum 34:110–117, 1991.
4. Boden SD: Rheumatoid arthritis of the cervical spine: Surgical decision making based on predictors of paralysis and recovery. Spine 19:2275–2280, 1994.
5. Cracchiolo A, Cimino WR, Lian G: Arthrodesis of the ankle in patients who have rheumatoid arthritis. J Bone Joint Surg 74(A):903–908, 1992.
6. Harris WH, Sledge CB: Total hip and total knee replacement (parts I and II). N Eng J Med 323:725–731 and 801–807, 1990.

7. Livesley PJ, Doherty M, Needoff M, et al: Arthroscopic lavage of osteoarthritic knees. J Bone Joint Surg 73B:922–926, 1991.
8. Mehloff MA, Sledge CB: Comparison of cemented and cementless hip and knee replacements. Arthritis Rheum 33:293–297, 1990.
9. Murray DW, Carr AJ, Bulstrode CJK: Pharmacological thromboprophylaxis and total hip replacement. J Bone Joint Surg 77(B):3–5, 1995.
10. O'Driscoll SW: Elbow arthritis: Treatment options. JAAOS 1(2):106–116, 1993.
11. Peppelman WC, Krause DR, Donaldson WF, Agarwal A: Cervical spine surgery in rheumatoid arthritis: Improvement of neurologic deficit after cervical spine fusion. Spine 18:2375–2379, 1993.
12. Weber H: Lumbar disc herniation: A controlled, prospective study with ten years of observation. Spine 8:131–138, 1983.
13. Wroblewski B: Cementless versus cemented total hip arthroplasty: A scientific controversy: Orthop Clin North Am 24:591–597, 1993.

93. DISABILITY

Scott Vogelgesang, M.D.

1. What options are available for an individual who can no longer perform his or her job satisfactorily because of a musculoskeletal problem?
1. Adapt the workplace
    Obtain or modify special equipment or devices
    Modify work schedules
    Job restructuring
2. Consider switching jobs or reassignment to another position
3. Vocational rehabilitation
4. Apply for disability benefits.

2. What is disability?
Disability can be defined **as not being able to do something because of an illness or injury.** Most often, disability refers to an economic loss to an individual (by not being able to work at a previously acceptable level) because of a physical or mental condition. In insurance policies, laws, and regulations, the word *disability* has a more specific definition and needs to be distinguished from two similar, yet specific, terms: *impairment* and *handicap.*

3. Give a specific definition of disability.
Disability is *an alteration of an individual's capacity to meet personal, social, or occupational demands because of an impairment.* It is the gap between what an individual can do and what the individual needs or wants to do. The degree of disability is affected by the interaction between the individual's impairment and the economic and social aspects of that person's life (i.e., age, education, training). People with the same impairment do not necessarily have the same disability. Disability is assessed by nonmedical means.

4. Define impairment.
Impairment is a physical or mental **limitation to normal function** resulting from a disease process. Impairment is determined by a physician. An impairment does not necessarily mean that a person is disabled.

5. What is a handicap?
Handicap refers to the **social consequences** that relate to an impairment or disability. A handicap is present if an individual has:

(1) Impairment or disability that substantially limits one or more of life's activities or prevents the fulfillment of a role that is normal for that individual;

(2) Medical record of such an impairment;

(3) Barriers to accomplishing life's tasks that can be overcome only by compensating in some way for the effects of the impairment. Such compensation involves things like crutches, wheelchairs, prostheses, or even the amount of time necessary to complete a task.

6. List the important factors contributing to work disability in patients with a chronic musculoskeletal disease (or any chronic disease).

Disease
    Type of musculoskeletal disease
    Disease severity
    Impairment severity
Personal
    Age
    Sex
    Education
    Personality

Work
    Occupation
    Job autonomy
    Work experience
Social
    Social support
    Peer and social pressures for or against
      disability

Most physicians concentrate on trying to alleviate the "disease" factors to decrease disability. The other factors may be just as or more important in determining whether a patient considers himself or herself disabled.

7. What state and federal programs are set up to deal with disability?

There are two major programs to deal with a person's inability to work: Social Security Disability and Worker's Compensation. The Social Security Administration administers two programs that differ mainly in eligibility criteria: Social Security Disability Insurance (Title II) (SSDI, also called Disability Insurance Benefits) and Supplemental Security Income (Title XVI) (SSI). These programs currently provide benefits to over 4 million Americans.

8. Describe Social Security Disability Insurance (SSDI).

SSDI is a federally regulated program that was established in the 1950s. It is the largest disability insurance program in the world. In SSDI, employers and workers pay into a trust fund. Workers contribute through payroll taxes (FICA) and receive benefits (based on lifetime earnings) if they meet certain listed criteria.

The individual must be unable "to engage in any substantial gainful activity by reason of any medically determinable physical or mental impairment which can be expected to result in death or which has lasted or can be expected to last for a continuous period of not less than 12 months." It is expected that the individual cannot earn minimum wage because of the impairment. The Social Security Administration tries to take into account individual variations in impairment, vocational, and educational backgrounds. SSDI considers only global disability, so there are no partial awards. Persons may also qualify for Medicare to help cover medical expenses after receiving SSDI benefits for 24 months.

9. What is Supplemental Security Income (SSI)?

Individuals not qualifying for SSDI because of a lack of work experience may be covered by another program, SSI. SSI pays monthly sums to financially needy people who are either >65 years of age or qualified persons of any age with documented disabilities. SSI requires an evaluation of assets, sometimes called a "means" test. Usually, those who receive SSI are eligible to have some medical expenses covered by Medicaid.

10. Describe the workers' compensation program.

Workers' compensation is primarily a state-based system, although there is also a program for federal employees under the auspices of the U.S. Department of Labor. Any worker who incurs an illness or sustains an injury during and because of employment is entitled to protection against financial loss. It is a "no-fault" insurance system that provides benefits to all workers who are covered and who meet criteria. It removes the necessity to sue the employer. Workers' compensation deals effectively with work-related traumatic accidents but has more difficulty with occupational illnesses. Workers' compensation can award partial disability.

11. Who is eligible for disability?
- Any employee ≤65 years of age
- Unmarried sons or daughters <18 years old (can be 18 years of age if attending high school)
- Unmarried son or daughter disabled before age 22
- Spouse ≥62 years
- Spouse who is:
    Caring for a child who is <16 years
    Caring for a child who is disabled
- Disabled widow or widower
- Disabled, divorced widow or widower

12. What paperwork is necessary to apply for Social Security Disability?
    Social security number
    Birth certificate or other proof of age
    W2 forms or tax return from previous year
    Summary of work history for past 15 years
    Date employee stopped working
    Marital history (if spouse is applying)
    Dates of military service

13. For those who meet the eligibility criteria and assemble the required application items, the Social Security Administration then evaluates four major factors. Name them.
    1. **Inability to perform substantial gainful activity.** Gainful activity is defined as earnings which average >$300/mo, excluding the cost of disability-related work expenses (i.e., special equipment).
    2. **Work credits.** This encompasses how long the individual has worked, how recently the individual was employed, and the age at which the individual became disabled. Currently, workers >age 31 must have contributed to the Social Security fund for 20 of the preceding 40 quarters. For younger workers, fewer years of contributions are required.
    3. **Severity and extent of impairment.** Objective evidence of a physical or mental impairment is required, and symptoms alone are never sufficient for a determination of disability. There must be corroborating physical, laboratory, and/or radiographic findings.
    4. **Does impairment meet or exceed listed criteria for disability for that impairment.** The patient's individual physician does not determine if the person is disabled. The Social Security Administration has a list of defined impairments under each body system. If the patient's disease meets the listed measurements of disease severity, then the patient is assumed to have a disabling impairment. These listings make the system more objective and uniform.

14. What is residual functional capacity?
If an applicant's impairment fails to meet the listed criteria for automatic disability, a physician or vocational specialist employed by the Social Security Disability Determination Service must make a determination of the applicant's **residual functional capacity** (RFC). RFC is the degree to which the applicant has the capacity for sustained performance of the physical requirements of certain levels of work. The physical demands of work are divided into five categories: sedentary, light, medium, heavy, and very heavy.

15. Outline the physical requirements for work for each of the five categories of residual functional capacity.

Sedentary work
    Sitting
    Lifting of ≤10 lbs
    Occasional (up to one-third of an 8-hr day) lifting or carrying small objects
    Occasional walking or standing
    Fine dexterity
Light work
    Lifting of ≤20 lbs
    Frequent (up to two-thirds of an 8-hr day) lifting or carrying of ≤10 lbs
    Frequent walking or standing
    Sitting with push/pull arm or leg controls
Medium work
    Lifting of ≤50 lbs
    Frequent lifting or carrying of ≤25 lbs
Heavy work
    Lifting of ≤100 lbs
    Frequent lifting or carrying of ≤50 lbs
Very heavy work
    Lifting of >100 lbs
    Frequent lifting or carrying of >50 lbs
Other factors taken into account when determining a person's RFC are fatigue; ability to see, hear, and speak; adequate mental capacity; ability for social interaction with coworkers; and skills to adapt to changes in work routine.

16. How does the Social Security Administration use the RFC in determining disability?

The disability examiner determines the physical demands of the work previously done by the applicant and judges whether the individual has the RFC to do such work. If not, then the examiner considers whether the applicant's RFC, coupled with the individual's age, education, and previous work experience, makes it possible for the applicant to do any work. If not, then the applicant can be declared disabled, even though his or her impairment did not meet listed disability criteria.

17. How is an application for disability benefits evaluated? Can a decision be appealed?

An application to the Social Security Administration for disability benefits is first evaluated by a physician-panel without a personal appearance by the applicant. Approximately one-third of applications are approved at this point. However, an individual has the option of appeal at many stages, while the Social Security Administration does not.

After initially being denied, an individual may have the application reviewed again by a separate physician-panel. However, about 15% of these appeals are granted benefits.

A denial at this stage may be appealed to a third level, an administrative law judge, where a personal appearance may first take place. Approximately 60% of the cases appealed to administrative law judges are subsequently approved, making this application step very important.

Applications denied by the administrative law judge can be appealed to the Social Security Appeals Council and ultimately to a U.S. District Court. Few of these cases (< 5%) are ultimately approved. Overall, approximately 50% of all applications to the Social Security Administration are ultimately approved.

18. If an individual who is receiving disability benefits returns to work, will their benefits be stopped?

Disability recipients continue to receive full disability benefits for up to 9 months after returning to work. This 9-month period is called a **trial work period.** The 9 months need not be continuous, and only months count in which the individual earns >$75.00 or works >15 hours.

Disability benefits are reassessed after the trial work period. If it is decided that disability benefits are no longer needed, the individual receives 3 more monthly checks. Subsequently, benefits are paid for any month the individual is disabled and unable to perform substantial gainful activity for up to 36 months after the trial work period ends. If disability payments end but the individual continues with impairment, the Medicare benefit can be continued for up to 39 months, even though the person is no longer receiving disability payments.

19. What is vocational rehabilitation?
Vocational rehabilitation (VR) is a service provided for by the Federal Rehabilitation Act of 1973. Funded by both state and federal governments, VR agencies assist people with disabilities to find and keep employment. Every state is required to have a VR program, although the range of services varies among states. Private vocational rehabilition agencies also provide a wide array of services to disabled and injured individuals.

Any person applying for disability is referred to and considered for vocational rehabilitation. The participating agencies provide counseling, interest/skills evaluation, basic living expenses, education expenses, transportation costs, purchase of special equipment, job training, and placement. These agencies may also acquire services from other public programs. Not all VR services are provided free of charge, but in some cases, VR does pay for all expenses when an individual has very limited resources. Disability benefits may be continued while an individual receives VR services, but refusal of VR services will stop disability benefits. If a person recovers while participating in VR services, disability benefits continue if they are likely to enable the person to work.

20. What is the primary physician's role while the patient is applying for disability?
The primary physician may be asked to fulfill several roles:
- Information source for the patient
  Details of the disability insurance system
  Options to be pursued if the request is denied
- Information source for the agency by documenting the impairment
  Prior health status
  Objective evidence of impairment (physical findings, radiographs, laboratory abnormalities)
  Progression of symptoms
  Impact the impairment has on the patient's activities of daily living
  Response to therapy
- Patient advocate, supporting the patient during the process of application
- Monitor of on-going therapy
- Independent validator of an impairment
- Expert witness for litigation

Difficulties arise for both the physician and patient when these roles become contradictory. A physician who tries to be an effective patient advocate and an impartial adjudicator at the same time may be risking a strain of the physician-patient relationship.

21. What are "activities of daily living"?
Usual activities that need to be assessed and documented when evaluating or documenting impairments. Over 60% of patients with chronic musculoskeletal disorders report some limitation with one or more of these activities of daily living.

Activities of Daily Living

CATEGORIES	SPECIFIC ACTIVITIES
Self-care and personal hygiene	Bathing, dressing, brushing teeth, combing hair, eating, toileting
Communication	Writing, speaking, hearing
Ambulation, travel, and posture	Walking, climbing stairs, driving, riding, flying, sitting, standing, lying down
Movement	Lifting, grasping, tactile discrimination
Sleep, social activities, and sexual function	—

22. Does the Americans with Disabilities Act of 1990 apply to musculoskeletal conditions?
Yes. This Act makes it unlawful to discriminate in employment against a qualified individual with a disability. It also outlaws discrimination against individuals with disabilities in state and local government services, public accommodations, transportation, and telecommunications. To be protected, one must have a "substantial" impairment (one that significantly limits or restricts a major life activity) and must be qualified to perform the essential functions or duties of a job with or without reasonable accommodation.

23. What is the impact and/or "cost" of musculoskeletal disorders to the patient and society?
Musculoskeletal disorders are the most common cause of chronic health problems, long-term disability, and health-care utilization. These conditions are the second leading cause for patients to apply for and receive disability allowances. In fact, over 17% of all workers receiving disability payments have a musculoskeletal disorder.

The costs to the patient and society are enormous. Studies show that lost wages have a far greater economic impact for the disabled person with a musculoskeletal disease than the direct costs of medical care and medications associated with treating the illness. Approximately $118 billion is "spent" annually on health care costs, lost wages, and lost productivity.

Additionally, individuals with musculoskeletal conditions account for:

7% of the noninstitutionalized population

14% of visits to physicians

19% of hospital stays

BIBLIOGRAPHY

1. Badley EM, Rusooly I, Webster GK: Relative importance of musculoskeletal disorders as a cause of chronic health problems, disability and health care utilization: Findings from the 1990 Ontario Health Survey. J Rheumatol 21:505, 1994.
2. Carey TS, Hadler NM: The role of the primary care physician in disability determination for Social Security Insurance and Worker's Compensation. Ann Intern Med 104:706, 1986.
3. Liang MH, Daltroy LH, Larson MG, et al: Evaluation of social security disability in claimants with rheumatic disease. Ann Intern Med 115:26, 1991.
4. Meenan RF: Work disability in rheumatoid arthritis: An approach to the problem. In Utsinger PD, et al (eds): *Rheumatoid Arthritis*. Philadelphia, J.B. Lippincott, 1985, 829.
5. Straaton KV, Harvey M, Maijiak R: Factors associated with successful vocational rehabilitation in persons with arthritis. Arthritis Rheum 35:503, 1992.
6. Yelin E: The economic impact of arthritis. In Schumacher HR Jr (ed): Primer on the Rheumatic Diseases, 10th ed. Atlanta, Arthritis Foundation, 1993, pp 322.
7. Yelin EH, Felts WR: A summary of the impact of musculoskeletal conditions in the United States. Arthritis Rheum 33:750, 1990.
8. Yelin E: The economic cost and social and psychological impact of musculoskeletal conditions. Arthritis Rheum 38:1351–1362, 1995.

XVI. Final Secrets

Repeition is the key to good pedagogy. Read this book again.
Thomas Brewer, M.D.
Senior resident who supervised
the editor during his first
month of internship
(July 1976)

94. UNCONVENTIONAL REMEDIES
AND FOLK MEDICINE

Alan R. Erickson, M.D.

1. What is the definition of unconventional or unproven remedies?
The term "unconventional or unproven remedies" describes therapies that have not been proved scientifically to be beneficial. This is not to be confused with quackery or fraud, which is a false claim made deliberately to promote a product or treatment.

2. Just how widely used are unconventional remedies?
Looking at all unconventional remedy use in all aspects of health care, the estimates are staggering. In 1990, Americans made an estimated 425 million visits to providers of unconventional remedies, which exceeds the number of visits to all U.S. primary care physicians (388 million). Expenditures for these unconventional therapies amounted to approximately $13.7 billion, three-quarters of which were paid out-of-pocket ($10.3 billion). This figure is comparable to the $12.8 billion spent out-of-pocket annually for all hospitalization in the United States. For patients with arthritis, over $3 billion are estimated to be spent annually on unconventional remedies. As many as 90% of arthritis patients may have used unconventional remedies.

3. Who uses unconventional therapies and why?
There is no "typical patient profile" to predict who will be tempted by the promises of unconventional remedies. Despite our scientific advances toward the understanding and treatment of rheumatic diseases, many of our therapies are empirical. Additionally, rheumatic illnesses are associated with significant pain. This, coupled with a lack of understanding by the lay public, psychosocial factors, and cultural practices, allows this huge market to succeed.

4. Why should physicians care if patients use unconventional remedies?
Rheumatic diseases are confusing to both the medical community and lay public. Unconventional remedies often return to the patient a sense of understanding, responsibility, and hope. Unfortunately, not all unconventional therapies are safe. Additionally, expenditures on unconventional remedies can divert scarce health-care resources.

5. List seven categories of unconventional remedies and philosophies.
Unconventional philosophies

Holistic medicine	Homeopathy
Naturopathy	New Age therapy

Diet therapies
  Dong diet   Elimination diet
  Low-fat diet   Macrobiotic diet
  Unpasteurized milk   Vegetarian
Nutritional supplements
  Amino acids   Antioxidants
  Cod liver oil   Evening primrose oil
  Fish oil   Green-lipped mussel
  Propolis, royal jelly, bee pollen
  Megavitamins and supplements
Herbal remedies
  Alfalfa   Chinese herbs
  Garlic   Kelp
Procedures
  Acupuncture   Biofeedback
  Chiropracty   Colon cleansing
  Hypnotherapy   Massage
  Mineral baths   Hydrotherapy
Diagnostic tests
  Cytotoxic testing   Hair analysis
  Iridology   Kinesiology
Miscellaneous
  Copper bracelets   Dimethyl sulfide
  Snake oil   Venoms
  Antimicrobials   Exercise

6. Define holistic medicine, homeopathy, and naturopathy.

Holistic medicine holds that people should try to maintain a balance between their physical and emotional processes while seeking harmony with the environment. Disease occurs when this balance is disrupted.

Homeopathy principles were set forth in the 1800s by German physician Samuel Hahnemann. They use dilute preparations of substances that cause the same symptoms the patient is experiencing to stimulate the body's natural defenses to fight disease.

Naturopathy claims that disease is an imbalance in the body that results from the accumulation of waste products. Natural therapies are said to remove the body's "poisons."

7. Is there any evidence that diet affects arthritis?

The subject of diet has attracted many claims of cures for patients with arthritis. This interest stems from various known facts. (1) Autoimmune disease is a relatively current phenomenon and seems to correlate with our changing diet. In the late paleolithic period, the human diet was rich in protein, as opposed to our current diet, which is rich in fat. This increase in dietary fat can affect the composition of cellular membrane fatty acids. These membrane fatty acids are the source of arachidonic acid-derived prostaglandins and leukotrienes, which contribute to inflammation. (2) It has been noted that some patients with inflammatory arthritis may be deficient in zinc, selenium, and vitamins A and C, which are involved in the scavenging or inactivation of oxygen free radicals. Though no convincing scientific evidence indicates that diet causes or cures arthritis, there are observations that diet may modulate the immune system.

8. Can fatty acid ingestion alter our inflammatory response to rheumatic disease?

Yes. Fatty acids (FA) are essential to the human diet, with ω-3 and ω-6 FAs being the two major groups. FAs are responsible for the composition of the phospholipids in cellular membranes, and thus these membranes can be altered by dietary intake of ω-3 or ω-6 FA. Additionally, FA are the precursors for **leukotrienes** (LT) and **prostaglandins** (PG), the agents (among many) responsible for our inflammatory response. ω-3 FAs are the precursors of PGE_3 and LTB_5, a less inflammatory prostaglandin and leukotriene than PGE_2 and LTB_4, which come from ω-6 FA.

9. How do fish oils and evening primrose oil affect rheumatic diseases?

It is known that ethnic cultures with diets rich in **fish oils,** which are primarily ω-3 FA, tend to have less autoimmune disease. ω-3 FA diets can reduce arachidonic acid levels by 33% and increase eicosapentaenoic acid levels in cellular membranes by 20 times. This results in production of PGE_3 and LTB_5, which have less inflammatory potential than those agents made from ω-6 FA.

Evening primrose oil is γ-linolenic acid (GLA), which is an ω-6 FA. In experimental animal models, excess dietary GLA results in more prostaglandin-1 compounds (PGE_1) and less leukotriene production, leading to less inflammation. This conclusion has not been supported in human studies.

10. What is the theory behind the use of antioxidants?

Antioxidants interfere with the production of free radicals, compounds with an unpaired free electron that takes electrons from others, potentially affecting the immune system or cell membranes. One well-known free radical is superoxide (O_2^-), which is formed using NADPH:

$$NADPH + O_2 \longrightarrow NADP^+ + O_2^- + H^+$$

Superoxide is both a reducing and oxidizing agent and can spontaneously undergo a reaction to form hydrogen peroxide (H_2O_2) and oxygen (O_2):

$$2H^+ + O_2^- + O_2^- \longrightarrow H_2O_2 + O_2$$

Hydrogen peroxide can also react with superoxide to produce a hydroxyl radical (the most reactive of the oxygen products) or chloride ions to form hypochlorous acid (the active ingredient in chlorine bleach).

A variety of antioxidants exist—including vitamins A, C, D, and E and the trace elements copper, zinc, iron, and selenium—which scavenge free radicals and protect cells against oxidation:

$$O_2^- + O_2^- + 2H^+ \xrightarrow{Cu, Zn} H_2O_2$$

$$H_2O_2 + H_2O_2 \xrightarrow{Fe-Catalase} 2H_2O + O_2$$

11. The theory that arthritis is caused by an allergy to certain foods is the basis of several popular diets. What are the scientific studies to support this claim?

Several anecdotal reports have described certain foods causing or worsening arthritis. Many of these are single case reports.

Food Allergy

Rheumatoid arthritis	Dairy products
	Wheat and corn
	Beef
Behçet's disease	Black walnuts
Lupus in monkeys	Alfalfa
Palindromic rheumatism	Sodium nitrate

There have been animal models of chronic synovitis induced with dietary changes. Additionally, carefully performed human studies in small groups of patients have documented inflammatory arthritis associated with the ingestion of certain foods. The best advice to patients with autoimmune disease is to eat a well-rounded and balanced diet.

12. American Indians have used natural remedies and folk medicine for years to treat all sorts of ailments. What are two recipes for "rheumatism"?

(1) Take 1 oz of cayenne pepper, 4 oz of ginger, 2 oz of cinnamon, 2 oz of clove, 1 oz of gum guaiacum, 1 oz of gum myrrh, and 1 gal "spirits." Let them stand by the fire 10 days before bottling, and then place them in a corked vessel. Take one wine glass full three times each day before meals.

(2) You must boil on the fire a glass of the urine of the person afflicted, and bathe the afflicted part. Afterward, dip a linen folded double in the urine, apply it on the pain, and tie it up. This remedy consumes and dissipates the humours entirely.

Though not specifically recommended, you may want to recommend the use of the first remedy prior to the second, in hopes that there is enough alcohol in the first recipe to allow compliance with the second.

13. Propolis, royal jelly, and bee venom have been claimed to cure arthritis. What is the science behind these claims?

Propolis is a resin made by bees to seal the hives and is reportedly high in bioflavanoids. **Royal jelly** is a sticky substance secreted by the worker honeybees and fed to larvae; it is supposedly high in pantothenic acid. Both bioflavonoids and pantothenic acid are in the B-complex vitamin family, one of many vitamins said to cure and/or treat arthritis.

Bee venom has been said to cure arthritis in anecdotal reports. Patients receive the bee venom from bee stings or from a local injection in an affected joint. Adequate treatment of rheumatoid arthritis (RA) may require as many as 2,000 or 3,000 stings over the course of a year. Bee venom is rich in phospholipase and other anti-inflammatory agents. As expected, these remedies may lead to serious allergic reactions. None of these agents has been shown scientifically to be useful.

14. A popular unconventional remedy uses raisins and gin. What is the recipe and the origins?

Recipe
1. One box of golden raisins
2. Cover the raisins with gin
3. Let stand uncovered until the liquid disappears
4. Eat 9 raisins per day

Supposedly, as far back as biblical times the healing properties of juniper berries have been noted, and gin is made from juniper berries. Several of my patients with arthritis, both RA and osteoarthritis, have tried this remedy with mixed results.

15. Many patients with rheumatoid arthritis wear copper bracelets. Why?

Copper bracelets were used by the ancient Greeks for their healing powers. Copper salts have been used for the treatment of RA, achieving generally favorable responses, unfortunately along with significant side effects. Copper in bracelets is absorbed through the skin (turning the skin green) and is said to improve arthritis symptoms in some patients, perhaps by binding oxygen free radicals. Interestingly, D-penicillamine, a proven therapy for RA, binds copper, which would suggest that copper is not a useful therapy.

16. Why is there so much interest in using antimicrobials for the treatment of rheumatic disease?

For years it has been thought that arthritis, particularly RA, is caused by an infectious organism. Tetracycline was proposed for treating RA many years ago because it was thought that RA was caused by mycoplasmas. More recent research has shown that minocycline may be useful for RA, not because of its antimicrobial actions but because of its antiproliferative and anti-inflammatory properties. Yesterday's unconventional remedy may be tomorrow's new therapy. The following is a list of antimicrobials used for RA:

Metronidazole	Minocycline
Clotrimazole	Ceftriaxone
Rifampin	Ampicillin
Tetracycline	

17. Describe two popular Chinese remedies for the treatment of arthritis.

Chinese herbs are claimed to cure arthritis and other diseases. Chinese medical theory holds that a treatment plan is devised individually for each patient based on his or her complaints. Common herbal compounds include:

Chuifong Toukuwan	Stephania
Ginseng	Ma-huang
Rehmannia	Tang-kuei
Clematis	Ho-shou-wu

Much research has been completed on herbal therapy in China, and more is being completed in the United States and other countries. Some of these preparations have nonsteroidal and steroid-like properties, which may partially explain their effectiveness.

Acupuncture is thought to relieve pain and correct disorders by restoring the balance of vital energy (Qi) to the body. According to traditional Chinese medicine, the Qi runs through the body in 12 channels. Proper balance is restored by stimulating acupoints. Acupuncture has been shown to stimulate the release of serotonins and endorphins, natural pain modulators. Controlled studies on acupuncture have been impressive in some studies and not in others. In general, scientific studies on acupuncture have been of poor quality. The role of acupuncture therapy for arthritis is unclear, and it may be best viewed as an adjunct to standard pain modalities.

18. How does one report a potentially unsafe unconventional remedy?
The Office of Consumer Affairs publishes the *Consumer's Resource Handbook* that explains how to file a complaint. The publication is free by writing to Consumer's Resource Handbook, Pueblo, CO 81009.

19. In summary, how should unconventional remedies be approached?
Unconventional remedies are widely used by patients with rheumatic diseases. Some are safe and harmless and others can be deadly. Some remedies have therapeutic potential and may unlock the door to the next treatment for rheumatic disease; these deserve the attention of the medical community.

BIBLIOGRAPHY

 1. Eisenberg DM, Kessler RC, Foster C, et al: Unconventional medicine in the United States: Prevalence, cost and patterns of use. N Engl J Med 328:246–252, 1993.
 2. Cronan TA, Kaplan RM, Posner L, et al: Prevalence of the use of unconventional remedies for arthritis in a metropolitan community. Arthritis Rheum 32:1604–1607, 1989.
 3. Gertner E, Marshall PS, Filandrinos D, Smith TM: Complications resulting from the use of Chinese herbal medications containing undeclared prescription drugs. Arthritis Rheum 38:614–617, 1995.
 4. Panush RS: Refletions on unproven remedies. Rheum Dis Clin North Am 19:201–206, 1993.
 5. Panush RS: Nontraditional remedies. In Schumacher HR (ed): Primer on the Rheumatic Diseases, 10th ed. Atlanta, Arthritis Foundation, 1993, pp 323–327.
 6. Kremer JM: Nutrition and rheumatic disease. In Kelley WK, Harris ED, Ruddy S, Sledge CB (eds): Textbook of Rheumatology, 4th ed. Philadelphia, W.B. Saunders, 1993, pp 484–498.
 7. Doanne NL: Indian Doctor Book. Aerial Photography Services, Inc., 1985.
 8. Tilley BC, Alarcón GS, Heyse SP, et al: Minocycline in rheumatoid arthritis: A 48-week, double-blind, placebo-controlled trial. Am Intern Med 122:81–89, 1995.
 9. Zurier RB: Prostaglandins, leukotrienes, and related compounds. In Kelley WK, Harris ED, Ruddy S, Sledge CB (eds): Textbook of Rheumatology, 4th ed. Philadelphia, W.B. Saunders, 1993, pp 201–212.
10. Unproven Remedies Resource Manual. Atlanta, Arthritis Foundation.

95. HISTORY, THE ARTS, AND RHEUMATIC DISEASES

James S. Louie, M.D.

1. What is the derivation of the word *rheuma*?

Rheuma is derived from the Greek term indicating "a substance which flows," a humor which originates in the brain and causes various ailments. Guillaume Baillou claimed that "what arthritis is in a joint is what rheumatism is in the whole body," raising the idea that arthritis is but one manifestation of systemic processes. In 1940, Bernard Comroe coined the term *rheumatologist,* and in 1949, Hollander used the term *rheumatology* in his textbook of *Arthritis and Allied Conditions.* Most lay persons, including five out of seven mothers of rheumatologists, do not know what a rheumatologist is by training or expertise.

2. Who described and named rheumatoid arthritis?

Augustin-Jacob Landre-Beauvais (lahn-dray boh-vay) is credited with the first clinical description in 1800. He called it a variant of gout—"goutte asthenique primitif." Benjamin Brodie described the slow progression from a synovitis and bursal and tendon sheath involvement. A.B. Garrod (gair-roh) coined the term *rheumatoid arthritis* (RA) in 1858 and differentiated RA from gout in 1892.

3. Which famous French painters were afflicted with RA?

Pierre Auguste Renoir (1841–1919), the popular French impressionist, developed a severe form of RA beginning about 1890. Despite his increasing disabilities, he continued to paint, supported his family, and devised his own exercises and adaptive equipment. By 1912, he was bedridden and unable to transfer (Class 4B). Just before his death, he developed vasculitis in his fingertips. Because he had rheumatoid nodules and vasculitis, one would guess his genotype was HLA-DRB 1*0401, homozygous.

Raoul Dufy (1877–1943), the talented Fauvist who explored "the miracle of imagination in color" in paintings, watercolors, ceramics, tapestries, and stage and mural designs, exhibited his first attack of RA at age 60. Within 13 years, when he became dependent on his crutches and wheelchair, he was invited to Boston to participate in one of the first drug studies which utilized different steroid preparations for the treatment of RA. He underwent a remarkable recovery, returned to his painting with vigor, but also suffered the consequences of the steroids, including a buttock abscess and a gastrointestinal bleed prior to his death.

4. What other famous people had RA?

Performers who developed rheumatoid arthritis include Edith Piaf, the French chanteuse, and motion picture actresses Rosalind Russell and Katherine Hepburn. The cardiac surgeon Sir Christian Barnard had RA, as did U.S. Presidents Thomas Jefferson, James Madison, and Theodore Roosevelt.

5. Who is credited with the early descriptions of systemic lupus erythematosus (SLE)?

1845 Ferdinand von Hebra described the butterfly rash on the nose and cheeks.
1895 Sir William Osler described the systemic features under the name exudative erythema.
1948 William Hargraves described the LE cell in bone marrow aspirates.
1956 Peter Miescher described the absorption of the LE cell factor by cell nuclei.
1958 George Friou described the method identifying anti-nuclear antibodies by labeling with fluorescent anti-human globulin.

6. Name some famous people who had SLE.
Famous persons who died from the complications of systemic lupus erythematosus include the Southern authoress, Flannery O'Connor, and the former Philippine President, Ferdinand Marcos.

7. Who is credited with the early descriptions of scleroderma?

c. 400 BC   Hippocrates described "persons in whom the skin is stretched, parched and hard, the disease terminates without sweats."

1842   English physician W.D. Chowne described a child with the clinical features.

1846   English physician James Startin described an adult with clinical features.

1860   French clinician, Elie Gintrac, coined the term sclerodermie.

1862   Maurice Raynaud described the vasospastic phenomenon of painful, cold-induced acrocyanosis.

1964   Richard Winterbauer, while a medical student, described the CRST syndrome of calcinosis, Raynaud's, sclerodactyly, and telangiectasia. The E for esophageal dysmotility was added subsequently (CREST).

8. What famous Swiss painter and printmaker had scleroderma?
Paul Klee (1879–1940), the complex and incredibly talented Swiss artist who completed more than 9000 works in diverse media, was stricken with scleroderma at age 56. His last paintings include "Ein Gestalter" (the Creator) as he recovered his desire and energy to paint, "Stern Visage" which described the skin changes, "Death and Fire" as he painted his requiem, and "Durchhalten" (Endure), a line drawing which described the dysphagia prompting his final admission to the sanitorium.

9. Who is credited with the early descriptions of the spondyloarthropathies?
In the late 1890s, the Russian physician, Vladimir von Bechterew, and the French physicians Adolf Strumpell and Pierre Marie described ankylosing spondylitis. The association with the Class I gene, HLA-B27, is credited to the Americans, Lee Schlosstein, Rodney Bluestone, and Paul Terasaki, and the Englishmen, Derrick Brewerton, Caffrey, and Nicholls. In the early 1900s, the German physician, Hans Reiter, and the French physicians, Fiessinger and Leroy, described the clinical characteristics of reactive arthritis or Reiter's syndrome.

10. Which famous personages had ankylosing spondylitis?

Olympic gold medalist swimmer, Bruce Furniss

Television emcee, Ed Sullivan

Renowned cellist, Gregor Piatigorsky

Motion picture actor, Boris Karloff (All of the stiff walking in his Frankenstein role may not have been acting!)

11. What persons are credited with the early descriptions of gout?

5th century BC   Although gout was reported in medieval medicine as gutta, Latin for "a drop" of a poisonous *noxa*, Hippocrates first described the clinical features of gouty arthritis following dietary excesses in sexually active men and postmenopausal women.

Late 1600s   Thomas Sydenham described the clinical features, and Anton van Leeuwenhoek described the microscopic appearance of uric acid recovered from a tophus.

1814   John Want reported the effectiveness of colchicine in the treatment of 40 patients with gout.

1857   A.B. Garrod developed an assay that detected uric acid in hyperuricemic states, demonstrated uric acid in cartilage of those with gout, and formulated the current hypotheses that lead to gouty arthritis.

1961   Joseph Hollander and Daniel McCarty demonstrated monosodium urate in the synovial fluid cells of those with gout.

1964   Michael Lesch, as a medical student, wrote the clinical description of a patient with neurobehavioral changes for his mentor, William Nyhan, who described the complete deficiency of hypoxanthine-guanine phosphoribosyl transferase (HGPRT), the enzyme which catalyzes the salvage reactions of purines (Lesch-Nyhan syndrome).

12. Which famous Flemish painter had gout?

Peter Paul Rubens (1577–1640), the portrayer of Baroque, developed attacks of fevers and arthritis which put him to bed at age 49. Within 10 years, his attacks were continuous, and he had difficulty painting and ambulating. He died of "ague and the goutte" at age 63. Some interpret the stylistic paintings of the hands as deformities which resembled rheumatoid arthritis.

13. Which American Presidents suffered from gout?

James Buchanan (1791–1868) and Martin van Buren (1782–1862).

14. What was Beethoven's disease?

Ludwig von Beethoven (1770–1827) noted hearing loss at age 26, was "stone deaf" at age 49, and died at age 57. His deafness is popularly attributed to otosclerosis, or 8th nerve compression from Paget's disease. More in-depth studies included records of attacks of rheumatism. A postmortem by Wagner and Rokitansky described "dense half-inch-thick cranial vault, shrunken auditory nerves, wasted limbs, with cutaneous petechiae, cirrhosis with ascites, a large spleen, and chalky deposits in the kidneys." These findings led to the differential diagnosis of meningovascular syphilis, sarcoidosis, and Whipple's disease.

15. What were the rheumatic diseases in the Civil War era?

Medical records of the American Civil War recorded 160,000 cases of "acute rheumatism", mainly acute rheumatic fever, perhaps infectious arthritis or gout. More than 260,000 cases of "chronic rheumatism" were recorded, probably chronic rheumatic fever and reactive arthritis, of which 12,000 were discharged. The validity of these clinical diagnoses on the war front may temper some of these data, and more recent data of war-related rheumatic syndromes gives a better perspective.

In 1863, General Robert E. Lee described paroxysms of chest pains radiating to the left shoulder and back, which was diagnosed as rheumatic pericarditis. He was given quinine. By 1870, because the pains occurred at rest, these attacks were probably advancing coronary atherosclerosis.

16. Did Abraham Lincoln have a genetic disease?

The debate on whether the American President Abraham Lincoln had **Marfan's syndrome**, the autosomal dominant disorder of connective tissue, reached national proportions when an advisory committee ruled on proposed molecular genetic testing of his tissue, which is preserved at the National Museum of Health and Medicine at the Armed Forces Institute of Pathology. Actually, the FBN1 gene on chromosome 15, which codes for fibrillin, the main component of extracellular fibrils, is the locus for mutations that result in a spectrum of true connective tissue diseases, including classical Marfan's syndrome. Because > 20 different FBN1 mutations or abnormal fibrillin metabolism have been described in Marfan's and even in healthy relatives and normal controls, genetic testing will not be definitive for the diagnosis.

BIBLIOGRAPHY

1. Appelboom T, de Boelpaepe C, Ehrlich G, Famaey JP: Rubens and the question of antiquity of rheumatoid arthritis. JAMA 245:483–486, 1981.
2. Ball GV: The world and Flannery O'Connor, in Appelboom T (ed): Art, History and Antiquity of Rheumatic Diseases. Brussels, Elsevier Librico, 1987, pp 82–83.
3. Benedek T: History of the rheumatic diseases. In Schumacher HR (ed): Primer on the Rheumatic Diseases, 10th ed. Atlanta, Arthritis Foundation, 1993, pp 1–4.

 4. Bollet AJ: Rheumatic diseases among Civil War troops. Arthritis Rheum 34:1197–203, 1991.
 5. Brewerton D, Caffrey M, Nicholls A: Ankylosing spondylitis and HLA-27. Lancet i:904–907, 1973.
 6. Francke U, Furthmayr H: Marfan's syndrome and other disorders of fibrillin. N Engl J Med 330:1384–
    1385, 1995.
 7. Homburger F, Bonner CD: The treatment of Raoul Dufy's arthritis. N Engl J Med 301:669–673, 1979.
 8. Louie JS: Renoir—His art and his arthritis. In Appelboom T (ed): Art, History and Antiquity of
    Rheumatic Diseases. Brussels, Elsevier Librico, 1987, pp 43–45.
 9. Mainwaring RD: The cardiac illness of General Robert E. Lee. Surg Gynecol Obstet 174:237–244, 1992.
10. Marx R: The Health of the Presidents. New York, G.P. Putnam's Sons, 1960.
11. Palferman TG: Beethoven: Medicine, music, and myths. Int J Dermatol 33:664–671, 1994.
12. Parish LC: An historical approach to the nomenclature of rheumatoid arthritis. Arthritis Rheum
    6:138–158, 1963.
13. Schlosstein L, Terasaki P, Bluestone R: High association of an HLA antigen, w27, with ankylosing
    spondylitis. N Engl J Med 288:704–706, 1973.
14. Sharma OP: Beethoven's illness: Whipple's disease rather than sarcoidosis? Int J Dermatol 87:283–286,
    1994.
15. Shearer PD: The deafness of Beethoven: An audiologic and medical overview. Am J Otol 11:370–374, 1990.

96. SIR WILLIAM OSLER, I PRESUME

Sterling West, M.D.

1. A patient with osteoarthritis of his hand joints wants to know if "popping" his knuckles when he was younger caused him to develop arthritis. What is your answer?

The joint cavity is a potential space with a negative pressure compared to ambient atmospheric pressure. Joint synovial fluid acts as an adhesive seal that permits sliding motion between cartilage surfaces while effectively resisting distracting forces. During knuckle cracking or popping there is a fracture of this adhesive bond. A gas bubble is created within the joint, which cavitates with a cracking sound, liberating energy in the form of heat and sound. This radiologically obvious bubble of gas can require up to 30 minutes to dissolve before the synovial fluid adhesive bond can be reestablished and the joint can be "cracked" again. Although knuckle cracking looks and sounds obnoxious, there are no data to support that it leads to osteoarthritis of the finger joints.

2. A 39-year-old man presents to the emergency room with a 3-day history of right shoulder pain. The pain came on after he painted his house. Physical examination shows he is afebrile. He has full but painful range of motion of his right shoulder. There is no heat, erythema, or swelling. Palpation of the tendon anterior to the humerus elicits pain. Speed's test and Yergason's maneuver are positive. What is the diagnosis? What further tests, if any, are necessary to establish the diagnosis?

This patient has bicipital tendinitis following overuse. The full range of motion of the joint, lack of inflammatory physical examination findings, and increase in symptoms with stressing maneuvers confirms the diagnosis. No additional laboratory or radiographic tests are necessary to establish the diagnosis prior to treatment. (See chapter 66.)

3. A 62-year-old woman presents with a 5-year history of increasing left leg pain. Read the description and decide the diagnosis.

She describes the pain as a dull ache in her groin that radiates to her medial thigh. She also notes pain in her hands, feet, knees, neck, and low back, although to a lesser degree than in her leg. These pains have been present for about 10 years and have not been associated with swelling, redness, or warmth of the joints. Examination of her joints reveal bony swelling of DIP and PIP joints, limiting her ability to close her fist completely. She has a bony prominence at the base of her thumbs on both sides. Examination of the hips reveals normal right hip motion but pain when she flexes her left hip beyond 75°. Both hips externally rotate to 50° without pain. Internal rotation of the right hip to 15° is asymptomatic but the left hip has only about 5–10° of internal rotation that produces pain. Both knees have crepitus without effusion or warmth. Patellar grinding is present. Her feet reveal bilateral great toes that are angulated and overlap the other toes. The first MTP is prominent and slightly tender but not red or warm. Her gait is remarkable for a noticeable limp. CBC, electrolytes, liver transaminases, and urinalysis are normal. Hand and hip radiographs are shown below. **What is the diagnosis?**

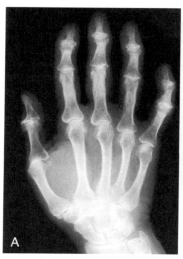
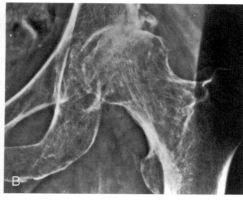

This patient has primary generalized osteoarthritis. Her major symptom is degenerative arthritis of her hip. The patient's noninflammatory symptoms, physical examination, unremarkable laboratory test results, and radiographs support this diagnosis. Hip radiographs are significant for joint space narrowing in the area of maximal stress accompanied by sclerosis and osteophyte formation. Hand radiographs reveal the classic "seagull" sign in the PIP and DIP joints. Physical examination would show Heberden's and Bouchard's nodes. (See chapter 55.)

4. A 60-year-old woman with long-standing rheumatoid arthritis presents for evaluation of a painful, swollen right knee for the past 2 days. Read the description and determine the diagnosis.

Her arthritis is moderately well-controlled on methotrexate, prednisone, and naproxen. The examination reveals a temperature of 38.5°C and chronic deformities of rheumatoid arthritis involving the hands, wrists, and feet without active synovitis. The right knee is swollen, warm, and erythematous. There is significant pain with movement and the knee is held in 30° of flexion. Aspiration of the synovial fluid reveals a synovial fluid white blood cell count of 85,000/mm³ with 95% neutrophils. **What is the diagnosis?**

Whenever a patient with rheumatoid arthritis presents with one joint much more symptomatic ("out of sync") than other joints, the clinician should suspect septic arthritis. The low-grade fever and extremely elevated synovial fluid white blood cell count are also compatible with this diagnosis. The most likely organism in this clinical situation is *Staphylococcus aureus*. (See chapter 42.)

5. You are asked to see a 72-year-old woman with right knee pain. She is recuperating from resection of a symptomatic parathyroid adenoma that was performed 3 days earlier. Read the description and make the diagnosis.

Her initial postoperative course was remarkable for transient hypocalcemia that responded readily to treatment. For over a year she has had mild right knee pain when she walks more than a block. Last night she developed pain and swelling of the right knee. Pain steadily worsened over the ensuing 12 hours and she is quite uncomfortable. There is no history of trauma and she has no systemic symptoms. She has never had any similar episodes previously. Her examination is normal except for the right knee. The knee is held in flexion. It is warm, swollen, and slightly erythematous. Any further flexion of the knee produces intense pain. A large effusion is present. Laboratory findings include a CBC with a hematocrit of 34%, WBC count of 12,300/mm³, platelets 256,000/mm³, erythrocyte sedimentation rate of 66 mm/hr, normal electrolytes, calcium 8.7 mg/dL, creatinine 1.5 mg/dL, albumin 3.3 mg/dL, and uric acid 8.2 mg/dL. Roentgenogram appears below. Arthrocentesis yields 48 cc of cloudy white fluid. Cell count of synovial fluid shows 28,000 WBC/mm³, with 83% neutrophils. Gram stain is negative with cultures pending. Polarized light microscopy of a specimen of synovial fluid reveals weakly positively birefringent rhomboid-shaped crystals. **What is the diagnosis?**

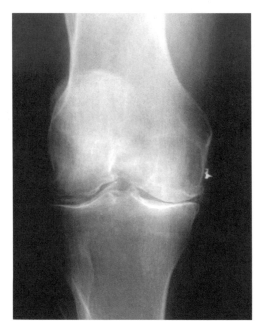

The diagnosis is acute pseudogout caused by calcium pyrophosphate dihydrate (CPPD) crystals. An elderly woman with a history of hyperparathyroidism who is postoperative, has chondrocalcinosis of the meniscus of her knee, and develops an acute monarthritis with weakly positively birefringent rhomboid-shaped crystals in the synovial fluid represents a classic presentation of acute pseudogout. (See chapter 50.)

6. A 50-year-old man is referred for evaluation of a rash of 1-month duration. Read the description and formulate the diagnosis. The rash is nonpruritic and involves his bilateral lower extremities. Recently he noted a small ulcer at the left medial malleolus. Review of systems was remarkable for Raynaud's phenomenon, arthralgias of the hands and knees, and severe paresthesias of the lower extremities. Past medical and surgical history were remarkable for coronary artery disease treated with bypass grafting 5 years previously and complicated by an episode of "jaundice" postoperatively. Examination revealed palpable purpura of the lower extremities extending to the thighs, with a small ulcer overlying the left medial malleolus. Moderate hepatosplenomegaly was noted. Tenderness of the wrists, MCPs, PIPs, and knees without swelling or warmth was noted. Neurologic examination was remarkable for decreased sensation to pinprick and light touch in the bilateral feet and ankles with absent Achilles reflexes. Laboratory results were re-

markable for a normocytic, normochromic anemia with a hematocrit of 34%. Neutrophil and platelet counts were normal. The erythrocyte sedimentation rate was elevated at 70 mm/hr. Serum chemistries revealed a normal creatinine (1.4 mg/dL) with mildly elevated liver associated enzymes. Urinalysis revealed 3+ proteinuria with urine sediment containing 5 white cells, 50 red cells, and rare red blood cell casts per high power field. Rheumatoid factor was positive in a titer of 1:2560 with a negative ANA (antinuclear antibody). Serum protein electrophoresis showed a polyclonal gammopathy. Complement levels revealed a markedly low C4 (8 mg/dL) and a normal C3 (85 mg/dL). Biopsy of one of the lower extremity skin lesions showed leukocytoclastic vasculitis. Nerve conduction testing demonstrated a diffuse symmetric sensorimotor polyneuropathy. **What is the diagnosis?**

Symptoms of palpable purpura, arthralgias, and polyneuropathy with liver enzyme transaminitis and an active urinary sediment on laboratory examination in a male is consistent with mixed cryoglobulinemia. Purpura is the most common presenting feature of cryoglobulinemia, with biopsies confirming leukocytoclastic vasculitis. The patient's history of postoperative jaundice and his elevated liver enzymes support a diagnosis of hepatitis C, which may be seen in over 50% of patients with mixed cryoglobulinemia. The positive rheumatoid factor suggests a mixed (type II or type III) cryoglobulin. The marked depression of C4 with normal C3 levels is a common complement profile in cryoglobulinemia. (See chapter 35.)

7. A 50-year-old woman is complaining of feeling tired and weak all over. Read the description and make the diagnosis.

She believes that her symptoms have progressively worsened over the past 2 months. She works in a grocery store where she has had difficulty lifting objects to the top shelves when restocking. Even more concerning to her is that within the past several weeks she has had difficulty brushing her hair and climbing stairs in her home. She relates having little problem walking on flat ground and little trouble performing tasks with her hands. She denies experiencing discomfort in her muscles or joints. Within the past 3 weeks, the patient has noticed a rash over her knuckles. She complains of feeling fatigued but has not experienced fever, chills, or weight loss. Past medical history is remarkable only for long-standing hypothyroidism. Her only medications are conjugated estrogens and thyroid hormone replacement. She drinks 2–4 glasses of wine per week. There are no muscle disorders or rheumatic diseases in her family members. Physical examination of the patient reveals symmetric proximal motor weakness quantified at approximately $4^-/5^+$. Distal strength is normal. No muscle tenderness is noted. Neurologic exam reveals normal and symmetric reflexes and normal cranial nerve function. No fasciculations are noted. Joint exam is normal. Examination of her skin reveals a raised, violaceous rash over the interphalangeal regions of the fingers and presence of periungual erythema. Otherwise examination revealed normal findings. Laboratory studies reveal: AST 100 U/L, ALT 150 U/L, total bilirubin of 0.8 mg/dL, normal creatinine and urinalysis, positive ANA 1:256 in a speckled pattern (ANA profile including anti-SSA, SSB, RNP, Sm, and dsDNA is negative); ESR 25 mm/hour; CPK 1050 U/L (normal <200 U/L). **What is the most likely diagnosis?**

The patient's complaints of painless symmetric proximal motor weakness is consistent with an inflammatory myopathy. The physical examination confirms the presence of weakness limited to the proximal musculature, and does not reveal findings to suggest a neuropathic etiology. Laboratory results suggest underlying muscle damage with elevated muscle enzymes (CPK, AST, ALT). Other potential etiologies need to be considered in this patient. With a history of hypothyroidism, noncompliance with her medication or under-replacement could result in motor weakness as well as an elevated CPK. Although presence of a positive ANA increases the possibility of an associated connective tissue disease such as SLE, MCTD, or systemic sclerosis, there is no historical, examination, or serologic evidence to suggest such. Myopathies caused by medications must always be a consideration, but this patient is not taking any that would put her at risk. The presence of a rash characteristic of dermatomyositis (Gottron's papules) makes this the most likely diagnosis. Neurodiagnostic studies and/or a muscle biopsy may be necessary to definitively confirm an inflammatory myopathy, although a characteristic presentation, rash, and elevated muscle enzymes may be adequate for diagnosis. Because dermatomyositis in adults is associated with the presence of cancer in approximately 15% of cases, a screen for neoplastic disease is indicated to complete this patient's evaluation prior to embarking upon appropriate therapy. (See chapter 24.)

8. A medical student shows you a radiograph of a patient whom he is evaluating for long-standing, severe arthritis. What is the diagnosis?

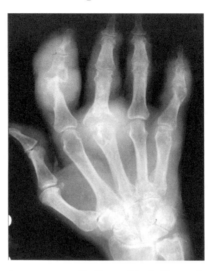

This patient has chronic tophaceous gout. Radiographic findings of erosions with sclerotic margins and overhanging edges (second PIP), cystic changes, expansile joint lesions (third MCP), and soft tissue lumps and nodules (tophi) are all classic for this disease. (See chapter 49.)

9. A 38-year-old woman presents with pain and swelling in her right calf. Read the description and decide the diagnosis.

The pain started 2 days previously in the posterior aspect of her calf and has been associated with increased swelling and edema over the past 24 hours. She denies fever, chills, sweats, any recent trauma to the leg, or changes in physical activity. She has a past history of two episodes of similar swelling in her leg—one 7 years and one 3 years previously. The first episode resolved spontaneously but the second was associated with shortness of breath and required hospitalization. At that time the diagnosis of thrombophlebitis was made and the patient was given Coumadin for 6 months. The patient has done well with regular checkups and no medical problems until the present episode. The patient denies skin rash, joint pain or swelling, excessive fatigue, hair loss, or photosensitivity. There is no history of kidney problems. There is no known family history of arthritis, connective tissue disease, or bleeding or clotting problems. The patient lives with her husband and one child, age 12. Obstetric history reveals the patient had a normal, healthy child 12 years previously but since that time has had three unsuccessful pregnancies with spontaneous abortions at 28, 14, and 30 weeks.

Examination reveals a healthy-appearing woman with normal vital signs. Skin shows a reticular "lace-like" vascular pattern over her thighs and upper arms. This rash blanches with pressure, and it is not pruritic or painful. The right calf is diffusely swollen and slightly red. It is tender to palpation and there is a palpable cord extending into the posterior aspect of the distal thigh. Her right foot shows 1–2+ pitting edema. The remainder of the examination is normal. Laboratory evaluation reveals normal CBC, chemistries, and urinalysis. Chest x-ray is clear. Serologic testing shows a weakly positive ANA (1:40) and negative rheumatoid factor. Clotting tests obtained prior to initiation of heparin therapy shows a prothrombin time of 12.9 seconds (normal 12.8–13.1), aPTT of 47 seconds (normal 33–35); a 1:1 mix with normal plasma yields an aPTT of 44.6 seconds. Anticardiolipin antibodies by ELISA shows an IgG of 48 units (normal <23) and an IgM of 6 units (normal <5). **What is the diagnosis?**

This patient has the primary antiphospholipid antibody syndrome (PAPS). She presents now with a deep venous thrombosis of her right leg. In addition to the acute DVT, the patient has a history of DVT and pulmonary embolism, and three fetal losses that occurred relatively late in pregnancy. The clinical constellation of recurrent thrombotic events and fetal loss in the face of clotting abnormalities makes the diagnosis of antiphospholipid antibody syndrome. This patient has a lupus anticoagulant as defined by the presence of a prolonged aPTT that does not correct with a 1:1 dilution with normal plasma. Additional testing should include a platelet neutralization procedure to ensure that the aPPT prolongation is corrected by the addition of frozen platelets, and a Russell viper venon time (RVVT), which should be prolonged. The patient also has anti-cardiolipin antibodies predominantly of the IgG type, as detected by ELISA. (See chapter 27.)

10. A 69-year-old woman presents with a 3-week history of a severe headache and a 30-second transient loss of vision in her right eye. Read the description and make the diagnosis.

Headache is characterized as a boring pain in her right temporal region. She also has pain and cramping in her jaw muscles when chewing, and arthralgias. Other complaints are low-grade fevers, 5-pound weight loss, and proximal muscle pain and stiffness. Examination reveals a temperature of 38°C, tenderness of her scalp and both temporal arteries, and breakaway weakness of the shoulders due to pain. Funduscopic examination is normal. There is a left carotid bruit. Laboratory findings include hematocrit 35%, white cell count 11,500/mm³, platelet count 522,000/mm³, and erythrocyte sedimentation rate of 110 mm/hr. **What is the diagnosis and initial management of this patient?**

This patient has giant cell arteritis. The new onset of headache, jaw claudication, and polymyalgia rheumatica symptoms coupled with scalp and temporal artery tenderness and an extremely elevated ESR is characteristic of this disease. Diagnosis should be confirmed with a right temporal artery biopsy. Because of the transient visual loss, she should be started immediately on high doses of corticosteroids even before the biopsy is obtained. (See chapter 31.)

11. A 40-year-old man presents with nonhealing leg ulcers on the left lower leg of 1-month's duration. Read the case presentation and discuss the diagnosis.

Review of systems shows he has had chronic sinusitis for the past year that has been worse recently. He also has experienced low-grade fevers, a nonproductive cough, and left hand numbness. Examination shows a temperature 38°C, blood pressure 150/90, left lower leg ulcer (figure), sinus tenderness, normal chest examination, and decreased sensation of the left hand. Radiographs show chronic maxillary sinusitis bilaterally and two nodular lung infiltrates. Laboratory findings include hematocrit 35%, WBC 12,000/mm³, platelets 490,000/mm³ and a sedimentation

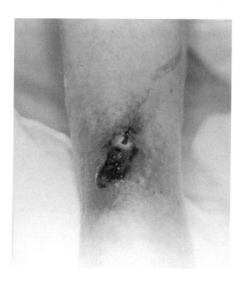

rate 92 mm/hour. Chemistries are normal but creatinine is 1.6 mg/dL and urinalysis shows 1+ protein and moderate blood. **What serologic test would help confirm your diagnosis?**

This patient has the triad of sinusitis, lung infiltrates, and glomerulonephritis characteristic of Wegener's granulomatosis. Fever, ulcerative skin lesion, neurologic involvement, and abnormal laboratory findings also may be seen in this disease. The antineutrophil cytoplasmic antibody (C-ANCA) test is likely to be positive and will help confirm the diagnosis. (See chapter 33.)

12. A 26-year-old white man comes to your clinic with a 1-year history of low back, buttock, and spine pain. He notes 2 hours of morning stiffness that improves by the afternoon with movement and exercise. Six months previously he had an episode of sudden pain in his right eye that was diagnosed as acute iritis and resolved after he was placed on steroid eye drops. His father had similar back pain problems. Examination reveals no joint swelling. Back range of motion is limited in flexion, extension, lateral rotation, and lateral bending. His Gaenslen's test is positive. What is the diagnosis?
This patient has ankylosing spondylitis. Chronic back pain with inflammatory features of prolonged morning stiffness that improves with exercise coupled with a global decrease in back range of motion is characteristic of this disease. Acute anterior iritis can also be a manifestation of this seronegative spondyloarthropathy. This disease occurs most commonly in young, white males, can occur in multiple family members, and is associated with the gene HLA-B27. (See chapter 38.)

13. A 65-year-old man was in good health until he developed dysesthesias in both hands. A diagnosis of carpal tunnel syndrome was made and his symptoms resolved following carpal tunnel release. He returns for evaluation 1 year later because of swelling in his wrists and hands and recurrence of dysesthesias. Read the description and provide the diagnosis.
The patient denies fever or anorexia but has been fatigued and experienced a 20-pound weight loss since the carpal tunnel release. The wrist swelling is persistent but not painful or associated with prolonged morning stiffness. He has noted some swelling in his hands and more recently his knees and shoulders. Examination reveals a chronically ill-appearing male with normal vital signs. Musculoskeletal examination reveals marked synovitis of both wrists with only minimal warmth and tenderness. There is similar but less marked involvement of bilateral metacarpophalangeal and proximal interphalangeal joints. Tinel's test is positive bilaterally. There is fullness of both shoulders and prominent synovitis of both knees, again with little associated warmth or tenderness. Laboratory studies show normal complete blood count, serum chemistries, and thyroid stimulating hormone. The urine has 2+ protein, the erythrocyte sedimentation rate is 65 mm/hour, and rheumatoid factor and ANA are negative. Serum protein electrophoresis reveals an IgG lambda monoclonal spike. Radiographs of the wrists show cystic changes. **What is the diagnosis?**
Primary systemic amyloidosis. A neuropathic presentation, usually carpal tunnel syndrome, is seen in about 20% of patients with primary amyloidosis. The onset of carpal tunnel syndrome in a male over the age of 40 years should raise the possibility of amyloidosis, as should the recurrence of symptoms following carpal tunnel release. Fatigue and weight loss, though nonspecific, are frequent in amyloidosis. A rheumatoid arthritis-like picture is seen in 7% of patients. Clinical findings that distinguish amyloid arthropathy from rheumatoid arthritis are the relatively mild joint symptoms and mild joint warmth and tenderness despite impressive synovitis, the absence of rheumatoid factor, and the cystic changes (not erosions) of bone seen on radiographs. (See chapter 77.)

14. A 45-year-old man returns to see you after your initial evaluation 1 week previously when he presented with a 6-month history of pain and swelling in his hands. Read the description and make the diagnosis.
At that time he denied morning stiffness, fever, weight loss, or repetitive trauma to the joints in question. He is otherwise healthy, although he did admit to some increased fatigue over the last 6 months. He is currently taking no medications and denies alcohol or tobacco use. There is a family history of "rheumatoid arthritis" in a brother and an uncle has hepatic cirrhosis. On physical examination you identified firm synovial swelling with mild tenderness of the second through fifth metacarpophalangeal and wrist joints bilaterally. Warmth and erythema were absent. The re-

mainder of the physical examination was unremarkable except for mild hepatomegaly. You ordered some routine laboratory tests and hand radiographs. The laboratory results include a normal complete blood count and chemistries. The erythrocyte sedimentation rate is 10 mm/hr. The liver panel reveals that both the SGOT (AST) and SGPT (ALT) are two time normal. The remainder of the liver panel is normal. Hand radiographs are shown below. **What is the diagnosis?**

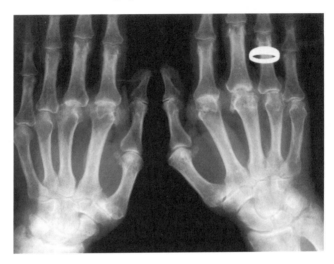

The clinical presentation and radiographs are characteristic for hemochromatosis. There is degenerative arthritis involving the second through fifth metacarpophalangeal joints (MCPs) with prominent joint space narrowing, subchondral cyst formation, sclerosis, and large hook-like osteophytes. Chondrocalcinosis is absent in this case, but can be seen on radiographs in 30–60% of cases, as can degenerative arthritis of the radiocarpal joints.

Hemochromatosis needs to be considered in the differential diagnosis of a seronegative polyarthritis, particularly in middle-aged men with MCP joint involvement. Other joints that may be involved are wrists, knees, ankles, and interphalangeal joints. The typical findings on physical examination are firm joint swelling with only mild tenderness without warmth, erythema, or morning stiffness. The diagnosis in this case is supported by the presence of hepatomegaly, abnormal liver function tests, and the family history of arthritis and cirrhosis; hemochromatosis is inherited as an autosomal recessive trait. Iron studies and a liver biopsy for iron quantification will confirm the diagnosis of hemochromatosis. (See chapter 61.)

15. A 32-year-old woman presents with a two-year history of pain and color changes in the fingers of her hands when she is exposed to cold weather. The fingers first turn white, then blue and eventually red with pain. Examination shows a few telangiectasias on her face and dilated capillaries with dropout around her nailfolds. What serologic test would help confirm your clinical diagnosis?
This patient has Raynaud's phenomenon characterized by the classic tricolor changes in her fingers on cold exposure. The facial telangiectasias and abnormal nailfold capillary examination suggest that she may develop limited scleroderma (CREST) in the future. A positive anticentromere antibody would help confirm this clinical diagnosis. (See chapters 22 and 78.)

16. A 35-year-old white woman is referred to you for evaluation of diffuse aches and pains of at least 5 years' duration that seem to be getting worse. Read the description and determine the diagnosis.
The patient also has fatigue, stiffness, headaches, cold intolerance, irritable bowel syndrome, and difficulty sleeping. She is under considerable stress at home with an abusive husband and is

chronically behind at work. Examination is completely normal except for bilateral tender points in the occipital region, trapezius muscles, rhomboid muscles, lateral epicondylar area of the elbows, low back and gluteal areas, trochanteric bursal regions, and medial knees. Laboratory and radiographic findings are normal. Specifically a CBC, sedimentation rate, chemistries, thyroid function tests, and creatine phosphokinase are within normal limits. **What is the diagnosis? What further workup is necessary?**

The patient has fibromyalgia. The prolonged duration of symptoms, multisystem complaints, normal examination except for tender points in characteristic locations, and normal laboratory results help confirm this diagnosis. This is a clinical diagnosis with no specific laboratory test being diagnostic. No further workup is necessary. (See chapter 65.)

17. A 45-year-old woman is referred with a 1-year history of swelling and pain in the MCPs, PIPs, wrists, left knee, ankles, and MTPs. Read the description and make the diagnosis.

The patient reports hours of morning stiffness, fatigue, and malaise. She has taken ibuprofen with some help. Physical examination reveals normal vital signs, soft tissue swelling, warmth, tenderness, and limitation of motion of the involved joints. Nodules are seen on the extensor surface of both forearms near the olecranon area. Laboratory findings include a hematocrit of 35%, WBC count 7200/mm³, and platelet count 480,000/mm³. Chemistries, liver enzymes, and uric acid levels are normal. Rheumatoid factor is positive at a titer of 1:640, ANA is negative, and erythrocyte sedimentation rate is elevated at 45 mm/hr. Radiographs of the hands show early MCP and PIP erosions. **What is your diagnosis?**

This patient has rheumatoid arthritis. The gradual onset of a symmetric polyarthritis involving the small joints of the hands, wrists, and feet associated with prolonged morning stiffness and rheumatoid nodules satisfies criteria for this diagnosis. Additional findings of a positive rheumatoid factor and erosions on hand radiographs support this diagnosis. The elevated sedimentation rate, anemia of chronic disease, and elevated platelet counts are reflections of the systemic inflammation caused by the rheumatoid arthritis. (See chapter 19.)

18. A 44-year-old man is admitted to the hospital complaining of abdominal pain, a 15-pound weight loss, fevers, fatigue, and right foot drop. He has a history of intravenous drug abuse. An abdominal angiogram is obtained. What is your diagnosis?

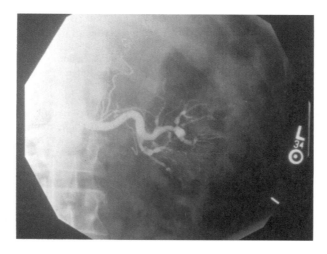

Polyarteritis nodosa. The presentation of multisystem disease coupled with an abdominal angiogram showing aneurysms in the abdominal and renal vessels is characteristic of this vasculitis. Because of his intravenous drug abuse history, you would expect him to be hepatitis B antigen positive. (See chapter 32.)

19. A 56-year-old woman presents with a complaint of a swollen right cheek. Read the description and formulate the diagnosis.

She was well until 5 years previously when she experienced a sensation of "sand" in her eyes and a dry mouth that has become progressively worse. She also has had multiple dental caries. Three months previously she experienced painless swelling of her right cheek as well as diffuse arthralgias. Examination reveals extreme dryness of the eyes and oral mucosa, poor dentition, and a swollen, nontender right parotid gland. A Schirmer's test and rose bengal test are positive. Laboratories are remarkable for hematocrit 35%, white blood cell count of 3,200/mm³, normal urinalysis, erythrocyte sedimentation rate 107 mm/hr, elevated IgG and IgM immunoglobulin levels, a positive rheumatoid factor at 1:640, and a positive antinuclear antibody at 1:256 with a speckled pattern. **What is your diagnosis?**

This patient has primary Sjögren's syndrome, which is the most common autoimmune disease in middle-aged women. The combination of sicca symptoms, dental caries, parotid swelling, and serologic abnormalities is characteristic of this disease. You would expect this patient to have antibodies against SS-A and/or SS-B antigens. (See chapter 26.)

20. A 24-year-old male construction worker comes to you for evaluation of a painful, swollen knee and "scabby" feet for over 2 months. Read the description and make the diagnosis.

There is no prior history of knee injury and a review of systems is unremarkable with two exceptions. First, he recalls having a brief bout of "pink-eye" 3 weeks previously that was "hardly noticeable." Second, he remembers having pain with urination on two occasions. He is sexually active with several female partners. As he limps to the examining table, you are told that his vital signs are normal, except for a temperature of 38.2°C. His general appearance is consistent with that of a manual laborer. Inspection of his eyes reveals no inflammation. Examination of his pharynx, however, reveals a desquamated hard palate. The knee is obviously swollen, warm to touch, and flexed at 30°. You are unable to fully extend the knee and the patella is ballottable. He has two diffusely swollen and tender toes on his right foot. The remainder of the musculoskeletal exam is normal, including the back. On the plantar surfaces of his feet, you observe multiple, papular lesions (figure). Despite their appearance, the lesions are asymptomatic. Inspection of his genitals reveals painless, superficial ulcers on the glans penis and urethral meatus. No discharge is noted. The rectal exam is unremarkable except for a slightly tender and enlarged prostate. Occult blood in his stool is not detected. **What is the diagnosis?**

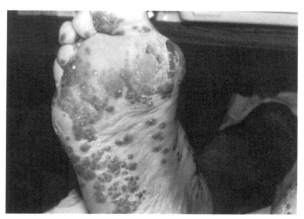

The clinical complex of conjunctivitis (pink-eye), urethritis and arthritis is classic for Reiter's syndrome. In this patient, the additional features of sausage digits, painless oral ulceration, keratoderma blennorrhagica (see figure), and circinate balanitis confirm the diagnosis. Furthermore, *Chlamydia*-induced urogenital disease is probable, given the history, the mild prostatitis, and the mucocutaneous lesions. (See chapter 40.)

21. A 26-year-old black woman presents with a 6-month history of polyarthritis involving the small joints of her hands, wrists, knees, and feet. Read the description and decide the diagnosis.

Two months previously she noted she was beginning to lose some of her hair. Four weeks previously she went to Hawaii on vacation and developed an erythematous rash over her face and upper body with sun exposure. Examination reveals a temperature of 38°C, pulse 120 beats/minute, and blood pressure 140/100 mm Hg. She has an erythematous rash over her cheeks and the bridge of her nose as well as spotty alopecia throughout the scalp without evidence of scarring. The remainder of the examination is normal except for synovitis of MCPs, PIPs, wrists, and MTPs. Laboratory findings include a hematocrit of 32%, white blood cell count 2,400/mm^3, platelets 110,000/mm^3, creatinine 1.8 mg/dL, and a urinalysis with 3+ protein and 5–10 red blood cells and white blood cells per high power field with a few granular casts. **What is your diagnosis?**

This patient has systemic lupus erythematosus. A young black woman presenting with a multisystem disease including polyarthritis, alopecia, photosensitivity, malar rash, nephritis, and hematologic abnormalities including leukopenia and thrombocytopenia is characteristic of this disease. You would expect her antinuclear antibody test to be positive, antibodies against double-stranded DNA to be elevated, and C3 and C4 complement levels to be decreased. (See chapter 20.)

22. A 28-year-old woman presents to the emergency room with a 2-day history of joint pain. Read the presentation and make the diagnosis.

The patient's pain started in her right ankle, migrated to her left knee, and then settled in her right wrist, which became tender, warm, and swollen. She has felt feverish and noted a few painless hemorrhagic skin lesions on her upper and lower extremities. She has no previous history of pelvic inflammatory disease but is sexually active. She began her menstrual cycle 3 days previously. Examination shows a temperature of 38.5°C, a severely swollen and painful right wrist with warmth and erythema along the extensor tendons as well as the true wrist joint. She has scattered discrete hemorrhagic papules over her hands and lower extremities. Laboratory results show a white blood cell count of 13,500/mm^3 with 93% neutrophils and 5% band forms. Radiograph of the wrist is remarkable for soft tissue swelling. **What is your diagnosis?**

This patient's presentation of migratory polyarthritis finally settling in one joint associated with fever and skin rash in a sexually active female is characteristic of disseminated gonococcemia. Onset within the first week of menstruation is also common. (See chapter 42.)

23. Who said "The secret of being a bore is to tell everything."?
Voltaire (1694–1778). This book undoubtedly has left out a "rheumatology secret" that the reader feels should be included in the next edition. Please write the book editor with any suggestions or additional "secrets".

INDEX

Page numbers in **boldface type** indicate complete chapters.

Arthritis (*Cont.*)
  familial Mediterranean fever-related, 462
  fungal, 68
  gonococcal, 76, 82, 83, 233, 237–239
    compared with reactive arthritis, 224
    diagnostic procedures for, 77
    differentiated from nongonococcal arthritis, 76
    polyarticular symptoms of, 81
  gouty. *See* Gout
  hypertrophic, 1, 301
  infectious, 83
    classification of, 1, 2
    synovial fluid findings in, 53
  inflammatory, 343
    bowel diseases associated with, 219–220
    differentiated from noninflammatory arthritis, 77
    of elbow, 513
    history of, 37
    juvenile, 407
    peripheral, 219–220
    radiographic features of, 56–58
  intermittent, periodic syndromes-related, 460–464
  juvenile
    chronic, **408–413**
    inflammatory, 407
    pauciarticular, 409
  Kawasaki's disease-related, 420
  lymphoma-related, 297
  meningococcal, 81
  monoarticular. *See* Monoarthritis
  multicentric reticulohistiocytosis-related, 463
  mutilans, 62
  ochronotic, 331, 332
  peripheral
    psoriatic arthritis-related, 232
    radiographic diagnosis of, 63
  polyarticular. *See* Polyarthritis
  polymyalgia rheumatica-related, 165, 166
  post-traumatic, 476, 514, 518
  prevalence of, 2
  pseudoneuropathic, 273
  pseudoseptic, 237
  psoriatic, 80, 102, 227, **229–232**
    drug therapy for, 482, 483
    extra-articular organ involvement in, 84
    in HIV-infected patients, 254, 255
    joint involvement pattern of, 82
    monoarticular symptoms of, 75, 76
    polyarticular symptoms of, 81
    radiographic features of, 65
    synovial fluid findings in, 53
    uveitis associated with, 443
  pyogenic, cancer-associated, 296
  reactive, 83, **222–228,** 460. *See also* Reiter's syndrome
    erythema nodosum leprosum as, 247
    juvenile, 413
  relapsing polychondritis-related, 209–210
  rheumatic fever-related, 262, 417
  sarcoid, 78, 446, 447
    extra-articular organ involvement in, 84
    joint involvement pattern of, 82
    polyarticular symptoms of, 81
  septic
    AIDS-associated, 254
    bacterial, **233–240**
    B-cell immunodeficiency-related, 339
    coexistent with acute crystalline arthritis, 274
    fungal infection-related, 247–249
    hemophilia-related, 291–292
    in HIV-infected patients, 256

Arthritis (*Cont.*)
  juvenile, 403, 407, 412
    radiographic features of, 58
  sickle cell anemia-related, 293
  staphylococcal, 341
  Sjögren's syndrome-related, 154, 155
  spinal, 219, 220–221
  spirochetal, 68
  Still's disease-related, 163, 164
  systemic lupus erythematosus-related, 80, 81, 110, 119
  systemic sclerosis-related, 130
  temporomandibular, 512
  viral, **249–254**
    extra-articular organ involvement in, 84
  Wegener's granulomatosis-related, 190
  Whipple's disease-related, 257, 258–259
Arthrocentesis, 52. *See also* Synovial fluid analysis
  "dry tap" in, 53
  for monoarthritis evaluation, 76–77
  for polyarthritis evaluation, 85
  postoperative, 99
  in warfarin-receiving patients, 290–291
  for Whipple's disease evaluation, 258
Arthrodesis, 514, 518
Arthrography, 55, 56
  of rotator cuff tears, 373
Arthro-ophthalmopathy, hereditary, 328–329
Arthropathy
  hemochromatosis-related, 333
  hemophilic, 291–293
  myxedematous, 286
  ochronotic, 335–336
Arthroplasty. *See also* Prosthetic joints
  of hip, 322, 512, 513, 515, 516, 517
  of knee, 307 512, 513, 515, 516, 517
  low friction, 515–516
  as osteoarthritis treatment, 307
  total, 512–513
    cemented, 516, 517,
    cementless, 516, 517
    hybrid, 516
    of multiple joints, 512
    revision, 516
Arthroscopy, 69, 79, 517
Aschoff, Ludwig, 260
Aspergillus, as arthritis cause, 248, 249
Aspiration, of joints, 37
  as pseudogout treatment, 274
Aspirin
  anti-inflammatory effects of, 19
  use during breast-feeding, 456
  development of, 465
  as hyperuricemia cause, 267
  as juvenile rheumatoid arthritis treatment, 411
  as preeclampsia-eclampsia prophylactic, 456
  preoperative discontinuation of, 96
  as Still's disease treatment, 164
Atherosclersosis, 269
Atlanto-axial subluxation, 95–96, 104
Australia antigen, 249–250
Autoantibodies
  in AIDS-associated rheumatic syndromes, 254
  in immunoglobulin A deficiency, 340
  in juvenile systemic connective tissue disease, 414–415
  myositis-specific, 144
  pathogenic roles of, 34
  in systemic lupus erythematosus, 112
  in tolerance, 29, 34